Table of Contents

Foreword

The treatment of individuals with spinal cord impairment (SCI) has evolved over time through changes in social, political, and cultural arenas; general health care practices; state-of-the-art technology; and legislation. Rehabilitation is a young specialty, and we are in the midst of making its history. This Core Curriculum, *Nursing Practice Related to Spinal Cord Impairment*, is a landmark publication likely to have a profound impact on nursing practice and on the lives of persons living with SCI.

SCI is a multifaceted, catastrophic experience for the individual and his/her family. Nursing, as an art and science, has a primary role in assisting persons with SCI to achieve and maintain an optimum level of function. SCI nurses are skilled practitioners, knowledgeable in the pathophysiological and psychological implications of SCI, who employ special techniques to deal with the impact of SCI on the individual, family, and society.

Research and technology hold much promise for the prevention, care, and cure of SCI. Movement into the twenty-first century is characterized by increasing complexity; rapid, continuous change; technological innovations; and advances in health care. Nurses play a critical role in health care and have a significant impact on the quality of care provided to persons with SCI in settings that include hospitals, outpatient centers, long-term care facilities, and home care.

It is a thrill to see this project come to fruition. The text fills a void that has been empty too many years. On behalf of the Eastern Paralyzed Veterans Association, I sincerely thank each contributing author, reviewer, and editor who contributed to the success of this project. We are grateful for this outstanding contribution.

James J. Peters
Executive Director, EPVA
Director, AASCIN

Preface

The scope of spinal cord impairment (SCI) nursing incorporates trauma care, stabilization after injury, rehabilitation, unrelated medical/surgical conditions, health maintenance, and long-term follow-up of the injured individual, as well as psychosocial support for the individual, his or her family, and significant others. *Nursing Practice Related to Spinal Cord Impairment: A Core Curriculum* is a comprehensive guide to the practice of SCI nursing. Developed under the auspices of the Eastern Paralyzed Veterans Association (EPVA), in collaboration with the American Association of Spinal Cord Injury Nurses (AASCIN), this core curriculum serves as an authoritative resource for nurses in this field.

The AASCIN is a nonprofit organization dedicated to promoting quality care for individuals with SCI. AASCIN is the only nursing organization devoted exclusively to promoting excellence in meeting the nursing care needs of individuals with SCI. In 1997, AASCIN broadened its focus to spinal cord impairment. While we have made a gallant effort to include impairment in this text, the expertise and experience of many of the authors and reviewers are historically more closely aligned with spinal cord injury. For readers who want a more in-depth review of spinal cord impairment, we refer you to a general rehabilitation text edited by Shirley Hoeman, Rehabilitation Nursing (Second Edition), published in 1995 and currently being updated (Third Edition).

This text was designed to meet the needs of nurses with varying years of experience in the specialty, as well as those in a variety of roles and practice settings. Settings in which SCI nurses are employed include private, public, and federal hospitals, as well as community, residential, or long-term care settings. SCI nursing roles include administrators, case managers, direct care providers, consultants, researchers, and educators. Nursing care is provided by a variety of professional and supportive nursing personnel. Student nurses, experienced nurses new to SCI, practical nurses, and nurses who have worked in this field for many years will find useful information to apply to their practice. A glossary is provided to help the less experienced nurse understand the complex terminology used throughout the text.

To supplement this Core Curriculum, readers are referred to additional references. One key source is a comprehensive text edited by Cynthia P. Zejdlik, Management of Spinal Cord Injury, Second

Edition, published by Jones and Bartlett in 1992. Clinical practice guidelines are now available through the Consortium for Spinal Cord Medicine, including such topics as neurogenic bowel, autonomic dysreflexia, thromboembolism, depression following SCI, and pressure ulcer prevention and management. You can access these guidelines through the Internet at http://www.pva.org/prof/healthcare.htm.

This book was written, reviewed, and edited by nurses with expertise in SCI nursing. Nursing experts in neurology, neurosurgery, SCI, rehabilitation, and orthopedics participated as contributing authors. To assure that this Core Curriculum addressed the myriad needs of nurses from a variety of clinical settings, roles, and levels of expertise, focus groups were held in conjunction with the AASCIN annual conference in Las Vegas. Twenty-nine nurses from the United States and Canada participated. Their suggestions for organization, topics and content were incorporated into this text. Furthermore, we recognize the contributions of many disciplines to effective health care, since nursing practice does not occur in a vacuum. Therefore, we included reviewers and co-authors from a variety of disciplines, including psychology, neuropsychology, urology, sociology, rehabilitation counseling, psychiatry, rehabilitation medicine, social sciences, dietetics, and physical therapy.

The organizing framework for this Core Curriculum comprises six sections: Background Information for Nursing Practice Related to Spinal Cord Impairment (SCI); Foundation for Nursing Practice Related to SCI; Functional Alterations: Physical Domain; Functional Alterations: Personal Domain; Trajectory of SCI Nursing Care; and Shaping SCI Nursing Practice. Section one provides background information for SCI nursing practice, including a historical overview of SCI and a brief description of AASCIN. Additional foundation for nursing practice is provided through presentations on philosophy, goals, and process of SCI nursing practice, diversity in nursing practice roles and settings, cultural issues, and collaboration in teams.

Section two provides the practicing nurse with a foundation, including brief presentations of anatomy and physiology of the spine and spinal cord and overview of the consequences of SCI. Familiarity with neuroanatomy and neurophysiology is essential in the management of individuals with SCI. An accurate identification of the physiological consequences of SCI provides a fundamental step in the delivery of comprehensive health care. Understanding the pathophysiology related to the type of SCI is necessary to appreciate varying functional outcomes. Guidelines are provided for comprehensive neurological assessment related to SCI. Lastly, we address special issues related to pediatric SCI care. Children with SCI require application of multiple management approaches implemented for adults. However, children have very specific growth and developmental needs, which create a constellation of unique needs in the pediatric population. The relationship of the child's age to onset of SCI, nutritional and metabolic needs, body mechanics and motor, cognitive and psychosocial development are key considerations.

Improving function and promoting independence are primary goals of rehabilitation. Section three addresses the myriad physical function alterations. These functional alterations are organized around body systems, including respiratory/pulmonary, cardiovascular and thermoregulatory control, bladder and bowel elimination and continence, nutrition, skin, musculoskeletal, sensation, and spasticity.

Section four continues the focus on functional alterations, but emphasizes the psychological / psychosocial rather than physical domain. Topics include sexuality and reproduction, body image, family, stress, and coping, and activity and exercise.

Rehabilitation is an ongoing process, beginning at the onset of impairment and extending throughout the entire episode of SCI and across the life span. Section five provides a trajectory of nursing care throughout this care continuum. Beginning with prevention of the initial injury, this section also includes trauma care, critical care, acute rehabilitation, caregiver training and support, and community reintegration and independent living. Since prevention continues throughout life, we added chapters on the prevention and management of secondary disabilities and aging with a disability.

Section six addresses topics that shape professional practice of nurses in this specialty field. Specifically, a chapter on quality improvement and outcome evaluation assists the nurse in program evaluation and quality enhancement. A chapter on research priorities addresses the evidence on which our practice is based and provides direction for the future.

The success of any task this large, undertaken by a nonprofit organization such as Eastern Paralyzed Veterans Association (EPVA) depends on the hard work, contributions, and critical analysis of many dedicated individuals. Clearly, James J. Peters, Executive Director of both EPVA and AASCIN, was the "driving force" responsible for this project. EPVA provided financial support for the project; without this support, this endeavor would not have been possible. Two Associate Editors, Cynthia P. Zejdlik and Linda Love, provided insightful assistance in shaping the final book organization as well as careful, painstaking reviews of many chapters. Both of these dedicated SCI nurses are nationally known and respected for their expertise. I am deeply indebted to them for their assistance. This Core Curriculum would not be possible at all, of course, without the extraordinary effort of the multitude of authors and reviewers. In particular, Lisa Pollich, MS provided an extensive review of the manuscript.

Movement into the twenty-first century is characterized by increased complexity and rapid, continuous change as a result of technological innovations in information systems and advances in health care. While the material presented in this text was current at the time it was written, it is the nurse's professional responsibility to verify information and apply current findings from research to practice.

Audrey Nelson, PhD, RN, FAAN
Editor

Contributing Authors

Ellen Barker, MSN, RN, CNRN
President/ Consultant
Neuroscience Nursing Consultants
Greenville, DE

Constance Captain, PhD, RN
Associate Chief, Nursing Service for Research
South Texas Veterans Health Care System
San Antonio, TX

Theresa M. Chase, ND, RN
Patient Education Clinical Specialist
Craig Hospital
Englewood, CO

Laureen Doloresco, MN, RN, CNAA
Assistant Chief, SCI/Rehabilitation Nursing
James A. Haley Veterans Hospital
Tampa, FL

Mary H. Gardenhire, MS, RN, CIC
Infection Control Practitioner
VA Medical Center
Augusta, GA

Jan Giroux, MSN, RN, C, CURN
Case Manager, SCI
VA Palo Alto Health Care System
Palo Alto, CA

Andrea Kaye Hixon, MS, RN, C, CNAA
Executive Assistant for CQI Programs & Quality
Improvement Coordinator
James A. Haley Veterans Hospital
Tampa, FL

Fina Canave-Jimenez, M.Ed., RN
Nurse Educator
Vancouver Hospital & Health Sciences Centre
George Pearson Centre
Vancouver, BC

Kelly Johnson, MSN, RN, CFNP, CRRN
Vice President, Nursing
Craig Hospital
Englewood, CO

Margaret Ross Kraft, MS, RN, CRRN
Chief, SCI/Rehabilitation Nursing
Edward Hines Veterans Hospital
Hines, IL

Cynthia Kraft Fine, MSN, RN, CRRN
Director of Respiratory Services &
Special Projects
Magee Rehabilitation Hospital
Philadelphia, PA

Kathryn M. La Favor, MSN, RN, CRRN
SCI Clinical Nurse Specialist
Froedtert Memorial Lutheran Hospital
Milwaukee, WI

Connie J. Mattera, MS, RN, TNS
Emergency Flight Nurse/Trauma
Chicagi, IL

Denise Miller Lemke, BSN, RN, CNRN
Neurosurgical Nurse Clinician
Medical College of Wisconsin
Milwaukee, WI

Audrey Nelson, Ph.D., RN, FAAN
Associate Chief, Nursing Service for Research
James A. Haley Veterans Hospital
Tampa, FL

Grace Nolde-Lopez, MS, RN, CRRN
SCI Clinical Nurse Specialist
Craig Hospital
Englewood, CO

Janet M. Paarlberg, MS, RN, CRRN
Clinician, Kluge Children's
Rehabilitation Center
University of Virginia Hospital
Charlottesville, VA

Pat Quigley, Ph.D., ARNP, CRRN
Rehabilitation Clinical Nurse Specialist
James A. Haley Veterans Hospital
Tampa, FL

Anne Scott, BSN, CRRN, COHN-S
Staff Rehabilitation Nurse
North Suburban Medical Center
Thorton, CO

Barbara Simmons, MSN, RN
Project Director, SCI
James A. Haley Veterans Hospital
Tampa, FL

Sheila M. Sparks, DNSc, RN, CS
Associate Professor, Nursing
Shenandoah University
Winchester, VA

Joan Stelling, MSN, RN, CRRN
Director of Rehabilitation Nursing
Spain Rehabilitation Center
Birmingham, AL

Donna Stultz, MS, RN
Program Administrator/
Executive Director of Nursing
The Institute for Rehabilitation Research
Houston, TX

Mimi Watson Sutherland, MS, BSN, RN, CNRN
Neurosurgical Coordinator
University of Miami/Jackson Memorial Medical
Center
Miami, FL

Marilyn Ter Maat, MSN, RN-C, CRRN-A, CNAA
Rehab/Restorative Nurse Consultant
The Evangelical Lutheran
Good Samaritan Society
Sioux Falls, SD

Susan S. Thomason, MN, RN, CS, CETN
Coordinator, SCI/D OPC
James A. Haley Veterans Hospital
Tampa, FL

Linda Love, MS, RN, CRRN
Clinical Nurse Specialist, SCI
VA Palo Alto Health Care System
Palo Alto, CA

Nahid Veit, MSN, RN
Clinical Nurse Specialist, SCI
James A. Haley Veterans Hospital
Tampa, FL

Holly Watson-Evans, MS, RN
Product Line Director Orthopaedics &
NeuroSpine Services & International Business
Development
Central DuPage Hospital
Winfield, IL

Reviewers

Craig J. Alexander, PhD
Director of Psychology
Kessler Institute for Rehabilitation, Inc.
West Orange, NJ

Margaret Amato, RN, BSN, CRRN
SCI Outpatient Services Coordinator
VA Medical Center
Milwaukee, Wisconsin

Joseph E. Binard, MD, FRCS(C), FICS
Associate Clinical Professor
University of South Florida
Director, Urological Research
Diagnostic Ultrasound Corporation
Tampa, FL

Helen Bosshart, MSSW, LCSW
Coordinator SCI Home Care
VA Medical Center
Augusta, GA

Harriett A. Bowers, BS, RN-C, CRRN
SCI Nurse Manager
VA Medical Center
Miami, FL

Rose S. Butler, MS, RN, C, CRRN, CCM
Clinical Nurse Specialist
Brooks Rehabilitation Hospital
Jacksonville, FL

J. Caminha-Bacote, Ph.D., RN, CS, CTN
President
Transcultural C.A.R.E. Associates
Cincinnati, OH

Fina Canave-Jimenez, MEd, RN
Nurse Educator
Vancouver Hospital & Health Sciences Centre
George Pearson Centre
Vancouver, British Columbia

Lise M. Casady, MS, RN, CRRN
Advanced Registered Nurse Practitioner
Tampa General Rehabilitation Center
Tampa, FL

Theresa M. Chase, ND, RN
Patient Education Clinical Specialist
Craig Hospital
Englewood, CO

Bonnie Closson, MSN, RN
Clinical Nurse Specialist, Rehabilitation
Mayo Foundation
Rochester, MN

Nancy Crewe, Ph.D.
Professor, Rehabilitation Counseling
Michigan State University
East Lansing, MI

Dennis Crowley, MD
Medical Director SCI Program
The Rehabilitation Hospital of The Pacific
Honolulu, HI

Janet Deneselya, PhD, RN
Coordinator, Research and Development Service
VA Medical Center
Butler, PA

Kathleen L. Dunn, MS, RN, CRRN
Clinical Nurse Specialist, SCI Service
VA San Diego Healthcare System
San Diego, CA

Michael Dunn, PhD
Staff Psychologist, SCI
VA Palo Alto Health Care System
Palo Alto, CA

Lauraine T. Dwyer, MS, RN, CRRN
Director, Ambulatory Care Services
VA San Diego Healthcare System
San Diego, CA

Mary H. Gardenhire, MS, RN, CIC
Infection Control Practitioner
VA Medical Center
Augusta, GA

Katherine A. Gilliland, MSN, RN, CNRN, TNCC
Clinical Nurse Specialist, Neuro/Ortho
Holmes Regional Medical Center
Melbourne, FL

Jan Giroux, MSN, RN, C, CURN
Case Manager, SCI
VA Palo Alto Health Care System
Palo Alto, CA

Tonnie Glick, MEd, RN, CCRN, CRRN
Coordinator, SCI Department
Kessler Institute for Rehabilitation
West Orange, NJ

Margaret C. Hammond, MD
Chief Consultant, Spinal Cord Injury and
Disorder Strategic Healthcare Group
VA Puget Sound Health Care System
Seattle, WA

Marcia Hanak, MA, RN, CRRN
Nursing Rehabilitation Consultant
Private Practice
San Francisco, CA

Patrick Inniss, PhD
Social Worker
Mount Sinai Medical Center
New York, NY

Angela Joseph, MN, RN, CURN
SCI Urology Nurse Coordinator
VA San Diego Health Care System
San Diego, CA

Elizabeth P. Juntilla, BS, RN
Facilitator, Subacute Program
St. Lukes Hospital
San Francisco, CA

Penniford Justice, MD
Chief, SCI Service
VA Medical Center
Memphis, TN

Brenda Kelley, MSN, RN, CRRN
SCI Clinical Nurse Specialist
James A. Haley Veterans Hospital
Tampa, FL

Debrann Kidwell, BSN, RN, CRRN
Staff Development Coordinator
Enloe Rehabilitation Center
Chico, CA

Rosemarie B. King, PhD, RN
Research Assistant Professor
Northwestern University Medical School
Department of PM&R
Chicago, IL

Karen Klemme, BSN, RN, CRRN
Rehabilitation Specialist
Interim Health Care
Kailua-Kona, HI

Steven D. Klemz, MS, MSW, LICSW
Social Worker
James A. Haley Veterans Hospital
Tampa, FL

Margaret Ross Kraft, MS, RN, CRRN
Chief, SCI/Rehabilitation Nursing
Edward Hines Veterans Hospital
Hines, IL

Judi Kuric, MSN, RN, CRRN, CNRN, CCRN
Clinical Nurse Specialist
Neuro-Rehab Solutions
Evansville, IN

Kathryn M. La Favor, MSN, RN, CRRN
SCI Clinical Nurse Specialist
Froedtert Memorial Lutheran Hospital
Milwaukee, WI

E. Jason Mask, MSW, LCSW
SCI Home Care Coordinator
VA Medical Center
Hines, IL

Jeanne Mervine, MA, RN, CRRN, PNP
Clinical Specialist
Rehabilitation Institute of Chicago
Chicago, IL

Stephanie Metzger, MS, RN, CS, PNP
Coordinator, Children's Hospital Rehabilitation
Richmond, VA

Mary Montufar, MS, RN
Nurse Manager, SCI
Palo Alto Health Care System
Palo Alto, CA

Janet M. Paarlberg, MS, RN, CRRN
Clinician
Kluge Children's Rehabilitation Center
University of Virginia Health Sciences Center
Charlottesville, VA

Deanna Persaud, MSN, RN
Professor, School of Nursing
California State University
Chico, CA

Barbara Rines, RN
Sexual Health Clinician
British Columbia Rehabilitation Society
Vancouver, BC

Diana Rintala, PhD
Director of Research
The Institute for Rehabilitation and Research
Houston, TX

Kathleen Sawin, DNS, RNC, FAAN
Associate Professor
School of Nursing, Commonwealth of Virginia
Midlothian, VA

Audrey J. Schmerzler, MSN, RN
Nurse Clinician, SCI
Mount Sinai Medical Center
New York, NY

Anne Scott, BSN, CRRN, COHN-S
Staff Rehabilitation Nurse
North Suburban Medical Center
Thorton, CO

Milena Segatore, MSN, RN, CNRN, CCRN
Clinical Nurse Specialist, Neurology
St. Joseph's Hospital
Milwaukee, WI

Marca Sipski, MD
Chief, SCI Service
VA Medical Center
Miami, FL

Sheila M. Sparks, DNSc, RN- CA
Associate Professor
Shenandoah University
Division of Nursing
Winchester, VA

Marilyn Ter Maat, MSN, RN-C, CRRN-A, CNAA
Rehab/Restorative Nurse Consultant
The Evangelical Lutheran Good Samaritan
Society
Sioux Falls, SD

Anaise O. Theuerkauf, M.Ed., RN, CRRN
Private Consultant
Education and Sports Consultants, Inc.
Shreveport, LA

Nahid Veit, MSN, RN
Clinical Nurse Specialist, SCI
James A. Haley VAMC
Tampa, FL

Martha Vidal, RD
SCI Dietitian
James A. Haley VAMC
Tampa, FL

Holly Watson-Evans, MS, RN
Product Line Director Orthopaedics and
NeuroSpine Services & International Business
Development
Central DuPage Hospital
Winfield, IL

Carol J. Wichman, MN, RN
Chief Flight Nurse
Penrose- St. Francis Healthcare System
Englewood, CO

Candace Wittenberg, BPT
SCI Physical Therapy Coordinator
Rehabilitation Hospital of the Pacific
Honolulu, HI

Nursing Practice Related to Spinal Cord Impairment: A Core Curriculum

Focus Group Participants

Margaret Amato, RN, BSN, CRRN
SCI Outpatient Services Coordinator
Clement Zablocki Department of Veterans
Affairs Medical Center
Milwaukee, WI

Ruth Baker, RN, BSN
Coordinator, SCI Home Care
VA Medical Center
Cleveland, OH

Sally Breen, BSN, RN
Sexual Health Clinician
George Pearson Centre
Vancouver, BC

Jane A. Boyd. BS, RN, CRRN
Director of Rehabilitation / Transitional Care
Methodist Medical Center of Illinois
Peoria, IL

Anita B. Cordova, MSN, RN, CRRN
SCI Clinical Nurse Specialist
VA Medical Center
Long Beach, CA

Elaine E. Detwiler, RN, BSN, CRRN
Head Nurse, SCI
VA Puget Sound Health Care System
Seattle, WA

Peggy Egan, RN, MSN
Clinical Nurse Specialist Rehabilitation
VA Medical Center
Indianapolis, IN

Gretchen M. Eichensehr, RN, BS
Staff Nurse
Shriners Hospital for Children
Philadelphia, PA

Carrie B. Fields, RN, BSN
Industrial Health Nurse
Department of Energy Westinghouse
Augusta, GA

Cindy Gatens, MN, RN, CRRN
Rehabilitation Clinical Nurse Specialist
Ohio State University Medical Center
Columbus, OH

Carol Ann Husted, RN
SCI Staff Nurse
VA Hudson Valley Health Care System
Castle Point, NY

Fina Canave-Jimenez, M.Ed., RN
Nurse Educator
Vancouver Hospital & Health Sciences Centre
George Pearson Centre
Vancouver, BC

Elizabeth P. Juntilla, BS, RN
Facilitator, Subacute Program
St. Lukes Hospital
San Francisco, CA

Debrann Kidwell, BSN, RN
Staff Development Coordinator
Enloe Rehabilitation Center
Chico, CA

Constance LaPorte, RN
SCI Staff Nurse
VA Medical Center
Hines, IL

Laura Leigh, MBA, MSN, RN, CRRN
Vice President, Patient Care
Rehabilitation Institute of Chicago
Chicago, IL

Nancy Lewis, MSN, RN, CRRN
SCI Case Manager
Health South Harmarville
Rehabilitation Hospital
Pittsburgh, PA

Elaine Lloyd, RN, MS
Clinical Nurse Specialist
Cupertino, CA

Janet Loehr, MN, ARNP
SCI Nurse Practitioner
VA Puget Sound Health Care System
Seattle, WA

Charlotte McDermott, RN, BSN, CRRN
Clinical Manager Spinal Cord Program
UPMC Rehab Hospital
Pittsburgh, PA

Sylvia Eichner McDonald, MS, RN, CRRN
Neuroscience Rehab Clinical Nurse Specialist
Mercy Medical Center
Oshkosh, WI

Mary Montufar, MS, RN
Nurse Manager, SCI
Palo Alto Health Care System
Palo Alto, CA

Veronica Morales, RN
SCI Nurse Clinician
Shriners Hospital for Children
Philadelphia, PA

Elma M. Padios, RN
SCI Clinical Manager
James A. Haley Veterans Hospital
Tampa, FL

Rob Rayner, RN, BSN, CRRN
Staff Nurse
VA Palo Alto Health Care System
Palo Alto, CA

Barbara Rines, RN
Sexual Health Clinician
British Columbia Rehab Society
Vancouver, BC

Ray Riska, RN
QA Coordinator
Froedtert Memorial Lutheran Hospital
Milwaukee, WI

Linda Love, MS, RN, CRRN
SCI Clinical Nurse Specialist
VA Palo Alto Health Care System
Palo Alto, CA

Judith L. Trotman, RN, BS, CCRN
SCI Clinical Manager
James A. Haley Veterans Hospital
Tampa, FL

CHAPTER

Historical Overview

Anne Scott, BSN, CRRN, COHN-S

I. Learning Objectives

A. Identify key areas that have impacted on the care of people with spinal cord impairment (SCI).

B. Identify landmark developments in history affecting treatment and rehabilitation of persons with SCI.

II. Introduction

The treatment of people with SCI has evolved over time through changes in social, cultural, and religious beliefs; health care practices; state-of-the-art technology; and legislation. Much of this progress was stimulated by war times and needs evidenced by wounded soldiers. This progress then spilled over into civilian services. Rehabilitation is a recently developed specialty, and we are in the midst of making its history. This chapter will include highlights of historical developments that have affected the care of individuals with SCI.

III. Advances In Health Care

A. **Historical References to Disability**
   1. 2600 B.C.: The Chinese recognized that disease was related to inactivity and used exercise (such as Kung Fu) as a way to promote health.
   2. 359 B.C.: Hippocrates recommended exercise for recovering patients and introduced traction to reduce deformities of the spine.
   3. In the 7th century, Paul of Aegina performed the "first surgical procedure for SCI" (Erico, Bauer, & Waugh, 1992).
   4. In the 9th century, the Mohemmedans established a hospital in Baghdad for those with disabilities.
   5. Spartans eliminated children with disabilities as a way of "upgrading the race" (Oberman, 1965).

6. Early examples of assistive aids are seen in the primitive walking stick and wheelchair.
7. Witchcraft reached its height in the 16th and 17th centuries and was often used as the explanation for disabilities.

B. **Colonial Development**
1. In the early hospitals, disabled people were "lumped with the poor, vagrants, sick and mentally ill" (Oberman, 1965). Later, efforts were made to segregate people with physical disabilities.
2. Many reforms of care and treatment were through the efforts of The Quakers. With the aid of Benjamin Franklin in 1752, the first general hospital, Pennsylvania Hospital, was opened near Philadelphia. The corner stone read "The saving and restoring useful and laborious members to a community is a work of Public Service and the Relief of the Sick Poor is not only an Act of Humanity, but a religious Duty" (Oberman, 1965).
3. 1798: Dr. Benjamin Rush, a signer of the Declaration of Independence, "advocated work as a remedial measure for patients in....hospital." He recommended "certain kinds of labor, exercise and amusements be contrived for them, which should act at the same time upon their bodies and their minds" (Hopkins & Smith, 1983, 4-5).

C. **The 19th Century**
1. Advances in the field of orthopedics and neurology
   a. 1810: Traction was developed by Dr. Scherger in Germany
   b. 1825: Similar traction beds and a traction chair were developed in France and England, although primarily used for treatment of scoliosis.
   c. 1863: The Hospital for the Ruptured and Crippled opened in New York.
   d. 1865: The New York Orthopedic Hospital and Dispensary opened.
   e. 1884: In Philadelphia, the Hospital for the Merciful Savior was established as the first institution to specialize in the care of disabled children.
   f. 1893: Russian neurologist, Berkhterev, published his method combining suspension and traction using a neck halter and weights.
2. Early legislation provided rehabilitation and training for children with disabilities.
   a. 1853: The Pennsylvania Training School for Feeble Minded Children opened, supported by state and private funds
   b. 1857: Both Connecticut and Ohio opened "schools for idiots".
   c. 1860: Kentucky Institute for the Education of Feebleminded Children and Idiots opened.
   d. 1897: Through the efforts of orthopedic surgeon Dr. Arthur Gillette, Minnesota provided the first legislative support for "treatment, care and education of crippled children" (Oberman, 1965).
3. Charity was accomplished through the churches in early colony years. Secular elements appeared in the mid-1700's through the development of "poor laws".
   a. 1840-1890: Many Family Service Societies were developed.
   b. 1881: The American Red Cross was organized.
   c. The Rockefeller Foundation and Carnegie Corporations were started at the turn of the Century.
   d. 1917: Jeremiah Milbank and the Red Cross donated funds for the Red Cross Institute for Crippled and Disabled Man, now known as the International Center for the Disabled.
   e. The Red Cross also established retraining programs for disabled veterans at Walter Reed Army Medical Center and other army hospitals.
4. Tuberculosis, a major cause of disability in the late 1800s, was the leading cause of death.
5. 1859: Guillian-Barré Syndrome was first described by Landry and again later, in 1916, by Guillian-Barré and Strohl.
6. 1868: French neurologist Charcot described multiple sclerosis as a distinct disease.
7. 1895: Roentgen discovered and named the x-ray.

D. **The Early 20th Century: 1900-1940**
   1. In the 20th century, the Easter Seal Society evolved to be a major provider of care to people with disabilities.
      a. 1907: The National Society for Crippled Children and Adults was organized in Elyria, Ohio.
      b. 1921: A Federation of State Societies was organized.
      c. 1934: The National Easter Seals Campaign was started to raise money through the sale of Easter seals.
   2. Development of occupational and physical therapy
      a. 1905: Nurse, Susan Tracy applied early therapy principles to bedfast orthopedic patients. She began a training program to develop physical activities at the Adams Nervine Asylum in Boston.
      b. 1910: The first occupational therapy text was published as a manual for nurses and attendants.
      c. Because of World War I, and the polio epidemic of 1916, there was tremendous development of the field then known as reconstruction therapy. The Surgeon General's Office formed the Division of Special Hospitals and Physical Reconstruction. Schools multiplied to meet the growing demand for reconstruction aides.
         (1) Physiotherapy aides treated wounded soldiers with "hydrotherapy, electrotherapy, mechanotherapy, muscle relaxation, active exercises, indoor and outdoor games and passive exercises in the form of massage" (American Physical Therapy Association, 1996).
         (2) Occupational therapy aides "furnished forms of occupation to convalescents" (Hopkins & Smith, 1983, p. 10).
      d. 1917: The National Society for the Promotion of Occupational Therapy was incorporated in Washington D.C. In 1923, the name was changed to the American Occupational Therapy Association.
      e. Many of these programs closed after the war; however, there continued a demand for reconstruction aides in civilian hospitals.
      f. 1921: The American Physical Therapy Association was formed with 274 charter members. By the end of the 1930's, there were 1000 members; and men were permitted to join.
   3. Post World War I activity
      a. State and Federal programs for vocational rehabilitation were initiated.
         (1) 1918: The Soldiers Rehabilitation Act was passed and the Federal Board for Vocational Education was established.
         (2) 1920: Woodrow Wilson signed the Smith-Fess Act extending vocational training to civilians with disabilities.
      b. 1923: The American Congress of Rehabilitation Medicine was formed.
   4. The Depression: The economic depression resulted in 33 percent reduction in health care spending causing obvious hardship for all medical areas and a halt in progress (Tunwar, 1994).
   5. 1933: Crutchfield tongs were introduced for skeletal traction.
   6. 1938: President Franklin Roosevelt established the National Foundation for Infantile Paralysis, now known as the March of Dimes.
   7. 1940: Advancements were made in techniques for surgical correction including open reduction and fusion of fracture-dislocations and use of plates for stabilization.

E. **The Rehabilitation Era: 1940 -1960**
   1. Post World War II: Once again, returning veterans spurred advancement of treatment programs.
      a. 1943: Dr. Howard Rusk and Dr. George Deaver developed a rehabilitation program for the Army Air Force and later for the Veterans Administration.
      b. Dr. Henry Kessler organized a rehabilitation program for the Navy and in 1948 formed the Kessler Institute in New Jersey. Dr. Kessler was also instrumental in the development of the workman's compensation program.

c. The first civilian rehabilitation unit was established at Bellevue Hospital under the direction of Dr. Rusk. At this time, Dr. Rusk was also an associate editor for the New York Times spreading his message to the public.

d. 1943: In England, Sir Ludwig Guttman developed a rehabilitation program at Stoke Mandeville Hospital.

e. Late 1930s and early 1940s: In Boston, with the aid of Liberty Mutual Insurance Company, Dr. Donald Munro opened a spinal injury unit at University Hospital.

f. 1944: Spinal Injury Centers were being developed through the Veterans Administration in the Bronx, New York and Hines, Illinois.

g. 1947 was the first registration exam for occupational therapists and two Masters degree programs in Occupational Therapy were created.

h. 1947: Physiatry was recognized as a specialty and the American Board of Physical Medicine and Rehabilitation was established.

i. In the late 1940s somatosensory evoked potentials were introduced to record nerve action.

j. 1950: What is now known as the National Institute of Neurological Disorders and Stroke was created by Congress.

k. 1952: Mary Switzer conducted the first survey of rehabilitation needs in the United States.

l. 1957: Physicians at the SCI Center in the Veteran's Administration Hospitals founded the American Paraplegia Society.

2. Advancements in medical and surgical practices

a. Early in the 1940s, penicillin was introduced, reducing the threat of previously lethal infections such as pneumonia and urinary tract infections.

b. 1941: Orthopedist and inventor, Dr. Homer Stryker, developed the Stryker Frame to facilitate care.

c. 1946: The National Multiple Sclerosis Society was formed and quickly launched three research projects.

d. The outbreak of polio also increased the need for rehabilitation services. The Salk vaccine, introduced in 1955, reduced the incidence of polio by over 90 percent. In 1965, the oral Sabin vaccine was introduced. Sister Kenny, an Australian nurse, revolutionized the care of patients with polio. The Sister Kenny Institute was opened in Minneapolis.

e. 1958: The circo-electric bed was introduced to facilitate turning patients on bedrest for prolonged traction.

f. 1958: The Harrington Rod was used to provide traction and stabilization for thoracolumbar fractures.

F. Period of Political and Social Change:1960-1980

1. Government programs reshaped care for persons with disabilities. Previous areas of care, such as polio, became obsolete; however others emerged such as motor vehicle accidents and injuries related to drug, alcohol, or crime activity.

a. 1966: The Association of Rehabilitation Centers (ARC) and the National Association of Sheltered Workshops and Homebound Programs (NASWHP) incorporated the Commission on Accreditation of Rehabilitation Facilities (CARF).

b. 1968: Dr.'s Kruzen, Rusk, and Freed spoke to Congress describing "the absolute disarray of service delivery" for persons with SCI (Thomas, 1990).

c. 1970: Dr. William Glenn of Yale University first applied his phrenic nerve pacemaker to a spinal cord injured patient.

d. The development of mandatory automobile passenger restraints evolved, responding to the growing numbers of motor vehicle accidents. Although available in most vehicles since the 1950s and 60s, restraints were not mandatory until a federal rule in 1972 required all American-made vehicles to include the "starter interlock," which required the occupant to buckle up before the ignition would start. This rule was later rescinded because of consumer dissatisfaction.

e. The Rehabilitation Services Administration (RSA), the branch of the government responsible for vocational rehabilitation, developed the Model Systems concept which was funded and implemented in 1970 in Arizona. This concept was designed to develop and provide quality care and stimulate basic and clinical research for spinal cord injury. In 1972, six additional centers were funded, providing an organized continuum of care from onset of injury through long-term follow-up, as well as a coordinated database. In 1973, statistical analysis of the Model Systems approach began.

   f. In the early 1970's a task force of the National Academy of Science and the National Research Council put together a curriculum forming the Emergency Management Systems: this resulted in improvements in pre-hospital care of people with disabilities.

   g. 1973: The Rehabilitation Act was passed providing civil rights for people with disabilities.

   h. In 1973, the American Spinal Injury Association and the Spina Bifida Association of America were formed.

   i. In 1974, the Association of Rehabilitation Nurses was founded and one year later, 143 rehabilitation nurses attended the first educational conference.

   j. 1975: The Education for All Handicapped Children Act was passed providing access to education and accommodations for children with disabilities.

2. Advances in technology: Technology has had effects throughout health care ranging from improved survival because of genetic testing; improved neonatal, emergency, and acute care; and improved quality of life afforded by assistive technology.

   a. Diagnostic technology

      (1) 1973: Computerized axial tomography (CAT) scan was added to the neuro-diagnostic artillery.

      (2) Electromyography (EMG) and somatosensory evoked potentials (SSEP) began use in rehabilitation and acute care.

   b. Assistive technology

      (1) The walking stick and wheelchair, used throughout history, continued to improve due to the availability of lightweight metals and plastics; these changes provided energy conservation, functional independence, and recreation opportunities previously not possible.

      (2) Functional aids were developed through new design, construction and materials such as Velcro.

      (3) Electronic technology was applied to rehabilitation in the 1970's; the environmental control unit was one of the first examples of technology allowing independent operation of television, telephone, and wheelchair.

G. **1980-1997:** Prominent issues in health care include funding and cost containment. Shortened hospital stays, entitlement programs, and managed care resulted in ethical dilemmas about eligibility and scope of services available.

1. Technology continued to develop at a swift rate.

   a. In the 1980s, microchip technology became available, creating a host of equipment that is either commercially available or was adapted for the rehabilitation arena.

   b. Other advancements included robotics and voice activated systems.

   c. Improvements in construction materials (lightweight, flexible, durable) enable new sport and recreation possibilities.

   d. Animal assistants were introduced to interface with severely disabled people.

   e. The Magnetic Resonance Imagery (MRI) became available in 1981 and revolutionized the diagnosis of diseases such as multiple sclerosis.

2. As length of stay in hospitals decreased, new models of care developed. Transitional or sub-acute rehabilitation units and comprehensive outpatient programs extended rehabilitation at reduced cost.

3. Early 1980s: Gardner-Wells tongs become available for cervical traction, reducing complications of cranial penetration.

4. Outcome measurement systems took hold as a means to validate the need for treatment, communicate with the payor source, and compete within the field. In 1983, a task force of the American Congress of Rehabilitation/American Academy of Physical Medicine and Rehabilitation developed the Functional Independence Measure (FIM).

5. Pharmacological developments have continued.
   a. Costs and use of antibiotics soared; almost one-third of all hospitalized patients were treated with antibiotics (Stein, 1990).
   b. 1990: High dose steroids were advocated to decrease the neurological deficit following SCI.
   c. 1992: Intrathecal drug delivery systems became available for management of spasticity and pain.
6. 1982: The first certification exam for nurses in rehabilitation was administered.
7. 1983: The American Association of Spinal Cord Injury Nurses (AASCIN) was founded and held their first annual conference.
8. Legislative changes continue.
   a. 1986: The Birth to Three Program began providing early intervention through rehabilitation services for infants and toddlers with disabilities.
   b. 1990: The Americans with Disabilities Act was passed.
   c. 1992: The reauthorization of the Rehabilitation Act provided phased compliance requirements for accommodation by employers and transportation providers, enforcing the original intent of the legislation.

H. **Future:** Research and technology hold much promise for prevention, care, and cure of SCI.

Personal Perspective: "That was Then, This is Now"

It may seem hard to believe but I am glad I was in rehabilitation in 1978. There have been substantial advancements in emergency medical service, diagnosis, acute care and rehab. But in my eyes there remains one major shortcoming and that is length of stay. First the advances.

When I was injured, I was transferred twice before landing at a large enough hospital to care for my injuries. Today, if you don't get on-site emergency care you will be airlifted to a regional trauma center. I went two weeks before a ruptured diaphragm and collapsed lung were found. Today's diagnostics would prI see the catch. After a two month acute stay plus a six month rehabilitation program, I was not ready to go home….my family was not ready to have me home. In fact, many health care funding sources want people discharged in the time it took me to learn to sit up on my own. This leads us to the question of in-patient versus out-patient services. Most important is the question, "…am I ready…..?"

Consider that up until that time in my life, I had little or no experience with disability— none with rehabilitation and therapy. I did have experience with my body, my career goals, and my self-concept. In an instant this ALL changed beyond my ability to comprehend, let alone participate in rehabilitation. So, as I look at then and now, yes there have been advances, many. However, the most important facet of the process, the wounded human being, is still basically the same and needs time to understand, adjust and hopefully eventually move on.

As for moving on, one of the best changes over the last twenty years has been the improvements in wheelchair design and other adaptive/assistive technology. Things have come a long way from the days of cannibalizing our everyday chairs with mail order add-ons. Today there are fluorescent pink chairs for tennis, racing and active lifestyles. Perhaps we can continue this process of technological and medical advances without forgetting the human being and provide them with the time they need to learn to live with the most traumatic event in their our lives.

John Bateman-Ferry, President
Disability Access Solutions
Syracuse, New York

References and Selected Bibliography

Adams, R.D., & Victor, M. (Eds.). (1993). *Principles of neurology* (5th ed.). New York: McGraw-Hill.

Apple, D.F., & Hudson, L.M. (Eds.). (1990). *Spinal cord injury: The model* (NIDDR Grant #H133C9014). Atlanta,GA Shepherd Center for Treatment of Spinal Injuries.

Breneman, J.C., & Hager, D. (1992). *The Stryker story: Homer Iliad*. Kalamazoo: Phil Schubert and Associates.

DeLisa, J.A., & Gans, B.M. (Eds.). (1993). *Rehabilitation medicine: Principles and practice* (2nd ed.). Philadelphia: J.B. Lippincott.

Errico, T.J., Bauer, R.D., & Waugh, T. R. (EDS). (1991). *Spinal trauma*. Philadelphia: J.B. Lippincott Co.

Goldenson, R.M. (Ed.). (1990). *Disability and rehabilitation handbook*. New York: McGraw Hill.

Goodgold, J. (Ed.). (1988). *Rehabilitation medicine*. St. Louis, MO: C.V. Mosby.

Guttman, L. (1976). *Spinal cord injuries: Comprehensive management and research* (2nd ed.). London: Oxford.

Holtzman, R., & Stein, B. (Eds.). (1985). *The tethered cord syndrome*. New York: Theime-Stratton.

Hopkins, H., & Smith, H. (Eds.). (1983). *Willard and Spakman's Occupational Therapy* (6th ed.). Philadelphia: J.B. Lipincott.

Kottke, F.J., & Lehman, J.F. (Eds.). (1990). *Krusen's handbook of physical medicine and rehabilitation* (4th ed.). Philadelphia: W.B. Sanders.

Livshits, A.V. (1991). Surgery of the spinal cord. Madison, WI: International University Press.

Oberman, C.E. (1965). *A history of vocational rehabilitation in America*. Minneapolis, MN: T.S. Denison.

Ohry, A., & Ohry-Kossoy, K. (1989). *Spinal cord injuries in the 19th century: Background, research, and treatment*. Edinburgh, Scotland: Churchill Livingstone.

Rowland, L.P. (Ed.). (1989). *Merritt's textbook of neurology* (8th ed.). Philadelphia: Lea and Fabiger.

Rusk, H. A. (1972). *A world to care for: The autobiography of Howard A. Rusk M.D.* New York: Random House.

Shterenshis, M.V. (1992). The history of modern spinal traction with particular reference to neural disorders. *Spinal Trauma, 35*, 139-146.

Stein, J. (Ed.). (1990). *Internal medicine* (3rd ed.). Boston: Little Brown.

Thomas, J.P. (1990). Opportunities for cooperation. *Paraplegia News, 48*(9), 34-39.

Tunwar, A.J. (1994). *Occupational therapy: Principles and practice* (6th ed.). Baltimore: Williams and Wilkins.

University of Alabama. (1996). *Spinal cord injury: Facts and figures at a glance*. Birmingham: University of Alabama at Birmingham.

Vinken, P.J., Bruyn, G.W., Klawans, H.L., & Frankel, H.L. (1992). *Spinal cord trauma*. Amsterdam: Elsevier.

CHAPTER

American Association of Spinal Cord Injury Nurses

Audrey Nelson, PhD., RN, FAAN

I. Learning Objectives

A. Describe the mission of AASCIN.

B. Appreciate the background, growth, and development of AASCIN since 1983.

C. Describe the major accomplishments of AASCIN.

D. Consider the future of AASCIN as a specialty nursing organization.

II. Introduction

The American Association of Spinal Cord Injury Nurses (AASCIN) is a non-profit organization dedicated to promoting quality care for individuals with spinal cord injury. This is achieved by advancing nursing practice through education, research, advocacy, health care policy, and collaboration with consumers and health care delivery systems. AASCIN is the only nursing organization devoted exclusively to promoting excellence in meeting the nursing care needs of individuals with spinal cord injury. In 1997, AASCIN expanded its focus to spinal cord impairment in addition to injuries.

A. **Mission Statement**
The mission of AASCIN is to advance, foster, encourage, promote, and improve nursing care of persons with spinal cord impairment (SCI); develop and promote education and research related to the nursing care of persons with SCI; and recognize nurses whose careers are devoted to the problems of SCI and promote the exchange of ideas.

B. **Philosophy**
The AASCIN believes that a spinal cord injury is a multifaceted, catastrophic experience for the person, his/her family or significant others. Nursing, as an art and science, has a primary role in assisting persons with SCI to achieve and maintain an optimum level of physical and

psychosocial function. SCI nurses are skilled practitioners, knowledgeable in the pathophysiological and psychological implications of spinal cord injury, who employ special techniques to deal with the impact of spinal cord disorders on the individual, family, and society.

Education and research are fundamental to professional growth, excellence in clinical practice, and facilitation of optimal health outcomes. Therefore, it is a primary goal of the Association to provide educational and research opportunities to its members through annual programs, workshops, research grants, and printed materials. Consumers, families, and significant others, as participating members of the health care team, should be included in the education process. Collaboration with colleagues, consumers, policy-makers, and other interested parties is central to appropriate patient outcome and the ability of nurses to optimize care and meet the needs of persons with SCI.

C. **Goals of AASCIN**
1. Promote and enhance the nursing care of individuals with SCI
2. Develop and promote education and research related to SCI
3. Provide educational opportunities for nurses who specialize in SCI
4. Facilitate the exchange of information and collaborate with other professionals involved in SCI care
5. Serve as a resource to individuals and organizations providing nursing and health care services, government agencies, educational facilities, and consumer groups
6. Recognize nurses committed to the care of individuals with SCI
7. Advance spinal cord injury nursing as a specialty practice

III. Historical Background

A. Ten founding members signed the articles of incorporation for the Association in 1983.

B. Thirty-seven charter members attended the first annual meeting of AASCIN in August, 1983. Susan Brady was the founding president.

IV. Membership

A. **Description of Members:** Members include registered and licensed practical/vocational nurses from the United States and Canada. These nurses practice in diverse settings such as: intensive care, acute SCI, rehabilitation, long term care, home care, and independent practice. AASCIN members serve in many professional roles including those of clinician, educator, administrator, and researcher.

B. **Membership Growth**
1. In the first year, membership grew to 368 members and doubled between 1985-86 to 800 members. In 1986, the membership exceeded 1,000. Membership peaked in 1988 at 1,869.
2. As of May 30, 1996 membership included 1,428 members. Of the 1,428 members, 1,194 were active members and 234 were associate members.

V. Board of Directors

A. A total of 10-15 Directors are elected from the AASCIN membership for a three-year term. Approximately one third of the Directors are elected each year.
B. All Directors are registered nurses, with the exception of the Executive Director.
C. The Board elects officers annually, including: President, Vice-President (President-Elect), Secretary, and Treasurer.

CHAPTER

Philosophy, Goals, and Process of SCI Nursing Practice

Barbara Simmons, MSN, RN

I. Learning Objectives

A. Describe the philosophy of rehabilitation.

B. Apply the concepts of rehabilitation to spinal cord impairment (SCI) nursing practices.

C. Describe the implications for nursing theories to SCI nursing practice.

II. Introduction

Movement into the twenty-first century is characterized by increased complexity and rapid, continuous change as a result of technological innovations in information systems and advances in health care. Nurses providing direct care to persons with SCI may experience this change as having a profound impact on the care they give and on the lives of persons with SCI. Changes in healthcare delivery are primarily driven by sources outside the influence of health care professionals and health care agencies. Financial concerns and diminishing resources are major factors influencing the provision of health care. Two longstanding roles of nurses have been that of advocate and of change agent. Exclusion from the process of change could result in nursing becoming a product of rather than an agent of change.

Exclusion could also minimize nursing's opportunity to advocate for humanistic care for people with SCI. Relying on nursing's rich heritage will assist nurses to cope with change and will provide the vision for the next century. Our heritage includes a nursing paradigm, nursing theories, philosophy, and use of scientific method.

This chapter presents a set of beliefs about nursing and rehabilitation that guide SCI nursing practice. Nursing process is the scientific method nurses use to provide quality care. Effective use of nursing process assumes theoretical knowledge. Nurse theorists have made significant and enduring contributions to the knowledge and practice of nursing two nursing theories will be described. Implications for the use of theories to guide the practice of SCI nurses will be offered.

III. Philosophy

A. **Definitions:** Philosophy may refer to a set of values, tenets, and premises; or it may also refer to the pursuit of knowledge. Values are the foundation of a philosophy. Tenets are beliefs held to be true. Premises held by an individual or the prevailing values, tenets, and premises of family, culture, community, or society may overly or covertly influence group. This philosophy provides the guiding principles that underlie goals and processes of practice.

B. **Philosophy of Science:** Philosophy as the pursuit of knowledge challenges academicians, scholars, philosophers, and disciplines to advance knowledge. Philosophies of science provide the structure for knowledge development and the direction for change within a discipline (Laudan, 1977; Reigel, Omery, Calvillo, Elsayed, Lee, Shuler, & Siegal, 1992). Philosophies of science may be developed by a discipline or borrowed from another discipline. According to Kuhn (1970), as disciplines or fields evolve they undergo shifts in paradigms where different theories compete for acceptance— some prevail while others do not. These paradigms provide the framework for scientific advancement and the manner in which a discipline conducts its practice.

C. **Tenets:** Philosophical values, tenets, and premises can also be gleaned from the literature. Independence and integration are values considered critical to the quality of the life of people with disabilities. The following tenets are interwoven in the literature:
   1. Each person with a disability is unique and exists synergistically within his/her environment.
   2. Each person with a disability is in possession of or has potential for self-worth, dignity, and transcendence.
   3. Each person with a disability is motivated when self-worth is recognized.
   4. Each person with a SCI has the right to accessibility.
   5. Each person with a disability has the right to improvement and autonomy.

D. **Premises of rehabilitation:**
   1. Rehabilitation begins at the onset of SCI.
   2. Rehabilitation minimizes the impact of social stigma.
   3. Rehabilitation promotes independence.
   4. Rehabilitation promotes integration.

E. **Guiding Principles:** Philosophical values, tenets, and premises provide guiding principles for SCI nurses. Zejdlik (1992) correlates philosophy with the goals for individuals with SCI and stipulates the nurse's role.

F. **Philosophical Underpinnings of Rehabilitation:** Philosophy as values, tenets, and premises is the primary focus of this discussion. Understanding the philosophical underpinnings of rehabilitation will assist the SCI nurse to participate in the development and implementation of a philosophy of SCI nursing.

IV. Rehabilitation

A. **Societal Attitudes:** Awareness of societal attitudes toward people with disabilities is crucial to understanding the philosophical underpinnings or rehabilitation. It can be said that the humanity of a society can be measured by the treatment and inclusion of its most vulnerable groups. Vulnerability may be a factor of age, race, gender, poverty, sexual preference, or religious belief. Vulnerability may also occur when an individual does not conform to society's ideal or is limited in ability to fulfill an expected role. Person's with SCI comprise a vulnerable group. Vulnerable groups possess characteristics that may provoke uncomfortable feelings in the general population and generate issues that are complex in nature.

B. **Classifications of Disablement:** The World Health Organization (1980) described three classifications of disablement:

1. Impairment is a loss or abnormality of psychological, physiological, anatomical and structure or function.
2. Disability is any restriction or lack (resulting from impairment) of ability to perform an activity in the manner or within the range considered normal for a human being.
3. Handicap is a disadvantage for given individual resulting from impairment or disability that limits or prevents fulfillment of a normal role for that individual.

C. **Interrelationships between Impairment, Disability, and Handicap:** It does not necessarily follow that a person with an impairment is also disabled, nor is a person with a disability always handicapped. Indeed, there are examples of athletes with impairments and disabilities who successfully complete with able-bodied athletes in professional sports. Patrick (1989) delineates interrelationships among impairment, disability, and handicap.
1. Impairment occurs at the intrinsic organ level and may result in a functional limitation and disability.
2. Disability occurs at the level of the personal behavior and is evidence in restricted activity.
3. A handicap occurs at the extrinsic social level when restricted activity impedes the person's ability to fulfill a designated role.

D. **Defining Rehabilitation:** Trieschmann (1988:26) describes rehabilitation as "the process of teaching people to live with their disability in their own home". Rehabilitation is an ongoing process beginning at the onset of injury or dysfunction and extending throughout the entire episode of SCI or across the life span.

E. **Settings for Rehabilitation:** Current literature consistently proposes that rehabilitation is best accomplished at home. However, rehabilitation and other services for persons with disabilities have historically taken place away from the home and community. Bradley & Knoll (1995) report that there has been a transition in the provision of services. They postulate that services have been provided within a theoretical perspective that they refer to as a paradigm. The paradigm has shifted from the medical model, to the developmental model then to the rehabilitation model.
1. Hallmarks of the medical model are institutionalization, separation from family and dependence. The public's growing concerns regarding the lack of standards, depersonalization, and segregation precipitated the shift for the medical model.
2. The developmental model followed and emphasized deinstitutionalization and community-based services, which continued to be provided away from the home setting. This model was impersonal and treated the person with disability as an object to be evaluated and trained to adjust to the community.
3. More recently, the shift was to the rehabilitation model assuring the person with disability control of their own life, and participation in decisions regarding services that are home or community based.

F. **Legislation:** Legislation assuring availability of rehabilitation services is evidence of societal commitment to people with disabilities. Fifield & Fifield (1995) report that legislation is drafted in political settings that are influenced by social values and economics.

G. **Goals of Rehabilitation:** Promoting function, independence, and autonomy are primary goals of rehabilitation.
1. Improving function includes all actions necessary to assure the person with SCI can live in the least restrictive setting of their choice.
2. Independence is achieved by compensating for the disability by learning alternative methods of accomplishing tasks and maximizing capabilities through an attitude of assertiveness, self reliance, and realism (Brummel-Smith, 1990; Kemp, 1990). According to Trieschman (1988), independence is behavior relating to activities a person can perform with minimal assistance. Autonomy is a critical element of independence.
3. Autonomy is the ability and right to make informed decisions. If a person with disability is denied the opportunity to make informed choices, even when those choices involve risk,

then independence is also denied. Allowing a person with disability the dignity to make their own mistakes and to experience the consequences of their mistakes can precipitate a breakthrough in rehabilitation. Accepting the right to risk and assuming the responsibility for the consequences is presumed equal among all rational persons.

H. **Habilitation:** Habilitation is both related to and part of rehabilitation. Habilitation involves the acquisition of new skills and abilities, whereas rehabilitation involves reacquisition of lost skills and abilities (Commission of Accreditation of Rehabilitation Facilities CARF, 1996).

"Not everyone with a disability needs rehabilitation, however, everyone can benefit from habilitation because everyone who has achieved a state of maturity can improve their capabilities. All people have a potential for improvement and things can always be done better. This philosophy helps us to maintain open, positive and dynamic through life's changes" P.A. Quigley (personal communication, January 9, 1997).

I. **Integration:** Integration refers to active participation in the individual's community of choice — a desired outcome of rehabilitation. The level of integration is correlated with the extent a person with disability adjusts to the community. Mutual adjustment by the community is required to achieve true integration. Adjustment by the community involves accessibility identified as the absence of architectural, attitudinal, social, economic, vocational, and communication barriers. The 1990 American Disabilities Act assured persons with disability the right to accessible services in the private sector. Fifield & Fifield (1995) provide summaries of legislation enacted to compensate veterans for disabilities obtained during service.

J. **Impairment:** Spinal cord impairment represents perhaps the most devastating disabilities a person can experience. Rehabilitation, a full range of services, and resources must be available for the successful community integration of the person with SCI. Rehabilitation is an ongoing process, which must be individualized. Rehabilitation is maximized when the individual participates in decisions, strives for independence, sets realistic goals, utilizes necessary resources, and remains in the community.

K. **Philosophy and Nursing Practice:** SCI nurses need to be knowledgeable of society's values and of the philosophical underpinnings of rehabilitation. This philosophy combined with the art and science of nursing provides a powerful mechanism in the rehabilitation process. See Table 3-1.

V. Nursing Process

A. Nursing process begins with data collection from which nursing diagnoses are formed. A plan is developed through collaboration and mutual goal setting among nurses, other health care providers, the person with SCI, and when possible, families. Goals represent intended outcomes of care. Strategies to implement the plan are identified and activated. Progress is evaluated at intervals to access outcomes and determines if goals are achieved.

B. Nursing process is the scientific method used by nurses to provide quality nursing care. With its scientific language and logical method, nursing process provided nurses further evidence that nursing is a science (Donnelly, 1987). As a science, nursing can claim a unique body of knowledge, rigor in method and the opportunity for parity with other sciences.

C. Nursing is more than a science, nursing is both art and science. Benner & Wrubel (1989) argue that while science is value free, the whole of nursing is not. They describe nursing as necessarily value laden, because of the human implications and essential connection of nursing practice to excellence.

D. Peplau (1988) defined nursing is both art and science. The art of nursing has three components: the medium, the process, and the product. The medium is the nurse as the instrument promoting change in the health of an individual. Process combines communication, skill,

Table 3-1: Correlating Philosophy with Goals of Care for Spinal Cord Injured Patients

Philosophy	Goals	Role Emphasized
1. Persons with a SCI are entitled to receive optimum care to meet their complex clinical, psychosocial, and economic needs.	To provide or secure the best health care possible for persons with SCI	Practitioner Advocate
2. Patients should be assisted to achieve and maintain and optimal level of physical and mental health and retain a sense of spiritual and social well-being.	To ensure that patients are cared for with respect as individuals and to help them reestablish their autonomy	Partner Counselor Educator
3. Families (or significant others) constitute an integral part of patients' lives and should be included in comprehensive health care for persons with SCI patients.	To provide psychosocial support to families and include them in assessing and meeting patients rehabilitative needs	Partner Counselor Educator
4. Nurses should develop expertise to apply a problem-solving process of assessment and diagnosis, goal setting, implementation, and evaluation skillfully and systematically to ensure individualized total patient care.	To promote physical and psychological well-being by minimizing risk factors, practicing preventive measures, recognizing onset of complications early, initiating immediate action, within the scope of nursing practice and policies, and evaluating care given	Practitioner Partner
5. Patient and family health education is an integral part of rehabilitation and must begin the moment of injury. Provision of an environment in which patients, families, and nurses can use their education, judgment, and individuality (creativity) is most conducive to a successful rehabilitation experience.	To provide a teaching/learning rehabilitation experience that actively involves patients (and families when appropriate) as participants and resource persons in the decision-making process, through which they can experience personal growth and independence	Partner Educator
6. Acute and concurrent rehabilitative care requires a skilled, well-integrated, interdisciplinary team.	To devise collaborative goals and provide coordinated care in a helpful, tolerable sequence for patients and families	Collaborator Coordinator
7. Nurses should coordinate and secure continuity of health care to facilitate transition (relocation) periods, especially on return to the community.	To determine patients' readiness for discharge and to initiate appropriate continuing health services	Coordinator Practitioner
8. Nurses should take responsibility for assessing and improving personal knowledge, attitude, and skills and should maintain awareness of current developments in the health care field.	To plan and participate in ongoing educational activities on a regular basis	Practitioner Advocate
9. Nurses must join forces with disabled people fighting to live independently in the community.	To participate in overcoming barriers—personal, social, financial—and obtain access to quality health care	Facilitator Supporter Advocate

From Management of Spinal Cord Injury (2nd ed., p. 12) by C.P. Zejdlik, 1992, Boston: Jones and Bartlett. Copyright 1992 by Jones and Bartlett. Reprinted with permission.

and knowledge allowing the expert nurse to practice in a fluid and competent manner. Product is the outcome experienced by the client.

E. The science of nursing is comprised of nursing's established knowledge and basic theories. Established knowledge is recognized by a discipline and accepted as true. Regarding the inseparability of the are and science of nursing, Peplau reported "There is a seamless quality, a graceful and delicately balanced movement between art and science portrayed by experienced, expert nurses that transcends as it uses the differences between these two forms"(Peplau, 1988:14).

VI. Nursing Theory

A. **Rationale for Theory:** Nursing requires unique knowledge and a logical structure. Without nursing knowledge, the nurse-client relationship would be imperiled. Without structure, the tasks of nursing would know no boundary. The over-arching framework of nursing is referred to as the metaparadigm of nursing. Metaparadigm represents the relationships of concepts and propositions for phenomena in a broad area and at a general level (Masternam, 1970). Nursing, person, health, and environment compose the metaparadigm of nursing. General or abstract concepts and propositions are difficult to apply in practice or research. Theories organized concepts and propositions with the goal of describing, explaining or predicting phenomena, (Chinn & Jacobs, 1987; Dickoff & James, 1986; Fawcett, 1989; Meleis, 1985.

B. **Scope of Nursing Theories:** The scope of nursing theories is on a continuum ranging from macro or grand to middle range to micro or partial theories (Chinn & Jacobs, 1987; Fawcett, 1989; Meleis, 1985):
    1. Macro or grand theories tend to be abstract, concepts are described in their broadest sense, and are more difficult to apply to practice or research because of the level of abstraction. Rogers' (1970; 1986) and Newman's (1979, 1986) theories are often cited as examples of macro theories of nursing.
    2. Middle range theories are more specific in describing concepts and propositions and interrelationships and are highly applicable to practice and research. The work of King (1995,1981, 1971) and Roy (1984, 1976) are examples of middle range theories. King's theory of goal attainment and Roy's adaptation model have clear implications for SCI nursing.
    3. Micro or partial theories tend to be narrowly focused or address specific nursing problems. Although micro theory is not general enough to apply to multiple areas of nursing, it has significant implications for application in a specific area. Further inquiry can expand micro theories into middle range theories. Nelson's (1990, 1992) work focusing on the process of reintegration of persons with SCI is an example of micro theory. While implications for this theory are obvious for SCI nurses, further study is needed to apply this model to other populations.

C. **Selecting a Theoretical Framework:** Multiple nursing theories exist and have implications for the practice of SCI nursing. Nurses are encouraged to evaluate several theories before choosing a theoretical framework. Education on nursing theories should be provided to all levels of nursing staff so they might also participate in the theory selection. Theories that best fit a specific nursing area support and reflect the philosophy of that area.

D. **Contribution to Nursing:** Many nurse theorists have dedicated their life's work to define nursing, validate nursing as a science, and promote autonomy within the profession of nursing. To ignore the utility of nursing theory is to diminish the stature of nursing as both are and science. Conversely, choosing and applying theories to the practice of nursing assures the continuance of nursing as a professional discipline.

VII. Theory of Goal Attainment

A. **Nursing:** According to King (1995, 1981, & 1971) nursing occurs within an open systems framework comprised of personal, interpersonal, and social systems. Health for individuals, groups and communities is the goal of the system. This open systems framework provided the structure for the theory of goal attainment. King (1995 & 1981) describes human beings as unique, open systems, rational, sentient, capable of thinking and making decisions. Human beings are in interaction with and inseparable from their environment. Nurses are human beings who perform a specific professional role. Nursing occurs in an interpersonal system which includes individuals and groups. Nursing is a process of action, reaction, interaction, and transaction (King, 1981).

B. **Health:** Health is described in holistic terms including physical, emotional and social aspects which are influenced by culture (King, 1971). "Health is defined as dynamic life experience which implies continuos adjustment to stressors in the internal and external environment through optimum use of one's resources to achieve maximum potential for daily living" (King, 1981:5). Environment is internal and external to human beings. The environment is constantly changing. Perceptions of the environment influence the individual's adjustment to life (King, 1981).

C. **Nurse/Patient Interactions:** Nurse-client interactions are the basis of the model of transactions. Through this process, nurse and client identify a situation, communicate with each other, set mutual goals, explore and agree on a means of attaining the goals. Goals are attained through these transactions. King (1995 & 1981) insists that individuals have the right to knowledge and to participate in decisions that affect them. This belief, coupled with the process of mutual goal setting, has clear implications for guiding SCI nursing practice. The theory provides a conceptual framework for research in SCI nursing.

VIII. Theory of SCI Nursing

According to Nelson (1992, 1990) rehabilitation is a process of reintegration whereby the individual is prepared to cope with physical limitations, architectural barriers, and prejudices while maintaining their integrity and sense of self worth. The process on reintegration is comprised of four phases: buffering transcending, toughening and launching.

A. **Buffering** is a nurturing and protective process that allows the individual to achieve the physical and emotional strength to cope with the ramifications of SCI.

B. **Transcending** is a life long process of identifying and rising above barriers and negative societal attitudes toward the person with SCI.

C. **Toughening** is the process of compensating for the disability, regaining independence, and maintaining social integration without "using the disability."

D. **Launching** is the process of providing real world experiences, exploring options for living following discharge, and facilitating discharge from the rehabilitation program.

IX. Application

A. **Applying King's Theory and Nelson's Phases of Reintegration:** Remaining a breast of clinical trends and findings is not enough. Spinal cord injury/dysfunction nurses are urged to include publications on philosophy and theory in their readings. "Theory is the poetry of science. The poet's words are familiar, each standing alone, but brought together they sing, they astonish, they teach" (Levine, 1995: 14). Interrelationships among the four philosophical premises. Nelson's phases of reintegration and King's theory of goal attainment in Table 3-2 reveal implications for nursing practice.

B. **Theory Integration:** The field of SCI nursing is emerging as a dynamic specialty area with a unique body of knowledge and skills. SCI nurses are challenged to incorporate nursing theory and philosophy into their practice not only to advance their standing among professional nursing specialties, but more importantly, to keep the promise of independence and integration for people with SCI.

Table 3-2: Application of King's Theory to Rehabilitatin Premises and Nelson's Phases of Reintegration

Rehabilitation Premises	Nelson's Phases of Reintegration	King's Theory of Goal Attainment
Rehabilitation begins at the onset of SCI.	**Buffering.** Nurturing & protecting to achieve physical & emotional strength to cope with the ramifications of SCI.	Mutual Goals-Interventions & education stabilize condition and assure safety (e.g. Nurse and client determine frequency of tracheotomy suction needed) to maintain patent airway).
Rehabilitation minimizes the impact of social stigma.	**Transcending.** Rising above limitations & negative attitudes toward persons with SCI.	Mutual Goals-Participation in rehabilitation program, responsibility for self, & interaction with persons with older injuries (e.g. Nurse and client agree that client will interact casually & formally in groups with other clients).
Rehabilitation promotes independence.	**Toughening.** Compensating for disability, regaining independence & social involvement.	Mutual Goals-Focus on activities essential to achieve maximal level of function (e.g. Nurse assists client with C5-6 quadriplegia to learn to feed self).
Rehabilitation promotes integration.	**Launching.** Exposing to the real world, exploring community living options, promoting autonomy, and preparing to leave the rehabilitation program.	Mutual Goals-Anticipate barriers, develop adaptation strategies & participate in discharge planning (e.g. Nurse and client develop plan for client to dress concealing urinary devices & to manage toileting problems in public facilities).

Practical Application

The following case study is of a person with a new SCI. It presents the phases of reintegration and new patient behaviors. Nursing interventions are presented and interactions with individuals with older injuries will be described.

Jim is a twenty nine year old C5-6 quadriplegic who sustained his injury in a motor vehicle accident. Following a fourteen-day stay in an intensive care unit, he was stable enough to be transferred to the SCI unit for rehabilitation. Jim was a construction worker, he is married with a five year old son. He enjoyed family activities, sports and his favorite hobby was building cars and drag racing. Upon arrival on the SCI unit, Jim was assessed to be dependent for all activities of daily living. He was quiet but responded appropriately when others initiated interactions. He verbalized that he would walk again and that he knew of another guy from his town who had "broken his neck but could walk." He talked about work and taking care of his family. Jim was in the buffering phase. The nurses were careful not to diminish his hope. They informed him that he was in "spinal shock" and could eventually get more return of functional ability but that his participation in the program was essential to his rehabilitation. The nurses described the rehabilitation program to him, they described their role and his role in the program. They were supportive, encouraged him to talk about his feelings, and they began to establish rapport. Jim's wife was given information about the programs and about her role. She was taken on a tour of the unit so that she could tell Jim about it. She was encouraged to tour the unit on her own and to talk to other patients and family members.

Jim began to accept that he was "currently" disabled and that he could return home. He was entering the phase of transcending. Nurses involved Jim in setting goals and developing a care plan. They demonstrated awareness of Jim's need for privacy and right to dignity. They were aware of their body language and avoided standing-over or talking down to him. Most importantly, the nurses made "dependency invisible" (Nelson, 1990: 51). Jim found dependency to be one of the most difficult aspects of his SCI. The nurses talked to Jim and joked with him. They treated him like he was an individual or one of the guys rather than treating him like a patient. Although Jim was attending therapies as scheduled and attentive when nurses provided patient education, he was perceived by the interdisciplinary team as not "working hard" and minimally involved with older injuries. Older injuries commented that Jim "needed to get with the program." Jim had also been resistive to a vocational rehabilitation referral. Experienced staff pushed Jim to do more for himself, such as, feeding himself and to set achievable goals. Older injuries shared their own experiences of alienating loved ones by using their own disability to manipulate others. One older injury, with quadriplegia, told Jim how he had completed school while living alone following his injury. Therapists challenged Jim to do as well as another new person who had a C3 level of injury. Jim began to push himself harder. He declined offers of assistance with tasks he could do for himself. His wife was pleased to report that Jim was not only feeding himself, but that he wanted to take her out to dinner on the weekend. Jim asked to see the vocational rehabilitation counselor. The toughening-up experience was leading Jim into the launching phase.

During the launching phase, Jim took full advantage of the resources and of his own skills. He collaborated with the home evaluation team to plan changes in his home to make it more accessible. He attended community outings, patient education and patient support groups. He was articulate and had strong interpersonal skills. He set a goal to use his knowledge of automobiles to pursue a career in car sales with the longer term goal of owning his own dealership. Jim and his wife attended the patient family workshop. Jim's wife was trained by the nursing staff to be his caregiver. Jim was overheard telling another new patient "This is a long and arduous process. You need to take advantage of what they offer here and make the most of what you have. It ain't easy but it's worth it."

References and Selected Bibliography

Americans with Disabilities Act Handbook. (1991). Washington DC: U.S. Equal Opportunity Office and the U.S. Department of Justice.

Benner, P., & Wrubel, J. (1989). *The primacy of caring: Stress and coping in health and illness.* New York: Addison-Wesley.

Bradley, V.J. & Knoll, J. (1995). Shifting paradigms in services to people with disabilities. In O.C. Karan & S. Greenspan, *Community rehabilitation services for people with disabilities* (pp. 5-19). Boston: Butterworth-Heinemann.

Brummel-Smith, K. (1990). Introduction. In B. Kemp, K. Brummel-Smith, & J.W. Ramsdell (Eds.), *Geriatric rehabilitation* (pp. 3-21). Boston: College-Hill.

Caramanica, L., & Thibodeau, J. (1987). Staff involvement in developing a nursing philosophy and the selection of a model for practice. *Nursing Management, 18*(10), 71.

Chinn, P. L., & Jacobs, M.K. (1987). *Theory and nursing: A systematic approach* (2nd ed.). Washington DC: C.V. Mosby.

Commission on Accreditation of Rehabilitation Facilities (CARF). (1996). *Standards manual and interpretive guidelines for medical rehabilitation.* Tucson, AZ: Author

Dickoff, J., & James, P. (1986). A theory of theories: A position paper. In L. H. Nicoll (Ed.), *Perspectives on nursing theory* (pp. 101-112). Boston: Little, Brown & Co.

Donnelly, G.F. (1987). The promise of nursing process: An evaluation. *Holistic Nursing Practice, 1*(3), 1-6.

Fawcett, J. (1989). *Analysis and evaluation of conceptual models of nursing.* Philadelphia: F.A. Davis.

Fawcett, J., & Downs, F.S. (1986). *The relationship of theory and research.* Norwalk, CT: Appleton-Century Crofts.

Fifield, B., & Fifield, M. (1995). The influence of legislation on services to people with disabilities. In O.C. Karan & Greenspan (Eds.), *Community rehabilitation services for people with disabilities* (pp. 38-70). Boston: Butterworth-Heinemann.

Gortner, S. (1990). Nursing values and science: Toward a science philosophy. *Image: Journal of Nursing Scholarship, 23*(2), 101-105.

Gregory, C.S. (1995). Creating a vision for a nursing unit. *Nursing Management, 26*(1), 38, 40-41.

Holton, G. (1986). *The advancement of science and its burdens.* New York: Cambridge University Press.

Kemp, B. (1990). The psychological context of geriatric rehabilitation. In. B. Kemp, K. Brummel-Smith, & J.W. Ramsdell (Eds.). *Geriatric rehabilitation* (pp. 41-57). Boston: College-Hill.

Kim, H.S. (1983). *The nature of theoretical thinking in nursing.* Norwalk, CT: Appleton-Century Crofts.

Kim, H.S. (1993). Identifying alternative linkages among philosophy, theory and method in nursing science. *Journal of Advanced Nursing, 18,* 793-800.

King, I.M. (1971). *Toward a theory for nursing*. New York: John Wiley & Sons.

King, I.M. (1981). *A theory for nursing: Systems, concepts, process*. New York: John Wiley & Sons.

King, I.M. (1995). The theory of goal attainment. In M.A. Frey & C.L. Sieloff (Eds.), *Advancing King's systems framework and theory of nursing* (pp. 23-32). Thousand Oaks, CA: Sage.

Kuhn, T.S. (1970). *The structure of scientific revolutions* (2nd ed. enlarged). Chicago: University of Chicago Press.

Laudan, L. (1977). *Progress and its problems: Toward a theory of scientific growth*. Berkeley, CA: University of California Press.

Levine, M.E. (1995). The rhetoric of nursing theory. *Image: Journal of Nursing Scholarship, 27*(1), 11-14.

Marriner, A. (1986). *Nursing theorists and their work*. St. Louis, MO: C.V. Mosby.

Masterman, M. (1970). The nature of a paradigm. In I. Lakatos & A. Musgrave (Eds.), *Criticism and the growth of knowledge* (pp. 59-89). New York: Cambridge University Press.

Meleis, A. (1985). *Theoretical nursing: Development & progress*. Philadelphia: J.B. Lippincott.

Nelson, A. L. (1990). Patients' perspectives of a spinal cord injury unit. *SCI Nursing, 7*(3), 44-63.

Nelson, A. (1992). Developing a therapeutic milieu on a spinal cord injury unit. In. C.P. Zejdlik, (Ed.) *Management of spinal cord injury* (2nd ed., pp. 213-227). Boston: Jones & Bartlett.

Nelson, A., Toth, L., Brady, S., Lynch, M.L., & Hanak, M. (1993). AASCIN strategic plan - 1993 - 1998. *SCI Nursing, 10*(4), 114-120.

Newman, M.A. (1979). *Theory development in nursing*. Philadelphia: F.A. Davis.

Newman, M.A. (1986). *Health as expanding consciousness*. St. Louis, MO: C.V. Mosby.

Patrick, D.L. (1989). A socio-medical approach to disablement. In D.L. Patrick & H. Peach (Eds.), *Disablement in the community* (pp. 1-18). New York: Oxford University Press.

Peplau, H.E. (1988). The art and science of nursing: Similarities, differences, and relations. *Nursing Science Quarterly, 1*, 8-15.

Reigel, B., Omery, A., Calvillo, E., Elsayed, N.G., Lee, P., Shuler, P., & Siegal, B.E. (1992). Moving beyond: A generative philosophy of science. *Image: Journal of Nursing Scholarship, 24*(2), 115-120.

Rogers, M.E. (1970). *An introduction to the theoretical basis of nursing*. Philadelphia: F.A. Davis.

Rogers, M.E. (1986). Science of unitary human beings. In V.M. Malinoski (Ed.), *Explorations on Martha Rogers' science of unitary human beings* (pp. 3-8). Norwalk, CT: Appleton-Century Crofts.

Roy, C. (1976). *Introduction to nursing: An adaptation model*. Englewood Cliffs, NJ: Prentice-Hall.

Roy, C. (1984). *An introduction to nursing: An adaptation model* (2nd ed.). Englewood Cliffs, NJ: Prentice-Hall.

Trieschmann, R.B. (1988). *Spinal cord injuries: Psychological, social and vocational rehabilitation* (2nd ed.). New York: Demos.

World Health Organization (WHO) (1980). *International classifications of impairments, disabilities and handicaps.* Geneva, Switzerland.

Zejdlik, C.P. (Ed.) (1992). *Management of spinal cord injury* (2nd ed.). Boston: Jones & Bartlett.

CHAPTER

Diversity in Nursing Practice Roles and Settings

Marilyn L. Ter Maat, MSN, RN-C, CRRN-A, CNAA

I. Learning Objectives

A. Identify three practice roles for spinal cord impairment SCI nurses.

B. Identify three practice settings for SCI nurses.

II. Introduction

SCI nursing provides care to individuals of all ages who have sustained damage to the spinal cord. Care is provided in private, public, and federal hospitals, as well as community, residential, or long-term care settings. Care is provided by a variety of professional and supportive nursing personnel. Spinal cord injury nursing roles include administrator, case manager, direct care provider, consultant, researcher, and educator. The scope of spinal cord injury nursing incorporates trauma care, stabilization after injury, rehabilitation, unrelated medical/ surgical conditions, health maintenance, and long-term follow-up of the injured individual, as well as psychosocial support for the individual, his or her family, and significant others. SCI nurses strive to prevent spinal cord injuries through public education programs, advocacy, and legislative process.

III. Practice Roles

SCI nursing is a speciality within the scope of professional nursing practice. Nurses serve in a variety of roles in the care of individuals with SCI.

A. **Clinical Educator:** The primary role of the nurse is to share information and help individuals develop skills necessary to achieve optimal independence (Willis-Sukosky, 1987). The nurse prepares individuals and significant others for the future and reinforces teaching done by other health care providers. The nurse provides verbal and written educational information for individuals, health care personnel, and the general public in a variety of areas such as activities of daily living, management of bowel and bladder, management of skin and personal hygiene, medication and diet, attendant care, community resources, and social and environmental conditions, especially accessability issues.

B. **Direct Care Provider:** The nurse is the primary care giver within the rehabilitation team. The nurse provides direct personal care to the individual until the individual is able to function independently or direct others regarding care. Direct care activities focus on prevention of complications, restoration, and maintenance of function.

C. **Coordinator of Care:** The nurse assists in coordination, throughout the continuum of care with the rehabilitation team, with other specialties, and the community.

D. **Counselor:** The nurse assists in anticipating challenges of community reentry. The individual is assisted with problem solving skills and the SCI nurse provides encouragement and praise for achievement of goals.

E. **Advocate:** The nurse views the person with SCI as a unique individual. Nurses bridge the gap between medical and nonmedical personnel. Nurses provide information and understanding to others about the rehabilitation process as well as individual needs progress and outcomes. SCI nurses support and initiate community and legislative activites that foster the rights of persons with disabilities.

F. **Consultant:** The nurse may be a consultant or expert witness providing specialized knowledge. Life care planning may be a service that a nurse provides clients, medical, and legal professionals.

G. **Researcher:** The SCI nurse may utilize the findings of research to improve practice, may participate in data collection for research studies, or may design and conduct research studies.

IV. Other Roles

A. **Administrator:** SCI nursing administrators provide leadership. Schroeder - Jaeger (1994) stated: "leadership is the facilitation of change through creative direction, motivation and guidance of others to achieve mutually accepted goals. Effective leadership is necessary since change requires the organized participation and cooperation of all persons involved in the process." The nursing administrator participates with colleagues from other disciplines to provide leadership. They engage in and support educational and research activities.

B. **Advanced Practitioner:** Advanced practitioners in SCI nursing include nurse clinicians, cinical nurse specialists, and nurse practitioners. Advanced practice nurses educate clients, staff, and the community. They use research findings in their practice and may conduct research studies. The advanced practice nurse serves as a clinical expert in complex clinical nursing situations, acts as a consultant, and collaborates with other interdisciplinary teams (Association of Rehabilitation Nurses ARN, 1994a). The nurse practitioner also functions in the area of health maintenance, evaluation, and management (DeJong and Batavia, 1992). This role is implemented based on the needs of the SCI populations and settings in which the nurse practices. The expertise needed for this role requires graduate level preparation.

C. **Home Care:** Home care nurses facilitate reentry into the home and community. The SCI home care nurse provides consumer driven care as part of a continuum between other health care settings and the home. The nurse may serve as a clinical resource, case coordinator, advocate, primary care provider, teacher, consultant, and team member (ARN, 1995a).

D. **Case Manager:** The SCI case manager practices in a variety of settings, primarily facility or agency based, insurance based, and independent practices. Nursing case management has been defined as a problem solving delivery model that facilitates continuity of care and cost effective appropriation of service. The case manager serves to coordinate and integrate services, and resources, among individuals with SCI, significant others, the treatment team, and the payor (Weed and Riddick, 1992). Current practice will need to incorporate movement toward community-based settings with logic that addresses not only preparation for life but support to deal with the realities SCI imposes (Zejdlik, 1995).

E. **Educator:** Nurse educators, function in both academic and institutional settings. The scope of the role may encompass: orientation, staff development, continuing and inservice education, student affiliation, and health education as it relates to SCI. The roles of the nurse educator may include program planner, instructor, role model, advocate, team member, and leader (ARN, 1995b).

F. **Manager:** Nurse managers provide accountability for the management of the SCI unit or program. Responsibilities typically include: staffing, budgets, quality improvement, and strategic planning. The manager needs strong clinical, leadership, and management skills, good interpersonal and interdisciplinary relationships, a creative problem solving ability, and a high level of initiative (ARN, 1994b).

G. **Researcher:** Nurse researchers develop SCI research programs within an interdisciplinary framework. The primary responsibilities include: theory development, research utilization, and the development of research programs that help to enhance and advance the quality of the life for the individual or improve the practice of SCI nursing.

H. **Staff Nurse:** Staff nurses assist the individual with SCI in adapting to an altered lifestyle while providing a therapeutic environment. The staff nurse provides direct nursing care, supervises ancillary personnel, coordinates health education, collaborates with the rehabilitation team, and acts as a resource and role model for staff and students (ARN, 1996a).

V. SCI Care Systems

Presently, in the United States, there are three distinct systems for providing spinal cord injury care: The Model Systems concept, Veterans Health Administration, and community facilities (Zejdlik, 1992). A wide variation exists within these systems in the ability to meet the complex needs of the SCI population.

A. **Model Regional Spinal Cord Injury System:** The Model Regional Spinal Cord Injury System was established in the early 1970's and is sponsored by the National Institute on Disability and Rehabilitation Research, U.S. Department of Education. The Model Systems utilize an interdisciplinary concept of comprehensive care from the time of injury through acute care, rehabilitation, community integration, and long term follow-up. The Model Systems also emphasize registry data collection, research, and education.

B. **Veterans Health Administration:** The Veterans Health Administration (VHA) has over twenty specialized SCI centers strategically located throughout the United States. The VHA has expertise in dealing with acute rehabilitation and lifetime care issues for persons with SCI. These centers also have support clinics that provide a continuum of primary care and specialized SCI hospital-based home care programs. The VHA offers a preventive health program including comprehensive SCI annual evaluation.

C. **Community Care:** Most individuals with SCI receive care within their own community. Although all require specialized care, typically only persons with complex needs, financial resources, veteran status, or who express a preference are referred to a specialized center.

VI. Practice Settings

The trend in health care has shifted from hospital to community based care. Practice settings include:

A. **Hospital based settings** may include emergency rooms, intensive and acute care units, rehabilitation units within hospitals, and freestanding rehabilitation hospitals. Most SCI nurses practice in one of these settings.

B. **Long term care settings** may include nursing homes, sub acute care units, and residential facilities. Approximately 2-5percent of the nurses practice in these settings. Traditionally the scheduled number of hours of therapy per week in the settings is reduced when compared to acute rehabilitation settings.

C. **Community based settings** include outpatient clinics, day treatment programs, independent living centers, community reentry programs, congregate living centers, and home care. This model emphasizes co-partnership among individuals with SCI, families and professionals to accomplish mutually established goals.

References and Selected Bibliography

Association of Rehabilitation Nurses. (1991). *Rehabilitation nurse case manager: Role description* [pamphlet]. Glenview, IL: Author.

Association of Rehabilitation Nurses. (1992). *Pediatric rehabilitation nursing: Role description* [pamphlet]. Glenview, IL: Author.

Association of Rehabilitation Nurses. (1994a). *The rehabilitation clinical nurse specialist: Role description* [pamphlet]. Glenview, IL: Author.

Association of Rehabilitation Nurses. (1994b). *Rehabilitation nurse manager: Role description* [pamphlet]. Glenview, IL: Author.

Association of Rehabilitation Nurses. (1995a). *The home care rehabilitation nurse: Role description* [pamphlet]. Glenview, IL: Author.

Association of Rehabilitation Nurses. (1995b). *The rehabilitation nurse educator: Role description* [pamphlet]. Glenview, IL: Author.

Association of Rehabilitation Nurses. (1996a). *The rehabilitation staff nurse: Role description* [pamphlet]. Glenview, IL: Author.

Bejciy-Spring, S., Neutzling, E., & Newton, C. (1994). Nursing case management: Enhancing interdisciplinary care of the spinal cord injured patient. *SCI Nursing, 11*(3), 70-73.

DeJong, G., & Batavia, A. (1992). Toward a health service research capacity in spinal cord injury. In C. Zedlik (Ed.), *Management of spinal cord injury* (2nd ed.). Boston: Jones and Barlett.

Faherty, B. (1991). The nurse legal consultant and disabling injuries. *Rehabilitation Nursing, 16,* 30-33.

Hoeman, S. (Ed). (1996). Conceptual bases for rehabilitation nursing. In *Rehabilitation nursing: Process and application.* St. Louis, MO: Mosby.

Johnson, K. (1994). *Spinal cord injury: Education content for professional nursing practice* (2nd ed.). Jackson Heights, NY: American Association of Spinal Cord Injury Nurses.

McCourt, A. (Ed). (1993). *The specialty practice of rehabilitation nursing: A core curriculum* (3rd Ed.). Skokie: Rehabilitation Nursing Foundation.

Mumma, C. (Ed). (1997). *Rehabilitation nursing: Concepts and practice - A core curriculum for rehabilitation nursing* (2nd ed.). Evanston, IL: Association of Rehabilitation Nurses, Rehabilitation Nurse Foundation.

Mumma, C., & Nelson, A. (1996). Models for theory based practice of rehabilitation nursing. In S. Hoeman (Ed). *Rehabilitation nursing: Process and application* (p.21). St. Louis, MO: Mosby.

Schroeder-Jaeger, K. (1994). President's message. *SCI Nursing, 11*(2), 36-37.

Spinal cord injury: Facts and figures at a glance. (1996, May). Birmingham: University of Alabama.

Weed, R., & Riddick, S. (1992). Life care plans as a case management tool. *Case Manager, 3*(1), 26-30.

Willis-Sukosky, N. (1987). Introduction to the field of rehabilitation and rehabilitation nursing. In C. M. Mumma (Ed). *Rehabilitation nursing: Concepts and practice - A core curriculum for rehabilitation nursing* (2ND Ed., pp. 1-25). Evanston: Rehabilitation Nursing Foundation.

Zejdlik, C. (Ed.) (1992). *Management of spinal cord injury* (2nd Ed.). Boston: Jones and Bartlett.

Zejdlik, C. (1995). Changes: Implications of spinal cord injury. *SCI Nursing, 12*(3), 71-72.

CHAPTER

Cultural Issues Affecting Care Delivery

Mary H. Gardenhire, MSN, RN, CIC

I. Learning Objectives

A. Discuss the ethnic distribution of persons with spinal cord injury as described by the National Spinal Cord Injury Statistical Center database.

B. Define culture and other relevant terms that apply to the cultural care of the individual with spinal cord impairment (SCI).

C. Discuss the relationship between culture and disability of the individual with an SCI.

D. Review the key points of a cultural assessment.

E. Identify nursing interventions that are culturally relevant.

II. Introduction

Culture is tightly interwoven into life and pervades ones thinking, actions, feelings, and health state (Leininger, 1967). Health and illness are strongly affected and often determined by the cultural background of an individual. SCI affects all cultures, presenting a challenge to nursing staff. Cultural assessments enhance nurses' ability to provide safe, efficient, and culturally relevant care. Research is needed to identify culturally unique aspects of nursing care specific to SCI.

"By the year 2000, more than one fourth of the U.S. population will consist of individuals from culturally diverse groups. Increasing numbers of international visitors and exchange students that will use the U.S. health care system, and U.S. nurses will engage in international exchanges with increasing frequency. To keep pace with these populations and health care trends, U.S. nurses will need to base their nursing care on a theoretically sound foundation that draws on knowledge from the physical, natural, and behavioral sciences, as well as on research-based theories from transcultural, cross cultural, and international nursing" (Andrews, 1992: 7).

Components of rehabilitation nursing and transcultural nursing can benefit the individual with an SCI during the rehabilitation process. The blending of the concepts and practices of transcultural nursing, the nursing process, and rehabilitation yields an all-inclusive dynamic concept called Multicultural Rehabilitation Nursing. History has brought to the rehabilitation setting many challenges for the rehabilitation nurse. He/she must be knowledgeable in all aspects of care that are secondary to a SCI. America is a pluralistic society, with many cultures and subcultures. Each culture has its own beliefs, philosophies, and practices. Rehabilitation nurses must examine their own beliefs and be able to interact with all individuals in a positive manner. Overall, when the nurse can better understand the factors that influence behavior, they can better meet the needs of individuals from various cultures.

A recent Chinese immigrant had major bladder surgery. He was told by the nursing staff to "force fluids". The client did not understand the "force fluid" expectation. He refused to drink the glasses of cold water from the big picture left on his bedside table. Each time the nursing staff entered the client's room, they reminded him that he needed to force fluids and drink many glasses of water. They threatened that the physician would order intravenous fluids if he did not drink more water. He refused to drink the water on his bedside. The staff said he was 'uncooperative,' 'strange' and a 'non-compliant' person. When the client's daughter came to see him, she told the nursing staff that he would drink hot herbal tea but not cold water. Finally, the nurses gave him the hot tea, and he drank several cups. The nurses did not understand why the hot tea was culturally acceptable as it was not what the nurses would drink. Later, a transcultural nurse explained the 'hot and cold' theory of the Chinese people and its importance in nursing care (Leininger, 1995: 86).

For increased comprehensibility and to decrease confusion, European (Anglo) American are umbrella terms for White and Caucasian; Black refers to African American, Haitians or of Dominican Republic descent; Native American refers to American Indians; Hispanics refers to Mexican Americans, Cuban, Puerto Ricans and other; and American Indian refers to Eskimo and Asian American or Pacific Islanders. Highlighted terms are those mostly used in this section. Other terms maybe used interchangeably depending on discussed topic and quotes from other references that used varying terminology.

A. **Scope**
This chapter links concepts related to culture, SCI, and nursing. Cultural phenomena affecting health care are presented for several dominant ethnic, racial, and religious groups. Cultural assessment tools and interventions are described.

B. **Demographics**
Of importance is the data gathered on ethnic groups pertaining to population growth or decline. Between 1980 and 1990 the proportion of Whites in the U.S. general population decreased from 83.1 percent to 80.3 percent; the African American population increased slightly from 11.7 percent to 12.1 percent, the proportion of Asian Americans almost doubled from 1.5 percent to 2.9 percent; and ethnic groups of Hispanic origin increased from 6.4 percent to 9.0 percent (U.S. Bureau of the Census, 1992).
1. Of the estimated 10.4 million people age 16-64 with severe disabilities, African Americans report highest percentage of severe disabilities (See Figure 5-1).
2. Hispanics have the second highest percentage of severe disability.
3. According to surveys done by LaPlante et al (1996):
   a. Thirteen million or 9.4 percent of Whites have health problems or disabilities that prevented or limited work activity (See Figure 5-2).
   b. By comparison 3.2 million of African Americans have the same limitations.
   c. Belgrave & Walker (1991) reported that transportation and social support were the strongest predictors of employment; health locus of control and self-esteem were minimally significant.
   d. Figure 5-3 depicts fewer limitations in work activity for Asians and Pacific Islanders.
   e. Native Americans report the highest limitations in work activity.

4. Females with disabilities constitute an area of concern, specifically if they are also from a different culture (Feist-Price & Ford-Harris, 1994).

   a. According to McNeil (1996), in the non-institutionalized population over the age of fifteen, 25.0 million (24.6 percent) females report disabilities compared to 21.0 million (22.4 percent) males.

   b. 14.0 million (13.8 percent) females report severe disabilities; while 9.6 million (10.2 percent) males report severe disabilities

   c. Disability rates for both sexes increase with age (McNeil, 1996).

   d. In a working hypothesis, Hanna & Rogovsky (1992) suggest that African American women with disabilities are especially disadvantaged, and that the disadvantage is linked to gender, race, and disability. Kolata (1991) reported that women are less likely to receive rehabilitation services.

   e. Women and African Americans have been underrepresented in research that shaped the services and practices in rehabilitation (Hanna & Rogovsky, 1992).

5. The incidence of traumatic SCI among various races has not been well studied. There are some data to suggest that nonwhites may have somewhat higher incidence rates than whites (Stover & Fine 1986). However information from the National Spinal Cord Injury Database, revealed the following (GO, DeVivo, & Richards, 1995):

   a. Racial distribution of SCI

     (1) SCI proportionately lower among Whites than seen in general population (70.1 percent versus 80.3 percent).

     (2) SCI proportionately higher among African Americans than in general population (19.6 percent versus 12.1 percent) (See Figure 5-4).

     (3) Comparison of recent trends for racial distribution for individuals enrolled in the SCI National Database:

Figure 5-1: Percentage of Severe Disabilities by Race/Ethnicity

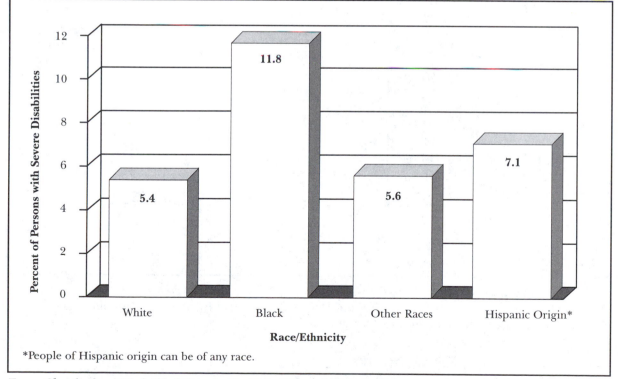

*People of Hispanic origin can be of any race.

From *Chartbook on Work Disabilities in the United States-1996: An info use report* (p. 43), by L.E. Kraus, S. Stoddard, & D. Gilmartin, 1996, Washington, D.C.: U.S. National Institute on Disability and Rehabilitation Research. Adapted with permission.

(a) 1973-1977: Whites 79.9 percent; African Americans 14.0 percent; Hispanics 6.2 percent; Native Americans 2.1 percent; and Asians 0.8 percent.

(b) 1990-1992: Whites 56.3 percent; African Americans 29.9 percent; Hispanics 11.2 percent; American Indians 1.6 percent and classified as others 0.6 percent (De Vivo et al., 1995).

b. Age at time of injury
  (1) Females: mean age 32.2 years
  (2) Males: mean age 30.3 years
  (3) Asians: 35.0 median years
  (4) Hispanics: 27.3 median years
  (5) African Americans: 33.2 median years
  (6) Whites: 30.3 median years (De Vivo et al., 1995)

Figure 5-2: Persons With Work Disability by Race/Ethnicity

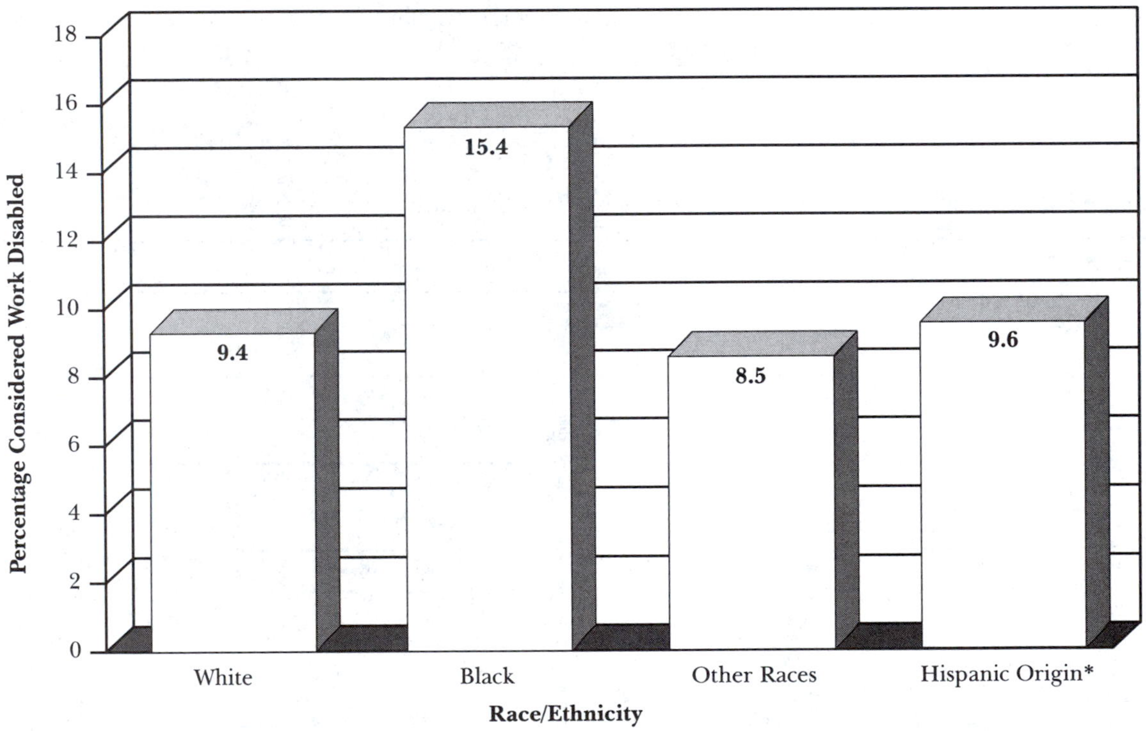

*People of Hispanic origin can be of any race.

From *Chartbook on Work Disabilities in the United States-1996: An info use report* (p. 38), by L.E. Kraus, S. Stoddard, & D. Gilmartin, 1996, Washington, D.C.: U.S. National Institute on Disability and Rehabilitation Research. Adapted with permission.

Figure 5-3: Percentage of Persons With Work Limitations by Race/Ethnicity

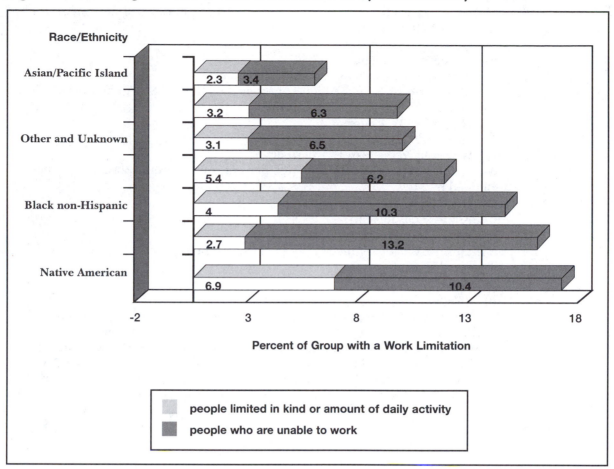

From *Chartbook on Work Disabilities in the United States-1996: An info use report* (p. 44), by L.E. Kraus, S. Stoddard, & D. Gilmartin, 1996, Washington, D.C.: U.S. National Institute on Disability and Rehabilitation Research. Reprinted with permission.

Figure 5-4: Comparison of Racial Distributions of Persons With SCI and General Population

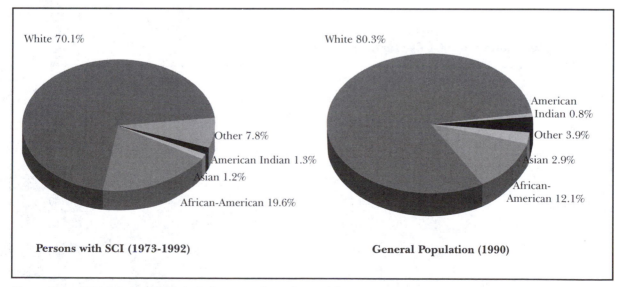

From *Spinal Cord Injury: Clinical Outcomes from the Model Systems* (p. 30), S.L. Stover, J.A. DeLisa, & G.G. Whiteneck (Eds.) 1995, Rockville, MD: Aspen. Reprinted with permission.

    c. Etiology and Racial/Ethnic groups (See Table 5-1)
      (1) American Indians have highest percentage (67.4 percent) of SCI from motor vehicle crashes (MVC), followed by:
         (a) Other 59.0 percent
         (b) Asian: 50.3 percent.
         (c) African American have the least (26.6 percent)
      (2) African Americans have the highest percentage (42.5) of SCI from acts of violence followed by:
         (a) Hispanics: 37.4 percent.
         (b) Other: 19.0 percent.
         (c) Whites have the least (7.1 percent)
      (3) Whites have highest percentage (16.0 percent) of SCI from sports related injuries followed by:
         (a) Hispanics: (7.5 percent)
         (b) Asians: (7.4 percent)
         (c) African American: (4.1 percent)
      (4) African Americans have highest percentage (19.6 percent) of SCI from falls followed by:
         (a) Whites: 18.4 percent
         (b) Asians: 17.7 percent
    d. The SCI Model Systems have reported interesting trends in data since its inception in 1973.
      (1) Decline in percentage of SCI from MVC and sports related injuries.
      (2) Increase in percentage of SCI from falls and acts of violence. Acts of violence seen in African-Americans, has increased from 39.5 percent prior to 1978 to 45.7 percent since 1990. The rate is 6-9 times higher among African Americans than Whites. Hispanics increase from 24.9 percent to 52.4 percent (De Vivo et al., 1995).
6. Distribution for level and extent of injury for Whites and African Americans
    a. Whites
      (1) Paraplegia 48.6 percent
      (2) Quadriplegia 51.4 percent
      (3) Complete 45.9 percent
      (4) Incomplete 51.4 percent
    b. African Americans
      (1) Paraplegia 48.0 percent
      (2) Quadriplegia 52.0 percent
      (3) Complete 43.9 percent
      (4) Incomplete 56.1 percent (James, DeVivo, & Richards, 1993)

Table 5-1: Distribution of SCI Etiologies by Race/Ethnic Group

Racial/ Ethnic Group	Motor Vehicle Crashes	Falls	Acts of violence	Sports	Other	Total
White	49.9%	18.4%	7.1%	16.0%	8.6%	100
African-American	26.6%	19.6%	42.5%	4.1%	7.2%	100
American Indian	67.4%	12.8%	9.1%	4.8%	5.9%	100
Hispanic	34.4%	13.3%	37.4%	7.5%	7.4%	100
Asian	50.3%	17.7%	17.7%	7.4%	6.9%	100
Other	59.5%	11.9%	19.0%	4.8%	4.8%	100

From *Spinal Cord Injury: Clinical Outcomes from the Model Systems* (p. 30), S.L. Stover, J.A. DeLisa, & G.G. Whiteneck Eds., 1995, Maryland: Aspen. Reprinted with permission.

III. Background Information

A. **1960's and 1970's:**The historical events of the 1960's and 1970's served to make North American society more aware of the gaps of cultural group identity, starting with African Americans, then followed by Hispanics, Asian Americans, Native Americans, and other ethnic groups. This aftermath of events forced society to examine and focus on inequality and its place in the health care arena. The 1965 Vocational Rehabilitation Act was broadened to include individuals with disabilities that considered their social status and culture (Atkins, 1988).

B. **1970's and 1980's:** The decades of the 1970's and 1980's signaled an era of immigration of refugees. Each individual brought along a system of traditional health and illness beliefs and practices. Nursing took the forefront in realizing that, with this influx of the culturally diverse immigrants, cultural sensitivity needed to be considered. Transcultural nursing took hold in the early 1970's with a goal of educating nurses on the importance of understanding different cultures and using cultural information to guide nursing practice. Blended with this goal was the awareness that cultural factors were important illness prevention, successful recovery, and maintenance of a healthy life style. Western medical culture has focused on cure. However, it has begun to fully accept rehabilitation as a specialty area and has incorporated it as an essential and logical step in the course of an individual's progress (Hoeman, 1989). Our nation, no longer referred to as the "melting pot", had begun to recognize that the diversity shared by cultures lends strength and uniqueness to the fabric of our society. The culturally diverse individual with an SCI represents a minority group which has been influenced by the civil rights movement, and has advanced with its own independent living movement.

C. **1990's:** The Disability Act of 1990 contributed greatly to the acknowledgement and advancement of individuals with disabilities. SCI, regardless of culture or race, is one group of many disabilities and the focus of this section. Cultural competence deals with the view that individuals from different cultural backgrounds respond differently to the rehabilitation process (Feist-Price & Ford-Harris, 1994). Culturally competent nurses will be able to work more efficiently with the individual with an SCI, and improve health outcomes.

IV. Key Concepts for Understanding Cultural Issues in Clinical Settings

A. **Culture**
   1. The sum of beliefs, practices, habits, customs, and rituals, that are shared and learned from family members and passed from generation to generation (Leininger, 1995).
   2. Culture has four basic characteristics: it is learned from birth, shared by all members of the same group, adapted to certain conditions and is a dynamic and severe changing process (Andrews & Boyle, 1995).
   3. A subculture is described as a smaller group within a culture and has unique ways of living that distinguish them from the dominant or larger culture (Dancey & Logan, 1994).

B. **Acculturation:** Members of a cultural group are not all alike. It is important to understand the diversity among members of various cultural groups and the degree to which they have immersed themselves into the dominant culture. Locke (1992) describes this degree of immersion in the following ways:
   1. Bicultural - Ability to function in the dominant culture as in their own, while holding on to certain parts of their own culture.
   2. Traditional - Ability to hold on to cultural values and customs from the culture of origin while rejecting many customs and values of the dominant culture.
   3. Marginal - Ability to have little to do with customs and values from dominant or culture of origin.
   4. Acculturated - Changing of one's cultural patterns to those of the host society, most likely the dominant cultural group or westernized culture.

C. **Ethnicity:** Pertaining to a social group within a cultural and social system that has status on the basis of specific traits including religion, language, ancestral, or physical characteristics (Leininger, 1995).

D. **Transcultural nursing:** In comparison to the term cross cultural, preferable terminology that better reflects how transcultural nursing expands across all cultures; terms are sometimes used interchangeably but, have different meanings (Leininger, 1995).

E. **Cultural nursing assessment:** Described by Leininiger (1978) as "...a systematic appraisal or examination of individual, groups, and communities as to their cultural beliefs, values, and practices within the cultural text of the people being evaluated" (pp. 85-86); a thorough assessment that addresses an individual's health practices, health beliefs, and lifestyles and will strengthen the nurse's judgment and decision making process when providing care (Andrews & Boyle, 1995); other terms used to describe a transcultural assessment are culturalogical assessment and culture care assessment.

F. **Western:** "...cultures that are usually highly industrialized and tend to depend on modern technologies with their lifeway practices" (Leininger, 1995, P. 63).

G. **Non-western (Eastern):** "...cultures that have existed for thousands of years and have generally strong philosophical ideologies and usually rely less on modern technologies and other Western values" (Leininger, 1995, p. 63).

H. **Ethnocentrism** is a universal phenomena that refers to a belief that one's own behavior or beliefs is superior or even morally correct ; rigid ethnocentric nursing practices can lead to stress, clashes, and non-compliance (Leininger, 1995).

I. **Cultural bias** is closely related to ethnocentrism; "...a firm position or stance that one's own values and beliefs govern the situation or decision (Leininger, 1995, p. 66).

J. **Cultural relativism:** The uniqueness of a culture and the need for that culture to be evaluated by its own values and standards (Leininger, 1995).

K. **Culture bound illness** is the feature of an illness that differs from culture to culture; may be viewed in Western medicine as psychiatric problems (Yap, 1977). Some examples of culture bound illness include Voodoo, Latah, and Susto.

L. **Cultural diversity:** Differences and variations between and among cultural groups secondary to differences in lifeways, language, norms, values, and other cultural issues (Leininger, 1995).

M. **Racism** "...derived from the concept of race, and is usually defined as a biological feature of a discrete group, whose members share distinctive genetic traits inherited from a common ancestor" (Leininger, 1995, p. 70). The following term are closely related to racism. "Prejudice refers to preconceived ideas, beliefs, or opinions about an individual, group, or culture that limit a full and accurate understanding of the individual, culture, gender, race, event, or situation" Discrimination generally refers to the limiting of opportunities, choices, or life experiences because of prejudices about individuals, cultures, or social groups. Stereotyping refers to placing people and institutions, mentally or by attitudes, into a narrow, fixed trait, rigid pattern, or with inflexible 'boxlike' characteristics (Leininger, 1995, p. 71).

N. **Enculturation:** Learning about a culture including values, beliefs, and practices; in preparation for living effectively in a particular culture (Leininger, 1995).

O. **Assimilation:** "…the way an individual or group from one culture selectively takes on and chooses certain features of another without necessarily taking on the total attributes of a particular culture" (Leininger, 1995, p. 73).

P. **Cultural Care-** "…the cognitively learned and transmitted professional and indigenous folk values, beliefs and patterned lifeways that can be used to assist, facilitate, or enable another individual or group to maintain their well-being or health or to improve their human condition or lifeways" (Leininger, 1995, p. 74); involves the following major principles:
   1. Cultural care accommodation
   2. Cultural care preservation
   3. Cultural care repatterning (See VII 3 a)

Q. **Cultural Competence:** "Being aware of your own cultural and ethnic background and its influences on your beliefs, behaviors, and interactions with others…" (Dancey & Logan, 1994, p. 339); To be culturally competent the nurse must be a patient advocate knowledgeable, empathetic, and communicate effectively (Dancey & Logan, 1994).

R. **Disability Culture -** Shared life experiences of the disabled; formation of kinship and bond among certain disabilities (Scheer, 1994). Stigma is "… a cultural pattern of undesired difference" (Scheer, 1994, p. 245); is used by social scientists to investigate the depreciation and marginality of people with disabilities in American society (Scheer, 1994).

S. **Cultural Pain** "refers to the suffering, discomfort, or unfavorable responses of an individual on group towards an individual who has different beliefs or lifeways, usually reflecting the insensitivity of those inflicting the discomfort" (Leininger, 1995, p.67); relatively new concept coined by Madeline Leininger; for example breaking a cultural taboo, hearing culturally offensive remarks about one's customs or practices can be just as painful as psychophysical pain (Leininger, 1995).

T. **Multicultural clinical interactions -** The greater the shared knowledge of each culture or cultural system among the participants of a clinical interaction, the less chance of misinterpretation, misunderstandings, or sense of disharmony and dissatisfaction; an interplay of three and sometimes four cultures and medical systems that include the personal culture of the provider, the culture of the individual with SCI, the culture of the principal medical system, and the conventional medical culture especially if a participant is from a non - Western background (Fitzgerald, 1992).

V. Models/Theories for Providing Culturally Competent Nursing Care

A. **Transcultural Care -** The Theory of Cultural Care Diversity and Universality focuses on a holistic view of the culture care involves being knowledgeable and respectful to individuals values (Leininger, 1983)
   1. Leininger's sunrise model embraces her theory on cultural care (See Figure 5-5).
      a. The "rising sun" symbolizes hope that nursing will be able to discover new and distinctive knowledge that could raise nursing to a glistening sunrise of cultures worldwide.
      b. "The model, therefore, serves as visual guide or a cognitive map to help nurses envision a holistic perspective of many influences on culture care with individuals, families, groups, institutions, communities, and different health care systems. The model is often used as a visual guide to help the researcher consider multiple potential aspects influencing nursing care" (Leininger, 1995, p.107).
      c. Leininger's sunrise model is also helpful in the performance of a culture care assessment and provides the foundation for culture care assessment (See Figure 5); the goal of performing a culturalogical assessment is to provide culturally congruent, meaningful care to individuals, families and special groups or subcultures

Figure 5-5: Leininger's Sunrise Model to Depict the Theory of Culture Care Delivery and Universality

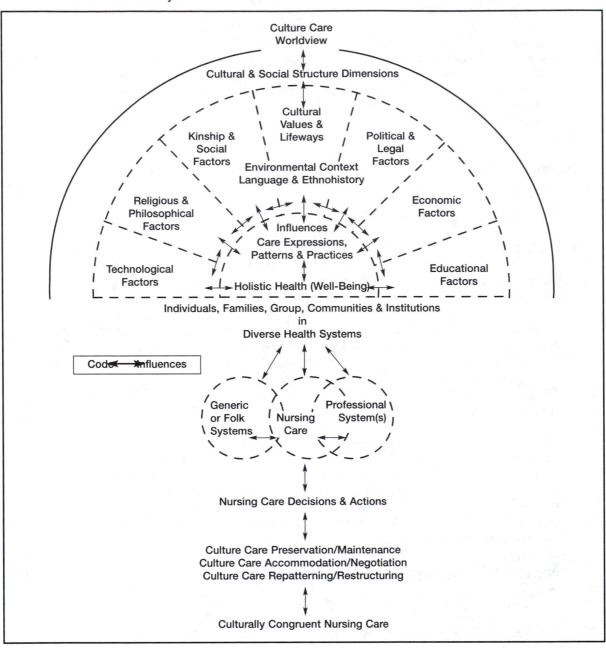

From *Culture Care Diversity and Universality: A Theory of Nursing* (p. 43), By M.M. Leininger (Ed.), 1991, New York: National League of Nursing. Reprinted with permission.

B. **Model of Multicultural Development.**

   Pedersen (1988) describes three stages of multicultural development that utilize the experiential and the didactic approach to learning (with emphasis on experiential learning); overall goal is to learn about the range of cultural awareness and differences; basically used at the college or university level but can be adapted to any clinical learning situation. The three stages are:
   1. Awareness of culturally learned assumptions; it's the beginning of change
   2. Knowledge about culturally relevant information
   3. Skill in taking the appropriate action and making "culturally correct" decisions

C. **Model of Multiculture Understanding.**

Locke (1992) describes a model of Multicultural Understanding that can be used to gain knowledge and understanding about the culturally diverse individual; provides a sound, solid foundation for examining cultural patterns, social relationships, and experiences of the cultural diverse individual; the model involves the following (See Figure 5-6):

1. Self awareness - "know thyself"
2. Global influences - know about world events and how these events are interpreted into personal meaning for the culturally diverse individual
3. Dominant Culture - know the characteristics and values of the dominant culture
4. Cultural Differences - know about the elements that characterize and make up different cultures

Figure 5-6: Multicultural Understanding

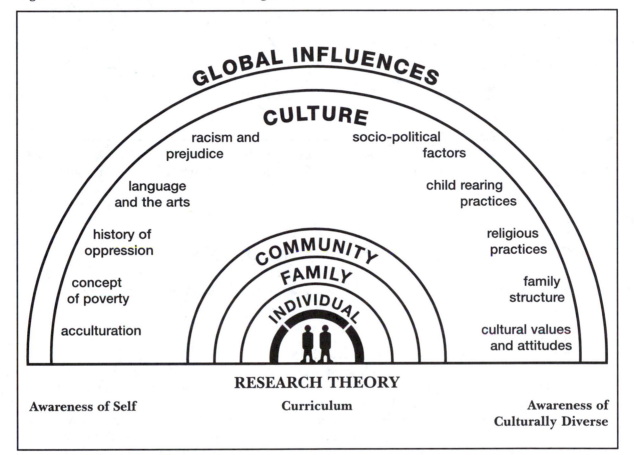

From *A Model of Multicultural Understanding: Increasing Multicultural Understanding* (p. 2), by D.C. Locke, 1992, Newbury, CA: Sage. Reprinted with permission.

D. **The Culturally Competent Model of Care** in Figure 5-7 outlines the components of cultural competence. "Cultural competence is viewed as" a process, not an end-point in which the nurse continuously strives to achieve the ability to effectively work within the cultural context of an individual or community from a diverse or ethnic background" (Campinha-Bacote, 1994d: 104-105).

1. Cultural awareness
2. Cultural knowledge

3. Cultural skills
4. Cultural encounters (See Figure 5-7)

Figure 5-7: Culturally Competent Model of Care

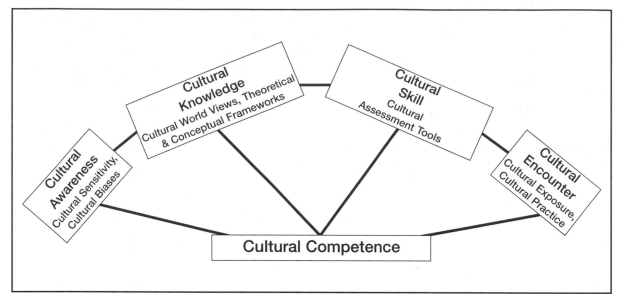

From *The Process of Cultural Competence in Health Care: A Culturally Competent Model of Care* (p. 7), by J. Campinha-Bacote, 1994, Ohio: Transcultural C.A.R.E. Associates. Reprinted with permission.

VI. Cultural Phenomena Affecting Health Care

A. **Ethnic/Racial:** Cultural variations include aspects of environmental control, biological variations, social organization, communication, and time orientation.

B. **Religion**
  1. Individuals from various cultures have different religious beliefs.
  2. Health care providers are also from various cultures and have different religious beliefs.
  3. The concept of spirituality, which is the totality of an individual's being, is widely acknowledged in the world's religions and beliefs.
  4. Meeting the spiritual needs go beyond just meeting the religious needs; spirituality is a much broader concept than religious practice or affiliation and is an important aspect of an individual's holistic care. Religion may serve as a method for expressing spirituality; most people satisfy spiritual needs through particular religious practices.
  5. Spiritual needs include those variables that inspire us to rise above the material world; the need to find purpose in life, illness and life situations, experiencing forgiveness, experiencing giving, the receiving of love, and the feeling of relatedness.
  6. Major religions: a good knowledge base of various religions and religious practices will help nurses in relating to an individuals' spiritual needs.

VII. Multicultural Rehabilitation Nursing Assessment

A. **Overview/Description Cultural Assessment**
  1. Requires cultural competence in order to elicit appropriate information
  2. Does not require information on every element of culture
  3. Elicits shared beliefs, values and customs relevant to health behaviors

   4. Performed to identify cultural patterns that help or interfere with nursing intervention or treatment regimen
   5. Elicits cultural factors necessary for appropriate nurse/patient relationship
   6. Integrates cultural assessment with the rehabilitation nursing assessment
   7. Examines and considers cultural orientation of patient and nurse
      a. Evaluates and decodes underlying patterns of belief and practices provided by patient.
      b. Looks for cultural patterns
         (1) Evaluates patterns that assist or may interfere with rehabilitation goals.
            (a) Some patterns have no effect on health outcomes.
            (b) Some provide security and comfort to patient.
         (2) Plan to identify disruptive patterns or those that interfere with optimizing rehabilitation goals.
            (a) Understand disruptive behavior and purpose in health outcome.
            (b) Patient may practice secretly or refuse to participate in planning, if behavior not understood by nurse and handled appropriately.

B. **Conducting the Assessment**
   1. Create non-judgmental atmosphere, so that individual with SCI feels as if cultural beliefs and background will be respected.
   2. Explain to the patient the reason why you are asking specific cultural questions.
   3. Verify assessment with patient and family member to avoid, misinterpretation, loss of trust, or errors secondary to stereotyping.
   4. According to Kleinman, Eisenberg & Good (1978) an explanatory model of illness postulates that all individuals have culturally based models for explaining symptoms; they use their own knowledge base to define the causes, mechanism of action, severity, and appropriate treatment; this explanatory model can therefore be useful in understanding beliefs and practices, illness behaviors, and treatment expectations, regardless of cultural background.
   5. Predictors cultural factors may have an important element one's healthcare:
      a. Emigration from a rural area
      b. Frequent returns to the country of origin
      c. Lack of limited formal education
      d. Little knowledge of English
      e. Inexperience with Western medicine and the health care delivery system
      f. Low socioeconomic status
      g. Major difference in dress and diet
      h. Recent immigration to the United States at an old age
      i. Segregation in an ethnic subculture
   6. Four points to be considered in the cultural assessment:
      a. "How the client's background influences the client's perceptions of health and illness, and treatment;
      b. How the client's background has influenced his or her help seeking process;
      c. How the client's background is likely to influence his or her interaction with professionals; and
      d. What impact the client's background will have on treatment, including treatment after discharge" (Dancy & Logan, 1994, p. 341).

C. **Cultural Assessment Tools**
   1. Basic premise of cultural assessment tool
      a. Individuals have a right to cultural beliefs, practices and values (Leininger, 1978).
      b. These rights should be considered, understood, and respected.
      c. The two guiding principals that assist the nurse in making a cultural assessment are:
         (1) Be objective and open minded about an individual's cultural practices and beliefs.
         (2) Do not judge all individuals the same, individuals have their own identity.
   2. Assessment tools:
      a. Tripp-Reimer, Brink & Saunders (1984) described an assessment tool that can help

separate individual-specific information from general normative data. The tool consists of the following components:

   (1) Phase 1 - Assessing culture content of patient's system; Screening assessment to determine if cultural conflicts exist; question regarding health beliefs and habit, including questions on illness and treatment.

   (2) Phase 2 - Placing culture content in context; seeks information on potential conflicts among health standards from individual with an SCI, The nurse, the caring facility, and how this may alter or hinder care.

b. Leininger (1995) used an ethnonursing guide that assists the user to enter the world of the individual and identify information to provide holistic, culture-specific care. The guide can be used with the Sunrise Model (previously depicted in Figure 5-5) to assess culture and health and involves the following areas:

   (1) Worldview: Questions that elicit how the individual sees the world around him/her

   (2) Ethnohistory: Questions that elicit information about heritage and background

   (3) Kinship and social factors: Questions that elicit information on family and significant others relationships and interactions

   (4) Cultural values, beliefs and lifeways: Questions that elicit "good caring" based on the individuals belief and practices

   (5) Religious/spiritual/philosophical factors: Questions that elicit information about the individual's religion and preferences on spiritual care

   (6) Technological factors: Questions that elicit information on the individuals feeling and use of technology

   (7) Economic factors: Questions that elicit how the individual feels about money and how money impacts on their health care

   (8) Political and legal factors: Questions that elicits how politics impact on the health of the individual

   (9) Educational factors: Questions that elicits level of education and how education impacts on health

   (10) Language and communication: Questions that elicits how individuals communicate, what language is used or preferred, and any communication problems

   (11) Professional and generic (folk or lay care beliefs and practices): Questions that elicit information about the individual's health care practices and views.

   (12) Generic and specific nursing care: Questions that elicit the individual's feelings about nursing, cultural care, and hospitalization (Leininger, 1995).

c. Bloch's assessment guide for Ethnic/Cultural Variations covers four major categories of data collection:

   (1) Cultural

   (2) Sociological

   (3) Psychological

   (4) Biological/Physiological (as cited in Camphina-Bacote, 1988)

d. Berlin & Fowkes (1983) suggest utilizing the following mnemonic for cultural assessment - LEARN

   (1) Listen to the individual with interest and without judgement

   (2) Explain how you perceive the problem

   (3) Acknowledge similarities and differences

   (4) Recommend interventions and treatments

   (5) Negotiate a plan of care including rehabilitation goals

e. Andrews & Boyle (1995) list the following components

   (1) Cultural affiliations

   (2) Value orientation

   (3) Health-related beliefs and practices

   (4) Nutrition

   (5) Organizations that provide cultural support

   (6) Educational background

   (7) Religious affiliations

   (8) Cultural aspects of disease incidence

3. Once the assessment is complete, the nurse needs to evaluate the information received and design a care plan.
   a. Use Leininger's Sunrise Model, especially the following components:
      (1) Cultural care accommodation - the intentional and cognitive steps taken into consideration to help a culture in expressing its beliefs, values, and practices
      (2) Cultural care preservation - the conscious push to maintain or preserve selected values, beliefs, or practices.
      (3) Cultural care repatterning -the way a person rearranges the different characteristics and peculiarities of a culture in order for new patterns of care to become evident.
   b. Example of potential nursing diagnosis related to the care of the culturally diverse individual with an SCI:
      (1) Decisional conflict related to perceived threat to value system
      (2) Noncompliance related to patient's value system
      (3) Knowledge deficit related to lack of exposure
      (4) Ineffective management of therapeutic regimen related to health beliefs
      (5) Fear related to unfamiliarity
      (6) Decisional conflict related to perceived threat to value system
      (7) Body image disturbance
      (8) Social isolation related to physiologic, environmental, or emotional barriers
      (9) Social isolation related to behavior that fails to conform to social norms
      (10) Social interaction impairment related to sociocultural dissonance
      (11) Social isolation related to inadequate personal resources.
      (12) Personal identity disturbance related to lowered self-esteem
      (13) Chronic low self-esteem (Sparks, 1995).

VIII. Culturally Competent Nursing Interventions

A. **Cultural factors that affect nursing merit attention.** To enable a more positive patient outcome nurses should examine their own cultural norms and values. Key questions important in exploring your ethnic and cultural background are outlined below:
   1. With what ethnic, social, or cultural group do you most closely identify?
   2. In what ways have your racial, cultural, and ethnic beliefs, perceptions, prejudices, and traditions influenced your reactions, behaviors, nursing diagnosis, and interventions?
   3. In what ways can you objectively assist ethnically diverse clients in achieving their optimal health status?
   4. Will you be able to respect the different perceptions and views of ethnically diverse clients as relevant and important?
   5. Can you accept ethnically diverse clients as active, valid participants in their health care?
   6. Will you be able to treat ethnically diverse clients with respect, that is, not belittle them by assuming that you understand their situation and that you know what the correct solutions are?
   7. In what ways can you create a respectful;, non threatening environment for the ethnically diverse client? This environment should foster open communication and optimal sharing (Bolander, 1994).

B. **Nurses' own ethnic background may affect their reaction responses and ultimately the cultural assessment.** Nurses should learn:
   1. Ways of avoiding assumptions and stereotypical judgments
      a. Be aware of various cultural beliefs.
      b. Be aware of the individual diversity and level of acculturation into western health culture
   2. That implementation of cultural assessment may be impeded because of nurses' belief that the individual will accept the rehabilitation goals and that he/she will work toward them.
      a. Nurse believes that the correct and important outcomes are rehabilitation nursing goals, which may be barriers to positive rehabilitation outcomes.
      b. Individual will come to conclusion that what is presented to him/her is expected to be acceptable and is the thing to do.
      c. Individual may be directed toward goals that are totally different from his/her own.

C. **Know about the various cultures and how they differ.** Members from several minority groups are demanding culturally relevant care that incorporates their beliefs and practices; these cultural diverse group members expect health care providers to respect their cultural health care rights (Leininger, 1984).

1. Principles for Culturally Relevant Care (Leininger, 1995):
   a. Understand and respect cultural differences; it is difficult to recognize cultural similarities and variations and not have cultural knowledge to reflect upon during the assessment period
   b. Understand one's own cultural heritage, views, values, beliefs, and lifeways
   c. Seek assistance from a culturally knowledgeable/educated professional, to serve as a mentor and consultant. Interpretation of verbal and non-verbal communication and the use of the three modes of cultural care theory (preservation and maintenance strategies, accommodation/negotiation/ and repatterning and restructuring) should be utilized for nursing interventions in the care of the SCI individual with a mental or psychiatric disorder.
   d. Understand the individual's cultural context, multiple social structure factors, and the world view all of which influence mental health behavior.
   e. Allow time and maintain sensitivity and patience while working with the culturally diverse individual.
   f. Know the various cultural illnesses and wellness of the cultures and know how to respond to these conditions appropriately.

2. Culturally relevant care for African Americans:
   Know and understand the different cultures. Know the various health and illness terms and references e.g. "I need to make water" refers to the need to urinate. Word expressions can also vary, e.g. "blood" can refer to high or low blood pressure, thick or thin (anemia) and sugar in the blood refers to diabetes. Most African Americans appreciate the use of and the power of words (an oral tradition), they may prefer someone talk to them rather than hand them a piece of paper to fill out. Set short term goals with constant reevaluation, allowing for individual and gradual movement toward long-term rehabilitation goals.

3. Culturally relevant care for Native Americans:
   Of utmost importance is knowledge and appreciation of the culture. Some Native Americans may have a hard time accepting help from non Native Americans. A good cultural assessment is important as there are several reactions to the dominant culture; i.e. the biculturalist emulates the host society, the traditionalist may distrust members from the dominant culture; marginalist may not try to compete with dominant culture. Be knowledgeable about their feelings about healing. Consider of options of involving the family, visiting the individual's home, and involving the tradition healer in the team.

4. Culturally Relevant Care for Mexican Americans:
   Mexican Americans are often present time-oriented. Therefore, set concrete short term goals; make appointments immediately rather than several weeks in advance. Value the appearance of agreeability, (disagreeability is rude). It may be best to be indirect until they get to know you; however if problems arise a directive approach may be appropriate. Being a cultural relevant nurse means greeting new admissions as soon as they arrive on the unit, acknowledging the importance of personalization, be sensitive by using first names when conversing, and introduce self using first name. Realize that Mexican Americans come from a diverse background and cannot be classified solely on their ability to speak either Spanish or English. The degree of acculturation into the dominant society and regional differences are important in understanding the Mexican American; therefore, a good cultural assessment is important. The goal in understanding Mexican-Americans is to make them feel comfortable in being bicultural.

D. **Ethnic diversity in staff nurse employment** in hospitals helps to achieve sufficient ethnic diversity "…at the service unit level to build cohesive work teams that can constantly challenge naïve or biased assumptions. Test innovative practices and tailor services to meet the unique needs of their clientele" (Minnick, Roberts, Young, Marcantonio, & Kleinpell, 1997: 35).

E. **Cultural Misunderstandings:** Problems do exist sometimes when persons from two cultural backgrounds with conflicting values meet, unless one is willing and able to adapt to the values and beliefs of the other.
   1. Nurse can mislabel individual behavior as resistive, non-compliant, difficult, or uncooperative (Leininger, 1984).
   2. Nurse may not be knowledgeable of individual customs, values, or beliefs.
   3. One way to reduce potential misunderstanding is to
      a. Sensitize nurses to their own biases
      b. Review outcome of the care delivered by the nurse (increased sensitive and effective care).

F. **Religion and Spirituality**
   1. Know the unique religious and cultural background of the individual
      a. Spiritual care and needs are sometimes overlooked, because of
         (1) Emphasis on advanced technology
         (2) Focus on cost savings
         (3) Need to scientifically evaluate and quantify information and treatment
      b. Nursing care must expand beyond the physical or biological care into the spiritual realm
      c. Different religious affiliations can affect health and illness (life events such as death, body image alterations and cause and effect of illness.
      d. It is important to understand the role of religious beliefs and practices.
      e. Know if there may behealing rituals that the individual believes will assist his/her well-being during illness.
      f. There may be recognized significant religious representatives that can be called on, e.g., Buddhist monk or preacher (Andrews & Boyle, 1995).
   2. Be aware how the individual with a SCI diagnosis may relate to cultural and religious beliefs.
   3. Be aware of interaction and commitment of family members during any difficult adjustment period.
   4. Make the distinction between religion and spirituality.

G. **Language and Communication**
   1. Individuals may or may not speak a different language; however, the following can affect communication:
      a. Differing customs
      b. Values
      c. Mores
      d. Social structures
   2. Cultural differences influence communication to the extent that you cannot take the meaning for granted without understanding the culture and the individual with an SCI and the way your own background influences the cues you give. Physical contact, physical closeness, and eye contact have various meanings to different individuals. You cannot know everything about every culture, but the more you are aware of and respond to cultural differences as you communicate, the better will be your rapport.
   3. *Awareness/Intervention*
      a. Learn as much as possible about the individual.
      b. Learn crucial words and sentences.
      c. Have translator write out cards that consist of useful bilingual sentences.
      d. Non-natives require more than just learning a few tips.
         (1) Self awareness of personal biases, avoid labeling.
         (2) Respect for individual experiences
         (3) Acceptance of the differences between individual and nurse

H. **Nutrition and Elimination**
   1. Food has many cultural and social functions and has many functions and uses with special symbols and meanings in different cultures. Culture strongly influences the use and beliefs about food in health and illness.

2. Altered elimination pattern is usually a consequence of SCI; however, elimination may be viewed differently by various cultures.
3. Assessment must be inclusive, yet respectful and sensitive.
4. Know about different cultural foods, individual likes and dislikes, how food is prepared served and eaten.
5. Know how foods are used at special events (weddings, births, religious, events and death).
6. Know about various cultural references and their meanings, e.g. hot/cold theory.
7. Know about the foods and nutrients, and how various foods can effect an individual's bowel regime.
8. American culture believes in daily bowel movements (BM).
   a. Older person preoccupied with scheduling BM
   b. Many individuals choose social isolation rather than risk cultural embarrassment by having an accident.
9. There are cultural beliefs about proper collection and disposal of any body waste, including fecal and urinary waste.
   a. Person wishing to cause harm can do so by obtaining something from individual's body.
   b. Personal items or body fluids can be used by spellcaster or root worker to hex or curse.
10. Modesty and privacy are important to Native-Americans
11. African Americans and Native Americans find incontinence most damaging to their self-esteem.

I. **Pain Management:** Pain is a universally recognized phenomenon, is an important area of consideration in nursing practice (Andrews & Boyle, 1995); the term is derived from the Greek word "penalty" which accounts for its long association between pain and punishment in Judeo-Christian belief (Andrews & Boyle, 1995).
1. There is a cultural and ethnic difference in perception of pain and response to pain. Pain perception differs from one individual and culture to the other. One individual/culture may embrace pain and that same pain may be denoted as intolerable in another (Andrews & Boyle, 1995).
   a. Measurement of pain - The literature reveals that pain threshold, pain tolerance and encouraged pain tolerance differ considerably among individuals. Sensation thresholds however are usually uniform among various cultural backgrounds.
      (1) Generally believed that humans normally experience comparable sensation thresholds
      (2) Cultural background does seem to have some effect on pain threshold (the point at which an individual reports that a stimulus is painful) as described in a study done by Clark and Clark, (1980). They found that Nepalese porters and Western guests were equally sensitive to electric shock; however, the Nepalese required greater intensities before describing the electrical stimuli as painful.
      (3) Encouraged pain tolerance refers to the amount of painful stimuli one accepts when encouraged to tolerate increasingly higher levels of stimulation. This type of measured pain can be compared to the increased amount of pain encouraged and tolerated by the so-called primitive tribes (Andrews & Boyle, 1995).
   b. Expressions of pain
      (1) A comparison of pain interpretation, significance of pain, and other specific aspects of pain including intensity, duration, and quality among four cultural groups; "...Zibrowski's research remains the classic study of cross-cultural pain responses" (Andrews & Boyle, 1995: 305).
      (a) Old Americans were stoic.
      (b) Italians and Jews complained more and preferred to be around others during episodes of pain; sought relief from pain and expressed pain through crying, moaning, and complaining.
      (c) Jews resisted medication more.
      (d) Italians were skeptical and suspicious of pain and concerned about implications of pain.
      (e) Irish Americans showed little emotion and denied pain.

(2) The way patients communicate pain is influenced by culture.

(3) Pain can be communicated as strength, character building, rituals for rites of passage, punishment for wrong doing, means of atonement, expression of grieving, and results of spell, or rootwork.

c. Present concept of pain for individual with an SCI: The individual is the authority on the pain.

   (1) May be a challenge to rehabilitation nurse because of neurological and physiological change.

   (2) Nurses from various cultures may assess pain differently.

d. Interventions

   (1) Confront personal beliefs about pain and suffering and explore how these beliefs affect paient care.

   (2) Establish an open relationship with individual with SCI

      (a) Respect the individual

      (b) Respect the individual's response to pain

      (c) Never stereotype based on culture

   (3) Establish an interpersonal competence by

      (a) Being available to the individual experiencing pain

      (b) Realizing the importance of the involvement of others, such as family

   (4) Assess pain.

      (a) Three major objectives for assessing pain are described by Fagerhaugh & Strauss (1977):

         - Let the nurse discern what the individual is feeling

         - Give the nurse the chance to evaluates the effect of the pain on the individual experiencing the pain

         - Sometimes helps with giving clues as to the physical nature of the pain

      (b) According to the National Institutes of Health (1987), self-report is the most reliable indicator for the existence and intensity of pain. Listen and react to what the individual is saying, do not depend totally on facial expressions (Beyer, McGrath, and Berde, 1990).

      (c) Know individual's ethnocultural background.

      (d) Correlate pain with level of injury.

      (e) Be aware of other signs and symptoms of pain.

      (f) Identify person's usual reaction to pain.

J. **Multicultural rehabilitation nursing** - The nurse should be able to integrate aspects of transcultural nursing to that of the rehabilitation process, utilizing the awareness, knowledge and skills in daily caring practices, giving an overall view and understanding of the cultural diverse individual with an SCI. Adapted from the rehabilitation counseling process endorsed by Atkins (1988); this process evolved as a category of the cross-cultural counseling discipline. It is used by the author to describe the following practices:

1. Utilizes the nursing process with principles of rehabilitation nursing for specific cultural groups.

2. Takes into consideration the dynamic methods in which cultural differences affect the rehabilitation and nursing process.

3. Identifies more specifically the rehabilitative clinical encounters seen on the rehabilitation unit interaction between nurse and the culturally diverse individual with SCI

4. Considers methods of how to properly assess and intervene with the individual.

References and Selected Bibliography

Alston, R., & Mngadi, S. (1992). The interaction between disability status and the African American experience: Implications for rehabilitation counseling. *Journal of Applied Rehabilitation Counseling,23* (2), 12-15.

American Nurses Association Expert Panel. (1992). ANA expert panel report: Culturally competent health care. *Nursing Outlook, 40*(6), 277-283

Andrews, M. (1992). Cultural perspectives on nursing in the 21st Century. *Journal of Professional Nursing, 8*(1), 7-15.

Andrews, M. M., & Boyle, J.S. (1995). *Transcultural concepts in nursing care* (2nd ed.). Philadelphia: J.B. Lippincott.

Andrews, M. M., & Hanson, P.A. (1995). Religion, culture, and nursing. In M.M. Andrews, & J.S. Boyle (eds.), *Transcultural concepts in nursing care* (2nd ed.), (pp. 353-409). Philadelphia: J.B. Lippincott.

Asbury, C.A., Walker, S., Stokes, A., & Rackley, R. (1994). Psychosocial correlates of attitudes toward disability and desire to work in African Americans with disabilities. *Journal of Applied Rehabilitation Counseling, 25,*(4) 3-7.

Atkins, B. (1988). An Asset-oriented approach to cross-cultural issues: Blacks in rehabilitation. *Journal of Applied Rehabilitation Counseling, 19*(4), 45-48.

Badwound, E., & Tierney, W. G. (1988). Leadership and American Indian values: The tribal college dilemma. *Journal of American Indian Education, 28*, 9-15.

Belgrave, F.Z., & Walker, S. (19901). Predictors of employment outcomes of black persons with disabilities. *Rehabilitation Psychology, 36*(2), 111-119.

Berlin, E., & Fowkes, W. (1983). A teaching framework for cross-cultural health. *The Western Journal of Medicine, 139*(6), 934-938.

Beuf, A.H. (1977). *Red children in white America*. University Park, PA: University of Pennsylvania Press.

Beyer, J.E., McGrath, P.J., & Berde, C.V. (1990). Discordance between self-report and behavioral pain measured between children age 3-7 years after surgery. *Journal of Pain and Symptom Pain Management, 5*(6) 350-356.

Boyle, J.S. (1995). Alterations in lifestyles: Transcultural concepts in chronic illness. In M. Andrews & Boyle, J.S. (Eds.), *Transcultural concepts in nursing care* (2nd ed., pp. 237-252). Philadelphia: J.B. Lippincott.

Campinha-Bacote, J. (1988). Culturalogical assessment: An important fact in psychiatric consultation-liaison nursing. *Archives of Psychiatric Nursing, 2*(4), 244-250

Campinha-Bacote, J. (1994a). Cultural competence in psychiatric nursing: A conceptual model. *Nursing Clinics of North America, 29*(1), 104-111.

Campinha-Bacote, J. (1994b). Ethnic pharmacology: A neglected area of cultural competence. *Ohio Nurse Review, 69*(6), 9-10.

Campinha-Bacote, J. (1994c). *The Process of cultural competence in health care: A culturally competent Model* (2nd ed.). Ohio: Transcultural C.A.R.E. Associates.

Campinha-Bacote, J. (1994d). Transcultural psychiatric nursing: Diagnostic and treatment issues. *Journal of Psychosocial Nursing, 32*(8), 81-86.

Campinha-Bacote, J. (1995). The quest for cultural competence in nursing. *Nursing Forum, 30*(4), 19-25.

Campinha, Bacote, J. (1996). A culturally competent model of nursing management. *Surgical Service Management, 2*(5), 22-25.

Capers, C.F. (Ed.) (1992). Culture and nursing practice: An applied view. *Holistic Nursing practice, 6*(3), 1-78.

Capers, C.F. (1994). Mental health issues and African Americans. *Nursing Clinics of North America, 29*(1), 57-64.

Clark, W.C., & Clark, S.B. (1980). Pain response in Nepalese porters. *Science, 209*, 410-412.

Champan, W.P., & Jones, C. (1944). Variations in cutaneous and visceral pain sensitivity in normal control subjects. *Journal of clinical investigations, 23*, 81-91.

Chan, F., Lam, C., Wong, D., & Fang, X. (1988). Counseling Chinese Americans with disabilities. *Journal of Rehabilitation Counseling, 19*(4), 25.

Cock, J. (1989). Hidden consequences of state violence: Spinal cord injury in Soweta, South Africa. *Social Science Medicine, 29*(10), 1147-1155.

Comas-Diaz, L., & Griffith E. E. (Eds.) (1988). *Clinical guidelines in cross-cultural mental health.* New York: Wiley.

Dancey, B., & Logan, B. (1994). Culture and ethnicity. In V. B. Bolander (Ed), *Sorensen and Luckmann's basic nursing a psychophysiologic approach* (3rd Ed., pp. 331-342). Philadelphia: W. B. Saunders.

Davitz, L., Sameshima, Y., & Davitz, J. (1976). Suffering as viewed in six different cultures. *American Journal of Nursing, 76*(8), 1296-1297.

Dejong, C. (1983). Defining and implementing the independent living concept. In Crew, N. & Zola, I. (Eds.)., *Independent living for physically disabled people*. San Francisco: Josey Press.

de Leon Siantz, M. L. (1994). The Mexican-American migrant farmworker family. *Nursing Clinics of North America, 29*(1), 65-79.

Deutsch, M. (1965). The role of social class in language development and cognition. *American Journal of Orthopsychiatry, 35*, 78-88.

DeVivo, M.J., & Fine, P. R. (1988). Spinal cord injury: Its short-term impact on marital status. *Archives of Physical Medicine and Rehabilitation, 66*(8), 501-506.

DeVivo, M.J., Hawkins, L. N., Richards, J. S., & Go, B.K. (1995). Outcomes of post-spinal cord injury marriages. *Archives of Physical Medicine and Rehabilitation, 76*(2), 130-138.

DeVivo, M.J., Rutt, R.D., Black, K.J., Go, B. K., & Stover, S.L. (1992). Trends in spinal cord injury demographics and treatment outcomes between 1973 and 1986. *Archives of Physical Medicine and Rehabilitation, 73*(5), 424-430.

DeVivo, M.J., Rutt, R.D., Stover, S.L., & Fine, P.R. (1987). Employment after spinal cord injury. *Archives of Physical Medicine and Rehabilitation, 68*(8), 494-498.

Dovidio, J.F., & Gaetner, S.L. (1986). *Prejudice, discrimination, and racism.* Orlando: Academic Press.

Fagerhaugh, S.Y., & Strauss, A. (1977). *Politics of pain management: Staff-patient interactions.* Menlo Park: Addison-Wesley.

Fee, F. (1994). An introduction to multicultural issues in spinal cord injury rehabilitation. *SCI Psychosocial Process, (7)*3, 104-108.

Feist-Price, S., & Ford-Harris, D. (1994). Rehabilitation counseling: Issues specific to providing services to African American clients. *Journal of Rehabilitation, 60*(4), 13-19.

Fernandez, M.S., & Freer, R. (1996). Application of an integrated model for counseling persons with spinal cord injury across ethnicities. *SCI Psychosocial Process, 9*(1), 4-9.

Fernandez, M., & Marini, I. (1995). Cultural values orientation in counseling persons with spinal cord injury. *SCI Psychosocial Process, 8*(4), 150-155.

Fitzgerald, M.H. (1992). Multicultural clinical interactions. *Journal of Rehabilitation, 58*(2), 38-42.

Francis, C.K., Oberman, A., & Saunders, E. (1994). Racial and ethnic differences in CVD: Managing risk factors. *Patient Care, 28*(1), 51-78.

Garrett, J.T. (1994). The path of good medicine: Understanding and counseling Native American Indians. *Journal of Multicultural Counseling and Development, 22*(3), 134-144.

Geissler, E.M. (1994). *Pocket guide to cultural assessment.* St. Louis: Mosby-Yearbook.

Giger, J.N., & Davidhizar,R.E. (1995). *Transcultural nursing: Assessment and intervention* (2nd ed.). St. Louis: Mosby-Yearbook.

Guy, E. (1988). Navajos' commitment benefits individual with disabilities. *Journal of Applied Rehabilitation Counseling, 19*(4), 26-28.

Hanna, W.J., & Rogovsky, E. (1992). On the situation of African American women with physical disabilities. *Journal of Applied Rehabilitation Counseling, 23*(4), 38-45.

Hautman, M. (1979). Folk health and illness beliefs. *Nurse Practitioner, 4*(4), 26-32.

Herbert, J., & Chetham, H. (1988). Africentricity and the black disability experience: A theoretical orientation for rehabilitation counselors. *Journal of Applied Rehabilitation Counseling, 19*(4), 50-54.

Hoeman, S.P. (1989). Cultural assessment in rehabilitation nursing practice. *Nursing Clinics of North America, 24*(1), 277-289.

Hopkins, V.L. (1994). Promoting spiritual health. In V. B. Bolander (Ed.), *Sorensen and Luckmann's basic nursing: A psychophysiologic approach* (3rd ed., pp. 1511-1512). Philadelphia: W.B. Saunders.

James, M., DeVivo, M.J., & Richards, S. (1993). Post injury employment outcomes among African-Americans and white persons with Spinal cord injury. *Rehabilitation Psychology, 38*(3), 151-164.

Jenkins, A.E., & Amos, O.C. (1983). Being black and disabled: A pilot study. *Journal of Rehabilitation, 49*(2), 54-60.

Johnson, M. (1994). Nursing care in a culturally diverse nation. In B. Bullough & V.I. Bullough (Eds.), *Nursing issues for the nineties and beyond* (pp. 187-189). New York: Springer.

Kalb, M. (1971). *An examination of the relationship between hospital ward behaviors and post discharge behaviors in the spinal cord injury patients* [Dissertation]. University of Houston.

Kavanagh, K.H., & Kennedy, P. (1992). *Promoting cultural diversity*. London: Sage.

Kleinman, A. (1980). *Clients and healers in the context of culture*. Berkley, CA: University of California.

Kleinman, A., Eisenberg, L., & Good, B. (1978). Culture illness and care: Clinical lessons from anthropologic and cross cultural research. *Annals of Internal Medicine, 44*(2), 251-258.

Kolata, G. (1991). Studies say women fail to receive equal treatment for heart disease. *The New York Times*, A1, B8.

Kraus, L. E., (1991). *Chartbook on work disabilities in the United States*. Washington, DC: U.S. Department of Education and National Institute of Health.

Kraus, L., Stoddard, S., & Gilmartin, D. (1996). *Chartbook on work disabilities in the United States - 1996: An info use report*. Washington, DC: U. S. National Institute on Disability and Rehabilitation Research.

Kunce, J., & Vales, L. (1984). The Mexican American: Implications for cross-cultural rehabilitation counseling. *Rehabilitation Counseling Bulletin, 28*(2), 97-107.

LaBrack, B., & Leonard, K. (1984). Conflict and compatibility in Punjabi-Mexican immigrants in rural California. *Journal of Marriage, 46*, 527-537.

LaPlante, M., Kennedy, J., Kaye, H., & Waegner, B. (1996). *Disability and employment, disability statistics* Abstract #11. Washington, DC: Disability Statistics Rehabilitation Research and Training Center National Institute on Disability on Disability and Rehabilitation Research.

Leininger, M. (1967). The culture concept and its relevance to nursing. *Journal of Nursing Education, 6*(2), 27-37.

Leininger, M. (1978). *Transcultural nursing: Concepts, theories, and practices*. New York: John Wiley & Sons.

Leininger, M. (1983). Cultural care: An essential goal for nursing and health care. *AANNT Journal, 10*(5), 11-17.

Leininger, M. (1984). Transcultural nursing an essential knowledge and practice field for today. *Canadian Nurse, 80* (11), 41-45.

Leininger, M. (1984). Transcultural nursing: An overview. *Nursing Outlook, 32*(2), 72-73.

Leininger, M. (1991) . *Culture care diversity and universality: A theory of nursing* (Ed.). New York: National League for Nursing.

Leininger, M. (1995a). African Americans cultural care. In M. Leininger (Ed.), *Transcultural nursing: concepts theories research & practice* (2nd Ed., pp. 383-400). New York: McGraw -Hill.

Leininger, M. (1995b). Anglo-American (USA) culture values and perspectives. In M. Leininger (Ed.), *Transcultural nursing: concepts, theories, research and practice* (2nd Ed., pp. 335-348). New York: McGraw-Hill.

Leininger, M. (1995c). Culture care assessment to guide nursing practice. In M. Leininger (Ed.), *Transcultural nursing: concepts, theories, research and practice* (2nd Ed., pp. 115-149). New York: McGraw-Hill.

Leininger, M. (1995d). Culture care of Mexican Americans. In M. Leininger (Ed.), *Transcultural nursing: concepts, theories, research and practice* (2nd Ed, pp. 93-114). New York: McGraw-Hill.

Leininger, M. (1995e). Transcultural foods functions, beliefs, and uses to guide nursing practice. In M. Leininger (Ed.), *Transcultural nursing: concepts, theories, research, and practice* (2nd Ed., pp. 187-204). New York: McGraw-Hill.

Leininger, M. (1995f). *Transcultural nursing: concepts, theories, research and practice*. New York: McGraw-Hill.

Leung, P., & Sakata, R. (1988). Asian Americans and rehabilitation: Some important variables. *Journal of Applied Counseling, 19*(4), 16-20.

Locke, D.C. (1992). *Increasing multicultural understanding: A comprehensive model*. Newbury Park London: Sage.

Locke, D. (1994). *A model of multicultural understanding*. Newbury, CA: Sage.

Marini, I. (1995). Spiritual and psychological correlates of adjusting to traumatic injury. *Journal of Religion in Disability & Rehabilitation, 2*(1), 65-71.

Marshall, C. A. (1992). The power of inquiry as regards to American Indian women with disabilities: Divisive manipulation or clinical necessity? *Journal of Applied Rehabilitation Counseling, 23*(4), 46-52.

Martin, W., Frank, L., Minkler, S., & Johnson, M. (1988). A survey of vocational rehabilitation counselors who work with American Indians. *Journal of Applied Rehabilitation Counseling, 19*(4), 29-34.

McNeil, J. (1996). *Household survey data on employment and disability*. Survey: CPS, 1995: Unpublished memorandum.

Meyerson, H. (1968). *Sense of competence in the spinal cord injury* [Dissertation]. University of Houston.

Minnick, A., Roberts, M.J., Young, W.B., Marcantonio, R., & Kleinpell, R. M. (1997). Ethnic diversity and staff nurse employment in hospitals. *Nursing Outlook, 45*(1), 35-40.

More, A. J. (1987). Reflected values: Sixteenth-century Europeans view the Indians of North America. *American Indian Culture and Research Journal, 11*, 31-50.

Morgan, C., Guy, E., Lee, B., & Cellin, H. (1986). Rehabilitation services for American Indians: The Navajo experience. *Journal of Rehabilitation, 52* (2), 25-31.

National Institutes of Health (1987). The integrated approach to the management of pain. *Journal of Pain and Symptom Management, 2*, 35-44.

Olson, J.S., & Wilson, R. (1984). *Native Americans in the twentieth century*. Provo: Brigham Young University Press.

Pedersen, P. (1988). *A handbook for developing multicultural awareness*. Richmond, VA: American Association for Counseling and Development.

Randall-David, E. (1989). *Strategies for working with culturally diverse communities and clients*. Rockville, Maryland: The Association for the Care of Children's Health.

Saravanabhavan, R.C., & Marshall, C.A. (1994). The older American Indian with disabilities: Implications for providers of health care and human services. *Journal of Multicultural Counseling and Development, 22*(3), 182-194.

Scheer, J. (1994). Culture and disability: An anthropological point of view. In J. Trickett (Ed.), *Human diversity: Perspectives on people in context* (pp. 244-260). San Francisco: Josey-Bass.

Smart, J., & Smart, D.W. (1993). Acculturation, biculturalism, and the rehabilitation of Mexican Americans. *Journal of Applied Rehabilitation Counseling, 24*(2), 46-51.

Sparks, S.M. (1995). *Nursing diagnosis reference manual 3rd ed*. Pennsylvania: Springhouse.

Spector, R.E. (1991). *Cultural diversity in health and illness*. Stamford, CT: Appleton & Lange.

Spector, R.E. (1993). Culture, ethnicity, and nursing. In A. Potter & A. Perrry (Eds.), *Fundamentals of Nursing* (3rd ed., pp. 95-116). St. Louis, MO: C.V. Mosby.

Spector, R.E. (1996a). *Cultural diversity in health & illness* (4th ed.). Stamford: Appleton and Lange.

Spector, R.E. (1996b). *Guide to heritage assessment and health traditions*. Stamford: Appleton Lange.

Stover, S. L., DeLisa, J. A., & Whiteneck, E. G. (1995). *Spinal cord injury: Clinical outcome from the model systems* (pp. 29-31). Rockville, Maryland: Aspen.

Stover, S., & Fine, P. (1986). *Spinal cord injury: The facts and figures*. Birmingham: University of Alabama.

Stripling, T., Fonseca, J.E., Tsou, V., Copperthite, A. (1983). A demographic study of spinal cord injured Veterans. *Journal of American Paraplegia Society, 16*(3), 62-66.

Suzuki, L.A., & Ponterotto, J.G. (Ed.). (1996). *Handbook of multicultural assessment*. San Francisco: Josey-Bass Publishers.

Tripp-Reimer, T., Brink, P., & Saunders, J. (1984). Cultural assessment: Content and process. *Nursing Outlook, 32*(2), 78-83.

U.S. Bureau of the Census. (1992). *Statistical abstract of the United States: 1992*. Washington, D.C.: U.S. Department of Congress.

Villarruel, A. (1995). Cultural perspectives of pain. In M. Leininger (Ed)., *Transcultural nursing: concepts, theories research and practice* (2nd ed., pp. 263-278). New York: McGraw-Hill.

Wallace, M. (1978). *Black macho and the myth of the superwoman*. New York: Dial.

Westbrook, M.T., Legge, V., & Pennay, M. (1995). Ethnic differences in expectations for women with physical disabilities. *Journal of Applied Rehabilitation Counseling, 26*(4), 26-32.

Yap, P. (1977). Culture-bound reactive syndromes. In D. Landy (Ed.), *Culture diseases and healing*. New York: MacMillan.

CHAPTER

Teams and Collaboration

Margaret Ross Kraft, MS, RN, CRRN

I. Learning Objectives

A. Identify several team models.

B. Discuss the process of team formation.

C. List the core members of a health care team.

II. Introduction

Restructuring of the health care system has placed an emphasis on primary care and the coordination of comprehensive services. In this era of limited health-care dollars, it is important to understand the workings of the team care delivery model and how it can impact costs and outcomes of care. Team care is recognized as the cornerstone of modern rehabilitation philosophy and practice (Strasser, Falconer & Martino-Saltzmann, l994). The team approach to Spinal Cord Impairment (SCI) rehabilitation distinguishes the rehabilitation model from the traditional medical model of care. Given the complexity and severity of SCI, appropriate care is seen as best provided through the health care team. Why teams? First, continuity of care is achieved over time despite changes in individual team members. Second, the need for continuous provision of comprehensive coordinated care has led to the realization that no single discipline can respond effectively in isolation. Team care for SCI patients was first documented in the l940s at the Stoke Mandeville Hospital in Britain (Wells & Nicosia, l992). The complexity of SCI necessitates a team approach to effectively address needs over the life span. Organizational and professional issues, staffing patterns, economic constraints, and interpersonal relationships impact development of successful teams. Health care providers have not always been educationally or experientially prepared to assume the collegial relationships required for successful team outcomes. Therefore, concepts of "team" must be taught.

III. The Team Concept

A. **Definition of Teams:** A team is defined as a number of persons associated together in work or activity; a group of specialists or scientists functioning as a collaborative unit (Webster, 1980). Teamwork is defined as work done by several associates with each doing a part but all subordinating personal prominence to the efficiency of the whole (Webster, 1980).

B. **Characteristics of Teams:** A team crosses the boundaries of various disciplines. A team has structure, definition, direction, identification, and group energy or synergy. Teamwork implies unified direction; commitment to achieving common objectives; focused on integrated outcomes.
   1. Coordinated team effort leads to effective utilization of time and facilities.
   2. Increases cooperation to meet needs.
   3. Concepts of teamwork can be taught.

C. **Decision-Making:** A team functions in accordance with the ethical principles of non-maleficence and beneficence; a team must not make paternalistic decisions; a team must consider individual life experiences and preferences. A group does not automatically create a team; teamwork does not mean automatic agreement.

D. **Holistic Care Approach:** A team follows the concept of holistic health care.
   1. Need for coordination of fragmented care is recognized.
   2. The increased complexity of individual lives is addressed.
   3. Individuals and caregivers have high expectations of quality of life.
   4. Maintaining and enhancing function is a common goal. Goals are the foundation of care interventions and are used to evaluate outcomes.

E. **Strengths of Teams:** A team addresses the costs of maintaining and restoring abilities. Advantages of teams include support for staff morale, reduced costs, earlier rehabilitation, and improved patient care. Team strengths include the ability reach consensus, provide of mutual support, and support of multiple leaders with the ability to adjust to changing demands.

IV. Team Models

Distinguishing factors of teams include membership composition, goal setting; team processes; degree of collaboration or interdependence in planning, problem solving, decision making, implementing and evaluating team-related tasks, and leadership.

A. **Unidisciplinary Team**
   1. One discipline with varying levels of expertise.
   2. Group of providers from one disciplinary background, who may be employed by different agencies but collaborate on occasion.
   3. Natural leader or person with highest rank provides leadership as needed.

B. **Intradisciplinary Team**
   1. Members come from different levels of expertise or different specializations within the same discipline e.g. registered nurses, practical nurses, nursing assistants working together.
   2. Members all employed by the same agency.
   3. Highest ranking professional assumes leadership.

C. **Multidisciplinary Team**
   1. Staff from a variety of disciplines working individually to enable patient to achieve goals.
   2. Each team member has knowledge of specific profession.
   3. Members have a single disciplinary perspective.
   4. Members come from a mix of health and social welfare professions.
   5. Members may share a common work site.
   6. Individual professional identities are more important than the team identity.

7. Members work independently.
8. Members do not implement a common plan but do share information about individual efforts and may consult with one another.
9. Highest ranking professional or person appointed by administration assumes leadership role.
10. Members do not attend to interactional processes.
11. Team is not primary vehicle for service delivery, and consultations are separate.
12. Little or no team communication; patient and family get recommendations from each specialty.

D. **Interdisciplinary Team**
1. Members from a mix of health and human service professions.
2. Staff provide coordinated rather than integrated services.
3. The team sets, coordinates, and shares common goals but individuals still function within own sphere of practice.
4. Members work toward the same goals at the same time.
5. Collective team identity is more important than the individual professional status of each member.
6. Members negotiate, collaborate, and work independently and interdependently.
7. Members share the right and responsibility for assuming leadership functions as needed to facilitate the team progress.
8. Attention is paid to internal interactional processes; members practice communication, role negotiation and other critical group process skills.
9. After individual assessments are completed, the team members meet to synthesize findings and reach agreement on recommendations and the appropriate means of ensuring that patients receive consistent information and integrated care.
10. Team members possess a shared reality; have reached a consensus on goals of treatment and share responsibilities for the team decisions.
11. Team members support each other's goals as the basis for team interventions.

E. **Trans-Disciplinary Team**
1. The most holistic team model.
2. Members have a patient-centered focus with interwoven communication.
3. Goals belong to the patient not the team.
4. Each member has an in-depth knowledge of own discipline and is continually expanding knowledge of the other disciplines.
5. Treatment approaches overlap. Sufficient trust and mutual confidence exists to allow members to engage in teaching and learning across disciplinary lines. Depending on the patient's needs, one team member may be selected as the primary therapist.
6. Members do more than collaborate; they also entrust, prepare, and supervise the shared disciplinary functions while retaining ultimate responsibility for services provided in their stead by fellow team members.

V. Team Development

An evolutionary process that may follow sequential phases as described by Tuckman (1965). Development phases are repeated when team functions, membership, and outcomes change.

A. **Forming:** Individuals enter a team relationship and begin to define themselves as a team. This has been described as the "honeymoon" phase of team development.
1. Expectations for behavior are set for the team and for it's members.
2. Opinions are expressed cautiously.
3. Efforts are unfocused.

B. **Storming:** Issues of leadership, power, and control are addressed. This phase could deteriorate into conflicts that sabotage team goals and team leadership. Disharmony could actually split the

team into opposition groups but with strong commitment, this phase can be survived and team development continued.
1. Alliances are formed.
2. Roles and relationships of team members are defined.
3. A team "language" is being developed.

C. **Norming:** Teams roles, functions, and goals are defined and "teamwork" can begin.
1. Leadership and control is determined.
2. A "we" identity emerges.
3. A level of comfort with member differences is reached.

D. **Performing:** The team is able to function appropriately and produce expected outcomes.
1. Members make honest disclosures and negotiate solutions.
2. Cohesiveness is developed.
3. Feedback is accepted.
4. Conflict, professional defensiveness, and dissent disappear.

VI. Team Membership

The size and composition of a team will vary according to the services and programs delivered to the person served (Commission on Accreditation of Rehabilitation Facilities (CARF), 1995). Factors influencing team size include needs of clients, care philosophy, availability of professional resources, financial resources, geographic location, and mandated requirements.

A. **Disciplines:** A single discipline cannot address the complex consequences of SCI, therefore current systems of care are placing emphasis on the "health team" to integrate care (Vinicor, 1995).

B. **Non-Traditional Team Members:** The current move to comprehensive and integrated care systems assumes that many persons can and should influence health care systems. Teams addressing systems of care now include non-traditional non-health professionals such as economists, sociologists, anthropologists, city planners, or political scientists.

C. **Core Members:** The individual and family are core members of the team. Outcomes are often directly related to the level of individual involvement with the team process. Advantages of involving the individual and family in the team are to:
1. Prevent morbidity and reduce the burden of care
2. Empower and support autonomy
3. Assign personal responsibility to attain optimal health
4. Obtain the knowledge necessary to manage personal health

D. **Constant Members:** The health care team in comprehensive hospital-based SCI programs may include but are not be limited to: physician, nurse, occupational therapist, physical therapist, psychologist, social worker, speech and language pathologist, and therapeutic recreation specialist (CARF, 1995).
1. Physicians who may be active team participants include: neurosurgeons, neurologists, psychiatrists, orthopedists, physiatrists, pulmonologists, and urologists.
2. Nurses on the team should have knowledge of SCI and rehabilitation.
3. Other therapists participating in treatment teams may include: kinesiotherapists, educational therapists, and respiratory therapists.

E. **Additional Team Members:** Additional membership arrangements should be made to provide: audiology, chaplaincy, chemical dependence counseling, diagnostic radiology, dietetics, driver evaluation and/or education, lab services, orthotics, pharmacy, prosthetics, rehabilitation engineering, and vocational rehabilitation.

F. **Case managers:** A relatively new member of the health care team is the case manager who is employed to function as an integrator of multiple services with a focus on cost containment.
  1. The case manager coordinates services throughout an entire episode of illness/care.
  2. The case manager may be responsible for:
     a. Selecting and coordinating services
     b. Monitoring care and participating in the review and decision process
     c. Maintaining communication with the health care team, payer, the individual, and family
     d. Reducing costs while maintaining quality of care standards of care delivery
     e. Providing an interface between hospital-based care and the community
  3. The case manager may be employed by the treatment facility, by industry, or by third party payers. Gust (1992) recommends that the case manager must have a professional degree and first hand experience with SCI. Well-informed consumers can function as their own case manager.

G. **Community-based teams** are a model of primary care and usually focus on prevention and health promotion. The community-based team membership includes all disciplines with continuing involvement based on individual needs. There may be membership transition from hospital-based to community-based teams.

VII. Team Functions and Roles

A. **Team functions** (CARF, 1995):
  1. Assessment
     a. Biological and psychosocial needs
     b. Functional abilities and evaluation
  2. Determination, modification, implementation, of the individual program plan.
     a. Interventions are based on problems and goals
     b. Interventions may be discipline specific
  3. Provision of direct services consistent with needs
  4. Education and training
  5. Discharge and life care planning
  6. Evaluation of the team care process

B. **Team membership responsibilities**
  1. Active participation in conferences
  2. Promotion of team functions
  3. Mutual support among all team members
  4. Communication and coordination within the team to facilitate service delivery
  5. Assessment of available resources
  6. Referral to other services/programs as needed

C. **Overlap in Roles and Functions:** No one member can assume all roles.
  1. Members need thorough knowledge of their discipline to see how that discipline can best contribute to the whole
  2. Members must appreciate the educational backgrounds, attitudes, personalities, and approaches to care of the other disciplines. Secure and competent professionals can communicate discipline strengths, limitations, and contributions
  3. Sources of role conflict:
     a. Role ambiguity, overlapping competencies and responsibilities
     b. Preconceptions that professionals have of their own role, stereotypic perceptions of specific disciplines
     c. Goal conflict from value differences
     d. Poor communication

    e. Confusion of assignment of responsibilities, prejudice, distrust
    f. Lack of confidence in other disciplines, reimbursement for specific disciplines, educational levels, and perceived status

VIII. Team Processes

A. **Communication**

B. **Collaboration**

C. **Coordination**

D. **Evaluation**

IX. Team Issues

A. **Leadership:** May be assigned by the status of the member, appointed by the organization, or determined by traditional practices. Should be based on competence, experience, and information.
1. Requires knowledge of group dynamics, organizational acumen, and interpersonal skills.
2. Must identify the talents of team members and use them appropriately.
3. Must support the right of members to disagree, clarify conflict, and negotiate compromises.

B. **Conflict Resolution**
1. The team must honor consumer preferences even if not consistent with societal or team values. The team must understand individuals within their own support systems.
2. Personal and professional disagreements can reduce the effectiveness of the team.
3. Respect of differences in beliefs and attitudes among members is essential to minimize conflict.

X. Clinical Pathways and Care Paths

The search for cost effective delivery of a continuum of care has led to the development of clinical pathways and care paths. Clinical pathways reflect the essential activities/interventions and outcomes that must be accomplished within specified time frames by various disciplines. Several SCI treatment centers have developed and implemented specific care pathways that clearly identify team goals and facilitate the team process. Clinical pathways are discussed further in a later chapter of this text.

Practical Application

H.J. is a 21 year old male with C-5 quadriplegia due to a diving accident. During surgery to stabilize his spine, he infracted at the C-1/brainstem junction. He presented approximately 14 days after injury to an acute SCI rehabilitation unit with C-1 ventilator dependent quadriplegia, able to communicate only by blinking or rolling his eyes. His wife of four months was extremely anxious, demonstrating disbelief, grief, and unrealistic expectations. In addition to his wife, the involved family support system included his parents, his in-laws and his sister-in-law. At the time of admission, his care team included his primary nurse, the nurse manager/rehabilitation clinical specialist, the physiatrist, and the attending physician. Within a few days, his treatment team expanded to include the physical therapist, occupational therapist, respiratory therapist, pulmonologist, dietician, psychologist, social worker, and chaplain. These team members did thorough assessments of H.J. and kept his family informed about the assessment process. It became very clear that the dynamics within the family support system required frequent communication from the SCI treatment team.

H.J.'s physical condition improved and stabilized but it became evident that his ability to participate in or direct his own care may not improve. With this information regarding his prognosis, Mr. J.'s wife began to go from team member to team member seeking a more positive prognosis and expressing her feelings about being unable to deal with the situation. When she was not satisfied with staff responses she began to complain about care and expressed anger at staff. The team realized the importance of helping Mrs. J. and other family members to cope and strategized on how to respond to this behavior in a productive way. Specific team members were charged with working directly with Mrs. J. on how to express her feelings and concerns. The team also helped the family to develop realistic goals for discharge, long term, and follow-up care. Two important goals agreed upon by the family and the team were to assess H.J.'s ability to be non-ventilator dependent and to develop some means for him to communicate. At this time, the educational therapist and the speech pathologist joined the SCI treatment team. Within a few weeks, H.J. was successfully weaned from 24 hour ventilator dependency and was able to spend up to ten hours off the ventilator, he continued to require ventilation at night. He received and learned to use an "eye-gaze" computer which allowed him to select letters to spell words to communicate with his wife and family. H.J.'s wife, mother, and sister-in-law all began to learn how to provide H.J.'s care. They were taught basic ADL care, bowel and bladder management, respiratory and skin care, management of the ventilator, and transfer techniques. H.J. began to join his family on "out" trips to the community and his time up in his special wheelchair was extended.

As the discharge date grew near, the SCI Home Care staff joined the treatment team. The nurse and therapist who would be assigned to M.J. for follow-up after discharge did home assessments at several locations. Since the home of M.J.'s parents was most accessible, the decision made by the extended family was to discharge to that location. In the mean time, home care staff also reviewed accessibility needs for a home which M.J. and his wife were interested in buying. The prosthetics department became active in the process of identification, purchase, and set up of home equipment which included back-up ventilation and suction support for possible emergencies. The special wheelchair had been secured early in the rehabilitation process to promote mobility. Throughout this entire planning process, the SCI treatment team maintained communication within the team to be sure all team members provided the family with consistent information.

On the actual day of discharge, the respiratory therapist and home care nurse met M.J. at home and reviewed the equipment and supplies again in the home setting. M.J.'s family reported high satisfaction with the education and training they had received and indicated a high comfort rate in providing care and solving problems related to ventilator dependency. Follow-up visits continued to reinforce the success of the team process in caring for this complex patient.

References and Selected Bibliography

Adler, S., Bryk, E., Cesta, T., & McEachen, I. (1995). Collaboration: The solution to multidisciplinary care planning. *Orthopaedic Nursing, 14* (2), 21-29.

Allred, C., Arford, P., & Michel, Y. (1995). Coordination as a critical element of managed care. *Journal of Nursing Administration, 25*(12), 21-28.

Anonymous. (1993). The rehabilitation team: Composition, models, functions, and issues. McCourt, A. (Ed.) In *The specialty practice of rehabilitation nursing: A Core Curriculum*. Skokie, IL: Rehabilitation Nurse Foundation.

Bair, J., & Greensan, B. (1986). TEAMS: Teamwork training for interns, residents, and nurses. *Hospital and Community Psychiatry, 37*(6), 633-635.

Becker-Reems, E. (1994). *Self-managed work teams in health care organizations*. Chicago: American Hospital Publishing.

Campbell, L. (1992). Team maintenance and enhancement. *American congress of rehabilitation medicine guide to interdisciplinary practice in rehabilitation settings* (pp. 173-187).

Capuano, T. (1995). Clinical pathways: Practical approaches, positive outcomes. *Nursing Management, 26*(1), 34-37.

Commission on Accreditation of Rehabilitation Facilities (CARF). (1995). *Standards manual and interpretive guidelines for medical rehabilitation*. Tucson.

Cosgrove, J. & Nicholas, J. (1986). Team treatment: Is a specialized unit more effective. *Archives of Physical Medicine and Rehabilitation, 67*, 632.

Czirr, R. & Rappaport, M. (1984). Tool kit for teams: Annotated bibliography on interdisciplinary health teams. *Clinical Gerontologists, 2*, 47-54.

Date', B., Grandquist, R., & Nettekoven, L. (1983). *Role clarification: Theory and practice for enhancing interdisciplinary collaboration on the rehab team*. Paper presented at the 45th annual meeting of the American Academy of Physical Medicine and Rehabilitation.

Dunn, M., Sommer, N., & Gambina, H. (1992). A practical guide to team functioning in spinal cord injury rehabilitation. In Zejdlik, C. (Ed.), *Management of spinal cord injury 2nd-ed.*, (pp· 229-239). Boston: Jones & Bartlett.

Halstead, L. (1976). Team care in chronic illness: A critical review of the literature of the past 25 years. *Archives of Physical Medicine and Rehabilitation, 57*, 507-511.

Gage, M. (1994). The patient-driven interdisciplinary care plan. *Journal of Nursing Administration, 24*(4), 26-35.

Griffin, B., Halstead, L., Healy, J. Higgins, L., Kanellos, M., Rheinecker, S., Rintala, D., & Whiteside, W., (1986). The innovative rehabilitation team: An experiment in team building. *Archives of Physical Medicine and Rehabilitation, 67*, 357-361.

Gust, T. (1992). Case management services. In Zejdlik, C.,(Ed.), *Management of spinal cord injury* (2nd ed., pp. 241-253). Boston: Jones & Bartlett.

Jaffe, K. & Walsh, P. (1993). The development of the specialty rehabilitation home care team: Supporting the creative thought process. *Holistic Nursing Practice, 7*(4), 36-41.

Keith, R. (1991). The comprehensive treatment team in rehabilitation. *Archives of Physical Medicine and Rehabilitation, 72,* 269-274.

Mariano C. (1989). The case for interdisciplinary collaboration. Nursing Outlook, 37 (6), 285-288

McCarren, M. (1990). Tough love for the rehab unit...no more nurse bashing. *Spinal Network Extra,* 12-14.

Moulder, T., Staal, A., & Grant, M. (1988). Making the interdisciplinary team approach work. *Rehabilitation Nursing, 13,* 338-339.

Mullins, L., Keller, J., & Chaney, J. (1994). A systems and social cognitive approach to team functioning in physical rehabilitation settings. *Rehabilitation Psychology, 39*(3), 161-178.

Neal, L. (1995). The rehabilitation nursing team in the home healthcare setting. *Rehabilitation Nursing, 20*(1), 32-36.

Nelson, A. (1992). Developing a therapeutic milieu on a spinal cord injury unit. In C. Zejdlik (Ed.), *Management of spinal cord injury.* (2nd ed., pp. 213-227). Boston: Jones and Barlett.

O'Toole, M. (1992). The interdisciplinary team: Research and education. *Holistic Nursing Practice,* 6(2), 76-83.

Phillips, S., & Elledge, R. (1989). *The team-building source book.* San Diego, CA: University Associates.

Purtilo, R., & Meier, R. (1993). Team challenges: Regulatory constraints and patient empowerment. *American Journal of Physical Medicine and Rehabilitation, 72*(5), 327-330.

Rintala, D., Alexander, J., Sanson-Fisher, R., Willems, E., & Halstead, L. (1986). Team care: An analysis of verbal behavior during patient rounds in a rehabilitation hospital. *Archives of Physical Medicine and Rehabilitation, 67,* 118-122.

Rothberg, J. (1981). The rehabilitation team: Future direction. *Archives of Physical Medicine and Rehabilitation, 62,* 407.

Scholtes, P. (1988). *The team handbook: How to use teams improve quality.* Madison: Joiner Associates.

Schut, H. & Stam, H. (1994). Goals in rehabilitation teamwork. *Disability and Rehabilitation, 16*(4), 223-226.

Strasser, D., Falconer, J., & Martino-Saltzmann, D. (1994). The rehabilitation team: Staff perceptions of the hospital environment, the interdisciplinary team environment, and interprofessional relations. *Archives of Physical Medicine and Rehabilitation, 75,* 177-182.

Tuckman, B. (1965). Developmental sequences in small groups. *Psychological Bulletin, 63*(6), 384-399.

Ulschak, R. (1995). *Team architecture: The manager's guide to designing effective work teams.* Health Administration Press.

Vinicor, F. (1995). Interdisciplinary and intersectional approach: A challenge for integrated care. *Patient Education and Counseling, 26,* 267-272.

Webster's new collegiate dictionary (1980). Springfield, Massachusetts: G. & C. Merriam.

Werlitz, P. & Potter, P. (1993). A managed care system. *Journal of Nursing Administration, 23,* 51-56.

Wells, J. & Nicosia, S. (1992). The effects of multidisciplinary team care for acute spinal cord injury patients. *Journal of the American Paraplegia Society, 16,* 23-29.

CHAPTER

Anatomy and Physiology of the Spine and Spinal Cord

Ellen Barker, MSN, RN, CNRN

I. Learning Objectives

A. Describe the structure of the spine, spinal cord, and spinal nerves.

B. Understand the function of the spine, spinal cord, and spinal nerves.

II. Introduction

Familiarity with neuroanatomy and neurophysiology is essential in the management of individuals with spinal cord impairment (SCI). It is necessary to understand the spinal cord and its role in the integration of body function and movement.

III. Anatomy and Physiology

A. **Spine**

The spine is a flexible column that consists of 33 bones called vertebrae, which are separated by intervertebral disks. The spine is approximately two feet long in the adult (See Figure 7-1). Spinal vertebrae are grouped into five areas:
1. Cervical (C 1-7)
2. Thoracic (T 1-12)
3. Lumbar (L1-5)
4. Sacral (S1-5 fused in adults)
5. Coccygeal (3)

B. **Components of Vertebrae** (See Figures 7-2, and 7-3, and Table 7-1)
1. Vertebrae consist of two major parts: the anterior body and the posterior arch
    a. The neural arch consists of a pair of anterolateral pedicles, a pair of posterolateral laminae, four articular processes, two transverse processes, and one spinous process that form a hollow cylinder to protect the spinal cord
    b. Protruding spinous process that separates two transverse processes, an anterior portion, the vertebral body and a posterior portion or neural arch

Figure 7-1: Anterior and Lateral Views of the Vertebral Column

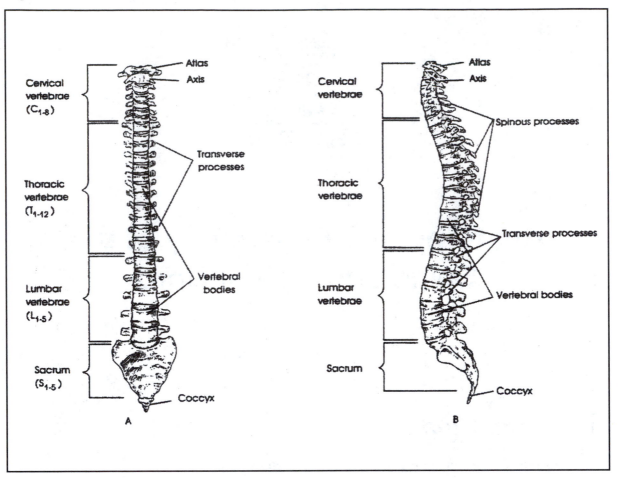

From *Management of Spinal Cord Injury* (2nd ed., p. 54), by C.P. Zejdlik, 1992, Boston: Jones & Bartlett. Reprinted with permission.

     c. Pedicles (2): short projections backward

     d. Laminae: broad plates that fuse together in the middle posteriorly, allow for attachment of the ligamenta subflava

     e. Spinous process: serves for the attachment of muscles and ligaments

     f. Transverse processes (2): serve for the attachment of muscles and ligaments.

     g. Articular processes (4): two on each side, from the junction of the pedicle with the laminae

     h. Body: largest portion

  2. Special characteristics

     a. A series of curves

        (1) Convex cervical curve

        (2) Concave thoracic curve

        (3) Convex lumbar curve

        (4) Concave pelvic curve

     b. Flexible for movement

     c. Atlas (C1): supports the "globe" or head, without body or spinous process, ring-like structure allows the head to rotate.

     d. Axis (C2): forms the pivot upon which C1 rotates. The odontoid (tooth-like) is a projection of C2. Instant death can result when the connection with the occipital bone via the lateral fasciculi ligament is disrupted. Allows for flexion and extension of the head.

Figure 7-2: A Lateral View and Cross-Section of A Vertebra Detailing Vertebral Arch

Figure 7-3: A Cross-Section of a Vertebra

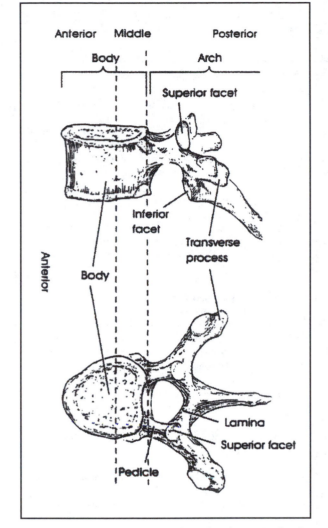

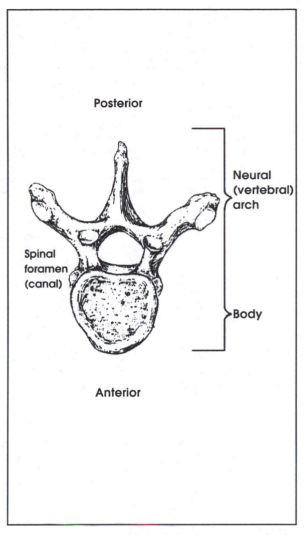

From *Management of Spinal Cord* Injury (2nd ed., p. 55), by C.P. Zejdlik, 1992, Boston: Jones & Bartlett. Reprinted with permission.

From *Management of Spinal Cord Injury* (2nd ed., p. 55), by C.P. Zejdlik, 1992, Boston: Jones & Bartlett. Reprinted with permission.

C. **Spinal Canal** - Vertebral foramina form the vertebral canal
   1. Large triangular cervical spinal canal
   2. Small and rounded thoracic region

D. **Supporting structures** (See Figure 7-4)
   1. Anterior longitudinal ligament (extends from C2 to the sacrum along the anterior surfaces of the vertebral bodies)
   2. Posterior longitudinal ligament (extends from C2 to the sacrum and descends along the posterior surface of the vertebral bodies)
   3. Ligamenta flava
   4. Supraspinal ligament
   5. Ligamentum nuchae
   6. Interspinal ligament
   7. Intertransverse ligament

Table 7-1: Spinal Vertebrae

The 33 Vertebrae	The Sacrum (S_{1-5}) [5 fused vertebrae]
	• Fused vertebrae in a solid triangular block; articulates with the fifth lumbar vertebra, the coccyx, and the two hip bones
C_1 (Atlas)	• Foramina allow for exit of lower lumbar and sacral spinal nerves
• Lacks a vertebral body; basically a ring-shaped arch on which the skull rests	• Unites the vertebral column with the pelvis (Forms the posterior wall of the pelvis)
• Lateral masses articulate with the skull (occipital condyle)	
• Allows flexion, extension, and lateral movement; no rotation	The Coccyx [4 rudimentary vertebrae]
	• Articulates with the sacrum superiorly and diminishes in size until reaches the lowest portion (apex) commonly called the tailbone
C_2 (Axis)	• Accommodates a division of the fifth sacral nerve
• Mainly a vertebral body and a large, strong, odontoid process (rising perpendicularly from the midportion) to fit inside the C_1 ring.	
• Articulates with C_1 vertebra at dens-atlas joint and two lateral (almost flat) facetjoints	**Intervertebral Connections**
• Allows rotation; no flexion or extension	
Movements controlled by alar and apical ligaments	Intervertebral Discs
	• Cartilaginous joints between discs with soft gelatinous substance (nucleus pulposus) forming the center, surrounded by a tough fibrous annulus that conforms to the size of discs between which they lie; extend from the axis to the sacrum
Lower Cervical Vertebrae (C_{3-7}) [5]	
• Articular facets oriented with superior facets facing posteriorly, slightly medially, and upwards	• Mainly function as a cushion between vertebrae to absorb stress although allow for greater mobility at the cervical and lumbar regions of the spine
• Small facet joints at each side of body	
• Allows flexion, extension, and rotation	
	Ligaments
Thoracic Vertebrae (T_{1-12}) [12]	• Strong fibrous bands that surrounded the vertebral column, holding it together
• Articular facets oriented with superior facets facing posteriorly, almost vertical, and slightly laterally	• Vary in width and strength depending on function performed; form various fusions and interconnections to enhance functions
• Joints for head of ribs on transverse processes and vertebral bodies	• Anterior and posterior longitudinal ligaments extend entire length of the spinal column
• Increase in size from above downward	• Ligamenta flava run between laminae
• Allows flexion and rotation of trunk	• Supraspinal and interspinal ligaments join the spinous processes
	• Ligaments of the sacrum and coccyx form a rich network to stabilize the pelvis and strengthen lower body stability and movement
Lumber Vertebrae (L_{1-5}) [5]	
• Articular facets oriented with superior facets facing medially, posteriorly, and almost vertically	
• Transverse processes large for lower body muscle attachment	
• Vertebrae are large and massive for their weightbearing function; lumbar curve is convex anteriorly for mobility	
• Movements mostly flexion and extension	

From *Management of Spinal Cord Injury,* (2nd ed., p. 57) by C. P. Zejdlik, 1992, Boston: Jones & Bartlett. Reprinted with permission.

Figure 7-4: Ligaments of Cervical Spine

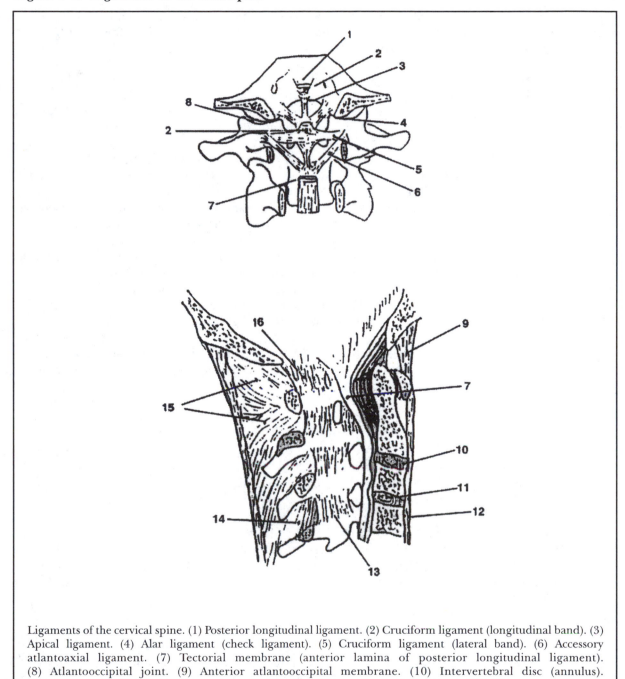

Ligaments of the cervical spine. (1) Posterior longitudinal ligament. (2) Cruciform ligament (longitudinal band). (3) Apical ligament. (4) Alar ligament (check ligament). (5) Cruciform ligament (lateral band). (6) Accessory atlantoaxial ligament. (7) Tectorial membrane (anterior lamina of posterior longitudinal ligament). (8) Atlantooccipital joint. (9) Anterior atlantooccipital membrane. (10) Intervertebral disc (annulus). (11) Intervertebral disc (nucleus pulposus). (12) Anterior longitudinal ligament. (13) Ligamentum flavum. (14) Interspinal ligament. (15) Nuchal ligament. (16) Posterior atlantooccipital membrane.

From Normal Adult Anatomy, in R. Winters, *The Cervical Spine* (p. 12), by H.H. Sherk & W. N. Parke, 1983, Philadelphia: J.B. Lippincott Co. Reprinted with permission.

E. **Disks** are nonsynovial joints and the largest avascular structures in the human body
   1. Serve as shock absorbers
   2. Made of three component structures:
      a. Vertebral end-plates
         (1) Function to disperse the load to the adjacent nucleus pulposus (NP) and annulus fibrosus (AF)
         (2) Permit fluid diffusion between vertebra sinsusoids and the NP and AF
         (3) The fluid exchange between the end-plates plays a major role in the nourishment of the avascular structures of the disc
         (4) Are the weakest structures of the three disc components
      b. Annulus fibrosus (AF) - outer region comprised of fibrocartilage or collagen fibers that form concentric lamellae or rings to contain the nucleus pulposus (NP)
         (1) The fibers in each lamella run obliquely 30 degrees to the end-plate. Thus two adjoining lamellae run in the opposite direction and cross each other at 120 degrees.
         (2) The interlamellar spaces are filled with abundant amounts of proteoglycan
         (3) Changes in the biochemical composition caused by aging produces susceptibility of the disk to trauma
         (4) The AF is the most important component in a spinal motion segment for biomechanical stability and for transmitting vertical weight-bearing forces.
         (5) The AF provides maximal stability against horizontal displacement.
      c. Nucleus pulposus (NP): inner region, contains no independent blood supply, no cells, and consists of a three-dimensional network embedded in a mucoprotein gel
         (1) Water content is approximately 80percent and decreases with age
         (2) Incompressible material that bulges out when the disc is incised
         (3) Compressed by the elastic properties of the ligamentum flavum to maintain the disk height
         (4) Acts like a ball bearing when the vertebral bodies roll in flexion and extension
         (5) The center of rotation within the disc changes instantaneously depending on the position of the spine during flexion and extension
         (6) Has no nocioceptive endings
         (7) Degeneration of the NP leads to loss of disc height and lateral load transmission across the disc and facet joints

F. **Facet joint**: is a true synovial joint and is richly innervated by nociceptive endings
   1. Function: to provide torsional stability of a motion segment
   2. In normal conditions bears < 20 percent of body weight

G. **Spinal cord** (medullar spinalis) (See Figure 7-5)
   1. An elongated, cylindrical continuation of the medulla oblongata and extends from the cranial border of the atlas and terminates at the level of the first lumbar vertebra (L1)
   2. Occupies most of the vertebral canal
   3. Average length in adult - 45 cm
   4. Average weight in adult - 30 gm
   5. Surrounded by three meninges (See Figure 7-6)
      a. Dura mater (outer layer): extends to S2
         (1) Epidural space - separates the dura from the vertebral column
         (2) Subdural space - separates the arachnoid from the pia
      b. Arachnoid mater: extends to S2.
         Subarachnoid space for approximately 75 ml of cerebrospinal fluid (CSF) to protect the cord.
      c. Pia mater: vascular and closely adhered to the surface of the cord
   6. Protected by CSF in the subarachnoid space
   7. Cervical region - gives origin to brachial plexus
   8. Lower thoracic region and lumbar regions - gives origin to lumbosacral plexus
   9. Tapers inferiorly into the conus medullaris (See Figure 7-7)
   10. Prolongation of pia mater tapers to become the filum terminale with attachment to the posterior surface of the coccyx (See Figure 7-5)

Figure 7-5: Spinal Cord

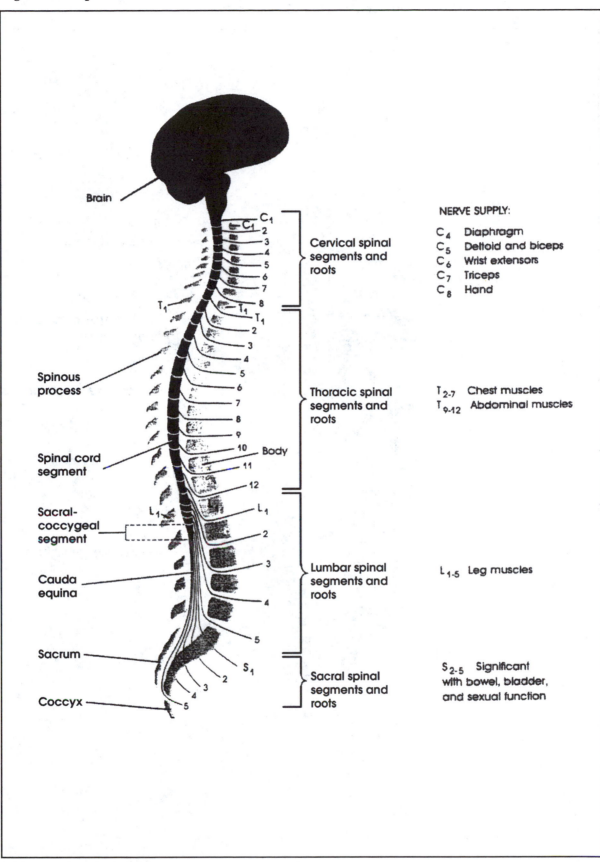

From *Management of Spinal Cord Injury* (2nd ed., p. 58), by C. P. Zejdlik, 1992, Boston: Jones & Bartlett. Reprinted with permission.

Figure 7-6: Meningeal Layers of Spinal Cord (Segment of Spinal Cord Viewed from Behind with Portions of Duramater and Arachnoid Removed)

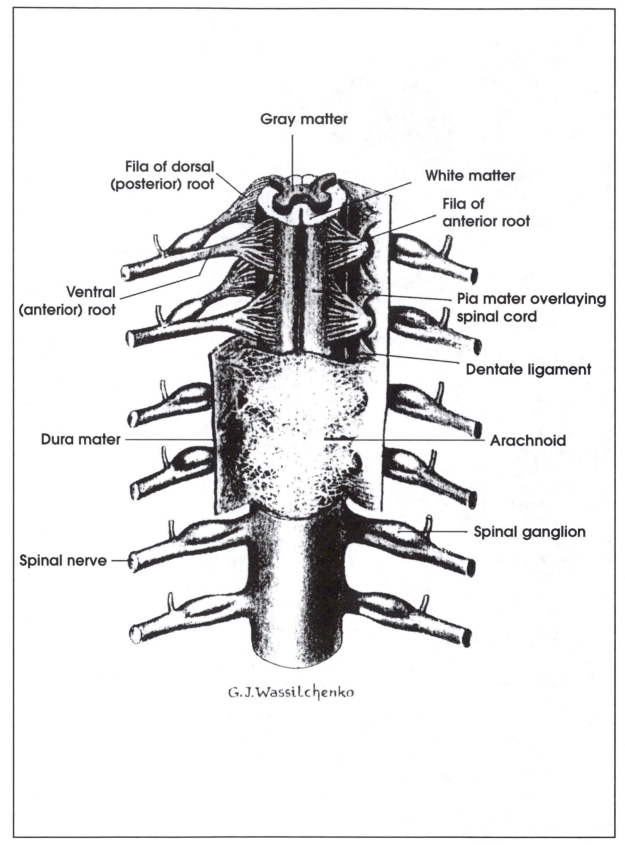

From *Advanced Neurological and Neurosurgical Nursing* (p. 94), by E. B. Rudy, 1984, St. Louis: Mosby. Reprinted with permission.

Figure 7-7: Conus and Cauda Equina In Relation to Thoracolumbar Junction of the Spine

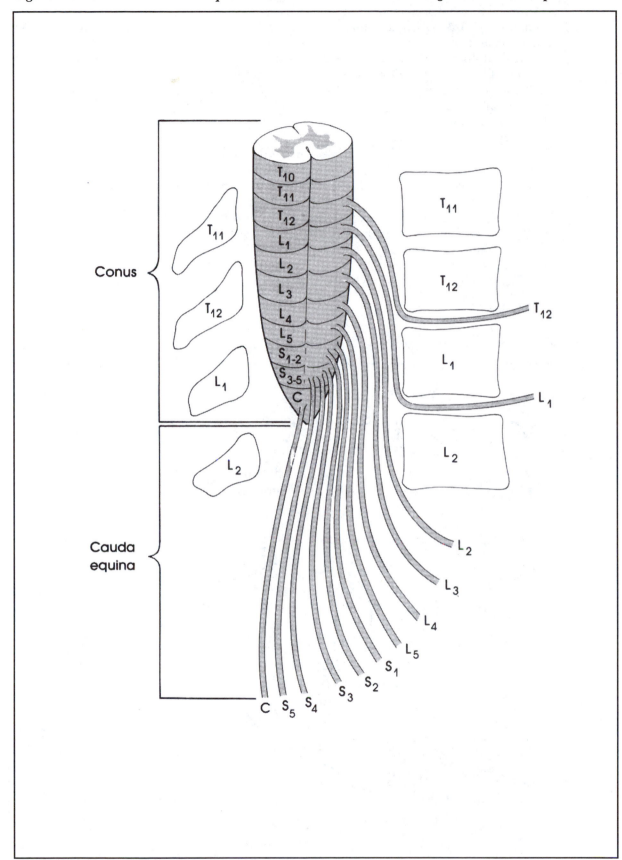

From *Management of Spinal Cord Injury* (2nd ed., p. 69), by C. P. Zejdlik, 1992, Boston: Jones & Bartlett. Reprinted with permission.

H. **Spinal nerves** (31 pairs) (See Figure 7-5) which leave the spinal cord and pass through intervertebral foramina or openings in the vertebral column.
   1. Spinal nerves are named according to the regions of the vertebral columns with which they are associated:
      a. Cervical - 8 pairs with short roots that are horizontal. First nerve exists above C1 and the second below C1 for a total of 8 nerves compared to only seven vertebra
      b. Thoracic - 12 pairs
      c. Lumbar - 5 pairs
      d. Sacral - 5 pairs
      e. Coccygeal - 1 pair
   2. Each spinal nerve is connected to the spinal cord by two roots: (See Figure 7-8)
      a. Anterior root
         Consists of bundles of nerve fibers carrying nerve impulses away from the central nervous system (CNS).
         (1) Efferent (motor) fibers innervate skeletal muscles to contract.
         (2) Located in the anterior gray horn of the cord - anterior horn cells (skeletal muscle motor cell bodies).
      b. Posterior root
         Consists of bundles of nerve fibers carrying nerve impulses to the CNS.

Figure 7-8: Diagram of a Typical Spinal Nerve

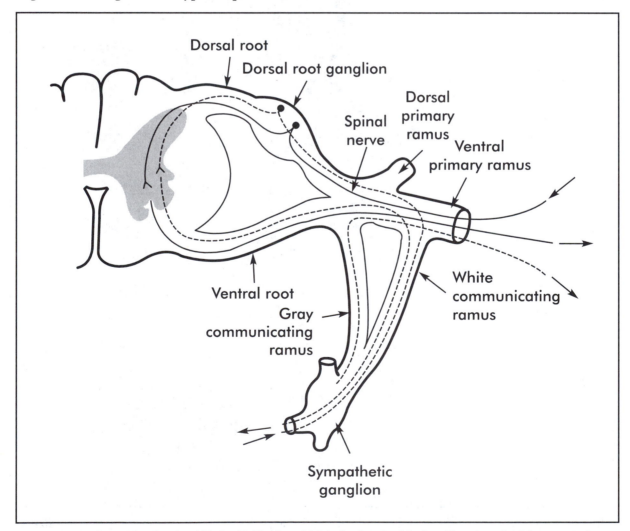

From *Neuroscience Nursing* (p. 17), by E. Barker, 1994, St. Louis: Mosby. Reprinted with permission.

(1) Afferent (sensory fibers) convey information about pain, touch, vibration, and temperature.

(2) Sensory cell bodies, located in the posterior root ganglion.

c. Spinal nerve roots unite to form a spinal nerve that is mixed with both motor and sensory fibers.

d. Each spinal nerve emerges from the foramen and divides into a ramus.

(1) Anterior ramus - large ramus that supplies the muscles and skin over the antero-lateral wall and muscles of the limbs.

(2) Posterior ramus - small rami that join at the root of the limbs to form nerve plexuses.

I. **Gray and White Matter of the Spinal Cord** (See Figure 7-9)

1. Gray matter (more abundant than white) contains cell bodies central to the cord in an "H" or butterfly shape (motor cell bodies)

2. White matter composed of bundles of nerve fibers that are primarily myelinated axons that surround the gray matter and are divided into funiculi or large bundles of fibers known as columns

a. Anterior column mediates motor function, posture reflexes, light touch, and pressure

(1) Descending motor tracts

(a) Corticospinal

(b) Anterior

(c) Vestibulospinal

(d) Tectospinal

(e) Reticulospinal

(2) Ascending sensory tracts

(a) Spinothalamic

(b) Spinoolivary

Figure 7-9: A Cross-Section of the Spinal Cord Detailing Major Motor and Sensory Tracts

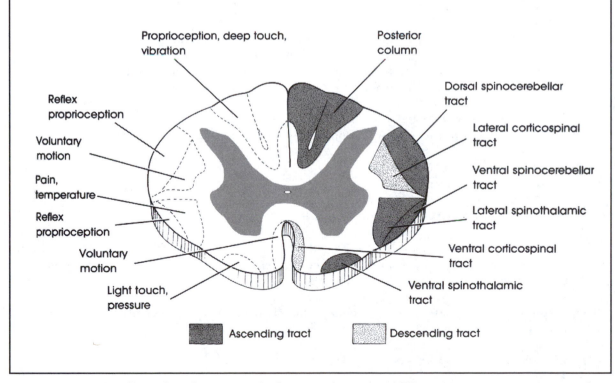

From *Management of Spinal Cord Injury* (2nd ed., p. 59), by C. P. Zejdlik, 1992, Boston: Jones & Bartlett. Reprinted with permission.

     b. Lateral white column mediates subconscious proprioception for control of locomotion, pain, temperature, and motor function
       (1) Descending motor tracts
         (a) Lateral corticospinal
         (b) Rubrospinal
         (c) Olivospinal
       (2) Ascending sensory tracts
         (a) Dorsal spinocerebellar
         (b) Ventral spinocerebellar
         (c) Lateral spinothalamic
     c. Posterior or dorsal column mediates proprioception, vibration, two-point discrimination, deep pressure and touch
       (1) Descending - motor tracts
         (a) Fasciculus interfascicularis
       (2) Ascending - sensory tracts
         (a) Fasciculus gracilis
         (b) Fasciculus cuneatus

J. **Central canal**: runs the full length of the cord from the fourth ventricle to the end of the conus medullaris and contains CSF to protect the cord.

K. **Neurons**: Neurons are the functional cells of the nervous system, consisting of a cell body, dendrites, and axons. Dendrites conduct impulses toward the cell body and axons convey impulses away from the cell body.
  1. Upper motor neurons (UMNs) - have their cell bodies in the brain and influence the activity of the lower motor neurons (LMNs) to facilitate or inhibit muscle contraction.
  2. Lower motor neurons - are the last neurons to carry information from the central nervous system out to the muscles to contract and are located in the anterior horns of the gray matter in the cord.
    a. Alpha motor neurons innervate most fibers in any given muscle.
    b. Gamma motor neurons are smaller in diameter and innervate small muscle cells within the muscle spindles.

L. **Spinal reflex arc**: An involuntary protective mechanism to prevent injury, requiring no cerebral intervention (See Figure 7-10). Composed of three parts:
  1. Sensory endings in the skin, joint, tendon, or organ detect stimuli and generate impulses in sensory neurons, enters dorsal horn of gray matter of cord via dorsal root of spinal nerve and synapses with an interneuron in the cord
  2. Interneurons activate LMNs of skeletal muscles
  3. Skeletal muscles react to stimuli from LMN (reflex response)

M. **Stretch reflex arc** (tendon reflex)
  1. Receptor tendon stretched by tap
  2. Neurons synapse with lower motor neuron
  3. Response with brisk contraction of muscle

N. **Dermatomes**: Dermatomes are areas on the surface of the body that are innervated by the afferent fibers from a single spinal root (See Figures 7-11, 7-12). They form a dermatome map that is useful in location of sensory changes or loss.

O. **Myotomes**: Myotomes are the collection of muscle fibers that are innervated by specific motor neurons.

P. **Circulation of the Spinal Cord** (See Figure 7-13)
  1. Arterial
    a. Anterior and posterior spinal arteries branch from the vertebral artery
      (1) Supply the upper cervical spinal cord

Figure 7-10: Pathway of the Lower Motor Neuron or Reflex Arc

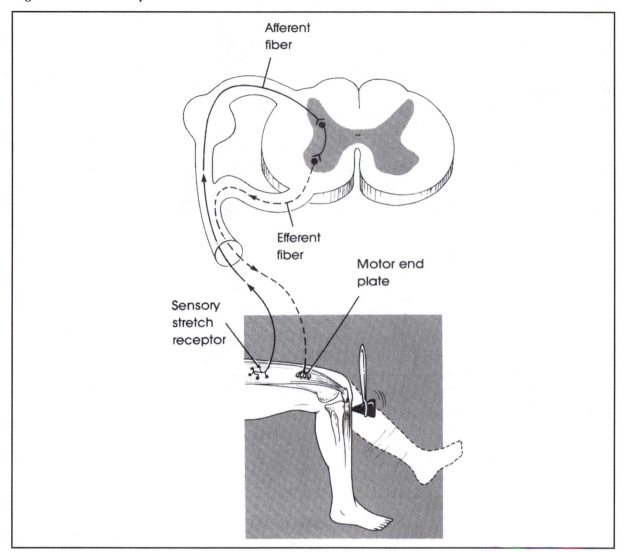

From *Management of Spinal Cord Injury* (2nd ed., p. 71), by C. P. Zejdlik, 1992, Boston: Jones & Bartlett. Reprinted with permission.

> (2) Enter the vertebral canal through the intervertebral foramina with one being larger (arteria radicularis magna) and may be major source of blood to the lower two-thirds of spinal cord.
> (3) Reinforced by radicular arteries
>
> b. Right and left anterior spinal artery unite to form a single anterior spinal artery
>> (1) Courses inferiorly in the anterior median fissure
>> (2) Perfuses the anterior two-thirds of the spinal cord
>
> c. Posterior spinal arteries divide to form two descending branches
>> (1) Run inferiorly along the side of the cord
>> (2) Supply blood to posterior third of cord

2. Venous
  a. Anastomose along cord
  b. Valveless
  c. Located in pia mater of meninges

Figure 7-11: Sensory Dermatomes

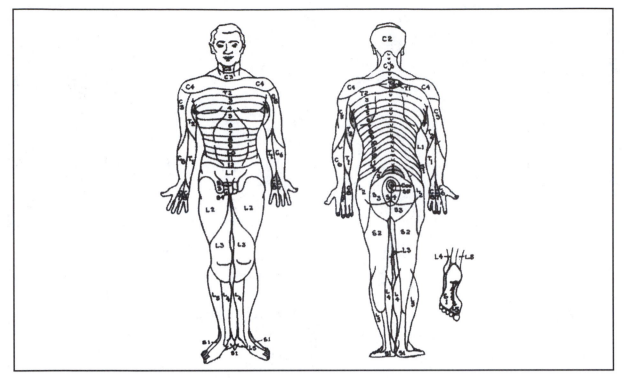

From *Management of Spinal Cord Injury* (2nd ed., p. 80), by C. P. Zejdlik, 1992, Boston: Jones & Bartlett. Reprinted with permission.

Figure 7-12: Arrangement of Dermatomes By Level of Injury

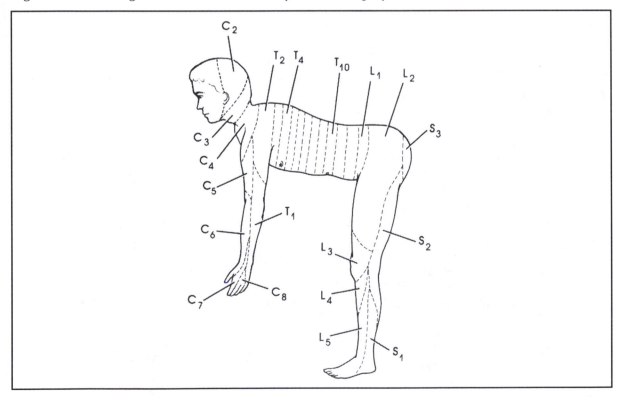

From *Management of Spinal Cord Injury* (2nd ed., p. 80), by C. P. Zejdlik, 1992, Boston: Jones & Bartlett. Reprinted with permission.

Figure 7-13: Spinal Cord Blood Supply

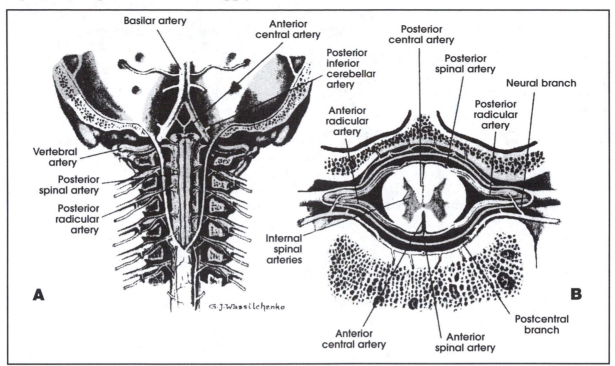

From *Neuroscience Nursing* (p. 397), by E. Barker, 1994, St. Louis: Mosby. Reprinted with permission.

References and Selected Bibliography

Alspach, J. (1991). *Core curriculum for critical care nursing*. Philadelphia: W.B. Saunders.

Barker, E. (1994). *Neuroscience nursing*. St. Louis, MO: Mosby.

Buchanan, L.E. & Nawoczenski, D.A. (1987). *Spinal cord injury*. Baltimore, MD: Williams & Wilkins.

Cammermeyer, M. & Appeldorn, C. (1990). *Core curriculum for neuroscience nursing (3rd ed.)*. Chicago, IL: American Association of Neuroscience Nurses.

McCourt, A.E. (1993). *The specialty practice of rehabilitation nursing: A core curriculum (3rd ed.)*. Skokie, IL: The Rehabilitation Nursing Foundation of the Association of Rehabilitation Nurses.

Raimondi, A.J. (1987). *Pediatric neurosurgery*. New York: Springer-Verlag.

Rudy, E.B. (1984). *Advanced neurological and neurosurgical nursing*. St. Louis, MO: Mosby.

Sherk, H.H. & Parke, W.N. (1983). Normal adult anatomy. In R. Winters, *The cervical spine*. Philadelphia: J.B. Lippincott.

Swaiman, K.F. (1994). *Pediatric neurology, volume I & II, (2nd ed.)*. St. Louis, MO: Mosby.

White, A.H., Rothman, R.H., & Ray, C.D. (1987). *Lumbar spine surgery*. St. Louis, MO: Mosby.

Winters, R. (1983). *The cervical spine*. Philadelphia: J.B. Lippincott.

Zejdlik, C.P. (Ed.) (1992). *Management of spinal cord injury (2nd ed.)*. Boston: Jones and Bartlett.

CHAPTER

Consequences of Traumatic Spinal Cord Injury

Ellen Barker, MSN, RN, CNRN

I. Learning Objectives

A. Identify mechanisms of traumatic spinal cord injuries.

B. Describe types of spinal cord injuries (SCI) as described in the American Spinal Cord Injury Association (ASIA) Impairment Scale.

II. Introduction

Injury to the spinal cord results when the delicate spinal cord is compressed, contused, severed, distracted, transected, dissected, or suffers an interruption of the blood supply. Manipulation during surgery may even cause the cord to swell. The results of SCI interrupt normal functioning of the cord with some degree of motor and/or sensory deficit. Vital pathways and autonomic functions may be lost depending on the location and extent of the injury.

An accurate identification of the physiological consequences of SCI provides a fundamental step in the delivery of comprehensive health care. Understanding the pathophysiology related to type of SCI is necessary to appreciate varying functional outcomes.

III. Incidence and Demographics

A. **Spinal Cord Injury**: Although the National Institute on Disability and Rehabilitation Research (NIDRR) - funded Model Systems furnish the largest database, it is estimated to represent only 15 percent of new traumatic spinal cord injuries. As of May 1996, the database included 16,799 people with SCI (University of Alabama-Birmingham, 1996):
1. Incidence: 30-40 per million or between 7,600-10,000 new SCI cases per year based on the 1992 census population.
2. Prevalence: 721-906 per million in the U.S. or 183,000-203,000 people.

3. Age at injury: 57 percent are between 16-30; the average age is 31.1. Between 1970 and 1990, the over-sixty SCI age group has increased from 4.7 percent to 9 percent reflecting the same trend in the general population.

4. Gender: 82.1 percent of the patients are male.

5. Etiology: Trends show a decline in injuries from motor vehicle crashes and sport injuries and an increase from acts of violence.
   a. Motor vehicle crashes: 35.9 percent
   b. Acts of violence: 29.5 percent
   c. Falls: 20.3 percent
   d. Recreational sporting activities: 7.3 percent

6. Neurologic level
   a. Tetraplegia: 52 percent
   b. Paraplegia: 46.7 percent

7. Martial status: 53.7 percent are single

8. Ethnic group: The injury rate for Caucasians has decreased while African American and Hispanic groups here have increased.
   a. Caucasian: 55.2 percent
   b. African American: 29 percent
   c. Hispanic: 12.8 percent
   d. American Indian: 0.5 percent
   e. Asian: 1.9 percent
   f. Other: 0.6 percent

9. Length of stay: From 1973 to 1994, the average length of hospitalization time including acute care and rehabilitation has decreased from 137 days to 63 days.

10. Life expectancy: Because of improved management, life expectancy is improving although still slightly below life expectancies for those with no spinal cord injury.

11. Cause of death: In the past, the cause of death was from renal disease; however, with improved urological management, this has changed. Cardiopulmonary problems are the threats on life expectancy today.

12. Lifetime costs: Lifetime costs vary according to the level and severity of the injury with high tetraplegia being the most costly at $417,067 for the first year and $74,707 for each subsequent year. Paraplegia costs are lower at $122,914 for the first year and $15,505 for each year. Not included in these figures are indirect costs such as lost wages of the individual and family, which could average almost $38,000 but may vary based on education, severity of injury and pre-injury employment.

IV. Pathophysiology

Any force, or combination of forces, exerted on the cord results in injury as illustrated with the following:

A. **Acceleration/deceleration** when the force generated to the spine whips the head backwards (hyperextension) then abruptly forward (hyperflexion)

B. **Rotation with the head turning on its axis,** which may disrupt ligaments, vessels, tissue, bone, and related organs

C. **Axial loading with vertical compression** that may result in such force on the vertebral body to cause a "burst" fracture with fragments that impinge on the cord

D. **Penetration injury** that may partially or completely sever the vertebra, cord, ligaments, and blood supply or indirectly cause injury by heat or shock wave

E. **Compression with flattening of the cord** from a tumor, stenosis, and/or edema

F. **Distraction with separation of structures** such as the occiput from the vertebra with stretching and disrupting the cord

G. **Infarction or ischemia** with decreased absent blood supply to the cord

V.   Types of Spinal Cord Injury (See Table 8-1 ASIA Impairment Scale)

A. **Complete SCI** (See Figure 8-1): Total disruption of the cord with complete loss of motor and sensory function below the level of injury.
   1. Irreversible spinal cord damage
   2. Tetraplegia in lesions in the cervical regions
   3. Paraplegia in lesions in the thoracic, lumbar, or sacral region

B. **Incomplete SCI**: Preservation of motor and sensory functions below the level of the lesion as defined by the International Standards for Neurological and Functional Classification of Spinal Cord Injury (1992).

C. **The ASIA Impairment Scale** (See Chapter 10, Table 10-1):
   A= No motor or sensory function is preserved in the sacral segments S4-S5
   B= Sensory but not motor function is preserved below the neurological level and includes the sacral segments S4-S5;
   C= Motor function is preserved below the neurological level, and the majority of key muscles below the neurological level have a muscle grade less than 3;
   D= Motor function is preserved below the neurological level, and the majority of key muscles below the neurological level have a muscle grade greater than or equal to 3;
   E= Motor and sensory function are normal.

D. **Clinical Syndromes** (as described by ASIA (1992):
   1. Anterior Cord Injury: A lesion that produces variable loss of motor function and of sensitivity to pain and temperature, while preserving posterior column functions of proprioception, pressure and vibration (See Figure 8-2).
      a. Etiology/Precipitating factors - fall, motor vehicle crashes with flexion injury, herniated intervertebral disc, or thrombosis of the anterior spinal artery
      b. Pathophysiology - acute compression of the anterior portion of the spinal cord that may also cause decreased circulation to the anterior spinal artery. The individual has motor paralysis and retains only deep pressure sensation and proprioceptive sense in the lower extremities without the ability to distinguish sharp-dull discrimination
      c. Focused nursing considerations
         (1) Signs and symptoms of immediate motor loss below the level of injury
         (2) Loss of pain and temperature below the level of injury
         (3) Sensation of touch, proprioception, and vibration remain intact
   2. Brown-Séquard Syndrome: A lesion that produces relatively greater ipsilateral proprioceptive motor loss and contralateral loss of sensitivity to pain and temperature, hemisection of the cord with spinothalamic tract involvement (See Figure 8-3).
      a. Etiology/Precipitating factors: penetrating injury to one-half the cord from gunshot wound, knife wound, or sharp objects
      b. Pathophysiology: the injury is lateralized to one-half the cord with the motor paralysis distal to the injury on the same side (ipsilateral) and loss of sensation distal to the injury on the opposite (contralateral) side of the body. There is greater motor strength with less sensory function on one side and greater weakness but better sensory function on the opposite side of the body.
      c. Focused nursing considerations
         (1) Motor and sensory deficits below the level of injury.
         (2) Bowel, bladder, and sexual functions.
         (3) Ambulation and functional recovery potential.

Figure 8-1: Spinal Cord Damage Causing a Complete Transverse Syndrome

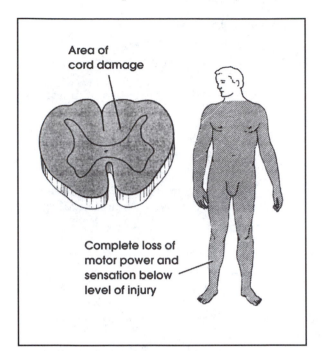

From *Management of Spinal Cord Injury* (2nd ed., p.68), by C.P. Zejdlik, 1992, Boston: Jones & Bartlett. Copyright 1992 by Jones & Bartlett. Reprinted with permission.

Figure 8-2: Cross-Section of Spinal Cord Depicting Damage That Causes an Anterior Artery Syndrome

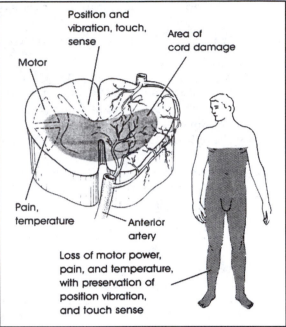

From *Management of Spinal Cord Injury* (2nd ed., p.68), by C.P. Zejdlik, 1992, Boston: Jones & Bartlett. Copyright 1992 by Jones & Bartlett. Reprinted with permission.

Figure 8-3: Cross-Section of Spinal Cord Depicting Damage That Causes Brown-Séquard Syndrome

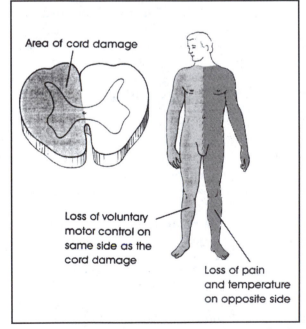

From *Management of Spinal Cord Injury* (2nd ed., p.68), by C.P. Zejdlik, 1992, Boston: Jones & Bartlett. Copyright 1992 by Jones & Bartlett. Reprinted with permission.

Figure 8-4: Cross-Section of the Spinal Cord Depicting Damage That Causes Central Cord Syndrome

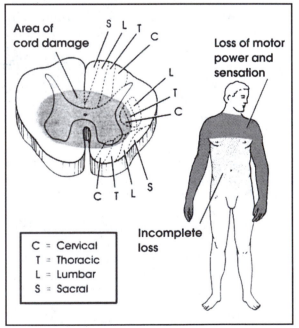

From *Management of Spinal Cord Injury* (2nd ed., p.68), by C.P. Zejdlik, 1992, Boston: Jones & Bartlett. Copyright 1992 by Jones & Bartlett. Reprinted with permission.

3. Central Cord Syndrome: A lesion occurring almost exclusively in the cervical region, that produces greater sensory loss and weakness in the upper limbs than in the lower limbs (See Figure 8-4).
   a. Etiology/Precipitating factors: usually follows a hyperextension injury in an individual with cervical spondylosis or stenosis; common in the elderly population following a fall or a motor vehicle crash.
   b. Pathophysiology: partial motor paralysis distal to the level of injury but with preservation of some sensory and motor function with sacral sparing. Characterized by microscopic hemorrhage and edema in the central gray matter of the cord.
      (1) Since the motor tracts are near the spinothalamic tracts, sacral sparing indicates potential for recovery of the sacral segments.
      (2) Return of function may follow a pattern with return of motor function, usually beginning with toe flexors; lumbar innervated muscles with plantar, extensor, and dorsal flexors of the ankle; flexors and extensors of the knee and hip.
      (3) Lower extremity spasticity due to upper motor neuron injury in the cervical long tracts may cause spastic gait.
      (4) Central gray matter damage with lower motor neuron paralysis of the muscles of the arms and hands that may cause loss of fine motor function.
   c. Focused nursing considerations
      (1) Motor and sensory changes to include sacral sparing
      (2) Degree of spinal tract damage and/or recovery
      (3) Bowel, bladder, and sexual function
      (4) Resolution of edema during recovery with progressive return of function
      (5) Supportive care in recognition of loss of hand and arm function
      (6) Safety factors and prevention of injury during ambulation due to spasticity and inability to guard with upper extremities in a fall
4. Cauda Equina Syndrome: Injury to the lumbosacral nerve roots within the neural canal resulting in areflexic bladder, bowel, and lower limbs. Refers to the lower portion of the spinal cord at the level of first lumbar vertebra and to the bundle of peripheral nerve roots that continue as the cord tapers. The roots emerge from the cord and descend through the spinal canal before reaching the foraminal openings.
   a. Etiology/Precipitating factors
      (1) Hematoma following lumbar surgery
      (2) Spinal tumors
      (3) Herniated disc
      (4) Edema and swelling of the lower cord secondary to trauma
      (5) Penetrating injury
   b. Pathophysiology: lower motor neuron injury with interruption of the spinal roots and compression or disruption of one or more nerve roots.
   c. Focused nursing considerations
      (1) Subjective complaints of pain, tingling of the legs
      (2) Changes in bowel, bladder, and sexual functioning
      (3) Sacral paresthesia
      (4) Hematoma at site of lumbar surgery
      (5) Sudden loss of function below the level of a herniated disc
      (6) Absent or diminished reflexes
      (7) Peripheral nerves regenerate, making some recovery possible under ideal situations
5. Conus Medullaris Syndrome: Injury to the sacral cord (conus) and lumbar nerve roots within the neural canal, which usually results in areflexic bladder, bowel, lower limbs, and sexual dysfunction (See Figure 8-5). Sacral segments may occasionally show preserved reflexes, e.g., bulbocavernosus and micturition reflexes.

VI. Vertebral Injuries

A fracture may occur in any anatomical part of a vertebra. The very shape, construction, and composition of the vertebrae makes them vulnerable to fracture and damage from trauma and the aging process as well as the combination of the two.

A. **Types of Vertebral Fractures:**
 1. Simple fracture: without displacement or neural compression
 2. Wedge Fracture: characterized by the vertebral body being compressed anteriorly secondary to a hyperflexion injury that may cause neural compression
 3. Comminuted fracture: results in a "burst" of the vertebra often driving fragments of bone into the cord
 4. Jefferson's fracture: a "burst" fracture of the first cervical vertebra (C-1)
    a. Axial loading directly downward on C-1 which may cause multiple fractures of C-1 with outward spread of lateral atlantal masses
    b. Widening of the distance between the odontoid and C-1, tearing of the transverse ligament if severe
    c. Symptoms range from cervical pain and cervical muscle spasm, to death if the fracture is displaced
 5. Odontoid fracture (See Figure 8-5): fractures of C-2 are classified as three types (see Figure 8-6):
    a. Type I: an oblique fracture line through the upper part of the odontoid process that may follow an avulsion fracture.
       (1) Type I vertebral fractures rarely occur.
       (2) Usually stable
       (3) Good prognosis
       (4) Minor treatment

Figure 8-5: Odontoid Fracture

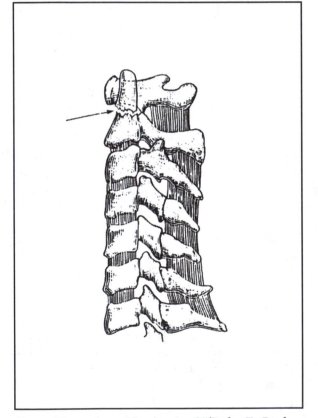

From *Neuroscience Nursing* (p. 357), by E. Barker (Ed), 1994, St. Louis, MO: Mosby. Reprinted with permission.

Figure 8-6: Three Types of Odontoid Fractures

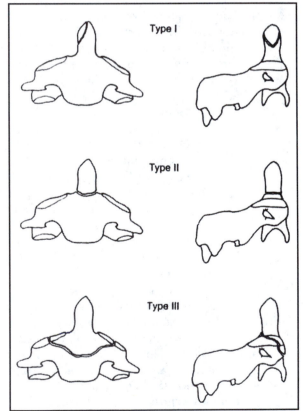

From *Neuroscience Nursing* (p. 207), by E. Barker (Ed), 1994, St. Louis, MO: Mosby. Reprinted with permission.

    b. Type II: occurs at the junction of the odontoid process and the body
       (1) The most common type of vertebral fracture
       (2) Usually unstable
       (3) Potential for nonunion
    c. Type III: the fracture extends down into the cancellous bone of the body of C-2
       (1) Tends to be more stable due to large surface area
       (2) Greater potential for union
6. Hangman's fracture (See Figure 8-7)
    a. Fracture through the pedicles of C-2
    b. Referred to also as "traumatic spondylolisthesis"
    c. May result from a front-end automobile collision if the person is thrown forward striking the windshield with axial loading and extension involving the neck creating a bilateral fracture with disruption of ligaments and possible subluxation, widening of the vertebral canal
    d. May be asymptomatic

Figure 8-7: Hangman's Fracture

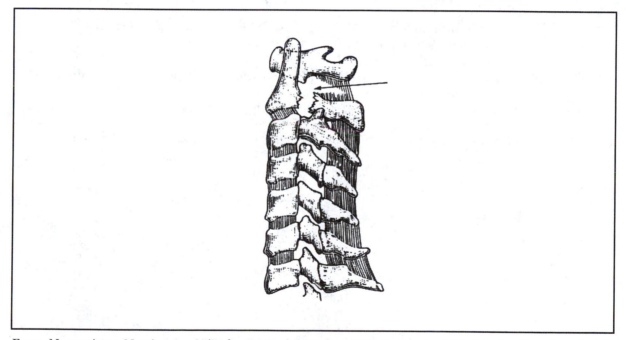

From *Neuroscience Nursing* (p. 357), by E. Barker (Ed), 1994, St. Louis, MO: Mosby. Reprinted with permission.

References and Selected Bibliography

Alspach, J. (1991). *Core curriculum for critical care nursing*. Philadelphia: W.B. Saunders.

American Spinal Injury Association (ASIA) International Medical Society of Paraplegia. (1992). *International standards for neurological and functional classification of spinal cord injury*. American Paralysis Association.

Anderson, L. (1983). *Fractures of the odontoid: Process of the axis*. In R. Winters (Ed.). *The Cervical Spine*. Philadelphia: J.B. Lippincott.

Barker, E. (1994). *Neuroscience nursing*. St. Louis, MO: Mosby.

Buchanan, L.E. & Nawoczenski, D.A. (1987). *Spinal cord injury*. Baltimore, MD: Williams & Wilkins.

Cammermeyer, M. & Appeldorn, C. (1990). *Core curriculum for neuroscience nursing (3rd ed.)*. Chicago: American Association of Neuroscience Nurses.

McCourt, A.E. (1993). *The specialty practice of rehabilitation nursing: A core curriculum (3rd ed.)*. Skokie: The Rehabilitation Nursing Foundation of the Association of Rehabilitation Nurses.

Raimondi, A.J. (1987). *Pediatric neurosurgery*. New York: Springer-Verlag.

Swaiman, K.F. (1994). *Pediatric neurology, volume I & II, (2nd ed.)*. St. Louis, MO: Mosby.

University of Alabama, Birmingham (1996, May). *Facts and Figures at a glance*. Birmingham: National Spinal Cord Injury Research Data Center, University of Alabama.

White, A.H., Rothman, R.H., & Ray, C.D. (1987). *Lumbar spine surgery*. St. Louis, MO: Mosby.

Winters, R. (1983). *The cervical spine*. Philadelphia: J.B. Lippincott.

Zejdlik, C.P. (Ed.) (1992). *Management of spinal cord injury (2nd ed.)*. Boston: Jones and Bartlett.

CHAPTER

Consequences of Spinal Cord Disorders

Ellen Barker, MSN, RN, CNRN
Janet Paarlberg, MS, RN, CRRN

I. Learning Objectives

A. Describe common categories of non-traumatic spinal cord disorders.

B. Identify spinal cord disorders related to congenital and developmental anomalies.

C. Describe types of spinal cord tumors.

D. Describe three spinal cord demyelination disorders.

II. Introduction

Spinal cord disorders secondary to spinal cord tumors, infectious processes, vascular interruption and cord ischemia, or congenital anomalies are presented in this chapter. The incidence and characteristics specific to these disorders are addressed. Health care management of individuals with spinal cord disorders is discussed in Chapter 11.

III. Spinal Cord Tumors

Many spinal cord tumors are benign; neurological consequences are due to the location of the tumor.

A. **Incidence**:
1. Spinal cord tumors are less prevalent than intracranial tumors (ratio 1:4).
2. Gender incidence is according to tumor type.
3. Occur predominantly in young and middle years.

B. **Tumor Location**:
1. Extradural lesions outside the dura mater
a. Account for 20 percent to 50 percent of spinal cord tumors.

      b. Usually malignant.

      c. Rapid onset.

      d. Pain occurs at site before spinal dysfunction.

  2. Intramedullary: lesions within the spinal cord

      a. Account for 29 percent of spinal cord tumors.

      b. Signs and symptoms develop slowly.

      c. Progressive signs and symptoms in relationship to cord compression.

      d. Pain is less common as vertebral structures are unaffected.

  3. Extramedullary: lesions outside the cord or in structures surrounding the cord, such as meninges, nerve roots or bone.

      a. The most common of spinal cord tumors account for 71 percent of the total.

      b. Early sign may be radicular pain that follows a nerve root.

      c. Neurologic dysfunction is a later sign.

  4. Intradural: lesions within or under the dura mater

      a. Initial symptoms may be loss of temperature and pain sensation.

      b. Symptoms develop as the center fiber tracts of the cord are compressed.

  5. Extravertebral

C. **Tumor Types**

  1. Neurilemma

      a. Most common intradural and are also found extramedullary.

      b. Arise from the nerve root sheaths.

      c. May appear in the lumbar canal more often than other sites.

  2. Meningioma

      a. Well circumscribed intradural or extramedullary primary tumors.

      b. Found more frequently in the thoracic area and in greater ratio of women to men.

  3. Sarcoma

      a. Usually malignant.

      b. Intradural or extramedullary.

  4. Astrocytoma

      a. Usually intradural and intramedullary.

      b. Greater ratio of men to women.

      c. Graded I to IV.

      d. Most are benign.

      e. Higher grades usually follow a short illness with deterioration and death.

  5. Ependymoma

      a. Usually intradural and intramedullary.

      b. May arise at any level in the spinal cord.

  6. Metastatic

      a. May account for up to 50 percent of spinal tumors.

      b. May metastasize to the vertebra.

      c. Short course of illness.

  7. Less common spinal cord tumors

      a. Lipoma

      b. Hemangioblastoma

      c. Dermoid and epidermoid cysts and teratoma

      d. Chordoma

IV. Infections

Spinal cord disorders secondary to infections processes are now less common and lethal due to antibiotic treatment.

A. **Osteomyelitis**

  1. Infection of the bone.

  2. Pyogenic infection often associated with staphylococcus aureus.

  3. Elevated sedimentation rate.

4. Little or no fever or malaise.
5. May occur after chest tube insertion during trauma resuscitation.

B. **Abscess**
   1. Localized collection of pus.
   2. May present with a history of progressive weakness, sensory loss, back pain, nuchal rigidity, and incontinence.
   3. May be blood-borne from another area of infection in the body.

C. **Other**
   1. Transverse myelitis
      a. An inflammation of the spinal cord that may result in an abrupt onset of progressive weakness and sensory disturbances.
      b. A history of a preceding viral infection accompanied by fever and malaise is documented in most instances.
   2. Poliomyelitis: virus invades the anterior horn cells of the spine with potential destruction of the neurons, causing motor but not sensory impairment.
   3. Pott's disease: tuberculous spondylitis, a rare and grave form of tuberculosis caused by mycobacterium tuberculosis that invades the spinal vertebrae
   4. Acquired immunodeficiency syndrome (AIDS)

V. Spinal Cord Arteriovenous Malformations (AVMs)

Occur as dural (most common form) or intradural arteriousnous shunt malformations in posterior thoracic segment from developmental anomaly or trauma. May be congenital.

A. **Incidence**
   1. Ratio of men to women is 10:1.
   2. Affects ages 20 to 40.

B. **Causes**: necrosis of the affected area by decreasing the blood supply and/or compression by the dilated vessels

C. **May be singular or multiple**
   1. Type I: extramedullary
   2. Type II: intramedullary
   3. Type III: juvenile AVM

D. **Signs and symptoms**: slow and may progress to include:
   1. Spasticity of legs.
   2. Diminished or loss of pain and temperature.
   3. Bowel/bladder incontinence.
   4. Sexual dysfunction.
   5. Nerve root pain.
   6. Back pain that is aggravated during activity.
   7. May progress from paraparesis to paralysis over time.

VI. Disc Disease

Cervical and lumbar disc diseases are a major health problem in the United States. Disc disease is second to the common cold as a cause of lost productivity. Herniated nucleus pulposus (HNP) (See Figure 9-1), also known as a ruptured disc, occurs more frequently in areas where a mobile part joins a relatively immobile part. Examples are the cerviothoracic and lumbosacral junctions where the annulus fibrosus ruptures and the central nucleus pulposus is forced out causing pressure on a spinal nerve or its roots.

Figure 9-1: Herniated Nucleus Pulposus (HNP)

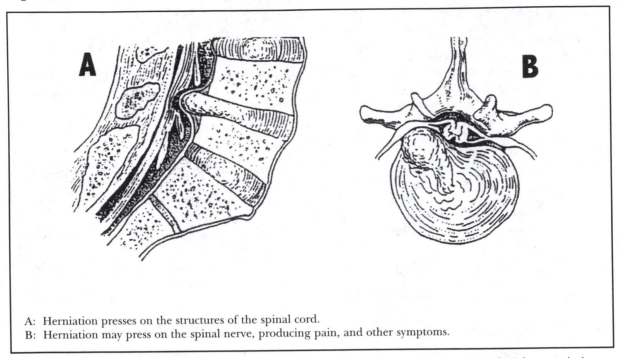

A: Herniation presses on the structures of the spinal cord.
B: Herniation may press on the spinal nerve, producing pain, and other symptoms.

From *Neuroscience Nursing* (p.396), by E. Barker, 1994, St. Louis: Mosby. Reprinted with permission.

A. **Cervical Disc Disease**
1. Less common than lumbar herniated discs; affecting women more than men.
2. C5-C6 and C6-C7 discs are the most likely to herniated.
3. Pain in the lower part of the back, the neck, and shoulders along the distribution of the affected nerve or root.
4. Central disc protrusion may compress the cord, the anterior spinal artery, and spinal tracts.
5. Headache radiating upward from the cervical area to the posterior region, along the distribution of the trapezius muscle and its attachment.
6. Spasms involving neck muscles.
7. Pain, paresis, paresthesia along affected cervical nerve distribution.
8. Diminished or absent affected reflexes, e.g., triceps and biceps.
9. Positive Spurling test: the examiner approaches the seated patient from above and presses down on the head with both hands, putting added pressure on the spinal nerve roots. Pain suggests nerve root impingement.

B. **Lumbar Disc Disease**
1. Disc problems affect 75 percent of the adult population at some time in their lives with an estimated impact at $21 billion per year to society.
2. Majority of disc problems occur between the ages of 30 to 60 years affecting men more than women.
3. Strenuous occupations that involve heavy lifting may correlate with disc disease.
4. LH, L5, and S1 are the most likely discs to herniate.
5. A large posterior herniation directly backward may compress the cauda equina producing paraplegia.
6. Herniation may be at one or more levels.
7. Pain is referred down the leg and foot following the path of the affected nerve(s).
8. Sciatica or injury to the sciatic nerve may cause foot-drop, pain, and sensory loss.
9. Aging of the spine creates degenerative changes as the disc and annulus lose their hydraulic and elastic properties and osteophytes develop.

10. Combinations of stenosis, spondylosis, subluxation, and ruptured intervertebral discs compound disc disease.

C. **Thoracic Disc Disease**
   1. Thoracic area is less mobile than other areas of spine.
   2. Affected in only 1.96 percent of disc cases.
   3. Account for approximately 3 percent of spine disc operations.

VII. Syrinxes

A syrinx is the formation of an abnormal cavitation in the central cord canal. A syrinx may be primary (occurring alone) or secondary following neoplasms, congenital malformations, or from a previous history of spinal cord trauma. The condition interrupts the lateral and anterior spinothalamic tracts as they cross the spinal cord in the anterior gray and white commissures.

A. **Incidence:**
   1. Familial link, with higher incidence in males.
   2. Occurs generally in fourth and fifth decades.

B. **Characteristics:**
   1. History may be positive for Chiari malformation (in primary Syringomyelia)
      a. Syringomyelia: a central cavitation of the spinal cord that develops gradually resulting in sensory changes, weakness, and muscle wasting.
      b. Syringobulbia: a cavitation in the medulla that may result in respiratory compromise and death.
   2. Characteristic lower motor neuron findings in the upper extremities with atrophy, fasciculation, spasticity, and weakness in the lower extremities.
   3. Sensory loss may be "capelike" involving the upper extremities and upper chest.
   4. Pain and temperature sensation are lost in affected region with preservation of light touch in posterior columns.
   5. Motor loss usually follows sensory loss. Symptoms may occur years post injury.
   6. A post-traumatic syrinx may be characterized by sensory or motor changes such as pain or weakness, which presents months or years following initial injury.

VIII. Infarction

A. **Vascular disease of the spine is rare**. An infarction is an interruption of the blood supply to an area of the spinal cord.

B. **Causes**: trauma, tumors, the "bends" (decompression sickness), clamping of the aorta during surgery, stenosis, infections, emboli, and hypotension.
   1. Anterior spinal artery occlusion
      a. Initial flaccid paralysis with diminished or absent reflexes.
      b. Reflexes later usually become hyperactive.
      c. Symptoms: weakness, muscle atrophy, paresthesia, aching, cramping, loss of bowel and bladder function, pain.
      d. Unless quickly corrected, may result in permanent paralysis.
   2. Other
      a. Iatrogenic - e.g., secondary to myelogram.
      b. Transverse myelitis

IX. Demyelination Disorders that Affect the Spine

A. **Guillain-Barré Syndrome** or acute inflammatory polyradiculoneuropathy, is an acquired inflammatory disease that results in demyelination of the peripheral nerves. The progressive ascending paralysis is usually reversible.

1. Incidence/Etiology:
   a. 0.6-1.9 cases per 100,000; incidence increases slightly with age, Hodgkin's disease, pregnancy, or general surgery.
   b. Most frequently occurring demyelinating disease.
   c. Etiology unknown but thought to be autoimmune.
   d. Recovery generally occurs after 3-6 months.
2. Characteristics:
   a. May be a cell-mediated immunologic reaction directed against a component of peripheral nerve myelin.
   b. Precipitating factors include a viral infection one to two weeks prior to onset of symptoms.
   c. Onset of symptoms is a progressive bilateral muscle weakness with accompanying:
      (1) Falling
      (2) Footdrop
      (3) Difficulty walking
      (4) Pain and tingling in the legs
      (5) Distal extremities affected first in an ascending manner
      (6) Loss of deep tendon reflexes
      (7) Cranial nerve involvement
      (8) Impaired respiratory functions that may progress to respiratory failure
      (9) Autonomic manifestations
         (a) Postural hypotension
         (b) Heart block
         (c) Tachycardia
      (10) Bowel and bladder dysfunction
3. Types:
   a. Ascending: most common.
   b. Descending: begins with bulbar muscles and descends to extremities.
   c. Miller-Fisher: symptoms include ophthalmoplegia, areflexia, ataxia with no sensory involvement.
   d. Pure motor: ascending with no sensory loss.
   e. Inflammatory cranial neuropathies: involves only the cranial nerves.
   f. Relapsing or chronic: chronic inflammatory polyradiculoneuropathy (CIP) is associated with a relapsing course in approximately 10 percent of cases.

B. **Multiple Sclerosis** (MS) is a chronic demyelinating disease with a history of relapse and remission. The cause is unknown, but an abnormality of immune regulation has been proposed. Multiple plaques form in the central nervous system (CNS) to include the brain, cervical spinal cord and less frequently the lower cord. Progression of the disease will impact severity of consequences.
   1. Incidence (Multiple Sclerosis Foundation, 1996):
      a. Prevalence of MS is estimated at approximately 350,000 - 500,000 people in the U.S.
      b. Occurs more often in women and the Caucasian population.
      c. MS is inversely related to proximity to the equator. The closer to the equator, the fewer the MS cases.
      d. Most MS cases are diagnosed between ages 30-50; the life expectancy is at least 75 percent of normal life span.
      e. Two thirds of individuals with MS remain functional after 20 years and 75 percent never require a wheelchair.
   2. Characteristics:
      a. Affects motor functions via the pyramidal and extrapyramidal tracts.
         (1) Spasticity
         (2) Babinski
         (3) Hyperreflexia
         (4) Clonus
         (5) Abnormal gait

b. Affects sensory functions via the posterior columns and posterior spinocerebellar tracts.
   (1) Paresthesia
   (2) Lhermitte's sign: a sudden, transient, electric-like shock sensation that spreads down the body when the head is flexed forward.
   (3) Decreased proprioception
   (4) Decreased temperature perception
c. Affects cerebellar function
   (1) Tremor
   (2) Uncoordination
d. Affects bowel and bladder
   (1) Fecal urgency
   (2) Urinary frequency and incontinence
e. Affects sexual functions
   (1) Women: decreased libido and lubrication, decreased orgasmic ability and decreased genital sensation.
   (2) Men: decreased libido, dysfunctions of erection, orgasm, and ejaculation.
f. Temperature intolerance
g. Fatigue

C. **Amyotrophic lateral sclerosis** (ALS), motor neuron disease, Lou Gehrig's disease, or Maladie de Charcot are all the same disease. The pathogenesis may be related to glutamate toxicity, environmental toxicity, oxidative stress, or familial ALS. There are no laboratory studies to confirm the diagnosis; rather it can be a diagnosis of exclusion after other diseases have been ruled out.

1. Incidence:
   a. ALS affects approximately 30,000 people in the U.S.
   b. Familial relationship; inherited in 5 percent of cases.
   c. Most often occurs in middle age.
   d. Incidence slightly higher in men.
   e. Particularly high incidence in Guam, thought to be from the familial link.
   f. Average survival without ventilatory support: 3-4 years.

2. Characteristics:
   a. Changes that occur in the nervous system include:
      (1) Loss of motor neurons in the brain, brainstem and spinal cord.
      (2) As the motor neurons in the brain die, their tracts in the spinal cord deteriorate and form a scar (lateral sclerosis).
      (3) Lower motor neurons (LMNs) in the spinal cord are lost (anterior horn cells).
      (4) The muscles lose their nerve supply and atrophy resulting in fasciculations and twitching.
   b. Clinical signs and symptoms:
      (1) Upper motor neuron (UMN):
          (a) Spasticity and hyperreflexia
          (b) Pathological reflexes, e.g. Babinski
      (2) Bulbar:
          (a) Dysarthria
          (b) Dysphasia
          (c) Hypersalivation with swallowing difficulties
      (3) Lower motor neuron (LMN):
          (a) Muscle weakness
          (b) Muscle atrophy
          (c) Fasciculations
          (d) Hyporeflexia
          (e) Hypotonicity or flaccidity
      (4) Respiratory:
          (a) Respiratory insufficiency
          (b) Exertional dyspnea

95

(c) Positional shortness of breath (SOB)

(d) Hypersomnia

(e) Respiratory failure

(5) Other:

(a) Fatigue

(b) Weight loss with muscle wasting

(c) Ocular palsy

X. Noninfectious Inflammatory Diseases

A. **Characteristics**:

1. Atlantoaxial subluxation is the most common disease of rheumatoid involvement of the cervical spine.
2. C-1, C-2 subluxation is a significant manifestation.
3. History of long duration of rheumatoid arthritis in an older adults with neck symptoms.
4. Upward migration of the odontoid is related.
5. Long-term use of steroids may be significant.
6. Changes in bone, cartilage, muscle, and connective tissue with deossification of bone in rheumatoid disease contributes to pathology.

B. **Symptoms may include**:

1. Localized arthritic symptoms of the cervical spine.
2. Mechanical instability.
3. Pain in the cervical area.
4. Neurologic dysfunction involving brainstem, cord, and peripheral nerve with possible nerve entrapment.
5. Vertebral artery insufficiency:
   a. Dizziness
   b. Tinnitus
   c. Suboccipital headache
   d. Blurred vision
   e. Vertigo
   f. Nystagmus
6. Sensory changes, e.g., paresthesia of hands, Lhermitte's sign
7. Urinary dysfunction with frequency or retention

XI. Pediatric Congenital and Developmental Anomalies

A. **Spina Bifida**: a congenital neural tube defect (NTD) with defective closure of the vertebral column.

1. Incidence:
   a. One out of every 1,000 new borns in the U.S.; however, incidence varies by geographic location.
   b. Many who have spina bifida have little or no permanent impairment; for those with significant impairment, the incidence is estimated at 1 out of 4,000 births.
   c. Slightly higher incidence in females.
   d. There is a familial tendency.
2. Characteristics:
   a. Neurological involvement may or may not be present.
   b. Most frequently noted in the lumbosacral region of the spine, but may affect any portion.

B. **Tethered Cord Syndrome/Tethered Spinal Cord**: A syndrome in which the spinal cord is restrained at or below the L2 level by inelastic structures as a result of thick filum terminale, tumors, scar formations, boney abnormalities. Characteristics:

1. Two anatomical abnormalities may occur:
   a. An elongated spine, most often occurring in the lumbosacral area.

   b. Inelastic structures attached to the caudal end of the spinal cord. During normal growth, the growth of the spinal column is greater than that of the spinal cord. If the spinal cord is not allowed to move freely and becomes tethered, tension is placed on the cord with resulting neurologic deficits.

2. Children may be born with or without neurologic deficits and develop neurologic signs in the first decade of life.

3. Symptoms include motor and sensory impairment in the lower extremities, incontinence, diffuse pain in the lower extremities, and musculoskeletal deformities.

4. Associated with spina bifida in most cases.

5. Surgical transection of the thickened filum terminale tends to halt the progression of neurologic signs and to prevent the development of dysfunction in the asymptomatic child.

C. **Myelocele**: failure of closure of the neural tube (myeloschisis) with a saclike protrusion of the spinal cord through a congenital defect in the vertebral column, resulting in flattening of the spinal cord. Characteristics:

1. Defect is covered by granulation tissue.

2. Highly vascular

3. Surrounded by a translucent membrane that establishes continuity between it and the peripheral skin.

4. All roots exit from the ventral surface of the malformed cord.

5. On the dorsal surface there are glial scars, dysgenetic ependyma, ectopic islands of neural tissue and extensive areas of degenerative changes.

6. Simple myeloschisis: the flattened cord lays normally within the ventral aspect of the spinal cord (See Figure 9-2)

Figure 9-2: Simple Myeloschisis (Myelocele)

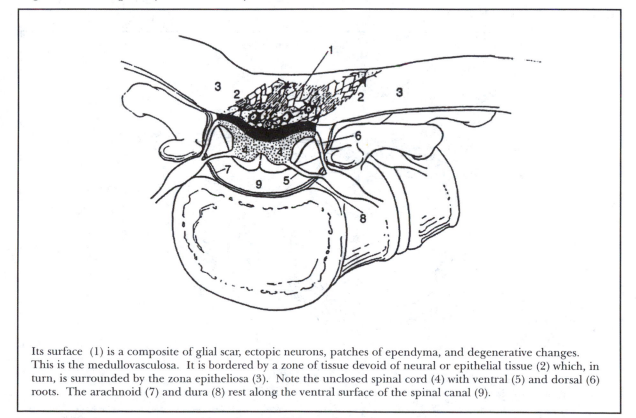

Its surface (1) is a composite of glial scar, ectopic neurons, patches of ependyma, and degenerative changes. This is the medullovasculosa. It is bordered by a zone of tissue devoid of neural or epithelial tissue (2) which, in turn, is surrounded by the zona epitheliosa (3). Note the unclosed spinal cord (4) with ventral (5) and dorsal (6) roots. The arachnoid (7) and dura (8) rest along the ventral surface of the spinal canal (9).

From *Pediatric Neurosurgery* (p.425), by A. J. Raimondi, 1987, New York: Springer-Verlag. Reprinted with permission.

Figure 9-3: Cystic Myeloschisis

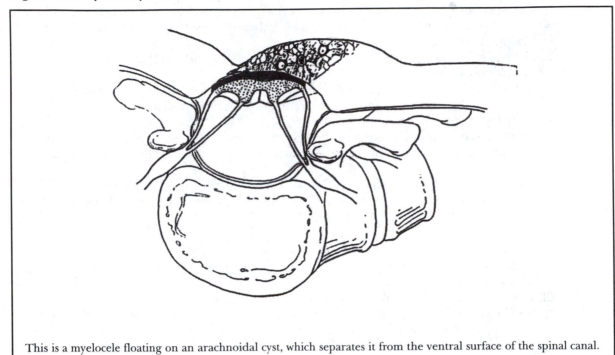

This is a myelocele floating on an arachnoidal cyst, which separates it from the ventral surface of the spinal canal.

From *Pediatric Neurosurgery* (p.425), by A. J. Raimondi, 1987, New York: Springer-Verlag. Reprinted with permission.

Figure 9-4: Scarred Myelocele

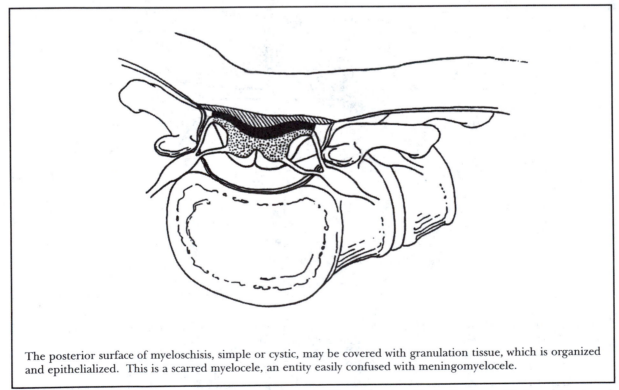

The posterior surface of myeloschisis, simple or cystic, may be covered with granulation tissue, which is organized and epithelialized. This is a scarred myelocele, an entity easily confused with meningomyelocele.

From *Pediatric Neurosurgery* (p.425), by A. J. Raimondi, 1987, New York: Springer-Verlag. Reprinted with permission.

7. Cystic myelocele: the cord is floating on an arachnoid cyst, which separates it from the ventral aspect of the spinal canal (See Figure 9-3)
8. Scarred myelocele: the vascularized granulation tissue covering the myeloschisis organizes and epithelializes (See Figure 9-4)

D. **Meningocele**: when the herniated sac protrudes through a congenital defect in the vertebral column. It consists of meninges covered by skin or epitheliallial tissue filled with cerebrospinal fluid (CSF). The posterior spinal arch defect is limited to one vertebra. Spina bifida cystica is the category for this type of lesion (See Figure 9-5). Characteristics:
1. Spinal cord is located normally within the spinal canal, resting upon its ventral surface.
2. Nerve roots may float into the hernia sac or be tethered to its neck.
3. Neurologic manifestations may be minimal.

E. **Meningomyelocele or Myelomeningocele**: a developmental defect where the spinal cord is herniated into a sac of intact meninges containing cerebrospinal fluid (CSF). Spinal cord and/or nerve roots located in the subcutaneous space results from failure of the neural tube to close during embryonic development or reopening of the tube from increased intracranial pressure (See Figure 9-6).
1. Incidence: Occurs in approximately 2 of every 1,000 live births.
2. Characteristics:
    a. Location may be at any point along the spinal column with three layers of meninges.
    b. Usually occurs in the low thoracic, lumbar or sacral region.
    c. May extend from 3 to 6 vertebral segments.
    d. The thin membranous covering is easily ruptured.
    e. Ruptured membrane may result in infection.
    f. Neurologic deficit correlates with the amount of neural tissue involved at the site.
    g. Infant usually has paralysis of the lower extremities.
    h. Deformities may also include clubfoot, joint deformity, hip dysplasia, bowel and bladder dysfunction, hydrocephalus related to Arnold-Chiari malformation.
    i. Surgical repair of neural tissue is usually not possible, only closure to seal cerebrospinal fluid and provide bony stability.
    j. Condition can be accompanied by a host of physical and potential psychosocial problems.

F. **Meningomyelohydrocele**: if the central canal is blown out into the hernia sac, the canal is disrupted. The dysgenic ependymal layer and the membranized dorsal protrusion of the spinal cord fuse with the arachnoid and dura to form a sac.

G. **Diastematomyelia**: the spinal cord is divided, usually almost equally, and cleft by a septum-like spur or fibrous band. This spur usually has bone at its base, cartilage at its tip, and connecting fibrous band, thus creating a septum, which is the point of division between the two spinal cord segments. Characteristics:
1. A lipoma may be present within the spur or attached to it.
2. Causes intermittent episodes of neurologic deficit or progressive spinal cord symptoms.
3. Septum commonly compromises the anterior horn cell column causing muscle atrophy, decreased or absent deep tendon reflexes, and moderate to severe weakness of the distal muscles of the legs and feet.
4. Septum transects nerve fibers as they cross, which may impair pain, temperature and light touch perception.
5. Corticospinal tracts may be compromised with corresponding signs.
6. Bilateral weakness of the lower extremities is usually the initial complaint.
7. Feet deformities include talipes equinovarus a deformity of the foot which is usually congenital, in which the foot is twisted. Refereed to as clubfoot, it is characterized by unilateral or bilateral deviation of the metatarsal bones of the forefoot with medial deviation and plantar flexion.
8. Spinal cord compression during growth.
9. Atonic bladder with urinary retention and incontinence may be present.

Figure 9-5 : Simple Meningocele

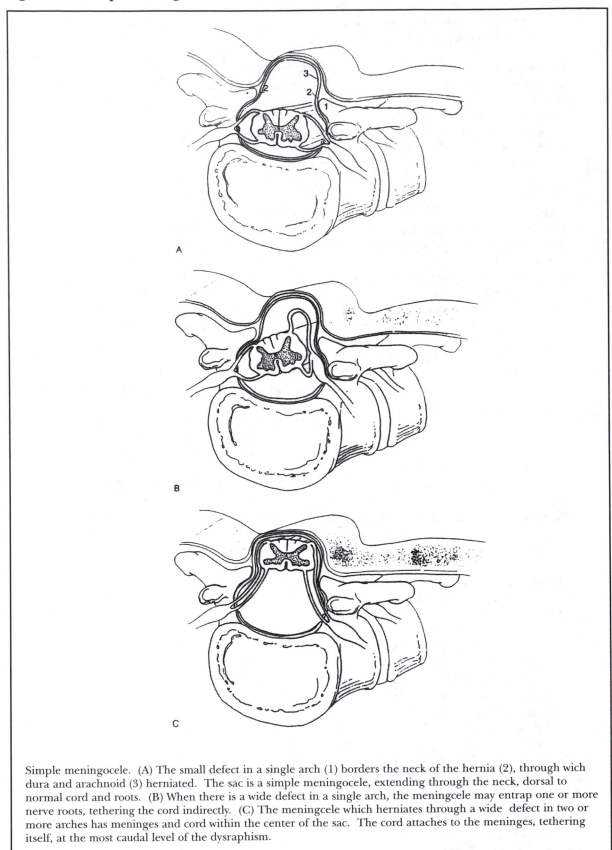

Simple meningocele. (A) The small defect in a single arch (1) borders the neck of the hernia (2), through wich dura and arachnoid (3) herniated. The sac is a simple meningocele, extending through the neck, dorsal to normal cord and roots. (B) When there is a wide defect in a single arch, the meningcele may entrap one or more nerve roots, tethering the cord indirectly. (C) The meningcele which herniates through a wide defect in two or more arches has meninges and cord within the center of the sac. The cord attaches to the meninges, tethering itself, at the most caudal level of the dysraphism.

From *Pediatric Neurosurgery* (p.430), by A. J. Raimondi, 1987, New York: Springer-Verlag. Reprinted with permission.

Figure 9-6: Meningomyelocele

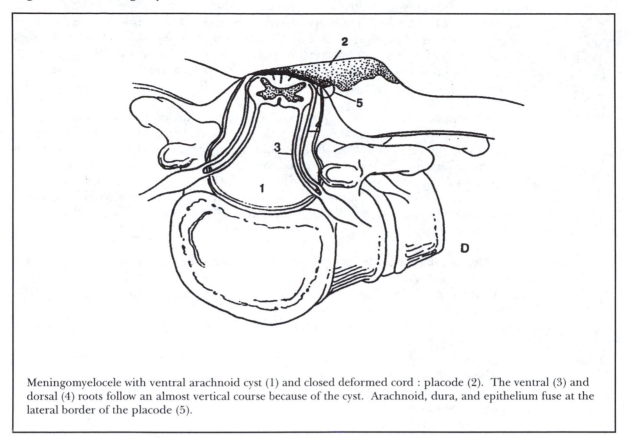

Meningomyelocele with ventral arachnoid cyst (1) and closed deformed cord : placode (2). The ventral (3) and dorsal (4) roots follow an almost vertical course because of the cyst. Arachnoid, dura, and epithelium fuse at the lateral border of the placode (5).

From *Pediatric Neurosurgery* (p.433), by A. J. Raimondi, 1987, New York: Springer-Verlag. Reprinted with permission.

    10. Kyphoscoliosis or scoliosis may occur.
    11. Should be resected immediately upon diagnosis.

H. **Hydromyelia**: consists of a dilation of the central canal that often complicates myelocele, meningomyelocele and meningocele, cause unknown. Characteristics:
  1. May cause minimally dilated central canal or a large chamber which expands to fill the entire spinal canal, compressing the cord.
  2. Anterior horn cell involvement.
  3. Found in more than 50 percent of patients with Chiari I malformations.
  4. More common in the cervical and lumbar cord enlargements.
  5. Distention may involve the entire length of the cord.
  6. Cavity is lined with ependymal cells.

I. **Chiari malformation**: Most common cerebellar anomaly and may lead to severe neurologic defects and even death. The Chiari malformation consists of two major subgroups.
  1. Incidence:
    a. Most often occurs with spina bifida.
    b. Incidence is estimated at 20 of 290 cases of spina bifida.
  2. Types/Characteristics:
    a. Chiari Type 1: The deformity consists of displacement of the cerebellar tonsils into the cervical canal. There is no associated myelomeningocele. It usually becomes symptomatic in first decade with onset of symptoms in late adolescence and adult years and is usually not associated with hydrocephalus. The symptoms include occipital and frontal

headaches, neck pain, urinary frequency, and progressive lower extremity spasticity, unsteady gait, progressive ataxia, and difficulty in swallowing.

    b. Chiari Type 2: Most frequent type encountered. The lesion represents an anomaly of the hindbrain resulting in an elongation of the fourth ventricle and kinking of the brain stem with displacement of the inferior vermis, pons, and medulla into the cervical canal. Associated with progressive hydrocephalus and myelomeningocele. There are associated abnormalities of the cord, brain stem, cerebellar and cerebral cortices and ventricular system.

        (1) Approximately 10 percent produce symptoms during infancy consisting of difficulties in sucking, swallowing, weak cry, vocalization, stridor and abnormal breathing patterns (or apnea). Bradycardia and apnea are often more apparent with feeding. This may be relieved with shunting or by posterior fossa decompression.

        (2) A subtler form consists of abnormalities of gait, spasticity, and increasing incoordination during childhood. The cerebellar tonsils protrude downward into the cervical canal with hindbrain abnormalities. The anomaly is treated by surgical decompression.

J. **Degenerative Conditions**: Muscular atrophies that are transmitted as an autosomal-recessive trait appear to be genetically determined.

  1. **Werdnig-Hoffmann Disease**: progressive infantile spinal muscular atrophy that manifests from infancy to two years. Characteristics:

    a. Involves the anterior horn cells in the spinal cord and the cranial nerve motor nuclei in the brainstem.

    b. Proximal weakness of the limbs and marked bulbar dysfunction.

    c. The earlier the onset, the more rapid the progression.

        (1) Group I: severe weakness of the proximal muscles of the limbs and the intercostal muscles, with more movement of hands and feet with a frog-leg position, and absent deep tendon reflexes preventing the infant from sitting.

        (2) Group II: Scoliosis is the most prominent symptom, other symptoms may develop later.

        (3) Group III: Initial symptoms appear between ages one and two with obvious weakness of the thigh and hip muscles, which may manifest with a waddling gait, lumbar lordosis, genu recurvatum and a protruding abdomen. By the second decade, the child is confined to a wheelchair. Scoliosis is seen late in the disease course.

  2. **Kugelberg-Welander Disease**: hereditary, juvenile proximal muscular atrophy. Characteristics:

    a. Results from anterior horn cell dysfunction

    b. Pattern of weakness is similar to infantile spinal muscular atrophy.

    c. Age of onset usually between the ages of 2 and 17.

    d. Weakness of the hip and thigh causes impaired gait

    e. Child develops a classic Gower's sign: inability to arise from a floor-lying posture without manual or sequential assistance/support.

    f. Protruding abdomen from weak abdominal muscles.

    g. Follows a slow progressive course.

K. **Cerebral Palsy (CP)**: refers to a group of disorders with an abnormality in the control of movement and the absence of recognized underlying progressive disease. Infants with low birth weight, newborns with neurologic deficits and infants with neurologic symptoms that appear later should be screened for CP.

  1. Incidence:

    a. Occurs in 1.2 to 2.5 children per 1000 by early school age.

    b. Approximately 5000 new cases in the U.S. every year; the most frequent permanent physical disability of children.

    c. Low birth weight or trauma account for most cases.

  2. Characteristics:

a. The pyramidal motor system that includes the motor cortex, basal ganglia, and the cerebellum is involved.

b. Children are expected to reach adulthood.

c. Spastic CP is evidenced by hyperreflexia, hypertonus (claspknife type) and clonus with abnormal postural reflexes, and possible hemiplegia in up to 40 percent of cases.

d. Categories:

    (1) Mild CP: consistent physical findings but no limitations in ordinary activities.

    (2) Moderate CP: definite difficulties in daily activities requiring assistive devices.

    (3) Severe CP: moderate to severe limitations in activities.

e. Mental retardation is not common.

f. Seizure disorders are seen in approximately 25 percent to 33 percent of cases.

g. Failure to meet early developmental milestones can alert caregivers to evaluate for CP.

h. Impaired vision or hearing.

i. The course of CP is one without progression.

j. Pathologic reflexes are present.

k. Four different forms:

    (1) Spastic CP: affects 70-80 percent of patients, muscles are stiffly and permanently contracted. If both legs are affected scissoring position is obvious.

    (2) Athetoid or dyskinetic CP: uncontrolled slow, writhing movements affecting the hands, feet, arms, legs, and sometimes the face and tongue resulting in dysarthria.

    (3) Ataxic CP: rare, affects balance and coordination resulting in gait disturbance.

    (4) Mixed forms of CP: individuals have more than one form; usually spastic and athetoid.

References and Selected Bibliography

Alspach, J. (1991). *Core curriculum for critical care nursing*. Philadelphia: W.B. Saunders.

Barker, E. (1994). *Neuroscience nursing*. St. Louis, MO: Mosby.

Buchanan, L.E., & Nawoczenski, D.A. (1987). *Spinal cord injury*. Baltimore, MD: Williams and Wilkins.

Cammermeyer, M. & Appeldorn, C. (1990). *Core curriculum for neuroscience nursing (3rd ed.)*. Chicago: American Association of Neuroscience Nurses.

McCourt, A.E. (1993). *The specialty practice of rehabilitation nursing: A core curriculum (3rd ed.)*. Skokie, IL: The Rehabilitation Nursing Foundation of the Association of Rehabilitation Nurses.

Multiple Sclerosis Foundation (1996). *MS Facts*. New York: Multiple Sclerosis Foundation.

Raimondi, A.J. (1987). *Pediatric neurosurgery*. New York: Springer-Verlag.

Stein, B. (1995). Vascular malformations of the spinal cord. In D. Pang (Ed.), *Disorders of the pediatric spine* (pp. 493-516). New York: Raven Press.

Swaiman, K.F. (1994). *Pediatric neurology, volumes I & II, (2nd ed.)*. St. Louis, MO: Mosby.

White, A.H., Rothman, R.H., & Ray, C.D. (1987). *Lumbar spine surgery*. St. Louis, MO: Mosby.

Winters, R. (1995). Spinal deformity. In D. Pang (Ed.), *Disorders of the pediatric spine* (pp. 309-348). New York: Raven Press.

Winters, R. (1983). *The cervical spine*. Philadelphia: J.B. Lippincott.

Yamada, S. & Iacona, R. (1995). Tethered cord syndrome. In D. Pang (Ed.), *Disorders of the pediatric spine* (pp. 150-173). New York: Raven Press.

Zejdlik, C.P. (Ed.) (1992). *Management of spinal cord injury, (2nd ed.)*. Boston: Jones and Bartlett.

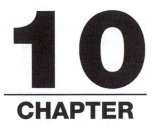

CHAPTER

Neurological Assessment Related to Spinal Cord Injury

Holly Watson Evans, MS, RN
Linda Love, MS, CRRN

I. Learning Objectives

A. Describe the purpose of the neurological assessment in spinal cord injury (SCI).

B. Identify neurological exams which assess level of consciousness.

C. Identify components of the motor and sensory neurological examinations.

D. Describe reflex activity examinations.

E. Identify common diagnostic tests to evaluate level and/or type of spinal cord injury.

II. Introduction

Neurological assessment involves examination of motor function, sensation, and reflex activity. A comprehensive neurological assessment is essential to provide a baseline neurological level of impairment as well as to determine realistic physiological and functional goals for the individual with SCI. General health status and any conditions that would affect movement or sensation, such as preexisting conditions or associated injuries are included in the assessment data. Physical examination of the spine is discussed in Chapter 27. Motor and sensory examination is a shared responsibility of health care team members. The nurse integrates the findings into the nursing process.

III. Neurological Assessment

A. **Level of Consciousness**: also consider cognitive impairment, head injury, chemical impairment, or hypothermia as sources of decreased level of consciousness.
1. Mental Status Exam: awareness, orientation.
2. Quantify responses with Glasgow Coma Scale.

B. **Cranial Nerve Assessment**: especially for SCI involving the cervical region or associated cognitive disorders. (Refer to Chapter 27 for cognitive and cranial nerve assessment).

C. **Neurologic Level of Injury/Impairment**:
   1. The purpose of a focused neurological exam is to establish level of injury, completeness of the lesion, and type of cord syndrome.

Table 10-1: Sensory Testing

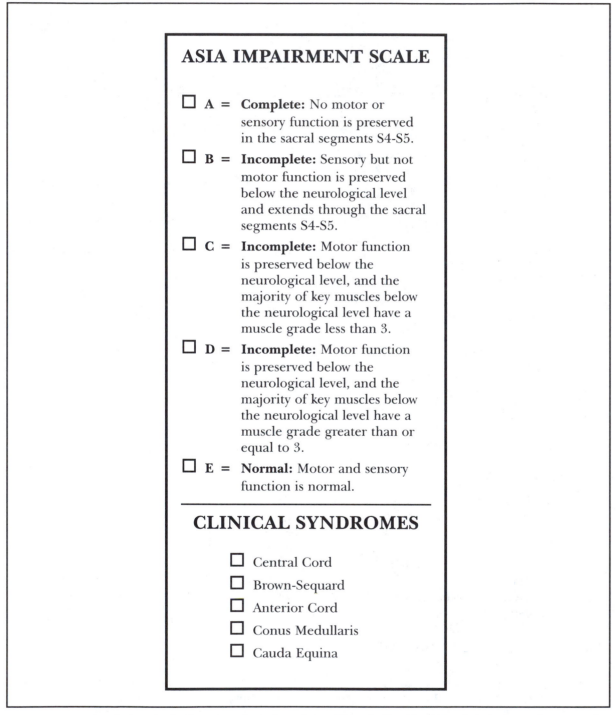

ASIA IMPAIRMENT SCALE

☐ **A** = **Complete:** No motor or sensory function is preserved in the sacral segments S4-S5.

☐ **B** = **Incomplete:** Sensory but not motor function is preserved below the neurological level and extends through the sacral segments S4-S5.

☐ **C** = **Incomplete:** Motor function is preserved below the neurological level, and the majority of key muscles below the neurological level have a muscle grade less than 3.

☐ **D** = **Incomplete:** Motor function is preserved below the neurological level, and the majority of key muscles below the neurological level have a muscle grade greater than or equal to 3.

☐ **E** = **Normal:** Motor and sensory function is normal.

CLINICAL SYNDROMES

☐ Central Cord
☐ Brown-Sequard
☐ Anterior Cord
☐ Conus Medullaris
☐ Cauda Equina

From *International Standards for Neurological and Functional Classification of Spinal Cord Injury,* by American Spinal Injury Association, 1992. Reprinted with permission.

2. In acute spinal cord injury conduct the exam every 2 hours during the first 48 hours, when reducing the fracture, or adjusting traction, and when serial films are being done. Follow-up exams are done on a regular basis to assess change in status in motor strength, or altered patterns of respirations or speech, especially in cervical lesions.

3. Motor Exam: Bilaterally assess each motor group from the head down using a scale of 0-5. Identify the lowest (most caudal) spinal cord segment associated with normal voluntary motor control, then determine the extent of function in segments below this level. This becomes the neurologic level of injury. The ASIA (American Spinal Injury Association, 1996) Impairment Scale is an assessment tool for grading muscle strength. (See Chapter 8, Consequences of Traumatic SCI). The ASIA neurological classification of motor and sensory status is presented in Table 10-1 and Figure 10-1.

4. Sensory Exam: Bilaterally assess sensory integrity from the feet up, making sure to touch the back of the patient's legs to evaluate for sacral sparing. The sensory exam should include an evaluation of the anterior spinothalamic tracts (touch and pain) and posterior columns (position and vibration). As with the motor exam, lowest level of sensation is assessed using the dermatome chart as well as any areas of intact "spared" sensation below this level (Refer to Anatomy and Physiology Chapter). Assess ability to differentiate between sharp and dull. Relative preservation of sensation in the rectum, buttocks, perineum or genitalia may be the only sign that the spinal cord lesion is incomplete.

Figure 10-1: Standard Neurological Classification of Spinal Cord Injury

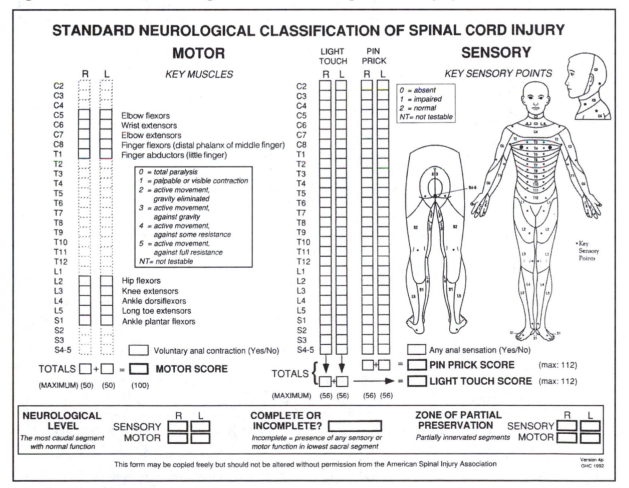

This form may be copied freely but should not be altered without permission from the American Spinal Injury Association.

5. Reflex Activity: Awareness of reflex activity below the level of injury, particularly the perianal reflexes, helps formulate diagnosis, prognosis, and the treatment plan. Management of bladder, bowel, and sexual dysfunction are specifically influenced by these findings.

    a. Rectal Examination: The presence of the bulbocavernosus reflex and the anal wink reflex are the first indications that spinal cord functional reorganization is occurring following acute spinal cord trauma and spinal shock.

        (1) Bulbocavernosus Reflex: is elicited by placing a gloved finger into the rectum and squeezing the glans penis or clitoris. Involuntary contraction of the rectal sphincter indicates a positive response and implies no physiological connection between the lower spinal cord and supraspinal centers. A positive reflex is indicative of a complete injury.

        (2) Anal Wink: a pinprick in the perianal skin causes an external anal sphincter contraction.

        (3) Rectal exam findings: usual prognosis
        Tone + Sensation = Incomplete injury
        Tone + No Sensation = Incomplete injury
        No Tone + No Sensation = Complete injury
        No Tone + Sensation = Possible incomplete injury

    b. Deep Tendon Reflex (DTR) Exam: Reflexes are initially absent following SCI but spinal neurons gradually regain excitability several hours to weeks post injury as spinal shock passes. If DTRs are present below the level of injury soon after injury, it can be a good prognostic sign of an incomplete injury. Useful reflexes in assessing spinal cord dysfunction are the DTRs of the biceps (C5), supinator (C6), triceps (C7), knee (L3) and ankle (S1) (Zejdlik, 1992).

    c. Proprioception: Evaluates ability to appreciate the position sense of extremities with eyes closed. Accompanying this, the posterior columns are assessed for vibratory response and deep pain.

IV. Diagnostic Procedures

A. **Radiographic Studies**: demonstrate level of bony injury and amount of anterior compression of a vertebral body.

1. Maintain spinal alignment by limiting any motion of the spine during procedures. The physician is responsible for applying/removing collar or traction device when moving the patient.

2. Treat all patients as if their spine is unstable until proven otherwise.

3. Plain Films:

    a. As soon as the airway is secure, a lateral cervical spine film is obtained to visualize all seven cervical vertebrae. In patients with large shoulders, a swimmer's view may be indicated.

    b. Because the vertebral fractures are often seen at multiple levels (20 percent), lateral and antero-posterior views of the thoracic and lumbar spine are taken. Lateral films usually disclose spinal fractures and may also show soft tissue swelling anterior to the spine. An antero-posterior view helps visualize disc spaces and evaluates lateral and rotatory dislocations.

    c. "Open-mouth" view visualizes the odontoid process and demonstrates the lateral atlantoaxial articulations.

    d. X-rays are examined for the following:

        (1) Contour and alignment of the vertebral bodies.

        (2) Displacement of bone fragments more than 3.5 mm or into the spinal canal.

        (3) Fractures or malalignment of the vertebral bodies laminae, pedicles, neural arches, or jumped facets.

        (4) Widening of the interspinous distance.

        (5) Widening of the atlantodental interval >3 mm, indirectly indicates the integrity of the transverse ligament.

    e. SCI may occur in the absence of radiographic changes. X-rays may not show the extent of bony displacement that occurred at the time of injury.

B. **Computerized Axial Tomography (CAT) Scanning**:
1. Outlines the spine and perispinal structures.
2. Assesses the middle spinal column in determining spinal ability.
3. Demonstrates neural canal impingement, posterior column injuries, and concomitant soft tissue injuries.
4. Is useful to obtain longitudinal cross-sections of the vertebral column, especially at C1-2 and C7-T1.

C. **Myelography**: an invasive procedure requiring spinal puncture for administration of contrast material. With the advent of magnetic resonance imaging, myelography is seldom indicated in the diagnosis of SCI. However, it may be used to rule out compressive pathology such as bony fragments that may be displaced and protruding into the canal space.

D. **Magnetic Resonance Imaging (MRI)**: a moninvasive imaging modality for assessing the amount of spinal cord compression and nature of injury that the cord has sustained primarily edema or hemorrhage. MRI can provide imaging of the soft tissues, namely the spinal cord, ligaments, and intervertebral discs, whereas CAT scanning gives better images of bony structure (Zejdlik, 1992).

E. **Magnetic Resonance Spectroscopy (MRS)**: a non-invasive procedure that offers a fingerprint of metabolic and biochemical change. Researchers have found a striking correlation between the loss of magnetism in tissue and the destruction of that tissue.

F. **Somatosensory Evoked Potentials (SSEPs)**: a procedure useful in determining prognosis for the individual with SCI. Scalp electrodes record cerebral cortex responses to peripheral nerve stimulation below the level of injury. If an injury is complete, SSEPs are absent because no messages can be conducted through the damaged cord. In an incomplete injury, altered responses are seen. Early persistence and gradual normalization of evoked potentials usually proceeds any clinical expression of improvement.

References and Selected Bibliography

American Spinal Injury Association (ASIA) (1996). *International standards for neurological and functional classification of spinal cord injury*. Atlanta, GA: ASIA.

Davis, A.E. (1991a). Acute care management of patients with spinal cord injuries. *Critical Care Currents*, 9 (1), 1-4.

Davis, A.E. (1991b). Acute care management of patients with spinal cord injuries. *Critical Care Currents*, 9 (2), 1-4.

Errico, T.J., Bauer, R.D., & Wauch, T. (1992). *Spinal trauma*. Philadelphia: Lippincott.

Fontanarosa, P.B. (1991). Avoiding the risks and repercussions of acute spinal cord injury. *Prehospital Care Reports*, *15*, 33-42.

Green, B.A. (1987). Spinal cord injury - A systems approach: Prevention, emergency medical services and emergency room management. *Critical Care Clinics, 3*(3), 471-493.

Mahon, J.C. (1992). Spinal cord injury. In E.W. Bayley & S.A. Turkle, *A comprehensive curriculum for trauma nursing* (pp. 285-306). Boston: Jones and Bartlett.

Przybylski, G.J. & Marion, D.W. (1996). Injury to the vertebrae and spinal cord. In Feliciano, Moore & Mattox (Eds.), *Trauma 3rd ed.* (pp. 307-323). Stanford, CA: Appleton & Lange.

Rothman, R.H., & Simeone, F.A. (1992). *The spine (Vol. 2) 3rd ed.* Philadelphia: Saunders.

Zejdlik, C.P. (Ed.) (1992). *Management of spinal cord injury (2nd ed.)*. Boston: Jones and Bartlett.

CHAPTER

Special Issues Related to Pediatric Care

Janet Paarlberg, MS, RN, CRRN

I. Learning Objectives

A. Describe measures to combine optimal spinal cord impairment (SCI) care with special considerations for pediatric rehabilitation.

B. Describe the importance of family-centered care.

II. Introduction

A. **Scope of the Chapter**
Children with SCI require the same application of multiple management approaches as those implemented for adults. However, children also have very specific growth and developmental needs. The relationship of the child's age to onset of SCI, nutritional and metabolic needs; body mechanics; and the motor, cognitive, and psychosocial development are key considerations.

To promote optimal outcomes, the health care team collaborates with the child and primary caregivers (parents, family, legal guardians, and/or foster family) to build self-esteem and maximize age appropriate functional independence. This chapter will highlight the concerns of children, adolescents, and their families.

B. **Spinal Trauma in Children**
1. SCI with major neurological involvement is relatively uncommon in infants and children. The estimated incidence is 3-5 percent in those under 15 years of age.
2. The incidence is higher in adolescence due to motor vehicle crashes, violence, and increased risk taking behavior.
3. Children younger than 10 years old are predisposed (>30 percent) to SCI without radiologic abnormalities (SCIWORA), delayed onset of neurologic deficits, and high level cervical injuries.

4. Multiple trauma co-exists with SCI in approximately 75 percent of children, especially traumatic brain injury and injury to the cord at separate levels (Zejdlik, 1992).

5. Injury is frequently related to anatomic and biomechanical considerations of the immature spine. The spinal column will stretch 2 inches before sustaining an injury whereas the spinal cord is able to stretch only one-fourth (?) inch before tearing.

6. Chapter 26, SCI Prevention, describes predisposing factors that place adolescents at risk and offers prevention strategies to optimize safety.

C. **Congenital Disorders: Prevention**

1. Good maternal nutrition is important.

2. Decreased maternal level of folic acid at time of conception is related to increased risk of neural tube defect (NTD).

3. Genetic counseling
   a. There is a 2.5 percent increased risk of subsequent children with NTD if the first child has NTD.
   b. Counseling should be offered when there is a family history of congenital spine disorders or an incidence in the immediate or extended family of disorders that may have an impact on the spine.

4. Congenital anomalies with spine and spinal cord involvement are presented in Chapter 9.

III. Special Considerations

A. **Family-centered Care** (Shelton & Stepanek, 1994)

1. The child needs to be considered a member of the health care team and participate in development of goals. Participation in decision making increases a child's sense of self-worth and autonomy.

2. The level of participation and decision making should be based on the child's developmental and cognitive age.

3. Team members should work collaboratively with the child and family and incorporate the elements of family-centered care into their practice (see Table 11-1).

4. Although adolescents are frequently referred to adult units for care, a pediatric facility may be more appropriate (up to age 18 or having completed high school). Personnel on adult units may be unfamiliar with the special needs of adolescents. Adolescents need to have a sense of control and need help in making good decisions about their care and future.

5. Previous behavior and cognitive level should be identified and used to develop treatment approaches, especially regarding behavior issues.

6. The caregivers need to be members of the health care team.

B. **Growth and Development**

1. An initial assessment should be completed, including the child's cognitive, emotional and social development.

2. All efforts should be made to promote normal development.

3. All members of the interdisciplinary team should have a working knowledge of normal growth and development.

4. Piaget's stages of cognitive development (see Table 11-2) and Erikson's stages of psychosocial development (see Table 11-3) provide an overview of cognitive and social development from birth to old age. The Growing Child Library (1987) is an ideal publication for the family and interdisciplinary team. It provides information on normal growth and development and age-appropriate behavior and activities.

5. All educational programs must be based on the child's and family's level of cognitive functioning.

6. Should the child have an associated cognitive delay, the rate of physical and cognitive recovery may be different. The Rancho Los Amigos Cognitive Functioning Scale (see Table 11-4) can be used to determine the level of cognitive recovery and the ability of the child to learn.

Table 11-1: Key Elements of Family-Centered Care

1. Incorporating into practice the recognition that the family is the constant in a child's life, while the service systems and support personnel within those systems fluctuate.

2. Facilitating family/professional collaboration at all levels of hospital, home, and community care
   - Care of an individual child;
   - Program development, implementation, evaluation, and evolution; and
   - Policy formation.

3. Exchanging complete and unbiased information between families and professionals in supportive manner at all times.

4. Incorporating into policy and practice the recognition and honoring of cultural diversity, strengths, and individuality within and across all families, including ethnic, racial, spiritual, social, economic, educational, and geographic diversity.

5. Recognizing and respecting different methods of coping and implementing comprehensive policies and programs that provide developmental, educational, emotional, environmental, and financial supports to meet the diverse needs of families.

6. Encouraging and facilitating family-to-family support and networking.

7. Ensuring that hospital, home, and community service and support systems for children needing specialized health and developmental care and their families are flexible, accessible, and comprehensive in responding to diverse family-identified needs.

8. Appreciating families as families and children as children, recognizing that they possess a wide range of strengths, concerns, emotions, and aspirations beyond their need for specialized health and developmental services and support.

From *Family-centered Care for Children Needing Specialized Health and Developmental Services*, (p. vii) by T. Shelton & J. Stepanek, 1994; Bethesda, MD: Association for the Care of Children's Health. Reprinted with permission.

Table 11-2: Piaget's Stages of Cognitive Development

AGE	STAGE	CHARACTERISTIC
Birth to 2 years	Sensorimotor	Develop a sense of cause and effect. Solve problems through trial and error. Begin to develop sense of self. Become aware of object permanence. Begin use of language. Imitate behaviors of others.
2 to 7 years	Preoperational	Intellectual development is egocentric. Thinking is concrete and tangible. Unable to make deductions or generalizations. Use imaginative play. Do not understand concept of reversibility.
7 to 11 years	Concrete operational	Begin logical thought. Develop new concept of permanence. Problem solve in a concrete systematic fashion. Use inductive reasoning. Become less self-centered. Thinking is socialized.
12 to 15 years	Formal operational	Become adaptable and flexible. Think in abstract terms and draw logical conclusions. Can deal with and resolve most contradictions.

Developed by Janet Paarlberg, based on *Nursing Care of Infants and Children*, by L. Whaley & D. Wong, 1991, St. Louis: Mosby Year Book.

Table 11-3: Erikson's Stages of Psychosocial Development

AGE	STAGE	CHARACTERISTIC
Birth to 1 year	Trust vs. Mistrust	Develop of basic trust. Mistrust develops when trust-promoting experiences are deficient or lacking. Central process is mutuality. Key agent is mothering person. Outcome: faith and optimism.
1 to 3 years	Autonomy vs. Shame and Doubt	Increasing ability to control body, self, and environment. Want to do things for self. Learn to conform to social rules. Doubt abilities and feel shame when forced to be dependent; make poor choices when shamed by others. Key socializing agent is parents. Central process is imitation. Outcome: self-control and will-power.
3 to 6 years	Initiative vs. Guilt	Strong imagination, like to explore, develop a conscience. Respond to an inner voice that warns and threatens. Sense of guilt develops when activities are in conflict with parents or others. Excessive guilt inhibits initiative. Key socializing agent is family. Central process is identification. Outcome: direction and purpose.
6 to 12 years	Industry vs. Inferiority	Ready to become workers and producers. Want to achieve. Attain a sense of mastery and self-assurance. Important time for social relationships. Feel inadequate or inferior when unable to meet standards set by others. Key socializing agents are teachers, peers. Central process is education. Outcome: competence.
12 to 18 years	Identify vs. Role Confusion	Preoccupied with the way appear to others as compared to self-concept. Struggle with own role, integration of concepts and values with those of society. Make decisions about occupation. Gain ability to sustain loyalties and commitments to others. Role confusion develops when unable to solve core conflict. Central processes are peer pressure and role experimentation. Key socializing agent is society of peers. Outcome: fidelity.
Early Adulthood	Intimacy vs. Isolation	Develop intimate love and interpersonal relationships. Feel isolated with intimacy. Central process is mutuality among peers. Key socializing agents are lovers, spouses, close friends. Outcome: love.
Young and Middle Adulthood	Generativity vs. Stagnation	Time of creation and care of next generation and of nourishing and nurturing. Become self-absorbed and stagnant if unable to nourish and nurture. Central process is person-environment fit and creativity. Key socializing agents are spouse, children, cultural norms. Outcome: production and care.
Old Age	Ego Identity vs. Despair	Have sense of integrity. Despair develops from remorse of what might have been. Central process is introspection. Outcome: renunciation and wisdom.

Developed by: Janet Paarlberg, Reference: Whaley, L.F., Wong , D.L (1991). *Nursing care of Infants and Children*.

7. Functional skill and cognitive assessment tools are available to document the progress the child makes during recovery (WeeFIM State University of New York at Buffalo, PEDI: Pediatric Evaluation of Disability Inventory).

C. **Mobility**
1. All children, regardless of the spine disorder, should be provided with the necessary equipment to maximize mobility.
2. Keeping mobile and active is important for normal growth and development; age-appropriate stimulation and activities; and good self-esteem.
3. Play is a child's work, and in order to play, a child needs to be mobile.
4. Mobility can be accomplished in a hospital bed, stretcher, stroller, travel chair, and manual or power wheelchair. Bed rest does not mean the child needs to be confined to a hospital room or home. Although it may be rejected for social reasons, a child with decubiti may attend school on a gurney. It may take some creativity, but mobilization can be accomplished regardless of the child's disability.
5. For the ventilator-dependent child, the wheelchair should be adapted to carry all necessary equipment to enable the child to attend school, community, and family activities.

D. **Psychosocial Considerations**
1. Child:
   a. Degrees of grief, guilt, denial, and anger may be experienced, regardless of the spinal cord disorder.
   b. The child may require short- or long-term psychosocial support to deal with the impact of the injury, such as the resolution of the cause of the SCI or death of others in a crash.
   c. Identification with others who have similar experiences may be helpful and aid in the recovery process and the long-term impact of the diagnosis.
   d. Independence
      (1) Driver's education and vehicular adaptation encourage normalization.
      (2) Academic and/or vocational training should be encouraged for the adolescent.
   e. Behavior
      (1) Behavior issues may develop as a result of the illness, injury, hospitalization, family issues, and the inability to attend school and participate in peer-related activities.
      (2) Interdisciplinary staff must be aware of age-appropriate behavior.
      (3) Inappropriate behavior should be addressed and a plan developed to encourage and reinforce appropriate behavior. Each developmental age has behaviors unique to that age group. For example, adolescent non-compliance should not be viewed as abnormal, but as characteristic of that age group.
      (4) Developmental and cognitive skill levels require assessment.
2. Family:
   a. Grief, guilt, denial, and anger may be experienced, regardless of the spine disorder.
      (1) Stress may cause the caregiver to express anger toward the child and providers.
      (2) Listening and collaborating with the parents may decrease the episodes of anger and help resolve minor issues before they become major issues.
   b. Factors such as marital conflict, work, injury or death of a spouse or sibling, sibling care, financial constraints, and individual abilities will influence the amount of time the caregivers are able to be with the child during hospitalization, as well as the amount of time available for learning about the child's care and when that learning will take place.
   c. Financial
      (1) Financial options should be investigated. Consult with social services regarding:
         (a) Supplemental Security Income (SSI).
         (b) Medicaid (benefits vary greatly from state to state).
         (c) State Department of Rehabilitation Services for children 16 years and older.
         (d) State services for disabled children.
         (e) Title 5.
      (2) Community fund raising may be considered for acquiring funds to purchase equipment.

Table 11-4: Rancho Los Amigos Cognitive Functioning Scale

I. **No Response** - Patient appears to be in a deep sleep, and completely unresponsive to any stimuli presented to him.

II. **Generalized Response** - Patient reacts inconsistently and nonpurposefully to stimuli in a nonspecific manner. Responses are limited in nature and are often the same regardless of stimulus presented. Responses may be physiological changes, gross body movements, and vocalization. Responses are likely to be delayed. The earliest response is deep pain.

III. **Localized Response** - Patient reacts specifically but inconsistently to stimuli. Responses are directly related to the type of stimulus presented, as in turning head toward a sound or focusing on an object presented. The patient may withdraw an extremity and vocalize when presented with a painful stimulus. He may follow simple commands in an inconsistent, delayed manner, such as closing his eyes, squeezing, or extending an extremity. Once external stimuli are removed, he may lie quietly. He may also show a vague awareness of self and body by responding to discomfort by pulling at nasogastric tube or catheter or resisting restraints. He may show a bias toward responding to some persons, especially family, and friends but not to others.

IV. **Confuse and Agitated** - Patient is in a heightened state of activity with severely decreased ability to process information. He is detached from the present and responds primarily to his own internal confusion. Behavior is frequently bizarre and nonpurposeful relative to his immediate environment. He may cry out or scream out of proportion to stimuli even after removal, may show aggressive behavior, attempt to remove restraints or a tube, or crawl out of bed in a purposeful manner. He does not discriminate among persons or objects and is unable to cooperate directly with treatment efforts. Verbalization is frequently incoherent and/or inappropriate to the environment. Confabulation may be present; he may be hostile. Gross attention to environment is very brief and selective attention often nonexistent. Being unaware of present events, patient lacks short-term recall and may be reacting to past events. He is unable to perform self-care without maximum assistance. If not disabled physically, he may perform automatic motor activities such as sitting, reaching, and ambulating, as part of his agitated state but not as a purposeful act or necessarily on request.

V. **Confused and Inappropriate, Non-agitated** - Patient appears alert and is able to respond to simple commands fairly consistently. However, with increased complexity of commands, or lack any external structure, responses are nonpurposeful, random, or at best, fragmented toward any desired goal. He may show agitated behavior, but not on an internal basis, as in Level IV, but rather as a result of external stimuli and in proportion to the stimuli. He has gross attention to the environment, is highly distractible and lacks ability to focus attention to a specific task without frequent redirection. With structure, he may be able to converse on a social-automatic level for short periods of time. Verbalization is often inappropriate; confabulation may be triggered by recent events. Memory is severely impaired, with confusion of past and present in reaction to ongoing activity. Patient lacks initiation of functional tasks and often shows inappropriate use of objects without external direction. He may be able to perform previously learned tasks when structured for him, but is unable to learn new information. He responds best to self, body, comfort, and often family members. The patient can usually perform self-care activities with assistance and may accomplish feeding with supervision. Management on the unit is often a problem if the patient is physically mobile, as he may wander off either randomly or with vague intention of "going home".

VI. **Confused and Appropriate** - Patient shows goal-directed behavior, but is dependent on external input for direction. Response to discomfort is appropriate and he is able to tolerate unpleasant stimuli; e.g. as NG tube when need is explained. He follows simple directions consistently and shows carryover for tasks he has relearned; e.g. self-care. He is at least supervised with old learning; unable to maximally assisted for new learning with little or no carry-over. Responses may be incorrect due to memory problems, but they are appropriate to the situation. They may be delayed to immediate, and he shows decrease ability to process information with little or no anticipation or prediction of events. Pat's memories show more depth and detail than recent memory. The patient may show beginning awareness of his situation by realizing he doesn't know an answer. He no longer wanders and is inconsistently oriented to time and place. Selective attention to tasks may be impaired, especially with difficult tasks and in unstructured settings, but is now functional for common daily activities. He may show a vague recognition of some staff, has increased awareness of self, family, and basic needs.

VII. **Automatic and Appropriate** - Patient appears appropriate and oriented within hospital/home settings; goes through daily routine automatically, but robot-like with minimal to absent confusion and with shallow recall of what he has been doing. He shows increased awareness of self, body, family, food, people and interaction in the environment. He has superficial awareness of but lacks insight into, his condition, has decreased judgment and problem solving and lacks realistic planning for his future. He shows carry-over for new learning at a decreased rate. He is independent in self-care activities and supervised in home and community skill for safety. With structure, he is able to initiate tasks or social and recreational activities in which he now has interests. His judgment remains impaired. Prevocational evaluation and counseling may be indicated.

VIII. **Purposeful and Appropriate** - Patient is alert and oriented, is able to recall and integrate past and recent events and is aware of and responsive to his culture. He shows carry-over for new learning if acceptable to him and his life role and needs no supervision once activities are learned. Within his physical capabilities, he is independent in home and community skills. Vocational rehabilitation, to determine ability to return as a contributor to society, perhaps in a new capacity, is indicated. He may continue to show a decreased response, relative to pre-morbid abilities, in quality and rate of processing, abstract reasoning, tolerance for stress and judgment in emergencies, or unusual circumstances. His social, emotional, and intellectual capacities may continue to be at a decreased level for him, but functional within society.

From Rancho Los Amigos Hospital, California.

3. Friends:
   a. Friends are supportive, are important to self-esteem, and help the child and family move forward and look to the future.
   b. Friends should be encouraged to visit if the child is hospitalized or not allowed to return to school for medical reasons.
   c. When possible, and with the approval of the child, friends may be taught proper handling of a wheelchair, lifting techniques, transfers, and how to handle emergency situations.

E. **Child/Caregiver Education**
   1. Child/caregiver education should begin on day one of admission.
   2. The child's education regarding SCI should be based on stage of cognitive development. Participation in actual care will be based on motor skills. Should motor skills be impaired, the child should be educated in how to direct a caregiver to do his or her care. Children as young as 3 or 4 years can to some extent direct their own care.
   3. Caregivers should be encouraged to participate in their child's care as early as possible. A gradual learning of their child's care needs increases their knowledge of their child and builds confidence. Delaying education and training to just prior to discharge puts a great deal of stress on the caregivers and child.
   4. Family-centered care encourages child and caregiver education and participation.
   5. Insurance policies typically have a cap, so it is important for families to plan for the future and to spend their child's insurance money wisely. Purchase of special equipment may need to be delayed or limited to extend the benefits of the policy over a longer period of time. Caregivers need to have a good understanding of what the insurance will and will not cover in regard to hospitalization, equipment, therapy, and home services.
   6. The caregivers should also look to the future and identify who will take responsibility and guardianship of their child should something happen to them. A trust can be established to protect the child's financial security.

F. **Community Re-entry**
   1. The discharge plan should be initiated upon admission and developed as early as possible with input from the child and family.
   2. The following is a summary of discharge needs:
      a. Home and school visits as early as possible, with child and family present.
      b. Community services in place prior to discharge (therapy services, emergency services, recreational plans, etc.).
      c. Child and family/parent/caregiver education completed.
      d. Local physician and other providers identified.
      e. Equipment for home and school use obtained with knowledge of how to operate.
      f. Home adaptation completed when possible.
      g. Home health and durable medical equipment company identified, if needed.
      h. Nursing care and attendant care needs identified.
      i. Community and center-based follow-up plans and appointments determined.
   3. Home:
      a. The rehabilitation team may make a home visit. The child and family should be present during the visit. The home should be assessed for architectural barriers, the ability to use special equipment in the home, fire exits, smoke alarms, telephone, power, water, etc..
      b. Therapeutic passes should be allowed prior to discharge to allow the family to identify barriers, to practice skills, and to gain confidence in their ability to care for themselves away from the hospital. Initially, passes should be only for a few hours. If allowed by the third party payers, overnight passes are recommended.
      c. Caregivers should be encouraged to provide care for the child for 48 hours prior to discharge, to promote a supervised and successful transfer of care.
      d. A local primary care physician should be identified prior to discharge, and the child seen within 48 hours of discharge for initial baseline exam.

e. Home health services will be needed based on the child's level of injury or illness. Efforts should be coordinated to provide the best and most efficient service with the least number of companies and people involved. The number of hours of nursing coverage will be determined by the third-party payers.

4. School:
   a. All children should enter or return to school.
      (1) Public Law 94-142, the Education for All Handicapped Children Act (EAHCA, 1975) and the Individuals With Disabilities Education Act (IDEA, 1990) are the laws that most frequently pertain to children with disabilities. The laws mandate that all children from birth to 21 years are entitled to a free and appropriate education in the least restrictive environment. The Technology-Related Assistance Act for Individuals with Disabilities (1988) and the amendments of 1993 (Public Law 103-218) recognize the importance of assistive technology in the lives of disabled persons (programs may vary from state to state).
         (a) Requires schools to provide an appropriate education for those already enrolled in school.
         (b) Allows infants and toddlers to receive services that promote normal development. Below age 2, services are provided in the home or at therapy centers. At age 3, services may be transferred to the school so the child may attend a centered-based school program.
         (c) Services include occupational, physical and speech therapy, audiology, therapeutic recreation, social work, counseling (including rehabilitation counseling), psychological services, transition services, medical services for assessment purposes, transportation, and developmental, corrective, and other supportive services designed to assist the child.
      (2) The child's program may include educationally based therapies, medically based therapies, or both. When the program has educationally based therapies the goal is directed toward education and function, with the school determines and pays for the therapies. In medically based therapies, the services are recommended and ordered by the physician. Frequently, the child will receive both educationally and medically based therapies. In this situation, the school and the third-party payers share the cost of the services.
      (3) The Individual Education Plan (IEP), required by the IDEA and EAHCA, may be written with a Health Services Plan (HSP) included. The IEP identifies the special education and the related and assistive-technology services that the child will receive and is reviewed annually. The HSP defines and builds health care needs into the IEP to define team member roles and to determine who is responsible for the health care of the child while at school. It is a contractual agreement.
      (4) The Individualized Family Service Plan (IFSP) is used for children receiving early intervention (0 to 2 years). It is developed and negotiated around the goals of the family for the child. Agencies that provide services for the child are included in the IFSP.
      (5) Depending on the child's medical status, home school may be considered for children under 5 years and for those with high spinal lesions during flu/cold season.
      (6) When possible, the child should return to the school he/she attended prior to the illness or injury.
      (7) Members of the interdisciplinary team should make a school visit prior to the child's discharge and return to school. The child and family should be present during the visit.
         (a) One or more room(s), depending on the size of the campus, should be identified to provide privacy for personal care needs.
         (b) Entrance/exit should be identified for easy access to the school.
         (c) Appropriate classroom assignment(s) and academic schedule should be discussed.

(d) Child should be mainstreamed unless there are cognitive and behavioral concerns.

(e) A fire drill (emergency) routine should be established.

(8) The school should provide a personal attendant for the child with a high-level lesion; that attendant's primary responsibility is to attend to the needs of that child.

(a) The attendant may be trained by the rehab facility while the child is still an inpatient or may attend outpatient therapy visits.

(b) In order to normalize the school experience, it is recommended that the parent not be the child's attendant.

(9) School staff should develop a protocol for emergency situations.

(a) A list of important telephone contacts should be readily available.

(b) School personnel should know how to respond to episodes of autonomic dysreflexia, elevated temperatures, and bowel and bladder concerns.

(c) Emergency services should be notified of the student(s) with special needs.

5. Community:

a. Should be alerted to the child's presence in the community.

b. The local rescue squad, utility companies (gas, electric, water, telephone), police, and fire department should be made aware of the child's disability and needs (i.e. ventilator dependent) and the need to restore service to this child's home following an electrical outage. The rescue squad/fire department should know where the child sleeps and/or spends the majority of his/her time should an emergency evacuation be necessary.

6. Recreational activities:

a. Recreation enhances physical strength and endurance, promotes cognitive development, and provides opportunities for socialization and the development of good self-esteem.

b. Recreational activities can be adapted to enable the child to participate.

c. Leisure activities that are appropriate to the child's functional level and the family's needs can be identified.

d. A recreational therapist can identify community recreational services for the child and make recommendations for the child's physical education class at school.

G. Health Maintenance and Promotion

1. The health care team must be aware of how pre-existing conditions can impact short- and long-term goals and therapeutic approach.

2. Guidelines identified by the American Academy of Pediatrics (AAP) should be followed for nutrition, growth and development, immunizations, preventive health maintenance exams, and dental care.

a. Immunizations:

(1) Status needs to be reviewed during initial admission, subsequent admissions, and at all well child visits.

(a) Follow recommendations of AAP in Table 11-5.

(b) The inpatient injectable form of polio vaccine (Salk) should be given. Sabin (oral from) is contraindicated because live virus will be shed in urine for weeks following administration and contact with immune-compromised individuals is possible.

(c) Yearly influenza vaccine should be given to the child with pre-existing chronic illness and with cervical or high thoracic injuries or lesions or other complicating respiratory problems.

(d) Pneumococcal vaccine should be given to children with a history of traumatic spleenectomy, functional asplenia, or a high respiratory risk.

b. Latex sensitivity and precautions:

(1) Children with spina bifida and congenital urinary defects have a known susceptibility to latex allergy and all efforts should be made to remove latex from their environment.

(2) Children with SCI who have frequent exposure to latex products are considered to be in the high-risk group for developing an allergy to latex.

Table 11-5: Recommended Childhood Immunization Schedule
United States, January - December 1997

Recommended Childhood Immunization Schedule
United States, January-December 1997

Vaccines[1] are listed under the routinely recommended ages. [Bars] indicate range of acceptable ages for vaccination. [Shaded bars] indicate *catch-up vaccination*: at 11-12 years of age, hepatitis B vaccine should be administered to children not previously vaccinated, and Varicella vaccine should be administered to children not previously vaccinated who lack a reliable history of chickenpox.

Age ▶ Vaccine ▼	Birth	1 mo	2 mos	4 mos	6 mos	12 mos	15 mos	18 mos	4-6 yrs	11-12 yrs	14-16 yrs
Hepatitis B[2,3]	Hep B-1									Hep B[3]	
		Hep B-2			Hep B-3						
Diphtheria, Tetanus, Pertussis[4]		DTap or DTP	DTap or DTP	DTap or DTP		DTap or DTP[4]			DTap or DTP	Td	
H. influenzae type b[5]		Hib	Hib	Hib[5]		Hib[6]					
Polio[6]		Polio[6]	Polio			Polio[6]			Polio		
Measles, Mumps, Rubella[7]						MMR			MMR[7] or MMR[7]		
Varicella[8]						Var				Var[8]	

Approved by the Advisory Committee on Immunization Practices (ACIP), the American Academy of Pediatrics (AAP), and the American Academy of Family Physicians (AAFP).

This schedule indicates the recommended age for *routine* administration of currently licensed childhood vaccines. Some combination vaccines are available and may be used whenever administration of all components of the vaccine is indicated. Providers should consult the manufacturers' package inserts for detailed recommendations.

---

[2] Infants born to HbsAg-negative mothers should receive 2.5 _g of Merck vaccine (Recombivax HB) or 10 _g of SmithKline Beecham (SB) vaccine (Engerix-B). The 2nd dose should be administered > 1 mo after the 1st dose. Infants born to HbsAg-positive mothers should receive 0.5 mL hepatitis B Immune globulin (HBIG) within 12 hrs of birth, and either 5 _g of Merck vaccine (Recomblvax HB) or 10 _g of SB vaccine (Engerix-B) at a separate site. The 2nd dose is recommended at 1-2 months of age and the 3rd dose at 6 months af age. Infants born to mothers whose HbsAg status is unknown should receive either 5 _g of Merck vaccine (Recomblvax HB) or 10 _g of SB vaccine (Engerix-B) within 12 hrs of birth. The 2nd dose of vaccine is recommended at 1 mo of age and 3rd dose at 6 months of age. Blood should be drawn at the time of delivery to determine the mother's HbsAG status; if it is positive, the infant should receive HBIG as soon as possible (no later than 1 wk of age). The dosage and timing of subsequent vaccine doses should be based upon the mother's HbsAG status.

[3] Children and adolescents who have not been vaccinated against hepatitis B in infancy may begin the series during any childhood visit. Those who have not previously received 3 doses of hepatitis B vaccine should initiate or complete the series during the 11-12 year-old visit. The 2nd dose should be administered at least 1 mo after the 1st dose, and the 3rd dose should be administered at least 4 months after the 1st dose and at least 2 months after the 2nd dose.

[4] DTaP (diphtheria and letanus toxoids and acellular pertussis vaccine) is the preferred vaccine for all doses in the vaccination series, Including completion of the series in children who have received 1 or more doses of whole-cell DTP vaccine. Whole-cell DTP Is an acceptable alternative to DTaP. The 4th dose (DTP or DTaP may be administered as early as 12 months of age, provided 6 months have elapsed since the 3rd dose. Td

(tetanus and diphtheria toxoids, adsorbed, for adult use) is recommended at 11-12 years of age if at least 5 years have elapsed since the last dose of DTP, DTaP, or DT. Subsequent routine Td boosters are recommended every 10 years.

[5] Three H. influenzae type b (Hib) conjugate vaccines are licensed for infant use. If PRP-OMP (PedvaxHIB (Merck)) is administered at 2 and 4 months of age, a dose at 6 months is not required. After completing the primary series, any Hlb conjugate vaccine may be used as a booster.

[6] Two poliovirus vaccines are currently licensed in the US: Inactivated poliovirus vaccine (IPV) and oral poliovirus vaccine (OPV). The following schedules are all acceptable by the ACIP, the AAP, and the AAFP:
- IPV at 2 and 4 months; OPV at 12-18 months and 4-6 yr
- IPV at 2, 4, 12-18 months, and 4-6 yr
- OPV at 2, 4, 6-18 months, and 4-6 yr

Parents and providers may choose among these schedules. The ACIP routinely recommends schedule 1. IPV is the only poliovirus vaccine recommended for immunocompromised persons and their household contacts.

[7] The 2nd dose of MMR is routinely recommended at 4-6 yrs of age or at 11-12 yrs of age, but may be administered during any visit, provided at least 1 month has elapsed since receipt of the 1st dose and that both doses are administered at or after 12 months of age.

[8] Susceptible children may receive Varicella vaccine (Var) at any visit after the first birthday, and thoses who lack a reliable history of chickenpox should be immunized during the 11-12 year-old visit. Children > 13 years of age should receive 2 doses at least 1 month apart.

(3) Non-latex products for ICP, bowel program, medication administration, and physical care should be obtained for use during hospitalization and at home.

(4) Child and family should be given a list of products that contain latex and of cross-sensitivity foods such as bananas, avocados, and tropical fruits.

(5) Child and family should be educated in the identification of latex-containing products and the emergent need for treatment of an allergic latex reaction.

IV. Transition to Adult-Based Services

A. **Transition from *pediatric*-based services to *adult*-based services** should begin as the child begins late adolescence or young adulthood (Peterson, P., Raun, K., Brown, J., & Cole, J., 1994; Rauen, K., 1995). This can be a very difficult process, especially if the child has limited cognitive abilities. It may also be difficult for the interdisciplinary providers, especially if the child began receiving services at a very young age. The move can be complicated if there are not established transition programs in place. Some factors that affect the transition process include the availability of physicians educated in pediatric acquired spinal cord related diagnoses, the cognitive and functional level of the adolescent, and the provider's knowledge of cognitive, functional, and growth and development related issues.

B. **Independent living services** may provide guidance and assistance (see Chapter 31).

Practical Application #1

T.A. was 13 months old when he was struck by the tailgate of his father's pick-up truck. He sustained a respiratory arrest at the scene of the accident and was given CPR by the parents. He was intubated at the scene, transported by rescue squad to a tertiary care hospital, and admitted to the pediatric intensive care unit. A diagnosis of a C3 fracture and spinal cord injury was made. He was placed on a ventilator and stabilized. T.A. was trached and had a gastric tube placed. He stayed at this facility for approximately 2 months.

Prior to transfer to a pediatric rehab center (approximately 150 miles from home), he was admitted to the pediatric intensive care unit (PICU) associated with the rehab center for a complete evaluation. He was severely malnourished. He had frequent episodes of bradycardia with a heart rate that would dip to the 20's. He had temperature instability with frequent spikes to 39 degrees. At the end of one month, he was placed on a portable home ventilator and transitioned from the PICU to an acute care unit and then to the rehab unit.

T.A. was initially seen in his room until he and the staff became comfortable. He was transitioned from his room to the playroom and finally to the therapy areas and school. A wheelchair was adapted to accommodate the vent and other respiratory equipment. He continued to have episodes of bradycardia and desaturation frequently associated with autonomic dysreflexia. T.A.'s energy level was low. He was diagnosed with a latex allergy.

Mother and father stayed locally during hospitalization. Mother visited during the day and actively participated in T.A.'s care. She was very alert to changes in T.A.'s behavior and medical status. Father found employment locally and usually visited after work, taking the more playful and entertaining role in his care. His 4 year-old sister visited daily when she stayed locally with her parents. When she returned to her home community, she stayed with her maternal grandmother.

1. Which medical services should be consulted and why?
2. Discuss the nursing care needs of this child and his family.
3. Develop a discharge plan for this child and his family and what needs to be in place in the community prior to discharge.
4. Discuss pertinent growth and development issues and how T.A.'s growth and development changed over the course of his admission.
5. Discuss the impact on his 4-year-old sister in light of *developmental age*. How can the sister be used as part of the interdisciplinary team?

Practical Application #2

J.T., presently 14 years old, was born with a lumbar myelomeningocele. At age 3 days his defect was closed and at 2 weeks of age a VP shunt was placed. His mother was single and unemployed at the time of his birth. Early surgeries included circumcision and bilateral club foot repair. J.T. was ambulating with crutches by age 3 years. At age 4, he experienced some changes in his swallowing and breathing requiring surgical intervention. At age 7 and again 9 years, J.T. experienced decreased sensation and strength and loss of function in his lower extremities. Surgical intervention was required at both age 7 and 9. He was unable to ambulate prior to each surgical intervention. Although limited to short distances, he was able to ambulate after each surgery.

J.T. was incontinent of urine but had some awareness of bladder fullness and the need to void. Bowel movements were irregular, and he was admitted on two occasions for bowel impaction. Behavioral problems developed at approximately age 8, with severe temper outbursts demonstrated. Mother received vocational training and became employed when J.T. was 10 years old. Father has never been involved.

1. Discuss what could be the cause of J.T.'s swallowing and breathing problems at age 4 and his inability to ambulate at age 7 and 9 years. Which medical and surgical services should be consulted and why?
2. Discuss pertinent growth and development issues, including behavioral impact.
3. Discuss psychosocial issues that affect this child.
4. Describe an appropriate bowel and bladder program for this child.

References and Selected Bibliography

American Academy of Pediatrics (AAP). (1997). *Guidelines on immunization practice*. Elk Grove: AAP.

American Spinal Injury Association (ASIA). (1992). *International Standards for neurological and functional classification of spinal injury patients* (rev. ed).

Apple, De.F., Anson, C., Hinter, J., & Bell, R. (1995). Spinal cord injury in youth. *Clinical Pediatrics, 34* (2), 90-95.

Betz, R., & Mulcahey, M. (Ed.). (1996). *The child with a spinal cord injury*. Rosemont, IL: American Academy of Orthopaedic Surgeons.

Farley, F., Hensinger, R., & Herzenbery, J. (1992). Cervical spinal cord injury in children. *Journal of Spinal Disorders, 5*(4), 410-416.

Hostler, S. (1994). *Family-centered care: An approach to implementation*. Charlottesville, VA: University of Virginia.

Johnson, K., Berry, E., & Wicker, E. (1991). Growing up with a spinal cord injury. *SCI Nursing, 8* (1), 11-20.

Johnson, K., & Persaud, D. (1993). *Spinal cord injury: Educational content for professional nursing practice*. Jackson Heights, NY: American Association of Spinal Cord Injury Nurses.

Lollar, D.(Ed) (1994a). *Preventing secondary conditions associated with spina bifida or cerebral palsy*. Washington, DC: Spina Bifida Association of America.

Lollar, D. (1994b). *Social development and the person with spina bifida*. Washington, DC: Spina Bifida Association of America.

Mahan, L.K. & Escott-Stump, S. (1996). Nutrition during pregnancy and lactation. In Krause, *Food, nutrition, and diet therapy*, (9th ed.), 181-212. Philadelphia: W.B. Saunders.

Mann, D. & Dodds, J. (1993). Spinal injuries in 57 patients 17 years or younger. *Spinal Injuries in Children and Adolescents, 16* (2), 159-164.

Massagli, T. & Jaffe, K. (1990). Pediatric spinal cord injury: Treatment and outcome. *Pediatrician, 17* (4), 244-254.

Molnar, S. (1992). *Pediatric rehabilitation*. Baltimore, MD: Williams and Wilkins.

Nelson, W., Behraman, R., & Vaughan V. (eds.) (1996). *Textbook of pediatrics (15th ed.)*. Philadelphia: W.B. Saunders.

Peterson, P., Rauen, K., Brown, J., & Cole, J. (1994). Spina bifida: The transition into adulthood begins in infancy. *Rehabilitation Nursing, 19* (4), 229-238.

Rauen, K. (1995). *Guidelines for spina bifida health care services throughout life*. Washington, DC: Spina Bifida Association of America.

Rauen, K., & Aubert, E. (1992). A brighter future for adults who have myelomeningocele - One form of spina bifida. *Orthopaedic Nursing, 11* (3), 16-26.

Riccardi, V. (1995). Neurofibromatosis and the pediatric spine. In D. Pang (Ed.), *Disorders of the pediatric spine* (pp. 467-480). New York: Raven Press.

Roberts, C., Clark, M., & Johnson, K. (1995). Rehabilitation of the child with spinal cord injury. In D. Pang (Ed.), *Disorders of the pediatric spine* (pp. 605-633). New York: Raven Press.

Safer, N. & Hamilton, J. (1993). Legislative context for early intervention services. In W. Brown, S.K. Thurman, & L. Pearl, *Family-centered early intervention with infants and toddlers*. Baltimore, MD: Brooks. HV888.5F34

Sawin, K. & Marshall, J. (1992). Developmental competence in adolescents with acquired disability. *Rehabilitation Nursing Research Journal, 1*(1), 41-49.

Shelton, T., & Stepanek, J. (1994). *Family-centered care for children needing specialized health and developmental services*. Bethesda, MD: Association for the Care of Children's Health.

Smithells, R.N., Sheppard, S., Schorah, C.J. (1980). Possible prevention of neural tube defects by periconceptional vitamin supplementation. *Lancet, 1(8164):339-40.*

Swaiman, K. (1994). *Pediatric neurology, principles and practice*. St. Louis, MO: Mosby.

Whaley, L., & Wong, D. (1991). *Nursing care of infants and children*. St. Louis, MO: Mosby Year Book.

Wilberger, J. (1986). *Spinal cord injuries in children*. Mt. Kisco, NY: Futura.

Zejdlik, C.P. (Ed.) (1992). *Management of spinal cord injury (2nd ed.)*. Boston:

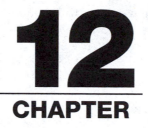

12
CHAPTER

Respiratory/Pulmonary
Kathryn M. La Favor, MSN, RN, CRRN

I. Learning Objectives

A. Explain neurological control of breathing.

B. Describe the effects of spinal cord impairment (SCI) on respiratory function.

C. Discuss health maintenance issues of the individual with respiratory compromise due to SCI.

D. Discuss the technology available to assist individuals with respiratory compromise due to SCI.

II. Introduction

A. **Demographics**
   1. Individuals with SCI affecting the cervical and/or thoracic spinal cord will experience some change in respiratory function due to loss of innervated musculature.
   2. About 50 percent of individuals with SCI will be tetraplegic with a complete or partial loss of respiratory muscle function (Singh, Suys & Villanueva, 1995).

B. **Etiology/Precipitating Factors**
   1. Depending on the level and completeness of the spinal cord lesion, there may be loss of innervation to the diaphragm, intercostal, and abdominal muscles.
   2. Individuals with complete lesions affecting the spinal cord above C3 will have no diaphragmatic or intercostal functioning.
   3. Lesions at C3-C5 level result in various degrees of diaphragmatic dysfunction and loss of intercostal and abdominal muscle functioning.
   4. Mid-cervical lesions spare diaphragmatic function, but the individual is at risk for respiratory complications and may need ventilatory assistance in the early period of the injury or illness. There is a loss of intercostal and abdominal muscle functioning.

5. Lesions of the lower cervical and thoracic cord result in full diaphragm functioning and absent or impaired functioning of the intercostal muscles. Abdominal muscle function is impaired or absent.

6. Retropharyngeal hematoma associated with injury of the upper cervical spine may impinge the airway.

C. **Anatomy/Physiology** (Bates, 1991; Guyton & Hall, 1996; Zejdlik, 1992)

  1. Normal structure and function of the respiratory system.

    a. There are four major events in the process of respiration:

      (1) Pulmonary ventilation: the flow of air in and out between the atmosphere and the alveoli of the lung.

      (2) Exchange of oxygen and carbon dioxide between the alveoli and the blood.

      (3) Transport of oxygen and carbon dioxide in the blood and body fluids to and from the cells.

      (4) Regulation of ventilation by control mechanisms of the body with regard to rate, rhythm, and depth.

    b. Muscles of the respiratory system:

      (1) Expansion of the lungs during inspiration can be accomplished in two ways:

        (a) Downward movement of the diaphragm; this is the major movement in normal quiet breathing.

        (b) Elevation of the ribs by the external intercostal muscles and the accessory muscles (sternocleidomastoid and scalene muscles).

      (2) Contraction of the lungs during expiration is accomplished in the following ways:

        (a) Relaxation of the diaphragm resulting in the elastic recoil of the lungs.

        (b) Depression of the ribs aided by the muscles of the anterior abdominal wall and the interior intercostal muscles.

    c. Nervous system control of breathing originates in the respiratory center of the brain and is mediated by the muscles of respiration (Zejdlik, 1992).

      (1) Respiratory center: arises from the medulla oblongata and pons.

      (2) Diaphragm: innervated by the phrenic nerve, which arises from C3-C5; A fully functioning diaphragm generates about 75 percent of the normal tidal volume (Singh, Suys & Villanueva, 1995).

      (3) Intercostal muscles: innervated by nerves exiting from T1-T12; intercostal muscles are responsible for a decrease in the antero-posterior diameter in forced expiration (Singh, Suys & Villanueva, 1995).

      (4) Accessory breathing muscles: the sternocleidomastoid muscle is innervated by cranial nerve XI and the scalene muscles are innervated by C2-C7; accessory muscles assist in elevating the upper rib cage during inspiration.

      (5) Abdominal muscles: innervated by T6-T12; during normal expiration, abdominal tone assists by pushing the diaphragm back to its resting position (Singh, Suys & Villanueva, 1995).

  2. Anticipated dysfunction after SCI (Table 12-1)

    a. Depending on the level and completeness of the SCI, the individual may have difficulty preserving neural control of the muscles of breathing and maintaining an airway.

    b. The diaphragm is supplied by the cervical nerves of C3, C4, & C5. Thus, cervical spinal cord injuries that cause damage to the C4 level and above produce almost total respiratory muscle paralysis. Individuals with complete injuries at this level cannot cough and require permanent ventilatory support (Zejdlik, 1992).

    c. Spinal cord lesions that occur below C4 will result in partial to full diaphragm functioning. Vital capacity will be decreased (see Table 12-1). With associated autonomic nervous system impairment, sleep-induced apnea may occur (Zejdlik, 1992).

    d. Complete low cervical and high thoracic injuries result in absent chest and abdominal muscle movement.

    e. If the cough reflex is impaired, bronchial secretions will accumulate. In individuals with high tetraplegia, where there is also an interruption in sympathetic pathways, bronchial secretions are increased (Singh, Suys & Villanueva, 1995).

f. Respiratory dysfunction may be present in individuals with non-traumatic spinal cord disorders (spinal cord tumors, abcesses, disc disease, spinal cord infarcts, and syrinxes), depending on the location and completeness of the lesion. For example, if an individual has a syrinx that invades the C3-C5 level of the cord, respiratory compromise similar to a C3-C5 level spinal cord injury can be anticipated.

g. Demyelination disorders of the spinal cord may result in loss of respiratory function.

(1) Guillain-Barre' syndrome (GBS) (Hickey, 1997; Morgan, 1991):

    (a) An autoimmune response which results in destruction of the myelin sheath surrounding the cranial and spinal nerves (see Chapter 9).

    (b) Respiratory dysfunction resulting from neuro-muscular weakness is common in GBS

    (c) Clinical indications of respiratory compromise in GBS include: decrease in vital capacity, weak cough effort, and ineffective airway clearance.

    (d) Monitoring vital capacity and comparing it with a predetermined optimal level for the patient (approximately 12-15mL/kg) will be necessary (Hickey, 1997, p. 692).

    (e) When the individual's vital capacity falls below the preset optimal level, elective intubation and mechanical ventilation may be necessary; thus careful assessment and planning process can prevent the emotional and physical trauma of an emergency intubation (Hickey, 1997).

Table 12-1: Neurological Control of Breathing and Anticipated Dysfunctions Following Spinal Cord Unjury

Muscles of Breathing		Segmental Nerves	Cough Function	Vital Capacity (VC)	
Inspiration	Expiration			Acute	Long Term
Accessory Muscles		CN XI / C1 / C2	Absent (non-functional)	5-10% of normal (500-600 ml)	Ventilator-dependent for life
Diaphragm		C3 / C4 / C5 / C6	Absent (non-functional)	20% of normal (1250 ml)	Most ventilator-free (especially C4 and C5) (some part-time) 50% of normal
External Intercostals	Internal Intercostals	C7 / C8 / T1 / T2 / T3 / T4	Weak	30-50% of normal	60-70% of normal
	Abdominals	T5 / T6 / T7 / T8 / T9 / T10	Fair	75-100% of normal	Nearly normal
		T11 / T12 / L1 / to / S5	Strong	Normal	Normal

From *Management of Spinal Cord Injury* (2nd ed., p.262), by C.P. Zejdlik, 1992, Boston: Jones & Bartlett. Copyright 1992 by Jones & Bartlett. Reprinted with permission.

       (f) The majority of individuals with GBS will require mechanical ventilation for about two weeks before the weaning process can begin (Hickey, 1997).

   (2) Multiple Sclerosis (MS):

       (a) A chronic, progressive neurological disease characterized by demyelinization of the central nervous system (Miller & Hens, 1993) (see Chapter 9).

       (b) The course of MS is varied and unpredictable. MS affects the white matter of the nervous system, and the lesions can be found in the brain and/or spinal cord; signs and symptoms vary from individual to individual but may include: sensory symptoms, motor symptoms (paresis, paralysis, spasticity, diplopia, bowel and bladder dysfunction), cerebellar symptoms, and other symptoms such as fatigue, optic neuritis depression, and impotence (Hickey, 1997).

       (c) When the respiratory system is affected by this disease process, it is usually a result of muscle fatigue and the complications of immobility; pneumonia accounted for a major cause of death in one large study (Sadovnick, Eisen, Ebers & Paty, 1991).

   (3) Amyotrophic Lateral Sclerosis (ALS):

       (a) A chronic, progressive motor neuron disease; also known as Lou Gehrig's disease (Tidwell, 1993) (see Chapter 9).

       (b) Signs and symptoms may include: progressive muscle weakness, muscle atrophy, fasciculations, decreased muscle tone, loss of tendon reflexes, dysarthria, dysphagia, and respiratory insufficiency (Tidwell, 1993).

       (c) Progression of this disease often results in degeneration of the motor neurons at the C3-C5 level of the spinal cord; this process weakens the diaphragm and intercostal muscles resulting in respiratory fatigue and eventually respiratory failure (Tidwell, 1993).

       (d) Respiratory management includes periodic assessment of respiratory function and parameters; aggressive pulmonary toilet, and potentially mechanical ventilation (Hickey, 1997; Tidwell, 1993).

  h. Congenital spinal disorders may result in distortion of underlying lung tissue (Bates, 1991).

   (1) Scoliosis: a structural lateral curvature of the spine.

   (2) Kyphosis: a structural deformity of the spine resulting in a rounded thoracic convexity.

   (3) Thoracic kyphoscoliosis: a curvature of the spine with corresponding deformities in the thorax.

3. Respiratory complications following SCI (Jackson & Groomes, 1994; Mansel & Norman, 1990; Singh, Suys, & Villanueva, 1995):

  a. Respiratory complications are the primary cause of death in the early stages of post-high cervical SCI (Jackson & Groomes, 1994; Mansel & Norman, 1990).

  b. The most frequent respiratory complications of cervical SCI (Jackson & Groomes, 1994):

   (1) Ventilatory failure: a PCO2 blood gas value greater than 50 and/or a PaO_2 of 50 or below on room air, and/or the necessity of ventilatory support.

   (2) Atelectasis: a state of airlessness within the lung; typically associated with decreased inspiratory capacity, rales, and arterial hypoxiemia without infection.

   (3) Pneumonia: a state of lung tissue inflammation.

  c. Other complications include:

   (1) Adult respiratory distress syndrome (ARDS): a state of pulmonary edema resulting from lung injury; characteristics include: reduced lung volumes, low pulmonary compliance, and normal pulmonary capillary pressures (Jackson & Groomes, 1994).

   (2) Pleural effusion: fluid in the pleural space (Jackson & Groomes, 1994).

   (3) Pulmonary thromboembolism: a pulmonary artery becomes acutely obstructed by a blood clot (Jackson & Groomes, 1994).

   (4) Neurogenic pulmonary edema: with mechanical trauma to the spinal cord, there is an associated short-lived increase in autonomic discharge causing an increase in total peripheral resistance with a shift of blood into the pulmonary circulation. The rise in pulmonary pressure and the loss of capillary integrity results in pulmonary edema (Singh, Suys, & Villanueva, 1995, p. 206).

(5) Associated pulmonary trauma (Singh, Suys, & Villanueva, 1995; p. 207):
    (a) Aspiration
    (b) Rib fractures
    (c) Flail chest
    (d) Pneumothorax
    (e) Hemothorax
    (f) Pulmonary contusion
    (g) Ruptured diaphragm

d. The incidence of atelectasis in thoracic SCI is similar to the incidence in cervical SCI; therefore, individuals with thoracic lesions require vigilant prophylactic pulmonary hygiene measures as well.

4. SCI with secondary musculoskeletal complications may further compromise respiratory function.

III. Initial Assessment

A. **Nursing History:** The sequence and length of the nursing history taking portion of a respiratory assessment may need to be modified for acutely ill patients. The ability to vocalize, and therefore participate in the history taking aspects of assessment, may be impaired by an artificial airway, poor endurance, and/or mechanical ventilation. Family members may be able to assist.
1. Chief complaint
2. History of present illness
   a. Spinal cord trauma
   b. Spinal cord disease
   c. Spinal deformities
3. Past health history
   a. Smoking history
   b. Preexisting cardiorespiratory conditions or diseases
   c. Age
4. Family history of cardiorespiratory disease

B. **Components of the physical examination portion of a respiratory assessment include:**
1. Inspection:
   a. Head and neck:
     (1) Airway difficulty: there is airway impairment if the patient is unable to talk, or is making gurgling, snorting, or grunting noises or is only able to speak 1-2 words. In the unconscious individual, the tongue may occlude the oropharynx.
     (2) Gasping
     (3) Cyanosis
     (4) Open mouth
     (5) Flared nostrils
     (6) Use of accessory muscles
     (7) Position of trachea
     (8) Central cyanosis: tongue or lips
     (9) Peripheral cyanosis: nose or ears
   b. Chest/Abdomen:
     (1) Respiratory rate
     (2) Depth of chest expansion if present
     (3) Presence of abdominal breathing
     (4) Breathing pattern
     (5) Symmetry of chest movements
     (6) Intercostal retractions
     (7) Effectiveness and frequency of cough, if present (Rinehart & Nawoczenski, 1987)
       (a) Functional: able to raise secretions by a normal, forceful cough without assistance

(b) Weak functional: able to clear secretions from the airway but unable to expel the secretions without assistance

(c) Nonfunctional: unable to inhale or exhale with any functional force and cannot move secretions out of the airways or expel secretions without major assistance

(8) Severe spasticity abdominal/thoracic area

(9) Gastrointestinal distention

c. Extremities:

(1) Clubbing of nails

(2) Peripheral cyanosis

d. Pulmonary secretions:

(1) Quantity: bronchial secretions may be increased in SCI due to loss of sympathetic control and unopposed vagus activity

(2) Quality

2. Palpation: The heel of the examiner's hand is held flat against the chest to determine whether the movements of each side of the chest are equal and symmetrical.

3. Percussion: Involves tapping the chest with a finger. The sounds produced provide information about the position, size, and density of underlying tissues.

4. Auscultation: using a stethescope, auscultate all four lobes of the lungs. Retained secretions cause: bronchial sounds, diminished breath sounds, increased or decreased fremitus, and adventitious sounds (Zejdlik, 1992, p. 263).

C. **Diagnostic Studies**

1. Chest radiograph

2. Pulmonary function tests:

a. Tidal volume (TV): the volume of air expired during normal ventilation.

b. Inspiratory reserve volume (IRV): the volume of forced inspiration over the tidal volume.

c. Expiratory reserve volume (ERV): the volume of forced expiration over normal expiration.

d. Residual volume (RV): the volume of air remaining following maximal expiration.

e. Vital capacity (VC): the volume of air that can be forcibly expired following a forced maximal inspiration; in the individual with SCI, this indicates the ability to take a deep breath and cough effectively; this can be measured at the bedside with a spirometer (Zejdlik, 1992).

3. Arterial blood gases reveal oxygenation status (Hickey, 1997: 212). These values are a reflection of:

a. Arterial oxygenation (PaO_2)

b. Alveolar oxygenation ($PaCO_2$)

c. Acid-base status (pH)

d. Oxygen delivery to the tissues

4. Pulmonary gas analysis:

a. Oxygen saturation (SaO_2); monitors the amount of oxygen bound to hemoglobin; normal readings are between 92 percent and 100 percent.

b. End tidal volume of carbon dioxide ($ETCO_2$)-analyzes CO_2 content in a sample of expired air.

IV. Nursing Process Applied to Airway Management

A. **Nursing Diagnosis: Ineffective airway clearance**

B. **Defining Characteristics** (Zejdlik, 1992):

1. Restlessness and agitation

2. Poor chest expansion

3. Abnormal or diminished breath sounds

4. Pale or dusky skin color, cyanosis of oral mucous membranes

5. Alterations in heart rate from baseline

C. **Expected Outcomes:**
1. Patent airway
2. Airway free of adventitious sounds
3. Effective oxygenation

D. **Interventions:**
1. Pulmonary secretion management
   a. Evaluate effectiveness of cough effort. Individuals with tetraplegia and high paraplegia usually do not have adequate innervated muscle (intercostals and abdominals) to produce an effective cough.
   b. If cough effort is too weak to adequately clear pulmonary secretions, consider the following interventions:
      (1) Suctioning: removal of secretions from the trachea and mainstem bronchi
         (a) Asotracheal, endotracheal or tracheostomy suctioning may be performed based on the individual's airway status
         (b) When suctioning an individual with high tetraplegia, be alert for an abnormal vasovagal response that may cause severe bradycardia or cardiac arrest (Zejdlik, 1992, p. 291)
      (2) Manual assisted cough maneuver
         (a) A procedure used to move secretions toward the trachea and the mouth of an individual with SCI who has absent or weak abdominal and intercostal muscles.
         (b) A caregiver applies firm pressure over the upper abdomen and diaphragm; after inspiration, even, firm pressure is directed inward and upward as the individual attempts to cough (Zejdlik, 1992). This procedure can also be coordinated with the ventilator breath or Ambu-bag breath (Johnson, Grant & Peterson, 1997). Caution: this practice may not be safe in individuals with spine fractures; always check with the orthopedic physician or neurosurgeon before initiating this intervention.
   c. Other bronchial hygiene procedures (Rinehart & Nawoczenski, 1987; Zejdlik, 1992):
      (1) Chest physical therapy (CPT): a technique that involves the use of gravity to aid flow of secretions to a point at which they can be expectorated with forceful coughing maneuvers or suctioned with a catheter; chest percussion may augment the procedure.
      (2) Intermittent positive pressure breathing (IPPB); positive pressure therapy administered during inspiration to aerate and humidify underventilated areas of the lungs in individuals with SCI who are unable to sigh or deep breathe regularly (Zejdlik, 1992).
      (3) Strength and endurance training:
         (a) Incentive spirometry: involves the repetitive use of a device used to measure sustained maximum inspiratory movements with the objective of strengthening the diaphragm and other respiratory muscles (Zejdlik, 1992).
         (b) Other inspiratory muscle training devices to control breathing resistence.
2. Artificial airways:
   a. Types:
      (1) Oropharyngeal airway: used to maintain airway by holding tongue anteriorly.
      (2) Nasopharyngeal airway: useful in facial or jaw fractures when oral airway cannot be used.
      (3) Endotracheal tubes: used for emergency or short-term intubation.
         (a) oral tracheal tubes
         (b) nasotracheal tubes
      (4) Tracheostomy: used for long-term airway maintenance.
   b. Potential complications of artificial airways:
      (1) Artificial materials (plastic or metal tubes) are foreign bodies which cause increased mucous production.
      (2) Chronic bacterial colonization
      (3) Impaired function of airway cilia
      (4) Impaired phonation

   (5) Mucous plugs which adhere to the tube

   (6) Impaired swallowing

   (7) The development of granulomas

  c. Impaired communication: Artificial airways bypass the vocal cords, making phonation difficult.

   (1) Some nonverbal methods of communication include:

    (a) Establish a means of indicating yes and no (blinking strategies are often successful; i.e. one blink for yes, two blinks for no)

    (b) Develop a word board. The board should include the letters of the alphabet and some common phrases or requests.

   (2) Consider special tracheostomies:

    (a) Fenestrated tracheostomy: has a removable inner cannula that exposes an opening on the upper surface of the outer cannula, which allows the individual to talk during expiration (Zejdlik, 1992).

    (b) "Talking" tracheostomy: has a port for an air supply to be attached; a caregiver can attach an air supply from a wall source to a port on the tracheostomy when having a conversation with the individual; forced air over vocal cords allows phonation to occur.

   (3) Deflating the trachestomy cuff and increasing the tidal volume (if the individual is on mechanical ventilation) is an option after the individual's respiratory status is stabilized and he/she is no longer at risk of aspirating secretions. This procedure allows air to pass over vocal cords and therefore allows phonation to occur (Chawla, 1993).

V. Nursing Process Applied to Ventilatory Insufficiency

 A. **Nursing Diagnosis: Ineffective Breathing Pattern**

 B. **Defining Characteristics** (Borel & Guy, 1995; Singh, Suys & Villanueva, 1995; Zejdlik, 1992):

  1. Dyspnea

  2. Apnea

  3. Nasal flaring, use of accessory muscles of respiration

  4. Clinical signs and symptoms of hypoventilation

   a. Reduced tidal volume

   b. Reduced vital capacity

   c. Elevated $PaCO_2$

 C. **Expected Outcomes:**

  The individual with SCI will be able to:

  1. Maintain respiratory parameters (tidal volume and vital capacity) in an adequate range.

  2. Maintain arterial blood gases in normal limits.

  3. Maintain clear breath sounds.

 D. **Interventions:**

  1. Position changes and bronchial hygiene techniques.

  2. Mechanical ventilation: positive pressure ventilators (Borel & Guy, 1995).

   a. Indications

    (1) High cervical cord injuries resulting in diaphragmatic paralysis

    (2) Ventilatory insufficiency

   b. Types of positive pressure ventilators

    (1) Pressure-cycled: delivers inspiratory flow until preset pressure has been reached

    (2) Volume-cycled: delivers inspiratory flow until preset volume has been delivered

   c. Modes of initiation of the inspiratory cycle

    (1) Assisted/controlled: a breath initiated by the patient will trigger the ventilator; if the patient fails to breathe, the ventilator will deliver a breath at a preset time interval.

(2) Assisted ventilation: the rate is triggered by the patient's inspiratory effort, which is augmented by the ventilator.

(3) Controlled ventilation: a preset volume is delivered at a preset interval; neither volume nor interval is affected by the patient's attempts to breathe.

d. Potential complications associated with the use of mechanical ventilation (Zejdlik, 1992) (see Table 12-2)

   (1) Hyperventilation

   (2) Hypoventilation

   (3) Increased airway pressure

   (4) Thick secretions, mucous plugs

   (5) Infection

   (6) Tracheal injury

   (7) Pneumothorax

   (8) Dislodged tracheostomy tube

e. Psychological care of the ventilator-dependent individual

   (1) Individuals who require ventilatory support are often subjected to extreme sensory overstimulation caused by alarms, and frequent, repetitious treatments. They often display signs of extreme anxiety. The nurse can play an integral role in providing for adequate rest periods.

      (a) Coordinate respiratory treatments with other activities to allow for periods of uninterrupted rest.

      (b) Eliminate as many extraneous noises as possible.

      (c) Dim the lighting at night to reduce day/night confusion.

   (2) Other interventions that may reduce anxiety and feelings of helplessness include:

      (a) Finding a reliable means to communicate with the patient, which includes taking the time necessary to understand what he or she is trying to say

      (b) Explain all procedures before they happen

      (c) Include family members in the teaching so that they will be available to reinforce the information

   (3) For individuals with SCI who will require long-term ventilatory support, it will be necessary to:

      (a) Involve the individual in all aspects of care planning

      (b) Obtain equipment that maximizes independence

      (c) Keep the individual informed of all options for ventilatory support and the right to discontinue ventilatory treatment

f. Weaning from mechanical ventilation

   (1) General principles:

      (a) Most individuals with conditions resulting in neuromuscular weakness will require a gradual withdrawal from ventilator support.

      (b) The longer the ventilatory support, the longer it will take to wean.

      (c) It is usually recommended that individuals with neuro-muscular weakness are weaned by gradually increasing time off the ventilator alternating with periods of complete rest on the ventilator (Johnson, Grant, & Peterson, 1997; Thomas & Paulson, 1994; Wicks, 1989).

      (d) Individuals with tetraplegia may find it easiest to wean in the supine position, as the abdominal contents provide some resistance for the diaphragm (Zedjlik, 1992).

   (2) General indications for weaning (Johnson, Grant, & Peterson, 1997):

      (a) Resolution of any underlying pulmonary pathology.

      (b) Stable and acceptable measurements of respiratory function.

      (c) Generally, a forced vital capacity (FVC) of 1,000cc or greater and a negative inspiratory force (NIF) of -30 to -50cm of water pressure are predictive of potential for weaning.

      (d) Stable metabolic and nutritional status.

      (e) Psychological readiness to wean.

Table 12-2: Common User- and Equipment-Related Problems with Mechanical Ventilation

User-Related Problems	Defining Characteristics	Equipment-Related Problems	Defining Characteristics (Indicators)
Hyperventilation (person ventilated too fast or with too much air)	• Increased respiratory rate • Low $PaCO_2$ • Dyspnea • Lightheadedness	Holes or tears in circuit tubing leading to leaks in the system	• Audible air leak coming from ventilator circuit • Ventilator gauge or dial does not register prescribed amount of volume • Low pressure alarm sounding
Hypoventilation (person ventilated with too little air)	• Dyspnea • Increased $PaCO_2$ • Decreased oxygen saturation and PaO_2 • Tachycardia • Lethargy and drowsiness • Anxiety and restlessness • Audible air leak	Blockage from kinks or water in tubing	• High pressure alarm sounding • Gurgling sound
Increased airway pressure	• Audible respiratory secretions • Airway pressure alarm sounding • Abnormal breath sounds	Disconnect between ventilator and patient	• Ventilator gauge or dial registering that no volume is being delivered • Low pressure alarm sounding
Thick secretions, mucus plugs	• Secretion thick, difficult to suction • Resistance in passing suction catheter • Low oral fluid intake and ventilator humidification	Ventilator failure	• Ventilator gauge or dial registers no volume delivered • Low pressure alarm sounding • Ventilator not cycling
Infection	• Changes in sputum— color, amount, and consistency • Fever • Positive laboratory data	Incorrect ventilator settings	• Ventilator gauges and controls register different readings from prescribed rates • Alarms may sound
Tracheal injury	• Blood-tinged mucus	Humidifier (cascade): decreased water supply, overfilling of reservoir, incorrect temperature, leaks	• Dry, hot gas when cascade humidifier becomes dry • Rain-out in tubing occluding gas flow • Pulmonary burns
Pneumothorax (barotrauma)	• Dyspnea • Diminished breath sounds • Weak, rapid pulse • Sudden increase in airway pressure or decrease in TV readings		
Dislodged tracheostomy tube	• Apnea • Bradycardia • Color changes • Anxiety and restlessness		

From *Management of Spinal Cord Injury* (2nd ed., p.300), by C.P. Zejdlik, 1992, Boston: Jones & Bartlett. Copyright 1992 by Jones & Bartlett. Reprinted with permission.

(3)   Guidelines should be established to direct weaning interventions. The following concepts should be addressed in institution protocol.
   (a) Criteria for beginning or increasing weaning times; examples are (patient agreement, clear or improving chest radiograph, stable ABGs or pulse oximetry)
   (b) Interval between changes in weaning schedule; example: each change should be maintained for 1-3 days.
   (c) An outline of how the weaning schedule is to progress; example: 2 minutes, 5 minutes, 10 minutes, 20 minutes, 30 minutes, 60 minutes TID.

(d) Directions for when weaning should take place (Example: between the hours of 0600 and 2200 if the patient is weaning 16 hours or less).

(e) Any specifics related to the tracheostomy; (Example: all weans are to be performed with the trach cuff deflated and with a tracheostomy talk device as tolerated).

(f) Criteria for holding or discontinuing weans; (Examples: oxygen saturation below 92 percent, respiratory rate above 35 breaths per minute, heart rate increased by 20 from baseline, blood pressure change of plus or minus 30 points from baseline, forced vital capacity less than half of documented patient baseline, patient request).

(g) Criteria for final discontinuation of ventilator; (Example: ventilator may be discontinued when the patient has been off the ventilator for 48 hours and is stable).

g. Ventilator dependence in individuals with SCI:

(1) The positive pressure ventilator is one option for the individual requiring permanent respiratory support. (See the following sections for alternative methods.) An individual may be ventilator dependent for 24 hours a day or may require the ventilator only during night hours.

(2) Once it has been determined that the individual faces long-term ventilator dependence, obtaining a portable ventilator should be considered. Portable ventilators allow for increased mobility and independence.

(3) Rehabilitation centers with expertise in managing individuals who require continued ventilation provide education programs to teach non-professionals, including patients and families, how to manage ventilator dependence in the home environment or at school (Bard, Jaminez, & Tornak, 1994; B.C. Rehab Society, 1995; Carter, 1993; Glass, 1993; Gipson, 1985; Splaingard, Frates, Harrison, Carter, & Jefferson, 1983; Zejdlik, 1992).

h. Ethical issues related to ventilator withdrawal:

(1) Individuals with SCI may request the withdrawal of medical interventions such as mechanical ventilators in order to allow the natural progression of the disease or condition to take place (Butt & Scofield, 1997; Maynard & Muth, 1987; Purtilo, 1986).

(2) A ventilator can legally be removed even when doing so will result in death (Hickey, 1997).

(3) In 1983, the President's Commission for the Study of Ethical Problems in Medicine and Biomedical and Behavioral Research reported that the principle of individual autonomy should guide treatment decisions.

(4) In order for an individual's request to be valid, the individual must have decision-making capacity (Hickey, 1992). The healthcare team may become involved in determining decision-making capacity. The factors of decisional capacity include (Butt & Schofield, 1997):

(a) the possession of a set of values and goals

(b) the ability to communicate and understand information

(c) the ability to reason and deliberate

(5) There still are no clear cut answers regarding all of the issues surrounding the discontinuation of ventilators. Other issues for the health care team to consider:

(a) Is the individual suffering from reactive depression? Does this condition limit decision-making abilities?

(b) Should individuals with SCI be encouraged to wait for a prescribed period of time in order to fully assess life with a ventilator?

(c) Should the individual's wishes to discontinue mechanical ventilation occur on the rehabilitation unit, or should policy mandate that the individual be transferred to another unit?

3. Alternative methods of ventilatory support:

a. Diaphragmatic pacemaker ventilation (Bach & O'Connor, 1991; Carter, 1993; Carter, Donovan, Halstead, & Wilkerson, 1987; Esclarin et al, 1994)

(1) Components
  (a) External transmitter and loop antenna
  (b) Internal receiver
  (c) Phrenic nerve electrode
  (d) Anode
(2) Description: surgically implanted electrodes are placed near the phrenic nerve; an external transmitter-antenna unit emits a signal that is converted into an electrical impulse which is carried by wires to the stimulating electrode on the phrenic nerve; the diaphragm contracts, pulling air into the lungs (Bach & O'Connor, 1991).
(3) Indications:
  (a) Chronic ventilatory insufficiency without significant impairment of the phrenic nerves, lungs, or diaphragm.
  (b) Respiratory paralysis without significant impairment of the phrenic nerves, lungs or diaphragm (example: being the SCI patient sustaining an injury at the C1-C3 level leaving the spinal cord free from trauma at the C4 segmental level) (Zedjlik, 1992).
(4) Advantages:
  (a) May have at least partial freedom from bulky ventilator equipment; phrenic pacer equipment is lighter.
  (b) May be some appearance/body image improvements using phrenic pacing as opposed to tracheostomy ventilation.
  (c) Less bronchial secretions (Esclarin et al, 1994).
(5) Disadvantages (Bach & O'Connor, 1991):
  (a) Requires surgery for placement.
  (b) Expensive equipment and training required.
  (c) No ability to program regular deep inspirations or to modify tidal volumes.
  (d) No internal alarms.
  (e) Still need back-up resuscitation and ventilation equipment.
(6) Potential complications:
  (a) Potential operative trauma to the phrenic nerve.
  (b) Phrenic nerve compression and infection.
  (c) Equipment failure.
  (d) Fatigue of diaphragm from excessive stimulation.
  (e) Aspiration related to asynchrony of laryngeal reflexes during phrenic pacing (Bach & O'Connor, 1991)>

b. Intermittent abdominal pressure ventilator (IAPV) (Bach, 1991; Miller, Thomas & Wilmot, 1988):
  (1) Pneumobelt: a corset-type device that produces artificial ventilation by assisting expiration rather than inspiration; the inflation of the bladder within the corset fills, compresses the abdomen and causes the diaphragm to move upward producing active expiration; when the bladder deflates, the abdominal contents and diaphragm move downward, resulting in passive inspiration (Wirtz, La Favor, & Ang, 1996).
  (2) Limitations (Miller, Thomas & Wilmot, 1988):
    (a) Must be sitting to use the pneumobelt.
    (b) Difficulty with fitting the scoliotic patient.
    (c) Minor skin abrasions.
    (d) May not be able to use in patients with extremes of body weight.
    (e) Significant obstructive apneas and oxyhemoglobin desaturations during sleep have been observed (Bach, Penek, 1991).
  (3) Advantages (Miller, Thomas & Wilmot, 1988):
    (a) Cosmesis
    (b) Improved speech
    (c) Increased independence and mobility
    (d) Comfort
    (e) Safety
    (f) Health

c. Noninvasive intermittent positive pressure ventilation (IPPV) (Bach, 1991):
   (1) Mouth IPPV: consists of a ventilator with a mouthpiece that is either kept in the patient's mouth or adjacent to the patient's mouth for assisted breaths as needed.
   (2) Nasal IPPV: consists of a ventilator that is connected to the patient via a nasal mask.
   (3) Advantages of noninvasive IPPV:
       (a) Tracheostomy not needed
       (b) Increased comfort and control
   (4) Potential disadvantages of noninvasive IPPV:
       (a) Airleaks
       (b) The development of allergies to the mouthpiece, lip seal, or nasal mask
       (c) Risk of aspiration during vomiting during the use of mouth IPPV with lip seal at night

d. Glossopharyngeal breathing (GPB) (Bach, 1991; Clough, 1983):
   (1) Characteristics:
       (a) The tongue, lips, soft palate, mouth, and pharyngeal muscles are used to project a bolus of air past the vocal cords, adding to the inspiratory effort.
       (b) The vocal cords close with each "gulp".
       (c) One breath consists of 6-14 gulps.
       (d) Also called "frog breathing".
   (2) Advantages:
       (a) Effective and inexpensive back-up for ventilator equipment failure.
       (b) Deeper GPB-assisted breaths are helpful for manual assisted coughing.
       (c) Can normalize the volume and rhythm of speech.
   (3) Disadvantages:
       (a) Rarely can be used long periods of time or while eating or sleeping.
       (b) Could cause a drop in blood pressure due to the high bronchial pressures produced, causing a decrease in venous return.

e. Education and anticipatory guidance related to the patient's respiratory status should be provided frequently and in terms that can be understood. An effort should be made to prepare the patient for respiratory interventions before they occur to minimize anxiety and feelings of loss of control.

f. Following respiratory crisis, when the individual and family are ready to learn, formal education should include the following components:
   (1) Review normal anatomy and function of respiratory system.
   (2) Describe functional changes in respiratory system after SCI.
   (3) Demonstrate interventions aimed at maintaining optimal respiratory health.
   (4) Allow frequent practice sessions for caregivers to practice skills relating to respiratory health.

VI. Reassessment

Once interventions have been initiated to stabilize respiratory status, it will be necessary to reassess the following aspects:

A. **Airway:** ensure that the individual is able to maintain an unobstructed airway, free of secretions.

B. **Assistive devices for respiratory support:** when mechanical support is needed, ongoing assessment of the equipment for proper functioning, and of the effects or potential complications of the equipment, is necessary.

C. **Ongoing measures of effective ventilation** should be assessed (Example: pulse oximetry to monitor SaO_2; ABGs).

D. **Auscultate the lung fields** at intervals appropriate for the individual's condition.

VII. Health Tips

A. **Education for individuals with respiratory compromise due to SCI:**
   1. Level of injury or disease process and how it affects respiratory function.
   2. Methods to clear airway, such as tracheal suctioning and assisted cough.
   3. Ways to prevent and treat upper respiratory infections.
   4. Strength and endurance exercises for respiratory muscles.
   5. The hazards of smoking.
   6. Cold and flu prevention techniques, including a review of flu vaccinations.
   7. Health care resources to contact in the event of illness.

B. **Education for individuals who are dependent on mechanical ventilation:**
   1. Use of the ventilator and all ventilator support equipment including: tracheostomy supplies, suction devices, and manual resuscitation bag.
   2. Safety practices related to mechanical ventilation including: back-up supplies, planning for power failures, manual resuscitation techniques, alerting the community fire department, hospital, paramedics, and local utility companies before discharge.

VIII. Special Issues Related to Pediatric Care

A. **Pulmonary complications** are a major cause of morbidity and mortality acutely following SCI, and are a major cause of death in children with tetraplegia under age 5 (Mansel & Norman, 1990). Rapid fatigue of the immature muscles of breathing necessitates immediate preventive measures to promote airway clearance, breathing patterns, and functional speech.
   1. Past health history:
      a. Smoking history in high-risk adolescent population
      b. Pre-existing conditions, especially bronchopulmonary dysplasia (associated with premature births) and asthma
   2. Pediatric population is at high risk of developing:
      a. Nosocomial infections
      b. Sleep-induced apnea

B. **Specific Interventions:**
   1. Early ventilatory support
   2. Airway management
      a. To encourage verbal communication, an uncuffed tracheostomy tube is used for almost all children under 8 years of age.
      b. Volume controlled ventilation is used with an uncuffed tracheostomy because of the risk for hypoventilation during sleep.
      c. Children as young as 3 years can be taught to breathe using accessory neck muscles, allowing some sense of security in case of accidental ventilator disconnection. Dr. Irene Gilgoff at Rancho Los Amigos has had excellent results with neck breathing for high spinal cord injuries, resulting in several hours off the ventilator in children over 3 years of age. Pharyngeal breathing is difficult for the young child to learn and is more effective with the older child (Gilgoff, Barras, Jones, & Adkins (1988)).

Practical Application #1

S.R., a 22 year old male, was admitted to the intensive care unit following a motor vehicle crash in which he sustained C5 complete quadriplegia secondary to a fracture. He arrived to the intensive care unit from the emergency room breathing on his own at a rate of 28 breaths per minute. An absence of chest expansion during respiration was noted; however, there was no history of chest trauma or lung disease. Auscultation of lung fields did not reveal any adventitious sounds. Three hours later, his respiratory rate was up to 34 breaths per minute, he appeared anxious and noted to be using his trapezius and sternocleidomastoid muscles with inspiration. Arterial blood gases: PO_2, 48; PCO_2, 56; pH 7.32. He was able to speak, but having difficulty completing sentences without stopping for breaths. A decision was made to intubate S.R. using a fiberoptic-assisted nasotracheal approach. He was placed on full mechanical ventilatory support. Two weeks later, S.R. was doing well on mechanical ventilation and demonstrating: spontaneous respirations, vital capacity of 1100mls, chest x-ray clear, arterial blood gases: PO_2, 88; PCO_2, 40; pH 7.41, vital signs and nutritional status stable. The treating team decided that he was ready to begin weaning from the ventilator.

Practical Application #2

P.M., a 20-year-old female college student, was admitted to a neurology floor with progressive quariparesis. She was alert and oriented. In addition to weakness, a workup revealed decreased nerve conduction, elevated cerebrospinal fluid, and loss of deep tendon reflexes. She was diagnosed with Guillain-Barre' (GB) syndrome. The team caring for P.M. knew that respiratory muscle weakness is the most serious potential complication of GB and developed a plan of care including close monitoring of vital capacity measurements. Three days later, P.M.'s paralysis ascended to include cranial nerves. Her vital capacity progressively deteriorated and the decision was made to intubate and mechanically ventilate her. The team developed a plan of care with interventions aimed at preventing respiratory complications of pneumonia, atelectasis, and pulmonary embolus. Within two days all respiratory muscle function was absent and a tracheostomy was done. In about 14 days, P.M.'s paralysis should show signs of receding. As her respiratory status improved, she was slowly weaned over a period of five weeks from mechanical ventilation. Seven weeks after admission, she was transferred to a rehabilitation facility to work on regaining strength and mobility. By the start of the next semester of college, P.M. was able to return to school using only a cane.

References and Selected Bibliography

Bach, J. R. (1991). Alternative methods of ventilatory support for the patient with ventilatory failure due to spinal cord injury. *The Journal of the American Paraplegia Society*, 14(4), 158-174.

Bach, J. R. & O'Connor, K. (1991). Electrophrenic ventilation: A different perspective. *The Journal of the American Paraplegia Society*, 14(1), 9-17.

Bach, J. R. & Penek, J. (1991). Obstructive sleep apnea complicating negative pressure ventilatory support in patients with chronic paralytic/restrictive ventilatory dysfunction. *Chest, 99*, 1386-93.

Bard, J., Jimenez, F. C., & Tornak, R. (1994). *Integration in the school setting. Outcome based health support program*. Vancouver, CAN: B.C. Rehab Society.

Bates, B. (1991). *A guide to physical examination and history taking* (5th ed.). Philadelphia: Lippincott.

B.C. Rehab Society (1995). *Attendant training manual: Care of ventilator dependent individual in the community*. Vancouver, CAN: Author.

Borel, C. O. & Guy, J. (1995). Ventilatory management in critical neurologic illness. *Neurological Critical Care, 13*(3), 627-644.

Butt, L. & Scofield, G. (1997). The bright line reconsidered: The issue of treatment discontinuation in persons with ventilator-dependent tetraplegia. *Topics in Spinal Cord Injury Rehabilitation, 2*(3), 85-94.

Carter, R. E. (1993). Experience with ventilator dependent patients. *Paraplegia, 31*, 1150-1153.

Carter, R. E., Donovan, W. H., Halstead, L. & Wilkerson, M. A. (1987). Comparative study of electrophrenic nerve stimulation and mechanical ventilatory support in traumatic spinal cord injury. *Paraplegia, 25*, 86-91.

Chawla, J. C. (1993). Rehabilitation of spinal cord injured patients on long term ventilation. *Paraplegia, 31*, 88-92.

Clough, P. (1983). Glossopharyngeal breathing: Its application with a traumatic quadriplegic patient. *Archives of Physical Medicine and Rehabilitation, 64*, 384-385.

DeVivo, M. J. & Ivie, C. S. (1995). Life expectancy of ventilator-dependent persons with spinal cord injuries. *Clinical Investigations in Critical Care, 108*(1), 226-232.

Esclarin, A., Bravo, P., Arroyo, O., Mazaira, J., Garrido, H. & Alcaraz, M. A. (1994). Tracheostomy ventilation versus diaphragmatic pacemaker ventilation in high spinal cord injury. *Paraplegia, 32*(10), 687-693.

Gilgoff, I., Barras, D., Jones, M., & Adkins, H. (1988). Neck breathing: A form of voluntary respiration for the spine injured ventilator-dependent child. *Pediatrics, 82*, 741-745.

Gipson, W. T. (1985). Mechanical ventilation in the home: The role of the physiatrist. *Cleveland Clinic Quarterly, 52*, 313-315.

Glass, C.A. (1993). The impact of home based ventilator dependence on family life. *Paraplegia, 31*, 88-92.

Guyton, C., & Hall, J.E. (1996). *Texbook of medical physiology* (9th ed.). Philadelphia: W.B. Saunders.

Hickey, J.V. (1997). *The clinical practice of neurological and neurosurgical nursing*. Philadelphia: Lippincott.

Jackson, A. B. & Groomes, T. E. (1994). Incidence of respiratory complications following spinal cord injury. *Archives of Physical Medicine and Rehabilitation, 75*, 270-275.

Johnson, K., Grant, T. & Peterson, P. (1997). Ventilator weaning for the patient with high-level tetraplegia. *Topics in Spinal Cord Injury Rehabilitation, 2*(3), 11-20.

Mansel, J. K. & Norman, J. R. (1990). Respiratory complications and management of spinal cord injuries. *Chest, 97*(6), 1446-1452.

Maynard, F.M. & Muth, J.D. (1987). The choice to end life as a ventilator-dependent quadriplegic. *Archives of Physical Medicine and Rehabilitation, 68*, 862-864.

Miller, C.M. & Hens, M. (1993). Multiple sclerosis: A literature review. *Journal of Neuroscience Nurses, 25*(3), 174-179.

Miller, J., Thomas, E. & Wilmot, C. B. (1988). Pneumobelt use among high quadriplegics. *Archives of Physical Medicine and Rehabilitation, 69*, 369-372.

Morgan, S.P. (1991, October). A passage through paralysis. *American Journal of Nursing*, 70-74.

Purtilo, R.B. (1986). Ethical issues in the treatment of chronic ventilator-dependent patients. *Archives of Physical Medicine and Rehabilitation, 67*, 718-721.

President's Commission for the Study of Ethical Problems in Medicine and Biomedical and Behavioral Research. (1983). *Deciding to forego life-sustaining treatment: A report on the ethical, medical, and legal issues in treatment decisions*. Washington, DC: U.S. Government Printing Office. 121.

Rinehart, M. E. & Nawoczenski, D. A. (1987). Respiratory care. In L. E. Buchanan and D. A. Nawoczenski (Eds.) *Spinal cord injury—Concepts, management and approaches* (pp. 61-80). Baltimore, MD: Williams and Wilkins.

Sadovnick, A.D., Eisen, K., Ebers, G.L. & Paty, D.W. (1991). Cause of death in patients attending multiple sclerosis clinics. *Neurology, 41*(8), 1193-1196.

Singh, R. V. P., Suys, S. & Villanueva, P. A. (1995). Prevention and treatment of medical complications. In E. C. Benzel & C. H. Tator (Eds.), *Contemporary management of spinal cord injury* (pp. 195-215). Park Ridge: American Association of Neurological Surgeons.

Splaingard, M.L., Frates, R. C., Harrison, G.M., Carter, E., & Jefferson, L.S. (1983). Home positive-pressure ventilation: Twenty years' experience. *Chest, 84*(4), 376-382.

Thomas, E. & Paulson, S. S. (1994). Protocol for weaning the SCI patient. *SCI Nursing, 11*(2), 42-45.

Tidwell, J. (1993). Pulmonary management of the ALS patient. *Journal of Neuroscience Nursing, 25*(6), 337-342.

Wicks, A.B. (1989). Ventilator weaning. In G. Whiteneck, C. Adler, R.E. Carter, D.P. Lammertse, S. Manley, R. Mentor, K.A. Wagner, & C. Wilmot (Eds.), *The management of high quadriplegia* (pp. 141-147). New York: Demos.

Wirtz, K. M., La Favor, K. M., & Ang, R. (1996). Managing chronic spinal cord injury: Issues in critical care. *Critical Care Nurse, 16*(4), 24-35.

Zejdlik, C. P. (Ed.) (1992). *Management of spinal cord injury.* (2nd ed.) Boston: Jones & Bartlett.

CHAPTER

Cardiovascular and Thermoregulatory Control

Linda Love, MS, RN, CRRN

I. Learning Objectives

A. Understand alterations in cardiovascular and body temperature control mechanisms related to spinal cord impairment (SCI).

B. Conduct a nursing assessment of the individual with altered cardiovascular and/or thermoregulatory control.

C. Describe nursing interventions in management of cardiovascular and thermoregulatory dysfunction.

D. Develop goals to assist the individual in preventing manifestations of altered cardiovascular and/or thermoregulatory control.

II. Introduction

A. **Scope of the Chapter**
This chapter focuses on the nature, character, prevention, and management of syndromes and complications associated with autonomic dysfunction: orthostatic hypotension, altered thermoregulation, autonomic dysreflexia (AD), and deep vein thrombosis (DVT). Cardiovascular instability related to spinal shock that occurs immediately following spinal cord injury is discussed in chapters 27 and 28.

B. **Demographics**
1. Preexisting cardiovascular disease or conditions further complicate the effects of autonomic dysfunction in individuals with SCI (Zejdlik, 1992).
2. Loss of ability to regulate body temperature is a problem related to autonomic nervous system dysfunction and loss of normal sweating mechanisms below the level of spinal cord injury.

3. Heat insensitivity is experienced by 60 to 80 percent of individuals with multiple sclerosis (MS) (Syndulko, Jafari, & Woldanski, 1996).

4. Autonomic dysreflexia, with its sudden and severe rise in blood pressure, is a potentially life-threatening crisis. AD may occur in up to 80 percent of neurologically impaired individuals with lesions at or above the T6 spinal cord segment (Chiou-Tan, Lenz, Robertson, & Grabois, 1994). Cases of AD in individuals with injuries as low as T10 have been reported (Lindan, Joiner, Freehafer, & Hazel, 1980). AD is considered a medical emergency, which, if left untreated, can lead to cerebral infarct, ischemia, hemorrhage, convulsions, or death (Givre & Freed, 1989; Yarkony, Katz, & Wu, 1986).

5. The incidence of deep vein thrombosis in acute SCI has been reported to be from 47-100 percent (Consortium for Spinal Cord Medicine, 1997b). DVT may embolize in up to 50

C. **Etiology/Precipitating Factors**

The autonomic nervous system (ANS) which provides regulatory control of heart rate, blood pressure, and body temperature, is disrupted after SCI. The higher the level of injury the more profound the effects of autonomic dysfunction. Injury to the spinal cord at the T6 level or above interferes with sympathetic function. Injury below T6 allows partial sympathetic outflow. In lower lumbar or sacral cord injuries, the sympathetic system remains intact; however, loss of reflex activity below the level of injury impairs vasomotor control to the lower extremities.

D. **Anatomy/Physiology**

The ANS regulates the activities of all smooth muscles, cardiac muscles, and glands. The two major subdivisions of the ANS are the sympathetic and parasympathetic systems. The sympathetic system is activated during stress situations such as fright, fight, or flight phenomena, resulting in increased heart rate and blood pressure as well as vasoconstriction of the peripheral blood vessels. The parasympathetic system stimulates those visceral activities associated with conservation, restoration, and maintenance of a normal functional level. The two branches of the ANS have opposing responses aimed at restoring balance; as one is activated, the other is suppressed. Sympathetic outflow arises from the intermediolateral cell columns between T1 and L2 spinal cord segments. Parasympathetic branches emerge with cranial nerves III, VII, IX, and X. The sacral portion of the parasympathetic system arises from the sacral segments of S2-S4. Autonomic effects of sympathetic and parasympathetic stimulation on various body organs is described in Table 13-1 (Guyton & Hall, 1997).

1. Orthostatic hypotension: Following SCI at T6 and above, interruption of the sympathetic outflow which controls vasopressor reflexes occurs resulting in a rapid and profound drop in blood pressure, that is exacerbated by position change, especially when assuming an upright position. Impaired vasomotor reflexes allow vasodilation, venous pooling, and decreased cardiac output, resulting in hypotension and decreased organ perfusion especially to the brain. Sympathetic impulses are blocked at the level of injury and vasoconstriction does not occur below the level of injury, resulting in syncope (Rehabilitation Nursing Foundation of the Association of Rehabilitation Nurses, 1995). Insufficient release of catecholamines in response to sudden positional change, slow release of antidiuretic hormone, cortisol, and aldosterone may also play a role (Freed, 1990). Lack of muscle contraction in the extremities and abdomen makes for sluggish venous return to the heart, resulting in further decrement in cardiac output, blood pressure, and cerebral blood flow.

2. Temperature regulation: Heat and cold receptors in the skin transmit impulses by way of the spinal cord to the hypothalamus to help control body temperature. SCI at T6 and above results in absence of vasoconstriction, loss of ability to shiver to conserve body heat, and loss of thermoregulatory sweating to dissipate heat. The loss of hypothalamic thermoregulatory mechanisms produces a poikilothermic state in which the individual assumes the ambient temperature. This puts the individual with SCI at risk for hypothermia or hyperthermia (Niederpruem, 1989). The exact mechanisms by which heat may exacerbate the symptoms of multiple sclerosis (MS) is unclear, but the increased susceptibility of demyelinated axons to elevated temperature is thought to be a primary factor (Syndulko, et al, 1996).

3. Autonomic Dysreflexia (autonomic hyperreflexia) is a hypertensive crisis, associated with significant cerebral morbidity and death. (See Figure 13-1). Stimulation of sensory receptors

Table 13-1: Autonomic Effects on Various Organs of the Body

Organ	Effect of Sympathetic Stimulation	Effect of Parasympathetic Stimulation
Eye		
Pupil	Dilated	Constricted
Ciliary muscle	Slight relaxation (far vision)	Constricted (near vision)
Glands	Vasoconstriction and slight secretion	Copious secretion (containing many enzymes for enzyme-secreting glands)
Sweat glands	Copious sweating (cholinergic)	Sweating on palms of hands
Heart		
Muscle	Increased rate Increased force of contraction	Slowed rate Decreased force of contraction (especially of atria)
Coronary arteries	Dilated ($\beta2$); constricted (α)	Dilated
Lungs		
Bronchi	Dilated	Constricted
Gut		
Lumen	Decreased peristalsis and tone	Increased peristalsis and tone
Sphincter	Increased tone (most times)	Relaxed (most times)
Liver	Glucose released	Slight glycogen synthesis
Kidney	Decreased output and renin secretion	None
Bladder		
Detrusor	Relaxed (slight)	Contracted
Trigone	Contracted	Relaxed
Penis	Ejaculation	Erection
Systemic arterioles		
Abdominal viscera	Constricted	None
Muscle	Constricted (adrenergic α) Dilated (adrenergic $\beta2$) Dilated (cholinergic)	None
Skin	Constricted	None
Blood		
Coagulation	Increased	None
Glucose	Increased	None
Lipids	Increased	None
Basal metabolism	Increased up to 100%	None
Adrenal medullary secretion	Increased	None
Mental activity	Increased	None

From *Human Physiology and Mechanisms of Disease* (6th ed.) (p. 499) by A. C. Guyton and J. E. Hall, 1997, Philadelphia: W. B. Saunders. Reprinted with permission.

below the level of injury (such as a distended bladder) sends noxious sensory input to the spinal cord. As these impulses ascend the spinal cord, sympathetic reflexes are stimulated, causing severe vasoconstriction in the peripheral arteries, producing a sudden and dramatic rise in blood pressure. Baroreceptors respond to the rise in blood pressure, and brainstem response is to slow the heart rate and dilate blood vessels. Because the SCI is at or above the major sympathetic outflow beginning at T6, the inhibitory sympathetic message is only effective above the lesion. Although heart rate is slowed, vasodilation below the level of injury cannot occur. Blood pressure remains elevated or continues to rise as long as noxious stimulus continues (Dunn, 1991).

4. Deep vein thrombosis: The following can precipitate formation of thrombi: alterations in hemostasis following SCI, venous stasis, immobility, age greater than 40, dehydration, poor nutritional status, obesity, smoking, heart disease, hip or long bone fractures, recent surgery, malignancy, congestive heart failure, use of oral contraceptives, estrogen therapy, pregnancy, and various inflammatory processes. A thrombus can partially or completely occlude a blood vessel, or break free (embolize) from the vessel wall and travel in the bloodstream. A pulmonary embolus occurs when the embolus enters the pulmonary circulation and obstructs blood flow to the lungs (Zejdlik, 1992).

III. Initial Assessment

A. Nursing History
1. Demographic information and cognitive status
2. Level, type, and completeness of SCI
3. Associated injuries
4. Previous medical/surgical history including cardiac and peripheral vascular problems
5. Functional ability/mobility, lifestyle, and living environment
6. Allergies and medications
7. Smoking history, alcohol and other drug use
8. Cardiovascular risk profile - hyperlipidemia, obesity, diabetes, tobacco use, hypertension
9. History of orthostatic hypotension, thermoregulatory problems, DVT, and AD
10. Bowel and bladder management/problems

B. Physical Exam
1. Check vital signs
2. Inspect, palpate, and auscultate heart and lungs
3. Assess pulses
4. Inspect and palpate upper and lower extremities for temperature, color, edema, skin lesions
5. Assess presence and degree of tone and spasticity
6. Inspect skin: color, temperature, moisture, pressure ulcers
7. Conduct abdominal, perineal, and rectal examination (see chapter 14 Bladder Elimination and Continence)
8. Check leg measurements to detect early swelling which may be indicative of DVT.

C. Diagnostic Studies
1. Hemodynamic monitoring: during the acute phase following injury (see chapter 28 Critical Care).
2. Electrocardiogram: identification of cardiac dysrhythmia
3. Chest Xray: evaluate heart and pulmonary status
4. Laboratory: blood analysis, urinalysis, urine culture and sensitivity
5. Oxygen saturation, vital capacity, arterial blood gas analysis for assessment of pulmonary compromise
6. Blood coagulation studies, doppler ultrasound, impedance plethysmography, and nuclear scanning to detect DVT
7. Urologic studies (see chapter 14 Bladder Elimination and Continence)

Figure 13-1: Autonomic Dysreflexia Pathophysiology

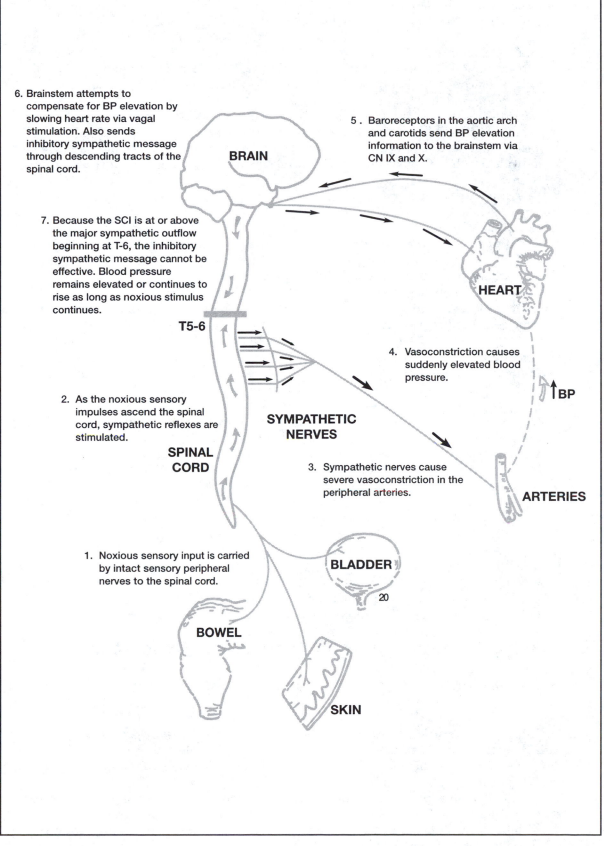

6. Brainstem attempts to compensate for BP elevation by slowing heart rate via vagal stimulation. Also sends inhibitory sympathetic message through descending tracts of the spinal cord.

5. Baroreceptors in the aortic arch and carotids send BP elevation information to the brainstem via CN IX and X.

7. Because the SCI is at or above the major sympathetic outflow beginning at T-6, the inhibitory sympathetic message cannot be effective. Blood pressure remains elevated or continues to rise as long as noxious stimulus continues.

BRAIN

HEART

T5-6

4. Vasoconstriction causes suddenly elevated blood pressure.

↑BP

2. As the noxious sensory impulses ascend the spinal cord, sympathetic reflexes are stimulated.

SYMPATHETIC NERVES

SPINAL CORD

3. Sympathetic nerves cause severe vasoconstriction in the peripheral arteries.

ARTERIES

1. Noxious sensory input is carried by intact sensory peripheral nerves to the spinal cord.

BLADDER

20

BOWEL

SKIN

From *"Autonomic Dysreflexia: A Nursing Challenge in the Care of the Patient with Spinal Cord Injury,"* by K. L. Dunn, 1991, *Journal of Cardiovascular Nursing, 5*(4), p. 58. Reprinted with permission.

IV. Nursing Process Applied to Orthostatic Hypotension

A. **Nursing Diagnosis:** Decreased cardiac output and cerebral blood flow, venous stasis, and associated alterations in mobility and knowledge deficits.

B. **Defining Characteristics:**
1. Critical clinical characteristics include lightheadedness, decreased thinking ability, blurred vision, syncope, weakness, and dizziness (Rehabilitation Nursing Foundation of the Association of Rehabilitation Nurses, 1995).
2. Decrease in systolic and diastolic blood pressure upon assuming an upright position; hypotension as low as 40 mm Hg systolic, 0 mm Hg diastolic.
3. Tachycardia may accompany hypotension as a compensatory mechanism, although an individual with high quadriplegia may be unable to generate compensatory tachycardia.
4. Nausea
5. Pallor above level of injury

C. **Expected Outcomes:**
1. Blood pressure maintained within normal limits for the individual. Baseline blood pressure for individuals with quadriplegia may be 90/60 mm Hg.
2. Pulse maintained within normal limits for the individual
3. Prevention and management of episodes of orthostatic hypotension
4. Individual and caregivers are knowledgeable regarding symptoms, prevention, and management of orthostatic hypotension.

D. **Interventions:**
1. In the early post-injury phase monitor blood pressure and pulse before and after significant position changes and compare with baseline data.
2. Adequate fluids - 2-3 liters/24 hours
3. Gradual elevation of head of bed and/or tilt table positioning as tolerated before progressing from bed rest to wheelchair following initial injury
4. Elastic stockings and abdominal binder before sitting to promote venous return
5. Reclining back wheelchair with elevating leg rests may be needed initially.
6. If symptoms of orthostatic hypotension:
   a. Immediately lower head of bed; recline or tilt wheelchair backward and elevate legs.
   b. Instruct individual to breathe deeply while gently compressing the abdomen with expiration.
   c. Hydrate
   d. Allay anxiety
7. Individual and caregiver instruction regarding symptoms, precipitating factors, and management of orthostatic hypotension
8. Ephedrine sulfate, per physician order, prophylactically in severe cases

V. Nursing Process Applied to Altered Body Temperature

A. **Nursing Diagnosis:** Ineffective thermoregulation secondary to SCI and associated knowledge deficits

B. **Defining Characteristics:** In addition to individuals use of SCI, elderly persons and individuals with diabetes mellitus, cardiovascular disease, obesity, and alcohol are at increased risk of adverse affects associated with excessively high or low environmental temperatures (Niederpruem, 1989).
1. Body temperature under 97° F or above 100° F. Due to inability to maintain a steady internal temperature, the individual may assume the temperature of the environment.
2. Inability to sweat below the level of injury to dissipate heat may result in profuse sweating above the level of injury.
3. Inability to effectively shiver to conserve heat

4. Hyperthermia - body temperature of 106° F (41.1° C) or above is caused by elevated body and environmental temperatures. Manifestations include:
   a. Heat Cramps - muscle spasms triggered by inadequate serum sodium levels
   b. Heat Exhaustion - weakness, nausea, lightheadedness
   c. Heat Stroke - Body temperature at least 40 percent above normal and a failure of all body cooling mechanisms. Symptoms include faintness, dizziness, headache, nausea, rapid pulse, and flushed skin (Niederpruem, 1989).
5. Hypothermia - Body temperature below 96.4° F (35.8° C), occurs when cold persists and heat loss exceeds heat production.

C. **Expected Outcomes:**
   1. Prevention and management of extremes in body temperature
   2. Prevention of complications related to extremes in body temperature such as hypothermia, hyperthermia, and dehydration
   3. Individual and caregivers are knowledgeable regarding symptoms, prevention, and management of temperature regulation

D. **Interventions:**
   1. Prevention:
      a. Monitor body temperature
      b. Maintain a desirable environmental temperature, approximately 70° F (21° C), whenever possible.
      c. Wear clothing appropriate to weather:
         (1) Lightweight, "breathable" clothing in hot weather
         (2) Warm layered clothing in cold weather
         (3) Hat to protect from heat and cold
      d. Use water spray bottle in hot weather to cool the body.
      e. Adequate fluid intake in hot weather
      f. Individuals with multiple sclerosis may find commercially available "cooling garments" helpful. These consist of cooled gel strips sewn into a vest.
      g. Avoid alcohol
   2. Management to conserve body heat during hypothermia
      a. Monitor vital signs frequently.
      b. Monitor closely for cardiac arrhythmias.
      c. Provide hot beverage, warm bath, warmed blankets.
      d. Keep the skin dry to prevent heat loss. Change bed linens or clothing as frequently as needed.
      e. Do not use hot water bottles or electric heating devices which may burn desensitized skin.
   3. Management to dissipate body heat during hyperthermia
      a. Monitor vital signs frequently.
      b. Provide cool beverages.
      c. Give cool sponge bath and apply cool moist compresses to neck, axilla, and groin areas
      d. Use fan or air conditioning
      e. Should shivering occur (generates heat), stop cooling measures.
      f. Replace fluids lost through profuse sweating to prevent dehydration and electrolyte imbalance.
      g. Monitor fluid and electrolyte balance
      h. Monitor urinary output
      i. Give O_2 as necessary due to increased tissue needs and metabolic rate
      j. Identify and treat cause of excessive diaphoresis.
      k. Differentiate cause of elevated temperature due to environmental factors from fever associated with infection, DVT, or emboli. (Zejdlik, 1992).

VI. Nursing Process Applied to Autonomic Dysreflexia (AD)

A. **Nursing Diagnosis:** Autonomic Dysreflexia and associated knowledge deficits

B. **Defining Characteristics:** Individuals with SCI, generally at or above the T6 level, may exhibit one or more of the following characteristics related to AD. Symptoms may be minimal or even absent, despite an elevated blood pressure (American Association of Spinal Cord Injury Nurses, 1996; Consortium for Spinal Cord Medicine, 1997a).
1. Headache which may become severe or pounding
2. Flushing and/or diaphoresis, usually above (or possibly below) the level of the spinal cord lesion
3. Elevated systolic and diastolic blood pressure, greater than 20 mm to 40 mm Hg above baseline
   Note: Normal blood pressure for persons with quadriplegia may be as low as 70/40; a BP of 130/80 would be considered hypertensive for these individuals.
4. Bradycardia
5. Goose bumps, usually above (or possibly below) the level of the spinal cord lesion
6. Chills without fever
7. Nasal congestion
8. Changes in vision - blurred, tunnel
9. Anxiety/apprehension
10. Bronchospasm

C. **Expected Outcomes** (American Association of Spinal Cord Injury Nurses, 1996; Rehabilitation Nursing Foundation of the Association of Rehabilitation Nurses, 1995):
1. Individuals who are at risk will be free of, or experience minimal, episodes of AD.
2. Prevention/management of AD episodes
3. Prevention of complications related to AD
4. Individuals at risk, family, caregivers are knowledgeable of and able to recognize signs and symptoms of AD.
5. Individual and family/caregivers are knowledgeable of causative factors, prevention, and management of AD.

D. **Interventions:** AD poses a serious threat to individuals with SCI, and without prompt intervention may lead to death (American Association of Spinal Cord Injury Nurses, 1996; Consortium for Spinal Cord Medicine, 1997a).
1. Awareness of risk factors/symptoms (include in initial assessment and reassessments)
   a. Level of SCI T6 or above
   b. Any recent episodes of AD and known causative stimulus
   c. Episodes of headache
   d. Systolic and diastolic blood pressure elevation greater than 20 mm to 40 mm Hg above baseline. Blood pressure elevation is usually associated with bradycardia.
   e. Altered bladder/bowel function or management. Bladder/urologic dysfunction accounts for 90 percent of the episodes of AD. The next most common cause is bowel overdistention (Dunn, 1991).
   f. Altered skin integrity
   g. Pain/pressure (identify location and source if possible)
   h. Current medications
   i. Females: labor and delivery (should be referred to an appropriate practitioner)
2. Awareness/detection of precipitating factors:
   a. Bladder/Genitourinary System:
      Bladder overdistention, urinary tract infection, bladder or kidney stones, invasive testing, urinary sphincter spasms, scrotal compression, epididymitis
   b. Bowel/Gastrointestinal System:
      Bowel distention/impaction, gallstones, gastric ulcers/gastritis, invasive testing, hemorrhoids, gastrocolic irritation, appendicitis, abdominal pathology/trauma.

    c. Skin:

       Pressure ulcers/treatment, ingrown toenail, burns/sunburn, blisters, insect bites, contact with hard or sharp objects

    d. Cardiovascular System:

       Deep vein thrombosis, pulmonary embolus

    e. Reproductive System:

       Menstruation, pregnancy (especially labor and delivery) (Wanner, Rageth & Zack, 1987), vaginitis, sexual intercourse, ejaculation

    f. Other Precipitating Factors:

       Constrictive clothes/shoes/appliances, heterotopic bone, fractures/trauma, surgical/diagnostic procedures, pain, temperature fluctuations

    g. Any stimuli that would cause pain or discomfort in an able-bodied individual with intact sensation (American Association of Spinal Cord Injury Nurses, 1996).

3. Prevention of AD episodes (American Association of Spinal Cord Injury Nurses, 1996).

    a. Monitor urinary output and make necessary changes to the bladder management program to prevent overdistention.

    b. Assess for urinary tract infection, acquire appropriate treatment, and evaluate effectiveness.

    c. Monitor bowel program and make necessary changes to the program to prevent constipation or impaction (Dunn, 1991; Erickson, 1980).

    d. Provide appropriate skin and wound care to prevent noxious stimuli (Erickson, 1980; Hall & Young, 1983).

    e. Provide other treatment measures as appropriate to alleviate the causes of noxious stimuli.

    f. Provide the individual and family/caregiver with educational information regarding AD.

    g. Assess the individual's, and family/caregiver's ability to prevent, recognize, and manage AD.

    h. Provide information regarding AD: medic alert bracelet or necklace, wallet card.

    i. Collaborate with physician regarding administration of nifedipine prior to genitourinary or gastrointestinal invasive diagnostic procedures.

4. Treatment of AD episodes (American Association of Spinal Cord Injury Nurses, 1996):

    a. Monitor blood pressure and pulse every 2-3 minutes throughout episode

    b. Elevate head to 90 degree angle; place legs in dependent position if practical.

    c. Loosen constrictive clothing, and/or appliances, remove all vascular support (ace wraps, elastic stockings, abdominal binder).

    d. The most common cause of AD is bladder distention. Beginning with the urinary system, assess and remove stimuli in this order until cause is found and eliminated:

    e. Individuals with indwelling foley catheter

       (1) Check for bladder overdistention

       (2) Remove any catheter or tubing kinks, mucous plugs, urethral constriction, or obstructions to urine flow; check for correct catheter placement.

       (3) If catheter blockage is suspected, gently irrigate with sterile fluid, such as normal saline at body temperature, (total volume not to exceed 30 cc), to prevent exacerbation of symptoms. Do not manually compress or tap the bladder.

       (4) If indwelling catheter remains plugged after irrigation, remove catheter and replace. If readily available, instill an anesthetic jelly into the urethra before inserting the new catheter.

    f. Individuals with an external collection device or no indwelling catheter.

       (1) Remove the external collection device

       (2) Catheterize, using anesthetic jelly if readily available. Empty the bladder by draining up to 500 cc of urine, clamping the catheter for 5 minutes, and repeating until bladder is emptied to prevent a rebound hypotensive effect.

    g. If systolic BP is greater than 140 to 150 mm Hg, apply one inch of nitropaste (15 mg) to the skin above the level of injury, per physician's order, to control BP as a temporary measure until the cause of AD can be identified.

    Note: Aggressive management of hypertension (use of antihypertensive agents) should not occur unless systolic pressure is above 140 to 150 mm Hg, to prevent rebound hypotension after the episode of AD is resolved.

h. Reassess blood pressure every 2 to 3 minutes, monitoring for hypertension as well as rebound hypotension, throughout the intervention process. Remove nitropaste and wash skin if the systolic BP is below 100 mm Hg

i. With a gloved, well-lubricated finger, insert anesthetic ointment or jelly into the rectal vault. Allow 3 to 5 minutes for anesthetic to work. Gently remove any stool from the rectal vault. If AD worsens, stop manual evacuation. Instill additional topical anesthetic and recheck for stool after approximately 20 minutes (Consortium for Spinal Cord Medicine, 1997a).

j. Reposition individual to alleviate twisted extremities and/or painful position.

k. Examine for pressure ulcers or other skin irritations. If open wounds are present, spray or apply an anesthetic ointment to open areas.

l. Observe for sensitivity to wrinkled sheets, ingrown toenails, or other noxious stimuli. Remove stimuli.

m. If systolic BP is greater than 150-160 mm Hg, per physician's order, administer antihypertensive agent, with rapid onset and short duration (American Association of Spinal Cord Injury Nurses, 1996; Consortium for Spinal Cord Medicine 1997a).

n. Evaluate for additional precipitating factors and follow-up as necessary if the above actions do not alleviate AD.

o. Refer individual to a monitored emergency specialty care area if the episode is unresolved.

5. Continuing care (American Association of Spinal Cord Injury Nurses, 1996; Consortium for Spinal Cord Medicine, 1997a):

a. Continue to monitor BP and pulse every 2 to 3 minutes until parameters have returned to baseline. Continue to observe and record BP and pulse every 15 minutes for minimum of one hour; then measure and record every 30 minutes for 2 to 3 hours.

b. Monitor for recurrence of any AD symptoms

c. Perform neurologic examination during and after any significant hypertensive AD episode.

d. Once the individual with AD has been stabilized, review the precipitating cause with the individual, family members, caregivers, and health care team in order to prevent future episodes.

e. Individuals who experience recurrent episodes of AD should be referred to SCI practitioners for further evaluation and health education as well as appropriate medical treatment.

VII. Nursing Process Applied to Deep Vein Thrombosis (DVT)

A. **Nursing Diagnosis:** Altered tissue perfusion (peripheral) and associated alterations in mobility and knowledge deficit.

B. **Defining Characteristics:**
1. Fever, frequently low grade (often occurring at night) and of unknown origin, may indicate thrombus formation.
2. Warmth, swelling, redness, pain, tenderness, or heaviness in an extremity, usually unilateral lower extremity presentation
3. An increase in the venous pattern of collateral veins in the affected extremity
4. Possible increase in spasticity of affected limb
5. Symptoms of pulmonary embolus include dyspnea, tachypnea, shortness of breath, feelings of chest compression or chest pain, crackles upon lung auscultation, unexplained fever, tachycardia, cough, hemoptysis, anxiety and/or apprehension.

C. **Expected Outcomes:**
1. Prevention of occurrence/recurrence of DVT/PE
2. Improved venous blood flow

3. Coagulation studies within desired range
4. Individual/caregiver are knowledgeable of risk factors and preventive measures associated with occurrence of DVT/PE

D. **Interventions:**
1. In addition to assessment measures as described in the initial assessment:
   a. Compare legs and closely observe for swelling, redness and/or warmth (usually unilateral).
   b. Obtain baseline lower-extremity measurements upon admission and continue serial leg (calf and thigh) measurements daily in patients at high risk of thrombophlebitis, especially during 3-5 weeks post-injury or if DVT is suspected (Zejdlik, 1992).
   c. Closely observe for symptoms of PE
   d. Be aware of food/drug interactions, which may potentiate or inhibit anticoagulants. Oral anticoagulants especially, tend to have interactions with many drugs.
2. Prevention to promote venous return and inhibit formation of thrombi:
   a. Range of motion exercises and early mobilization
   b. Compression hose or pneumatic devices should be applied to the legs of at-risk individuals as well as individuals during the first two weeks following acute SCI. If thromboprophylaxis has been delayed for more than 72 hours following acute SCI, tests to exclude the presence of thrombi should be performed prior to applying compression devices (The Consortium for Spinal Cord Medicine, 1997b). Compression modalities should be inspected for proper placement and removed every eight hours to check the underlying skin for evidence of abrasions, pressure ulcers, ecchymosis, or other injury.
   c. Avoid constricting urinary leg bag straps, garters, tight knee high boots, girdles, or overly tight socks, stockings, or slacks
   d. Correct positioning and turning to prevent gravitational edema and localized pressure on limbs and venous structures
   e. Prevention of dehydration, monitor intake and output as needed.
   f. Prophylactic low dose anticoagulants are administered per physician order. Baseline partial thromboplastin time, prothrombin time, and platelet count are obtained before coagulation therapy is initiated. Individuals should be monitored for thrombocytopenia, signs of bleeding including epistaxis, hematoma, hematuria, melena, and/or decrease in hemoglobin or hematocrit (Consortium for Spinal Cord Medicine, 1997b).
   g. No smoking
   h. Exercise and weight loss if applicable
   i. Birth control pills may be contraindicated.
3. If DVT is suspected or confirmed:
   a. Maintain bedrest and minimize lower-extremity movement until diagnosis is confirmed, appropriate therapy implemented, and further activity orders are obtained.
   b. Elevate affected limb with hip and knee extended, being careful not to exert pressure on popliteal space, to promote circulation.
   c. Prepare patient for diagnostic tests.
   d. Administer anticoagulant medication as ordered.
   e. Monitor coagulation blood studies as ordered.
   f. Observe closely for hematomas or signs of frank bleeding in sputum, nasogastric drainage, urine, and stool (Zejdlik, 1992).
   g. Vena cava filters may be indicated in some individuals (Consortium for Spinal Cord Medicine, 1997b).
4. Individual/caregiver education regarding:
   a. Risk factors, prevention, and symptoms of occurrence/recurrence of DVT/PE
   b. Medication management and monitoring of patient on long-term anticoagulation therapy
   c. Food and drug interactions with anticoagulants

VIII. Reassessment

In addition to initial assessment measures associated with cardiovascular function and body temperature regulation, important reassessment factors include the following:

A. In general, individuals with cervical and high thoracic complete lesions are at greatest risk for conditions related to cardiovascular disorders and body temperature alteration.

B. Although cardiovascular function does improve following spinal shock phase, the individual continues to be at risk of complications associated with cardiovascular and thermoregulatory dysfunction. Lifelong reassessment is a necessity.

C. Generally, a lower body temperature, lower blood pressure, and lower pulse rate often persist in SCI. A baseline blood pressure of 90/60, pulse rate of 60, or temperature of 97-98° F is common. Documentation of "normal" baseline vital signs for the individual and ongoing monitoring are necessary.

D. With aging, concomitant cardiovascular disorders, and increased cardiac demands, cardiac reserve may be compromised and venous elasticity may decrease, putting the older individual at greater risk of autonomic disorders and DVT as well as development of cardiac insufficiency. It is therefore of importance that particular emphasis be placed upon ongoing cardiovascular assessment of the aging individual with SCI, as well as those with concomitant or preexisting cardiovascular disease.

E. Ongoing reassessment of functional ability/mobility and lifestyle are necessary, as the individual whose lifestyle is inactive or sedentary is at greater risk of cardiovascular complications.

F. Monitoring of medication regimes and their relation to cardiovascular function should be part of ongoing reassessment.

G. Reassessment should include history of recent or remote occurrence of orthostatic hypotension, thermoregulatory problems, DVT, and AD symptoms.

H. Bowel and bladder management problems should be included in ongoing reassessment.

I. Risks associated with poor nutrition, obesity, and substance abuse should be part of the reassessment.

IX. Health Tips

Prevention, early symptom recognition, and prompt management of cardiovascular and thermoregulatory dysfunction are the key in regard to these complications. General health promotion strategies are of particular importance for the individual with SCI, these include:

A. Maintain an active lifestyle, which includes a regular exercise program to promote circulation and maintain existing tone.

B. Maintain a well-balanced diet that is rich in fiber and low in cholesterol and calories. Maintain a desirable weight. Individuals with diabetes should maintain blood sugar control.

C. Promote venous return through intermittent lower-extremity elevation, passive/active exercises, elastic stockings or hose, and abdominal binder if necessary.

D. Maintain adequate fluid intake to prevent dehydration, orthostatic hypotension, and hyperthermia.

E. Maintain appropriate and adequate bowel and bladder management programs to prevent AD.

F. Dress appropriately for the environment, and maintain indoor temperature at a comfortable level. Use effective and appropriate warming and cooling measures.

G. No smoking; avoid alcohol/drug abuse.

H. Annual health exams are of vital importance and should focus upon wellness and health promotion as well as factors specific to SCI.

X. Special Issues Related to Pediatric Care

A. **Nursing Process:** The nursing process applied to cardiovascular and thermoregulatory control in children is similar to that in adult care. The incidence of syndromes and complications may differ in the pediatric population.

B. **Special Considerations:** Children are particularly sensitive to the following:
   1. Bradycardia
      a. Acute bradycardia initially following SCI is frequent.
      b. Children may require placement of cardiac pacemaker (Gilgoff, Ward, & Hohn, 1991).
   2. Orthostatic Hypotension
      a. Common acute problem
      b. Orthostatic hypotension may recur after periods of illness.
   3. Altered Body Temperature
      a. Infants are at greatest risk because of increased body surface area.
      b. Children need to learn how to dress appropriately for the environment. All caregivers must be aware of overheating.
   4. Autonomic Dysreflexia
      a. Episodes may be more difficult to detect, as children demonstrate only vague complaints.
      b. Children may be limited in their ability to describe symptoms and express feelings.
   5. Deep Vein Thrombosis
      a. Children are less likely to experience DVT.
      b. Athletic adolescents are at greater risk.
      c. Prophylactic medication is generally not used for children under 12 years.

Practical Application

D.G. is a 24 year old male with T4 complete paraplegia who was injured in a motor vehicle accident six weeks earlier. He was progressing well in his rehabilitation program at a spinal cord injury center. D.G. was participating in his daily physical therapy program when his therapist noticed that D.G. was flushed and perspiring profusely about his face, neck, and shoulders. The physical therapist asked D.G. how he felt and he replied that he had a headache. The therapist checked D.G.'s blood pressure, which was 144/98. The therapist immediately returned D.G. to the rehab unit and alerted his nurse, who rechecked D.G.'s blood pressure which was 160/108, and a pulse rate of 58. She knew his baseline blood pressure generally ranged from 90-100/60-70 and a pulse rate that ranged from 70-80. He then described his headache as more severe and "pounding." D.G.'s nurse notified his physician that D.G. was having symptoms of autonomic dysreflexia. She put him in bed, removed his compression hose, raised the head of the bed to 90 degrees, and rechecked D.G.'s blood pressure, which was 156/100, and a pulse rate of 62. Per order of his physician, the nurse applied one inch of nitropaste (15 mg) to D.G.'s upper chest. D.G.'s bladder had been managed with intermittent catheterization, without any spontaneous voiding. His prior catheterization was four hours earlier. D.G. told his nurse that he had consumed more fluids than usual before he went to therapy that morning. The nurse immediately instilled anesthetic jelly into D.G.'s urethra and catheterized him. After obtaining 500 cc of urine she clamped the catheter and rechecked D.G.'s blood pressure, which was 134/88, and a pulse of 68. He stated the headache was subsiding, he was less flushed and diaphoretic. After 5 minutes, she unclamped the catheter and another 350 cc of urine was obtained. D.G.'s blood pressure was 108/72, and a pulse rate of 74. D.G.'s nurse removed the nitropaste and continued to monitor his blood pressure every 15 minutes for one hour and then every 30 minutes for the next two hours. His vital signs returned to baseline; headache, flushing, and diaphoresis subsided.

D.G. and his nurse discussed the possible cause of the dysreflexic event and decided that his fluid intake of greater than 800 cc that morning had precipitated the episode. D.G. agreed to maintain a fluid restriction of not greater that 2000 cc in 24 hours and to increment his fluids appropriately throughout the day. D.G. and his family participated in the SCI education program, which included a class and literature pertaining to autonomic dysreflexia.

References and Selected Bibliography

American Association of Spinal Cord Injury Nurses (1996). *Clinical practice guideline: Autonomic dysreflexia*. Jackson Heights, NY: American Association of Spinal Cord Injury Nurses.

Braddom, R.L., & Rocco, J.F. (1991). Autonomic dysreflexia: A survey of current treatment. *American Journal of Physical Medicine & Rehabilitation, 70*(5), 234-241.

Carabasi, R.A., Moritz, M.J., & Jarrell, B.E. (1987). Complications encountered with the use of the Greenfield filter. *American Journal of Surgery, 154,* 163-168

Chiou-Tan, F.Y., Lenz, M.L., Robertson, C.S., & Grabois, M. (1994). Pharmacologic treatment of autonomic dysreflexia in the rat. *American Journal of Physical Medicine & Rehabilitation, 73*(4), 251-255.

Cohen, J.A., Hossack, K.F., & Franklin, G.M. (1989). Multiple sclerosis patients with fatigue: Relationship among temperature regulation, autonomic dysfunction, and exercise capacity. *Journal of Neurologic Rehabilitation, 3*(4), 193-197.

Colachis, S.C. (1992). Autonomic hyperreflexia with spinal cord injury. *Journal of the American Paraplegia Society, 15,* 171-186.

Colachis, S.C., & Otis, S.M. (1995). Occurrence of fever associated with thermoregulatory dysfunction after acute traumatic spinal cord injury. *American Journal of Physical Medicine & Rehabilitation, 74*(2), 114-119.

Consortium for Spinal Cord Medicine. (1997a). *Clinical practice guidelines. Acute management of autonomic dysreflexia: Adults with spinal cord injury presenting to health-care facilities.* Washington, DC: Paralyzed Veterans of America.

Consortium for Spinal Cord Medicine. (1997b). *Clinical practice guidelines. Prevention of thromboembolism in spinal cord injury.* Washington, DC: Paralyzed Veterans of America.

DeVivo, M.J. & Stover, S.L. (1995). Long term survival and causes of death. In S.L. Stover, J.A. DeLisa, & G.G. Whiteneck (Eds.), *Spinal cord injury: Clinical outcomes from the Model Systems* (pp. 289-316). Gaithersburg, MD: Aspen.

Dunn, K.L. (1991). Autonomic dysreflexia: A nursing challenge in the care of the patient with spinal cord injury. *Journal of Cardiovascular Nursing, 5*(4), 57-63.

Erickson, R.P. (1980). Autonomic hyperreflexia: Pathophysiology and medical management. *Archives of Physical Medicine and Rehabilitation 61,* 431-440.

Fowler, S.B. (1995). Deep vein thrombosis and pulmonary emboli in neuroscience patients. *Journal of Neuroscience Nursing 27,* 224-228.

Freed, M.M. (1990). Traumatic and congenital lesions of the spinal cord. In F. J. Kottke & J. F. Lehmann (Eds.). *Krusen's handbook of physical medicine and rehabilitation* (pp. 717-748). Philadelphia: W. B. Saunders.

Gilgoff, I., Ward, S., & Hohn, A. (1991). Cardiac pacemaker in high spinal cord injury. *Archives of Physical Medicine and Rehabilitation, 72,* 601-603.

Givre, S., & Freed, H.A. (1989). Autonomic dysreflexia: A potentially fatal complication of somatic stress in quadriplegics. *Journal of Emergency Medicine, 7,* 461-463.

Grossman, E., Messerli, F.H., Grodzicki, T., & Kowey, P. (1996). Should a moratorium be placed on sublingual nifedipine capsules given for hypertensive emergencies and pseudoemergencies? *JAMA, 276*, 1328-1331.

Guyton, A.C., & Hall J.E. (1997). *Human physiology and mechanisms of disease* (6th ed.). Philadelphia: W. B. Saunders.

Hall, P.A., & Young, J.V. (1983). Autonomic hyperreflexia in spinal cord injured patients: Trigger mechanisms, dressing changes of pressure sores. *Journal of Trauma, 23*, 1074-1075.

Herzog, J.A. (1992). Deep vein thrombosis in the rehabilitation client. *Rehabilitation Nursing, 17*, 196-198.

Hickey, J.V. (1986). *The clinical practice of neurological and neurosurgical nursing* (2nd ed.). Philadelphia: J.B. Lippincott.

Laskowski-Jones, L. (1993). Acute SCI: How to minimize the damage. *American Journal of Nursing, 93*(12), 22-32.

Lee, B.Y., Karmaker, M.G., Hertz, B.L., & Sturgill, R.A. (1995). Autonomic dysreflexia revisited. *Journal of Spinal Cord Medicine, 18*, 75-87.

Lehmann, K.G., Lane, J.G., Piepmeier, J.M., & Batsford, W.P. (1987). Cardiovascular abnormalities accompanying acute spinal cord injury in humans: Incidence, time course and severity. *Journal of the American College of Cardiology, 10*(1), 46-52.

Lindan, R., Joiner, E., Freehafer, A.A., & Hazel, C. (1980). Incidence and clinical features of autonomic dysreflexia in patients with spinal cord injury. *Paraplegia, 18*, 285-292

Molitor, L. (1988). Triage decisions: An adult male with spinal cord injury and hypotension and bradycardia. *Journal of Emergency Nursing, 14*(5), 324-325.

Niederpruem, M. S. (1989). Controlling body temperature. In S. Dittmar (Ed.), *Rehabilitation nursing: Process and application* (pp. 120-133). St. Louis, MO: C.V. Mosby.

Nolan, S. (1994). Current trends in the management of acute spinal cord injury. *Critical Care Nursing Quarterly, 17*(1), 64-78.

Perkash, A., Sullivan, G.H., Toth, L., Bradleigh, L.H., & Linder, S. H . (1993). Persistent hypercoagulation associated with heterotopic ossification with spinal cord injury. *Paraplegia, 31*, 653-659.

Ragnarsson, K., Hall, K.M., Wilmot, C. B., (1995). Management of pulmonary, cardiovascular, and metabolic conditions after spinal cord injury. In S. L. Stover, J. A. DeLisa, and G. G. Whiteneck (Eds.), *Spinal cord injury: Clinical outcomes from the Model Systems* (pp. 79-99). Gaithersburg, MD: Aspen.

Rehabilitation Nursing Foundation of the Association of Rehabilitation Nurses (1995). Autonomic dysfunction. In Faculty manual for basic rehabilitation nursing practice, *Rehabilitation nursing: Directions for practice.* (pp. 201-207). Skokie, IL: Rehabilitation Nursing Foundation of the Association of Rehabilitation Nurses.

Sawka, M.N., Latzka, W.A., & Pandolf, K.B. (1989). Temperature regulation during upper body exercise: Able-bodied and spinal cord injured. *Medicine and Science in Sports and Exercise, 21*(5 Suppl), S132-140.

Spoltore, T.A., & O'Brien, A.M. (1995). Rehabilitation of the spinal cord injured patient. *Orthopaedic Nursing, 14,* 7-15.

Syndulko, K, Jafari, M, Woldanski, A., Baumhefner, R.W., & Tourtellotte, W. W. (1996). Effects of temperature in multiple sclerosis: A review of the literature. *Journal of Neurological Rehabilitation, 10*(1), 23-31.

Wanner, M.B., Rageth, C.J., & Zack, G.A. (1987). Pregnancy and autonomic hyperreflexia in patients with spinal cord lesions. *Paraplegia 25,* 482-490.

Wirtz, K.M., La Favor, K.M., & Ang, R. (1996). Managing chronic spinal cord injury: Issues in critical care. *Critical Care Nurse 16* (4), 24-37.

Yarkony, G.M., Katz, R.T., & Wu, Y. C. (1986). Seizures secondary to autonomic dysreflexia. *Archives of Physical Medicine and Rehabilitation, 67,* 834-835.

Zejdlik, C. P. (Ed.) (1992). *Management of spinal cord injury* (2nd ed.). Boston: Jones & Bartlett.

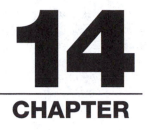

CHAPTER

Bladder Elimination and Continence
Jan Giroux, MSN, RN-C, CURN

I. Learning Objectives

A. Describe the anatomy and physiology of the urinary tract.

B. Describe the neurologic innervation of the urinary tract.

C. Describe laboratory, radiographic and urodynamic studies (UDS) utilized in assessment of urologic function in individuals with spinal cord impairment (SCI).

D. Describe prevention and management of urinary complications in individuals with SCI.

E. Identify nursing diagnoses for the individual with SCI.

F. Describe nursing interventions in bladder management techniques for individuals with SCI.

G. Describe management options for individuals with SCI including behavioral, pharmacologic, and surgical interventions.

II. Introduction

A. **Scope of the Chapter:** Urinary incontinence can be caused by pathological, anatomical, or physiological factors affecting the genitourinary tract (Agency for Health Care Policy and Research (AHCPR), 1996). Neurogenic bladder dysfunction caused by SCI affects the physiological functioning of the lower urinary tract. Dysfunctional voiding problems generally manifest clinically as either urinary incontinence (failure to store) or urinary retention (failure to empty) or a combination of both. Continence and normal micturition is a complex process that involves the bladder, urethra, the periurethral striated muscle, and the central and peripheral nervous systems. Any disorder that affects the normal physiological function of any of these systems can cause incontinence. The focus of this chapter is bladder dysfunction caused by SCI. Elements of the nursing process and the importance of nursing management to assist the individual with SCI to preserve the upper urinary tract will be discussed. If not managed properly, complications such as symptomatic bacteriuria, autonomic dysreflexia, hydronephrosis, and urinary calculi disease can compromise renal function in these individuals and lead to an increase in illness and death rates. Nurses in all care settings, working with individuals with SCI need to understand the importance of monitoring lower urinary tract function, as it determines the fate of the upper tracts (Steele, 1993). The successful outcome of a bladder retraining program depends on a realistic plan maximizing involvement of the individual with SCI, family, and the health care team. These individuals require regular, long-term follow-up to minimize complications associated with a neurogenic bladder. Autonomic dsyreflexia will be briefly mentioned as it relates to bladder involvement but will be extensively covered in Chapter 13.

B. **Demographics**
   1. 10-35 percent of adults have voiding disorders (AHCPR, 1996).
   2. Urinary incontinence imposes tremendous social and economic burden, annual cost estimated between 12 and 15 billion dollars (Tanagho, 1995).

C. **Etiology/Precipitating Factors:** Urinary continence is the ability to exert voluntary control over the urge to urinate. Individuals with neurological disease or injury may be unable to achieve urinary continence because they do not receive or are unaware of the signals indicating the need to urinate, or they are unable to control the urge until it is acceptable to empty their bladder. Incontinence is not a disease, but a symptom which represents a significant health problem and may indicate a serious underlying disease process. Such entities can affect the normal structures of the urinary system, afferent or efferent neural pathways, or the cortical control centers. Bladder dysfunction due to interruption of the neural pathways is termed neurogenic bladder.
   1. Neurogenic bladder represents one of the most common problems in individuals with a variety of neurologic disorders.
   2. Urinary incontinence increases risk of complications such as urinary tract infection (UTI), skin breakdown, and social isolation.
   3. Neurogenic bladder disorders include traumatic and non-traumatic lesions of the spinal cord, multiple sclerosis, stroke, demyelinating disease, tumor, and diabetes mellitus.
   4. Bladder dysfunction causes disturbances in the normal micturition process that affects either the filling and storage or emptying capability of the bladder.

D. **Anatomy**
   1. Kidneys: maintain internal homeostasis through fluid and electrolyte balance, serum pH levels and excretion of by-products of metabolism.
   2. Ureters: transport urine from kidneys to bladder through peristaltic action.
   3. Ureterovesical junction: muscular, one-way valve-like structure, which allows efflux of urine into bladder and prevents reflux of urine into the ureters.
   4. Bladder: hollow, smooth muscle organ, which stores and expels urine.
   5. Urethra: serves as conduit for urine expulsion during micturition and maintenance of continence during bladder filling.
      a. Internal sphincter: Located at the bladder neck, has function of closing off the bladder neck in the resting state and maintaining continence; is not under voluntary control.
      b. External sphincter: Striated skeletal muscle surrounding the urethra, which can be voluntarily relaxed and contracted.
   6. Urinary meatus: Opening of the urethra.

E. **Physiology:** The neurologic control of micturition involves the micturition reflex, sympathetic and parasympathetic nerve supply, and cerebral centers involved in voiding (Figure 14-1).
   1. Micturition reflex: Includes a sequence of events that lead to voiding in absence of voluntary inhibition. Normal voiding involves effective bladder contraction coordinated with relaxation of urethral sphincters. This sequence of events provides free flow of urine and prevents reflux. Bladder fills with urine and maintains low intravesical pressure with

increasing volumes. As bladder fills to 300-400 ml of urine, stretch receptors in the bladder wall send sensory impulses through the pelvic nerves to the sacral cord segments (S2-S4). Sensory messages are sent from spinal cord to higher centers in cerebral cortex through spinothalamic tracts and posterior columns. Inhibitory centers in frontal lobe can override micturition reflex by voluntarily contracting the external sphincter via pudendal nerve. Messages of fullness and urge to void are processed in pons and cortex. When appropriate to void, motor messages are sent through corticoregulatory tract to sacral reflex center. Peripheral nervous system relays messages via parasympathetic and somatic fibers, which stimulate detrusor contraction, external sphincter relaxation, and bladder emptying.

2. Central (cerebral) innervation: frontal cerebral cortex facilitates or inhibits pontine micturition center.

3. Parasympathetic innervation: S2-S4 segments provide motor stimulation to bladder and facilitate detrusor contraction and bladder neck relaxation via pelvic nerve.

4. Sympathetic innervation: originates in T11-L2 segments, allows bladder to fill while maintaining contraction of internal bladder neck sphincter via the hypogastric plexus (Emick-Herring, 1993).

F. **Classification of Neurogenic Bladder:** Several classifications of voiding dysfunction exist. The Wein classification describes voiding dysfunction as a storage problem, emptying problem, and/or combination of storage and emptying problems. Disruption of sensory or motor pathways in the central or peripheral nervous system will cause dysfunction in bladder filling and emptying. The classification of voiding dysfunction is formulated on a functional basis describing whether the deficit is primarily one of the filling/storage or of the emptying phase of micturition (Wein, 1981).

1. Bladder filling and urine storage requires:

Figure 14-1

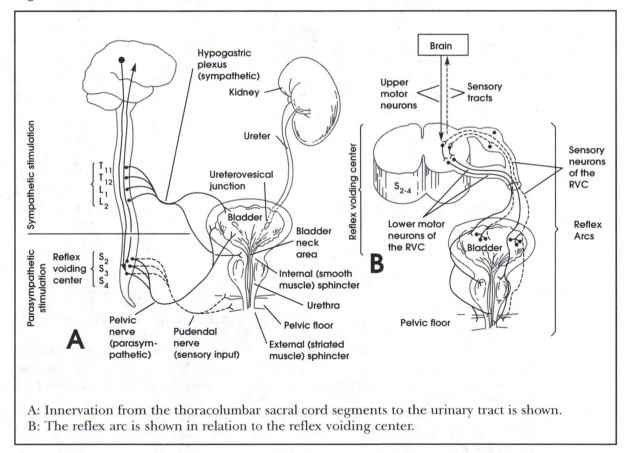

A: Innervation from the thoracolumbar sacral cord segments to the urinary tract is shown.
B: The reflex arc is shown in relation to the reflex voiding center.

From Management of Spinal Cord Injury (2nd ed., p. 355), by C.P. Zejdlik, 1992, Boston: Jones & Bartlett. Copyright 1992 Jones & Bartlett. Reprinted with permission.

    a. Accommodation of increasing volumes of urine at low intravesical pressure and with appropriate sensation.

    b. Closed bladder outlet at rest, which continues during increases in intra-abdominal pressure.

    c. Absence of involuntary bladder contractions.

2. Bladder emptying requires:

    a. Lowering of resistance in the proximal urethra and at the striated urethral sphincter, coordinated with

    b. Contraction by the bladder smooth muscle sufficient to generate a substantial increase in intravesical pressure and

    c. Absence of anatomic obstruction (Steers, Barrett & Wein, 1996).

III. Initial Assessment

A. **Nursing History:** Ascertain the individual's cognitive and affective status, level and completeness of injury, and any associated injuries. Inquire about past health status/history, preexisting urinary complications/surgeries or conditions, preexisting disease/medical condition, and any allergies. Medications, including over-the-counter, and drug or alcohol use are important to assess. Document present method of bladder management, awareness of bladder fullness, voiding pattern/diary, and dietary/fluid intake. Note the individual's living environment, mobility, manual dexterity, and age. In females, obtain the dates of the last menstrual period and a gynecological history.

B. **Examination**

1. Vital signs: May show signs of hypotension, bradycardia, or lowered body temperature (especially cervical injuries) due to spinal shock.

2. Inspection: lower abdomen observed for fullness, asymmetry, swelling, inflammation, lacerations, bruises, scars. Perineal/genital area observed for trauma, bruising, swelling, bleeding, lesions, maceration, excoriation. In females, assess for signs of hypoestrogenism such as atrophy of the vulvar skin, and for loss of the posterior portion of the labia, vaginal infection, or menstruation. In males, examine the penis and scrotal folds for skin ulceration. Retract the foreskin in uncircumcised males to expose the glans penis. Urethra is observed for: bleeding, discharge, meatal lesions/injury, position of meatus. Observe urine color, amount, clarity, odor, pH, hematuria, spontaneous voiding.

3. Auscultation: Of limited value to assess urinary function unless severe internal trauma or venous malformations are suspected. Bruits, swishing or blowing sounds are abnormal.

4. Palpation: Bladder is normally not palpable.

    a. When distended, bladder is felt as a smooth, round tense mass and can extend to umbilical region.

    b. Use caution in asensory patient, since gentle palpation may cause referred pain if area is traumatized internally.

5. Percussion of suprapubic area:

    a. Empty bladder produces tympanic sound.

    b. Distended bladder produces dull sound.

6. Vaginal/Rectal exam

    a. Vaginal exam: Assess for evidence of cystocele and presence of fistula.

    b. Rectal sphincter control: Assess for ability to contract or relax, presence of tumor, or fecal impaction.

    c. Bulbocavernous reflex: Tested by inserting a finger into the anus to detect anal sphincter contraction when the glans penis is squeezed in males. In females, the clitoris is pressed against the pubis, or indwelling foley catheter is gently pulled in order to elicit the reflex.

        (1) Positive reflex suggests voiding reflex is intact.

        (2) Absent in areflexic bladder and may be absent in spinal shock phase.

    d. Anal wink: Visible contraction of the anal sphincter immediately after a pinprick stimulus applied to the mucocutaneous junction of the anus.

    e. Palpation of prostate:
      (1) Enlargement
      (2) Consistency
      (3) Nodules
7. Sacral sparing/sensation
8. Intake and output
9. Post-void residual (PVR) urine
10. Observation of control, sensation, and voiding pattern
11. Assessment of functional abilities
12. Assessment and prompt treatment of autonomic dysreflexia (AD): Spinal cord injury individuals with level of injury at T6 and above are at risk. AD is considered a medical emergency and is most frequently related to bladder dysfunction (American Association of Spinal Cord Injury Nurses, 1996). With the return of bladder tone, bulbocavernous reflex, and beginning of spasticity, the potential for AD occurs (see Chapter 13 for an in depth review of autonomic dysreflexia). Causative factors for AD related to the genitourinary system include: bladder overdistension, urinary tract infection, bladder or kidney stones, invasive testing, urinary sphincter spasms, scrotal compression, and epididymitis.

C. **Diagnostic Studies**
1. Laboratory
    a. Urinalysis
    b. Urine culture and sensitivity
    c. Blood Urea Nitrogen (BUN) and Creatinine
    d. Creatinine clearance: 24-hour urine
2. Radiographic tests
    a. Intravenous urogram (IVU)
    b. Kidney, Ureter, Bladder (KUB) xray
    c. Cystoscopy
    d. Renal Ultrasound
    e. Voiding Cystourethrogram (VCU)
    f. Bladder ultrasound (bedside)
    g. Renal scan
3. Urodynamics studies (UDS): Diagnostic techniques to evaluate bladder and voiding problems. Generally performed after resolution of spinal shock. Focuses on the functions involved in bladder filling, storing, and emptying in terms of pressure of urine within the system, flow rate of urine, muscular activity, resistance factors calculated from pressure, and flow reading (Zejdlik, 1992). Urinary flow rate is a measure of the volume of urine expelled from the bladder via the urethra over a given period of time. It is calculated as milliliters per second. Calculation of flow rate may not be possible in an individual who is unable to spontaneously void.
    a. Cystometrogram (CMG): assesses how the bladder responds to filling and storage phase when gradually filled with water or carbon dioxide. Spinal cord injury individuals, T6 or above, must be assessed for any symptoms of autonomic dysreflexia. An individual with sensation is asked to indicate first sensation of bladder filling, first sensation of comfortable or moderate degree of bladder fullness, and definite fullness with need to void. CMG measures:
      (1) Sensation
      (2) Bladder capacity
      (3) Stability
      (4) Compliance (Gray, 1992)
    b. Urethral pressure profile (UPP):
      (1) Measures pressures along the length of urethra
      (2) Assesses competency of the urethra and sphincter
      (3) Demonstrates any weakness or hyperactivity in either the smooth or voluntary muscle
    c. Valsalva leak point pressure (LPP)
      (1) Test of outlet resistance

(2) Distinguishes intrinsic sphincter incompetence from pelvic descent

(3) May be assessed through intravesical or abdominal pressure (Gray & King, 1993).

d. Electromyography (EMG): Records electrical activity of striated muscles of pelvic floor. Evaluates the coordination of the external urethral sphincter and pelvic floor musculature with bladder activity during bladder filling and emptying. Two needles or wire electrodes are inserted into the periurethral muscle or anal sphincter for recording purposes. Surface electrodes can be used for individuals with perineal sensation. Detrusor-sphincter dyssynergia (DSD) can be assessed with EMG.

e. Videourodynamics:

(1) Simultaneous measurement of bladder and urethral pressures under fluoroscopic monitoring.

(2) Detrusor-external sphincter dyssynergia can be identified

(3) Bladder neck obstruction can be diagnosed (Watanabe, Rivas & Chancellor, 1996)

IV. Nursing Process Applied to Altered Patterns of Urinary Elimination Related to Failure to Empty.

A. **Nursing Diagnoses:**

1. Impaired skin integrity related to urinary incontinence
2. Risk for urinary complications related to method of bladder management
3. Alteration in self-concept
4. Risk for infection related to urinary obstruction and stasis
5. Knowledge deficit related to bladder management protocol

B. **Defining Characteristics:** Individuals with failure to empty may have suprasacral or sacral lesion, with or without incoordination of the voluntary external urinary sphincter muscle and the involuntary smooth muscle of the urethra and detrusor muscle (Dittmar, 1989). Motor paralytic bladder dysfunction (i.e., poliomyelitis, Guillain-Barre', trauma, and tumor) can affect failure to empty. Sensory paralytic bladder dysfunction (i.e., diabetes mellitus, spinal shock, and detrusor sphincter dyssynergia also cause failure to empty. Voiding maneuvers, intermittent catheterization, use of external collecting devices, absorbent products, indwelling catheters, pharmacologic management, behavioral strategies, surgical treatment options, and electrical stimulation are management techniques used to assist in bladder emptying. The method chosen depends upon the underlying neurologic dysfunction, as indicated by neurological/urological diagnostic testing, and the individual's functional status, preference, and level of cooperation. The individual with lower motor neuron bladder dysfunction, failure to empty, may exhibit some or all of the following characteristics:

1. Urinary retention, also seen in spinal shock phase
2. Suprapubic pain
3. Distended, palpable bladder
4. Overflow incontinence
5. Symptoms of autonomic dysreflexia in SCI individuals T6 or above
6. Frequency, urgency, nocturia
7. Frequent voiding in small amounts or absence of urine output
8. Sensation of bladder fullness
9. Dribbling
10. Increased bladder capacity with increased residual urine
11. Dysuria
12. Bladder bacteriuria
13. Unaware of normal bladder filling
14. Unable to initiate voiding
15. Intact or impaired saddle sensation (dependent on site of neurologic dysfunction)
16. Weakened detrusor
17. Spastic sphincter
18. Detrusor sphincter dyssynergia

C. **Expected Outcomes**
  1. Individual achieves acceptable bladder emptying by using appropriate bladder management techniques. The individual should be able to:
     a. Communicate an understanding of the signs, symptoms, and appropriate handling of urinary retention.
     b. Become free of urinary tract complications.
     c. Communicate an understanding of the signs, and symptoms, preventive and management actions of urinary tract infection (UTI).
     d. Communicate knowledge of prescribed medications and side effects.
     e. Understand cause of voiding dysfunction.
     f. Maintain skin integrity.
     g. Decrease or eliminate episodes of incontinence.
     h. Maintain renal function.
     i. Maintain self-esteem.
  2. Individual/family able to care for urostomy and appliance. The family unit/individual should be able to:
     a. Catheterize continent urinary diversion.
     b. Perform or direct intermittent catheterization (IC).
     c. Perform proper management of indwelling urethral/suprapubic catheter.
     d. Describe potential problems related to bladder management program and strategies for coping with these problems.
     e. Communicate need for regular urological follow-up care.
     f. Demonstrate sufficient knowledge concerning treatment options to enable them to participate in plan of care.
     g. Demonstrate application of external catheter and drainage system.
     h. Describe signs and symptoms of autonomic dysreflexia and appropriate actions to take.
     i. Demonstrate compliance and success with recommended management techniques for urinary incontinence and urinary retention.
     j. Describe goals and process of timed voiding schedule and fluid intake control.

D. **Interventions**
  1. Assess for bladder distention. Use of bladder ultrasound is beneficial and eliminates unnecessary catheterizations.
  2. Monitor intake and output (I & O).
  3. Assess/monitor voiding pattern.
  4. Establish a voiding schedule.
  5. Initiate bladder training or reconditioning program.
  6. Teach individual/family potential side effects of medication and strategies to counteract or eliminate these effects.
  7. Assist individual to minimize or reverse specific risk factors for urinary calculi.
  8. Assess for signs and symptoms of urinary tract infections/colonization.
     a. Urinary tract infection: bacteriuria with tissue invasion and resultant tissue response with signs and/or symptoms.
     b. Asymptomatic bacteriuria: colonization of urinary tract with no reference to signs or symptoms. (National Institute on Disability and Rehabilitation Research Consensus Statement, 1992).
     c. Symptoms can include:
        (1) Fever
        (2) Cloudy urine and/or sediment
        (3) Increase in spasms, especially in legs and abdomen
        (4) Dysuria
        (5) Urgency
        (6) Frequency
        (7) Malaise
        (8) Autonomic dysreflexia
        (9) Chills

      (10)   Hematuria

      (11)   Foul smelling urine

      (12)   Urine leakage between intermittent catheterization or around indwelling catheter

      (13)   Leukocytes in urine

      (14)   The individual may have no symptoms.

9. Maintain fluid intake of at least 2000ml daily unless contraindicated.

10. Assess for bladder retraining as soon as feasible after the resolution of spinal shock.

11. Educate individual/family regarding medications that can exacerbate retention (AHCPR, 1996).

   a. Antidepressants

   b. Sedatives, hypnotics, tranquilizers

   c. Anticholinergics

   d. Beta-adrenergic agonists

   e. Alpha-adrenergic agonists

   f. Over-the-counter cold medications

   g. Narcotics

   h. Calcium channel blockers

12. Maintain acidic urinary pH of around 5.

13. Initiate bladder program in consultation with physician, including one or more of the following strategies:

   a. Establish intermittent catheterization program (ICP) every 4-6 hours or volume directed per protocol. Use of bladder ultrasound beneficial for volume-directed management.

      (1)   Sterile or clean technique per institutional protocol.

      (2)   # 14-16 F size straight catheter. Coude catheter may be necessary for some male individuals.

      (3)   Maintain of at least 2,000ml daily fluid restriction, regulate based on urine volumes.

      (4)   Limit fluids in evening, e.g. after 8 PM.

      (5)   Maintain bladder capacity of less than 500ml.

      (6)   As residual urine decreases and spontaneous voiding increases, intervals between catheterizations can be lengthened. For males with spontaneous voiding, external catheter appliance is an option (wet management).

      (7)   For individuals with minimal urinary leakage, addition of an anticholinergic may be beneficial.

      (8)   ICP may be eliminated when effective bladder emptying is achieved. PVR is less than 20 percent of bladder capacity. Applies to individual with reflex voiding ability.

      (9)   Teach individual/family clean technique ICP for home and long term use.

    (10)   Teach individual about prescribed medications, indications, and any side effects.

   b. Introduce appropriate manual techniques to facilitate voiding prior to each catheterization. Voiding maneuvers differ according to type of neurogenic bladder dysfunction.

      (1)   Suprapubic triggering: For individuals with weak uninhibited bladder contraction (Linsenmeyer & Stone, 1993).

         (a) Suprapubic tapping

         (b) Pulling pubic hairs

         (c) Stroking or squeezing genitalia

         (d) Stimulating the anus digitally

      (2)   Crede method: Micturition reflex arc (S2-S4) absent. Strong, external pressure exerted over and around bladder to push urine out of bladder and override bladder neck and urinary sphincter resistance. May lead to rectal prolapse, hemorrhoids, or hernia. Contraindicated in individuals with hyperreflexic bladders (detrusor sphincter dyssynergia). Documented vesicoureteral reflux contraindicates this type of voiding (Linsenmeyer & Stone, 1993).

      (3)   Valsalva method: Straining to void by taking a deep breath and bearing down. Must have strong abdominal muscles. May lead to rectal prolapse, hemorrhoids, or hernia. Contraindicated in individuals with hyperreflexic bladders (detrusor sphincter dyssynergia). Documented vesicoureteral reflux contraindicates this type of voiding (Linsenmeyer & Stone, 1993).

c. Pharmacologic management: The following medications may be indicated in individuals with failure to empty (Table 14-1).

    (1)   Drugs that stimulate detrusor contraction and promote bladder emptying:

        (a) Cholinergics: Increase bladder contractility. Most useful in individuals with bladder hypocontractility and coordinated sphincter function (Finkbeiner, 1985). Contraindicated in mechanical outlet obstruction and DSD.

        (b) Prostaglandins (investigational): Noted to increase detrusor pressures in individuals with suprasacral lesions (Vaidyanathan, Rao et al, 1981).

        (c) Narcotic agonists: May block enkephalins which are believed to inhibit sacral micturition reflex (Booth, Hisamitsu, Kawatani, & deGroat, 1985).

    (2)   Drugs that decrease outlet or sphincter resistance:

        (a) Alpha-adrenergic blocking agents: Incidence of gastrointestinal (GI) tumors in rats reported. Increases relaxation of urethral smooth muscles and decreases outflow resistance.

        (b) External sphincter/striated muscle relaxants: Increase relaxation of striated external sphincter.

d. Indwelling urethral catheter: Used if other interventions are inadequate or individual has a preference.

    (1)   #14-16 F non-latex catheter with 5cc balloon to prevent meatal irritation or urethral diverticulum. Catheter selected should be smaller than external meatus.

    (2)   Aseptic technique for insertion. Prevent cross-contamination if switching from drainage bag to leg bag.

    (3)   Tape catheter to abdomen (males) to prevent peno-scrotal fistula or urethral diverticula.

    (4)   Tape catheter to upper thigh (females) to prevent urethral erosion or urethral diverticula.

    (5)   Fluid intake of at least 3,000ml daily unless contraindicated.

    (6)   Daily perineal hygiene and catheter care with mild soap and water.

    (7)   Pubic hair should be shaved or kept trimmed.

    (8)   May be only practical choice for females who cannot maintain continence or for the female with quadriplegia.

    (9)   Teach individual/family proper management of indwelling catheter, how and when to change catheter, and cleaning of drainage appliance.

  (10)   Maintain unobstructed flow of urine by proper tubing and drainage bag placement.

  (11)   Instruct individual/family regarding signs and symptoms of UTI.

  (12)   Teach individual/family about potential complications of calculi formation and signs and symptoms to monitor.

  (13)   Initiate periodic urine cytology and cystoscopy to rule out bladder cancer as directed by physician.

  (14)   Individuals may be on anticholinergic medication to decrease bladder spasms.

e. Suprapubic catheter: Used if other interventions are inadequate or individual has a preference.

    (1)   Smallest size catheter that will drain adequately, #14-16 F non latex.

    (2)   Tape to abdomen.

    (3)   Aseptic technique for insertion. Prevent cross-contamination if switching from drainage bag to leg bag.

    (4)   Fluid intake of at least 3,000ml daily unless contraindicated.

    (5)   Daily catheter care with mild soap and water.

    (6)   Shave hair around stoma.

    (7)   Teach individual/family proper management of suprapubic catheter, how and when to change catheter, and cleaning of drainage appliance.

    (8)   Maintain unobstructed flow of urine by proper tubing and drainage bag placement.

    (9)   Instruct individual/family regarding signs and symptoms of UTI.

  (10)   Teach individual/family about potential complications of calculi formation and signs and symptoms to monitor.

  (11)   Initiate periodic urine cytology and cystoscopy to rule out bladder cancer as directed by physician.

f. External collecting devices: Variety of male products available; female devices are rarely satisfactory.
 (1) Select appropriate size and brand.
 (2) Assess for comfort, adequate drainage, and adhesion to penile skin to prevent leakage.
 (3) Instruct individual/ family on proper application.
 (4) Instruct on importance of daily hygiene and perineal/penile skin inspection.
 (5) Instruct on proper cleaning of urinary drainage bag.
 (6) Maintain at least 3,000ml fluid intake unless contraindicated.
 (7) In female individual, assess history of pelvic radiation treatments. Irradiated tissue is more sensitive to adhesives, solvents, and pressure.
 (8) Instruct individual on proper bladder emptying technique.
 (9) Consult with physician concerning appropriateness of long-term prophylactic or suppressive anti-infective medications for recurrent UTIs.

g. Absorbent products:
 (1) Assess product for aborbency, comfort, ease of application, concealment, individual preference, and cost.
 (2) Instruct individual to change pad frequently.
 (3) Instruct to inspect skin with each pad change.
 (4) Perineal cleansing with each pad change.
 (5) Use moisture barrier creams or films as appropriate on buttocks/perineal skin.
 (6) Teach individual to inspect skin for rashes, lesions, inflammation, or infection.
 (7) Assess for urinary leakage around absorbent product.
 (8) Maintain at least 3,000ml fluids intake unless contraindicated.

h. Behavioral strategies
 (1) Timed toileting: Fixed voiding schedule in individuals with sensory paralytic neurogenic bladders (Emick-Herring, 1993). Not successful in individuals with DSD (Linsenmeyer & Stone, 1993).
  (a) Toilet individual every 2-4 hours.
  (b) No systematic effort is made to motivate individual to delay voiding or resist urge.
  (c) Encourage individual to monitor clock to promote awareness of schedule.
  (d) Decrease or eliminate bladder irritants:
   - Beverages with caffeine
   - Citrus drinks
   - Some bath preparations(bubble bath)
  (e) Encourage fluid intake of at least 2,000ml per day.
  (f) Limit fluids after evening meal.
  (g) If appropriate, try various techniques that assist with stimulation to void.
  (h) Instruct individual with sensory paralytic bladder not to wait for sensation of bladder fullness.
 (2) Electrical stimulation (neurostimulation): Direct electrical stimulation to bladder reported to be effective in individuals with hypotonic and areflexic bladders (Barrett & Wein, 1987). Stimulation also produces side effects of abdominal, pelvic, and perineal pain; defecation; and increase in intravesical pressure not coordinated with bladder neck opening. This type of stimulation not generally used. Electrical stimulation of nerve roots includes sectioning relevant posterior roots in order to abolish hyperreflexia and intradural identification of sacral roots responsible for voiding with electrostimulation and intraoperative urodynamics (Brindley, 1994; Tanagho, Schmidt, & Orvis, 1989). Stimulator is placed on anterior roots.
  (a) Appropriate candidate selection is important.
  (b) Male individuals need to be informed of possible adverse effect on erection.
  (c) Used when other conservative methods have failed.
  (d) Ensure pre- and post-operative teaching regarding type of neurostimulator used and proper operating procedure.
  (e) Establish bladder emptying schedule.

i. Ileal conduit (ileal loop): Ileum is bowel segment most commonly used.
    (1) Pre-op assess of proper placement of stoma to maximize individual self-care.
    (2) Post-op monitoring for signs and symptoms of bowel obstruction.
    (3) Assess for return of bowel program.
    (4) Monitor input and output, electrolyte balance.
    (5) Assess for anastomotic leaks:
        (a) Abdominal distention
        (b) Signs of peritoneal irritation
        (c) Drainage of feces or urine through drains or incisions
    (6) Assess for stomal ischemia: dark red or purplish tint or cyanotic hue.
    (7) Assess for stomal necrosis: brown or black discoloration of stoma.
    (8) Assess for mucocutaneous separation: check for stomal separation.
    (9) Assess urine output through stoma: initially blood tinged, then becoming straw colored; mucus shreds are normal.
    (10) Assess for patency of ileal conduit.
    (11) Instruct individual/family on proper care of ileal conduit, stomal inspection, and application of urinary appliance.
    (12) Provide appropriate pouching system with antireflux valve and spout.
    (13) Assess for signs and symptoms of infection.
    (14) Instruct individual/family on prevention and/or management of skin deterioration around stoma site.
        (a) Chemical damage: effluent in contact with skin.
           - Eliminate effluent contact.
           - Skin barrier or sealant if needed.
        (b) Mechanical damage: incorrect skin care.
           - Teach appropriate skin care with skin barriers or solid barrier.
           - Fungal rash: persistent skin moisture, antibiotics causing fungal overgrowth.
           - Keep skin dry.
           - Antifungal powder and sealant as indicated.
        (c) Allergic reaction: can be caused by any product.
           - Eliminate contact with allergen.
           - Corticosteroid agent if needed.
           - Use cream or spray, not ointment that interferes with pouch adherence.
    (15) Educate regarding problems with odor and diet management.
    (16) Discuss with individual and partner possibility of male impotence and infertility.
    (17) Instruct individual/family regarding procedure for obtaining medical-alert identification bracelet.

j. Continent urinary reservoir: Construction of internal pouch using segments of detubularized ileum or colon.
    (1) Pre-op assessment of proper placement of stoma to maximize individual self-care.
    (2) Immediate post-op regular irrigation needed to keep catheters that drain pouch free of mucus plugs.
    (3) Assess for stomal ischemia: dark red or purplish tint or cyanotic hue.
    (4) Assess for stomal necrosis: brown or black discoloration of stoma.
    (5) Instruct individual/family on proper irrigation of stoma while in hospital.
    (6) When pouch has healed (10-30 days post-op), instruct individual on proper catheterization and irrigation procedure.
    (7) Instruct individual/family to gradually increase interval of catheterizations, which allows pouch to hold larger amounts of urine.
    (8) Pouch capacity 400-800ml; catheterize 2-4 times per day.
    (9) Instruct on assessment and care of stoma.
    (10) Instruct individual/family on care and storage of catheters.
    (11) Instruct individual/family on potential long-term complications and signs and symptoms:
        (a) Pouchitis
        (b) Difficulty with catheter insertion
        (c) False passage

(d) Parastomal hernia

(e) Leakage from pouch

(12) Instruct individual/family regarding procedure for obtaining medical-alert identification bracelet.

k. Transurethral procedures: for obstruction at bladder neck and/or level of external sphincter or prostate. Indicated for individuals with upper tract changes with increased intravesical pressures and spastic external sphincters, areflexic bladders with inability to open bladder neck, persistent high residual urines, recurrent symptomatic UTIs, and/or autonomic dysreflexia. Procedure is performed in males due to resultant urinary incontinence and required use of external collection device.

(1) Sphincterotomy/Prostatectomy

(a) Pre-operative management:

- Assess for tolerance and proper fit of external catheter and appropriate drainage system.
- Educate individual on potential loss of erectile ability, retrograde ejaculation.
- Instruct on proper daily perineal hygiene and penile skin inspection.
- Instruct on daily external catheter change and drainage bag cleaning.

(b) Post-operative management:

- Assess for hematuria or signs of dysreflexia from clots, or irritation from indwelling catheter.
- Maintain patency of indwelling catheter.
- Assess for signs and symptoms of infection.
- Tape catheter securely to abdomen to prevent irritation from foley balloon, or dislodgement.
- Daily perineal and catheter care with soap and water.
- Maintain continuous irrigation if ordered.
- When foley discontinued, perform or instruct individual on ICP and triggered voiding techniques until residual urine volume is acceptable.
- Instruct on pharmacologic management as indicated.
- Reinstitute appropriate bladder retraining program

l. Endourethral Prosthesis (urethral stent): indicated for DSD, failure to empty. Placement of alloy mesh stent over the external urethral sphincter (Joseph, Juma & Niku, 1994).

(1) Candidate is male individual with normal bladder compliance and adequate detrusor contraction.

(2) Pre op assessment to evaluate ability to wear external catheter.

(3) Instruct individual to avoid pelvic congestion and prolonged pressure during post-op recovery.

(4) No urethral catheterization for 3 months post-operatively. Use of suprapubic catheter if necessary.

(5) Monitor urine output.

(6) Observe for signs and symptoms of AD.

(7) Observe for excessive bleeding post-operatively.

(8) Issue medical-alert bracelet.

E. **Evaluation**

1. Individual/family is able to manage bladder management program.
2. Individual is free of urinary complications or incidence of complications is reduced.
3. Individual exhibits no signs of perineal skin breakdown associated with urinary incontinence.
4. Episodes of urinary incontinence reduced or eliminated.
5. Individual's renal function is preserved.
6. Individual/family is knowledgeable regarding urological follow-up.
7. Socialization within the community is maintained.
8. Individual's self-concept is maintained.
9. Tissue perfusion is normal.
10. Urinary retention is adequately managed.

11. Body image is not disturbed.
12. Individual/family understands mechanism of incontinence.
13. Individual/family is able to describe long-term implications of neurogenic bladder dysfunction and preventive management techniques.
14. Individual is able to manage bladder for sexual activity.

V. Nursing Process Applied to Altered Patterns of Urinary Elimination Related to Failure to Store

A. **Nursing Diagnoses:**
1. Impaired skin integrity related to urinary incontinence
2. Risk for urinary complications related to method of bladder management
3. Alteration in self-concept
4. Risk for infection related to neurogenic bladder dysfunction
5. Knowledge deficit related to individual bladder management protocol

B. **Defining Characteristics:** Individuals with failure to store include those with uninhibited/reflex neurogenic bladders and stress incontinence. The failure to store could be due to bladder or outlet dysfunction. Loss of higher inhibition from higher centers results in spastic bladder and sphincter behavior (Tanagho, Schmidt, & Orvis, 1992). Common lesions include cardiovascular accident (CVA), multiple sclerosis (MS) and Parkinson's disease. Spinal cord lesions can also be the result of trauma, multiple sclerosis, or tumor. Voiding maneuvers, ICP, external collecting devices, indwelling catheters, behavioral strategies, surgical treatment options, absorbent products, and pharmacological management are techniques used to assist in bladder filling/storage. The method chosen depends upon the underlying dysfunction, individual's functional status, preference, and level of cooperation. The individual with failure to store may exhibit some or all of the following characteristics:
1. Urinary incontinence
2. Urgency
3. Frequency
4. Unihibited bladder contractions/spasms
5. Nocturia
6. Voiding small amounts
7. No awareness of bladder filling
8. Detrusor external sphincter dyssynergia
9. Reduced bladder capacity
10. Decreased bladder capacity and increased residual urine
11. High bladder pressures with emptying
12. Impaired or absent saddle sensation
13. Hyperactive bulbocavernous reflex
14. UTI
15. Spasticity of pelvic striated muscles.

C. **Expected Outcomes:** Are the same as for failure to empty, with the following exceptions:
1. Individual achieves acceptable level of continence.
2. Individual/family catheterizes continent urinary diversion.
3. Individual/family describes goals and process of timed voiding schedule and fluid intake control.

D. **Interventions**
1. Assess for bladder distention every 2-4 hours. Use of bladder ultrasound is beneficial and eliminates unnecessary catheterizations.
2. Monitor input and output.
3. Assess/monitor voiding pattern.
4. Establish a voiding schedule.
5. Initiate bladder training or reconditioning program.

6. Teach individual/family potential side effects of medication and strategies to counteract or eliminate these effects.
7. Assist individual to minimize or reverse specific risk factors for urinary calculi.
8. Assess for signs and symptoms of urinary tract infections/colonization.
   a. Urinary tract infection: bacteriuria with tissue invasion and resultant tissue response with signs and/or symptoms.
   b. Asymptomatic bacteriuria: colonization of urinary tract with no reference to signs or symptoms (National Institute on Disability and Rehabilitation Research Consensus Statement, 1992).
   c. Symptoms can include:
      (1) Fever
      (2) Cloudy urine and/or sediment
      (3) Increase in spasms, especially in legs and abdomen
      (4) Dysuria
      (5) Urgency
      (6) Frequency
      (7) Malaise
      (8) Dysreflexia
      (9) Chills
      (10) Hematuria
      (11) Foul smelling urine
      (12) Urine leakage between intermittent catheterization or around indwelling catheter
      (13) Leukocytes in urine
      (14) Or the individual may have no symptoms.
9. Maintain fluid intake of at least 2000ml daily unless contraindicated.
10. Assess for bladder retraining as soon as feasible after the resolution of spinal shock.
11. Reduce or eliminate factors contributing to incontinence.
    a. UTI
    b. Medications that can exacerbate incontinence
       (1) Diuretics
       (2) Sedatives, hypnotics, tranquilizers
       (3) Alpha-adrenergic blockers
12. Limit fluids after the evening meal.
13. Monitor input and output.
14. Decrease or eliminate fluids with diuretic, dehydrating, or irritating effects on bladder, such as: tea, coffee, colas, citrus drinks, drinks containing aspartame, and alcohol.
15. Assess for signs and symptoms of bladder infection.
16. Assess for bladder distention. Use of bladder ultrasound is beneficial and reduces unnecessary catheterizations.
17. Assess and monitor voiding pattern.
18. Maintain skin integrity.
19. Initiate bladder program in consultation with physician, including one or more of the following strategies:
    a. Establish ICP program every 4-6 hours per protocol (see failure to empty)
    b. Introduce appropriate manual techniques to facilitate voiding prior to each catheterization. Voiding maneuvers differ according to type of neurogenic bladder dysfunction.
       (1) Suprapubic triggering: For individuals with weak uninhibited bladder contraction (Linsenmeyer & Stone, 1993).
          (a) Suprapubic tapping
          (b) Pulling pubic hairs
          (c) Stroking or squeezing genitalia
          (d) Stimulating the anus digitally
    c. Pharmacologic management as directed by physician. Teach individual/family about prescribed medications, indications, and monitor for side effects. The following medications may be indicated in individuals with failure to store (Table 14-1).
       (1) Drugs that inhibit bladder contractility and facilitate storage:

176

    (a) Anticholinergics: Use with caution in individuals with bladder neck obstruction, as complete urinary retention may occur (Ghoneim, 1996). Use with caution with tricyclics.

    (b) Alpha-adrenergics: Increase urethral and bladder neck resistance.

    (c) Musculotropics/antispasmodics

    (d) Tricyclic antidepressants: Use of imipramine hydrochloride is contraindicated in individuals receiving monamine oxidase inhibitors (Barrett & Wein, 1987).

    (e) Calcium antagonist: Has both calcium antagonist and anticholinergic properties (Linsenmeyer & Stone, 1993).

    (f) Beta-adrenergic agonist: Used in urge and urgency incontinence (Barrett & Wein, 1987).

    (g) Prostaglandin inhibitors: Under investigation for bladder effects. Most fall under heading of nonsteroidal anti-inflammatory (Wein, 1992).

(2) Drugs that increase bladder outlet resistance:

    (a) Alpha-adrenergic agonist: Essential that detrusor hyperreflexia or poor bladder compliance be ruled out with urodynamic study prior to initiation of these agents. Use with caution in individuals with hypertension and cardiovascular disease.

    (b) Beta-adrenergic antagonists: Contraindicated in individuals with asthma.

    (c) Estrogen: Used exclusively in women with sphincter incontinence. Can be given in oral or topical form (Ghoneim, 1996). Increased risk of endometrial cancer.

    (d) Intravesical therapy: To control bladder over activity and avoid extra urinary side effects. Agents used include: Atropine, Terodiline, Oxybutynin, Phentolamine and Capsaicin (Ghoneim, 1996).

d. Indwelling Foley catheter: Because of the risk of infection, an indwelling catheter is used when other interventions have not been effective, or based on patient preference for convenience.

e. Suprapubic catheter: While typically not the first choice in bladder management, some patients prefer suprapubic catheters.

Table 14-1: Medications to Treat Voiding Disorders

DRUG CLASS	ACTION	ADVERSE EFFECTS	NURSING CONSIDERATIONS
Drugs That Inhibit Contractility and Promote Urine Storage			
Anticholinergics (propantheline bromide, hyoscyamine, methantheline bromide, dicyclomine hydrochloride, tincture of belladonna, atropine sulfate, glycopyrrolate)	Reduces spasm or smooth muscle contraction by blocking or inhibiting the effects of acetylcholine at the muscarinic receptor	Dizziness, drowsiness, blurred vision, dry mouth; increased HR; contraindictated in many disease states – check before administration	Give 30-60 min before meals and at bedtime; monitor vital signs and urine output; use gum or sugarless candies to relieve dry mouth
Antispasmodics/direct smooth muscle relaxants (oxybutynin chloride, flavoxate hydrochloride, belladonna & opium {B & O} suppositories)	Inhibits muscarinic action of acetylcholine on smooth muscle; direct antispasmodic effect on detrusor smooth muscle	Same as for anticholinergics	Same as for anticholinergics
Beta-adrenergics (terbutaline)	Increases bladder capacity through beta-stimulatory effect on bladder body	Palpitations, insomnia, hypertension	Monitor pulse and blood pressure

continued on page 178

Table 14-1: Continued

DRUG CLASS	ACTION	ADVERSE EFFECTS	NURSING CONSIDERATIONS
Tricyclic antidepressants (imipramine, doxepin)	Anesthetic-like action at nerve terminals; produces strong inhibitory effect on bladder smooth muscle	Weakness, fatigue, sedation, postural hypotension, rash, parkinsonian effect, fine tremors, abdominal distress, nausea and vomiting, headache, lethargy, irritability	Elderly require close observation; inform patient of possible side effects
Drugs That Increase Bladder Outlet Resistance			
Alpha-adrenergics (ephedrine sulfate, imipramine, phenylpropanolamine hydrochloride, pseudoephedrine)	Exaggerates alpha iresponsein the bladder neck and urethra to increase bladder outlet resistance	Tachycardia, precordial pain, cardiac arrhythmias, vertigo, headache	Used to treat stress urinary incontinence, postprostatectomy incontinence; monitor vital signs
Beta-adrenergic blocks (propranolol)	Blocks beta-adrenergic receptors in the urethra, thereby increasing urethral pressure	Bradycardia, lightheadedness	Used when alpha-adrenergics are contraindicated
Estrogens	Increases periurethral blood flow; strengthens periurethral tissues	Headache, nausea, edema, hypertension, weight changes, breast tenderness	Assess for vaginal bleeding, GU, or abdominal pain; monitor blood pressure and weight
Drugs That Stimulate Detrusor Contractility and Promote Bladder Emptying			
Cholinergics (bethanecol chloride, neostigmine methylsulfate, myotonachol, carbachol)	Stimulates muscarinic cholinergic receptors in the bladder to increase bladder tone and sensations to bladder filling	Increased GI motility; vasodilation; decreased HR	Used for postoperative and nonobstructive urinary retention; do not give bethanecol IM or IV; give oral bethanecol on empty stomach; monitor vital signs; contraindicated in many disease states - check before administering
Drugs That Decrease Bladder Outlet Resistance			
Alpha-adrenergic blockers (phenoxybenzamine hydrochloride, phentolamine, reserpine, prazosin, terazosin, doxasozin)	Blocks alpha-adrenergic receptors of the bladder neck, posterior urethra, and external sphincter	Postural hypotension	Have patient change positions slowly; give with food or milk; avoid use with alcohol; avoid cold products containing sympathomimetics
External sphincter/striated muscle relaxants (baclofen, diazepam, dantrolene sodium)	Relaxes the external sphincter by inhibiting postsynaptic reflexes of striated muscles	Weakness; sedation	Often used in patients with multiple sclerosis or high-cord lesions; implement safety precautions

Key: Heart rate (HR) Genitourinary (GU) Gastrointestinal (GI) Intravenous (IV) Intramuscular (IM)

From *Urologic Nursing Principles and Practice* (p. 391), by K. Karlowicz (Ed.), 1995, Philadelphia: W.B. Saunders Co. Reprinted with permission.

f. External collecting devices: Variety of male products available, female devices are rarely satisfactory (see failure to empty).

g. Absorbent products (see failure to empty).

h. Behavioral strategies
   (1) Timed toileting: Fixed voiding schedule in individuals with uninhibited neurogenic bladders (Emick-Herring, 1993). Not successful in individuals with DSD (Linsenmeyer & Stone, 1993).
       (a) Toilet individual every 2-4 hours.
       (b) No systematic effort is made to motivate individual to delay voiding or resist urge.
       (c) Encourage individual to monitor clock to promote awareness of schedule.
       (d) Decrease or eliminate bladder irritants.
           - Beverages with caffeine
           - Citrus drinks
           - Some bath preparations (bubble bath)
       (e) Encourage fluid intake of at least 2,000 ml per day.
       (f) Limit fluids after evening meal.
       (g) If appropriate, try various techniques that assist with stimulation to void.
   (2) Bladder training: Individual with unihibited neurogenic bladder.
       (a) Establish individual's voiding behavior by observing wetness and dryness pattern for several days.
       (b) Gradually increase time between toileting with encouragement to practice inhibiting urge sensation and postponing voiding.
       (c) Keep toileting schedule consistent.
       (d) Assess individual's access to toilet facility and any physical limitations.
       (e) Institute double voiding: Individual voids, waits a few minutes, and then voids again to enhance complete bladder emptying.
       (f) Encourage fluid intake of at least 2,000ml per day.
       (g) Limit fluids after evening meal.
   (3) Habit training: Used for individuals with uninhibited bladder (Emick-Herring, 1993).
       (a) Individualize toileting schedule to voiding pattern.
       (b) Assess baseline voiding pattern and episodes of incontinence.
       (c) Toilet individual every 2-4 hours and adjust as needed.
       (d) Progressively increase toileting time interval as continence is achieved.
   (4) Biofeedback: Individuals with stress incontinence. Used to assist individuals to identify pelvic muscles.
       (a) Assess individual's motivation.
       (b) Obtain baseline measurement to establish bladder capacity, interval between voids, and number of incontinent episodes.
   (5) Electrical stimulation: Increases outlet resistance and decreases bladder contractility. Performed by placing probe in rectum or vagina. Causes inhibition of pelvic plexus with ablation of unstable detrusor contractions. Percutaneous, transrectal, or transvaginal electrodes may be used. Limited to individuals with stress and urge incontinence. Maximal electrostimulation is non-invasive and often managed by a nurse in consultation with physician.
       (a) Assess individual's type of incontinence.
       (b) Assess individual preference.
       (c) Teach individual to use stimulation device effectively and safely.
       (d) Instruct individual in setting the proper intensity of current.
       (e) Instruct individual on use of frequency/volume chart.
       (f) Assess individual's ability to discern stimulation.
   (6) Pelvic muscle exercises: Generally combined with biofeedback.
       (a) Assess individual's motivation.
       (b) Obtain baseline measurements to establish bladder capacity, interval between voids, and number of incontinent episodes.

(c) Help individual to identify, isolate, and contract the pelvic muscles, and perform pelvic (Kegel) exercises.
  (1) Females: Instruct to stop flow of urine, or insert gloved finger into vagina and instruct her to tighten as if holding back urine.
  (2) Males: Instruct to stop flow of urine, or insert gloved finger into rectum and ask him to tighten anus.
(d) Instruct individual on frequency of exercises.
(e) Repeated contractions of pelvic floor muscles inhibit detrusor contractility (Blaivas & Oliver, 1991).

(7) Artificial urinary sphincter: Insertion of prosthetic device consisting of cuff, pump, and reservoir.
  (a) Assess individual's motivation and compliance.
  (b) Assess functional ability.
  (c) Teach individual proper use of artificial sphincter and its operating parts.
  (d) Teach individual regarding possible malfunction of equipment and when to seek medical advice.
  (e) Provide pre-op and post-op care.
  (f) Instruct individual/family regarding procedure for obtaining medical-alert identification bracelet.
  (g) Instruct individual/family on measures to prevent UTI.
  (h) Instruct individual on appropriate voiding frequency with artificial sphincter.

(8) Urinary diversion: Generally reserved for individuals with severe neurogenic bladder disease. Indications include unresolved upper tract obstruction with bladder instability, detrusor hypertrophy, vesicoureteral reflux with renal deterioration (Jonas & Truss, 1991). (see failure to empty).

(9) Augmentation cystoplasty: Surgical treatment to improve bladder capacity and lower intravesical pressure. Used for individuals with severe detrusor hyporeflexia who have failed conventional management (Linsenmeyer & Stone, 1993). Portion of bladder is removed and a larger segment of bowel is attached to remaining bladder. Emptying failure post-procedure is a possibility but can be generally predicted by careful pre-op urodynamic evaluation (Wein, 1992).
  (a) Detubularized segment of bowel used to achieve low-pressure storage.
  (b) Pre-op and post-op teaching needed.
  (c) Individual/family must be motivated to perform intermittent catheterization(IC).
  (d) May require long term IC after surgery.
  (e) Post op: assess drain and suprapubic catheter for patency.
  (f) Drain is usually removed prior to discharge.
  (g) Suprapubic catheter generally remains 3 weeks post-op.
  (h) Follow-up cystogram performed to confirm absence of leakage before individual is started on a bladder-emptying regimen with either valsalva maneuver, crede maneuver, or intermittent catheterization (IC) (Muller, et al, 1991).
  (i) Increased mucus in urine is expected.
  (j) Post-op bladder is partially filled twice daily to ensure that bladder does not heal in contracted state (B.W. Snow & Cartwright, 1996)
  (k) When doing IC, catheter should be passed only to point where urine returns, to avoid mechanical perforation (B.W. Snow & Cartwright, 1996).
  (l) Intermittent bladder irrigation may be necessary to prevent obstruction from mucus plug.
  (m) Long-term consequences of bowel attached to bladder are unknown.
  (n) Long-term follow-up is required.
  (o) Adenocarcinoma in bladder has been reported (Filmer & Spencer, 1990).

(10) Bulking agents (Teflon/Collagen): Indications are for failure to store and external sphincter deficiency. Periurethral injection of collagen increases urethral resistance.
  (a) Assess for urinary retention following procedure.
  (b) Procedure may have to be repeated in several months to achieve or maintain continence.
  (c) Potential long-term health risks associated with Collagen or Teflon are unknown.

VI. Reassessment

Two primary goals in urologic rehabilitation are prevention of life-threatening complications and preservation of renal function. These goals should be ever present as the nurse reassesses post-injury/onset individuals who present for follow-up evaluation. Long-term urological follow-up is mandatory for all SCI individuals because urologic status can deteriorate, often without overt clinical signs and symptoms, even many years after initial injury/onset. Even individuals with lower motor neuron function who may never develop spontaneous reflex bladder activity should be monitored periodically with UDS studies. Bladder can lose compliance, possibly due to increased adrenergic activity and mucosal fibrosis, which could increase bladder pressures greater than 40cm water (Wheeler & Walter, 1993). The nurse must also be aware of the normal aging changes that affect the urinary system and how this can affect the individual with SCI.

A. **Nursing History:** Assess any mental status changes since last evaluation. Due to the possibility of secondary complications, such as post-injury syrinx or post-polio syndrome, evaluate the current level and completeness of injury. Collect updated information on post-injury urinary complication or conditions, post-injury disease/medical condition, development of new allergies, current prescribed and over-the-counter medications, and any change in current drug or alcohol use. Assess the appropriateness of the current method of bladder management and the individual's compliance with the bladder management program.

B. **Examination:** Assess for increased incidence of autonomic dysreflexia due to urologic causes. Inspect the perineal/vaginal area, observing for any changes in baseline exam. Observe for atrophic changes in the vagina or penile retraction in the male, which may make present bladder management problematic. Palpate the prostate for benign prostatic hyperplasia (BPH), inflammation, or nodules. Reassessment of functional abilities is necessary in the aging individual with SCI.

C. **Diagnostic Studies:** In the individual who has done well during the first 5 years post-injury, intervals of 2-5 years may be appropriate unless clinical signs and symptoms warrant sooner evaluation (Lanig, 1992). Generally, annual evaluations are recommended.
1. Laboratory (during annual routine follow-up):
   a. Urinalysis
   b. Urine culture and sensitivity
   c. Blood urea nitrogen (BUN) and Creatinine
   d. Creatinine clearance: 24 hour urine
   e. Urine cytology: (age greater than 50, history of smoking, chronic suprapubic/urethral catheter)
   f. Prostatic-specific antigen (PSA)
2. Radiographic tests:
   a. IVU (when clinically indicated).
   b. KUB (when clinically indicated).
   c. Cystoscopy (when clinically indicated).
   d. Renal Ultrasound (every 2-5 years if baseline exam normal).
   e. Voiding Cystourethrogram (VCU): when clinically indicated.
   f. Urodynamics studies: when clinically indicated.
   g. Bladder ultrasound: to check for residual urine.
   h. Renal scan (every 2-5 years if baseline exam normal).

VII. Health Education Tips

A. **Educate individual to avoid over-the-counter medications without checking with health care provider.**

B. **Educate individual/family on prevention of urinary calculi.**
1. Calcium stones: Reduce intake of dairy products, and leafy green vegetables. Increase non-dairy fluids.

2. Oxalate stones: Reduce intake of asparagus, beets, cocoa, rhubarb, and raspberries.
3. Uric acid stones: Reduce intake of foods high in purines, such as organ and lean meats and whole grains.

C. **Problems with deflating foley catheter balloon.**
1. Contact urologist.
2. With instruction from physician:
   a. Inject 1 ml of lightweight mineral oil into lumen of catheter.
   b. The balloon will usually break within 5 minutes to 1 hour.
   c. Mineral oil should be washed out by irrigating catheter before removal.

D. **Foley catheter leakage.**
1. If large size foley in place, replace with smaller size 14-16 Fr., 5 cc balloon and reassess.
2. Use non-latex catheter; may be less irritating and avoid encrustation.
3. Keep urine acidic.
4. Keep catheter taped.
5. If urine leakage is not resolved with other measures, discuss anticholinergic medication with physician.

E. **Pouchitis in continent urinary diversion.**
1. Symptoms
   a. Malaise
   b. Elevated temperature.
   c. Pain in lower back.
   d. Increased mucus.
   e. Change in color or odor of urine.
2. Do not treat bacteriuria from pouch unless the individual is symptomatic.

F. **Difficulty catheterizing continent urinary diversion**
1. Use generous amounts of lubricating jelly.
2. Dilatation of stoma.
3. Coude catheter.
4. Change position of individual.
5. If unable to catheterize, instruct individual to seek emergent care.

VIII. Special Issues Related to Pediatric Care

A. **Critcal Problem.** Optimal management of bladder elimination and continence is critical for the pediatric population to prevent significant long-term disabilities associated with upper urinary tract dysfunction. SCI and spina bifida are predominant diagnoses.

B. **Age-Appropriate Expectations.** Normal continence occurs between 2 and 3 years of age with total independence by 5 years of age. Neurogenic bladder training should start at the same age toilet training would normally begin, or as based on urodynamic studies and urologist recommendations. ICP may start with the newborn or during infancy, depending on bladder dynamics and renal function.
1. Diapers are acceptable for infants and toddlers. When Crede (manual expression) is used, care must be taken to avoid pressure to the upper urinary tract. Documented vesicoureteral reflux contraindicates this type of voiding in adults (Lynsenmeyer & Stone, 1993). Usually requires fluid intake pattern and voiding/ICP every 3 hours.
2. At age 3, continence training may begin and the use of appropriate techniques may be initiated. The use of bladder training underwear may be introduced (usually requires fluid intake pattern and voiding/ICP every 3 to 4 hours, mostly dependent on bladder capacity and cognitive ability.

3. At age 5, a child may begin to perform a bladder training program including ICP, either independently or able to give instructions to caregivers (Sogal, et al, 1993). The use of a commode is helpful.

4. Whenever possible, diapers should be avoided for use by school-age children. Various high absorbency padding systems are available commercially.

5. Effective bladder management depends on the participation of the child and family. Whatever approach is chosen must be reasonable, acceptable to the family and child, and not cause major interruptions in the child's and family's schedule and lifestyle. The program should allow the child to attend school and recreational activities without constant interruptions. The program can change over time as the child grows and develops. Bladder augmentations (Kurtz, Van Zandt, & Sapp, 1996) and foley catheters (especially for teenagers) are options.

C. **Bladder Volumes** (Beger et al, 1983)
   1. Volumes are smaller in children
   2. Volumes may be calculated by: Volume in ounces equal (=) age in years plus (+) ounces (+/- 2 ounces standard deviation) or age in years plus 2 (x) 30. Example: 3 year old bladder volume = 3 ounces or 90 ml (age in years) + 2 ounces or 60 ml for a total of 150 ml.
   3. A normal newborn may have a normal bladder volume as small as 15-25 ml or as large as 60 ml.
   4. The maximum volume by the age of 16 years should be no greater than 500 ml.

D. **Urinary Tract Infection (UTI)**
   1. Although symptoms are similar to those of adults, children may exhibit a change in behavior or increased level of irritability because of their inability to describe their symptoms. Fever is usually the deciding factor when considering antibiotic treatment. Accepted practice is to treat UTI if associated with systemic symptoms.
   2. Urolithiasis is a potential complication of UTI more common in children.

E. **Reassessment.** Annual, or more frequent, reassessment is essential because a child experiences more rapid changes with growth and development.

Practical Application #1

B.A., a 50-year-old male was admitted to the rehabilitation unit with exacerbation of multiple sclerosis (MS). B.A. had been experiencing more episodes of urinary frequency, and urgency, with incontinence and occasional hesitancy. As part of his urinary workup, the cystometogram showed an uninhibited neurogenic bladder; VCU and renal ultrasound showed a stable upper urinary tract. The functional classification was failure to store. On physical examination, B.A. had a bulbocavernous reflex and intact bladder sensation. From this information, the nurse knew the reflex arc was intact. Nursing interventions included instituting intake and output records and planning a timed toileting schedule based on B.A.'s bladder capacity, post residual urine, and voiding pattern. To achieve an effective voiding technique, stimulation of trigger areas to induce reflex voiding was begun. For B.A., manual percussion or tapping of the suprapubic region facilitated maximum voiding. An every 3 hour voiding schedule was necessary initially to avoid incontinence. To decrease urinary hesitancy, B.A. was taught such methods as running water from the tap and relaxation techniques. Pharmacologic management included a trial of Propantheline bromide to reduce bladder contractility and increase bladder capacity. As bladder capacity increased, an every 4 to 5 hour voiding schedule was sufficient to effectively empty his bladder. Periodic checks with the bladder ultrasound confirmed his PVR's were less than 20 percent of his bladder capacity. Additional important teaching areas for the nurse to cover with B.A. included: potential side effects of Propantheline, monitoring urinary output and episodes of incontinence, adhering to a timed voiding schedule, and limiting fluids after dinner if nocturia was a problem.

Practical Application #2

L.J. is a 30-year-old female, developed urinary retention and overflow incontinence after acute transverse myelitis at the T12 level. Urodynamic studies showed an areflexic bladder with complete motor and sensory loss. Baseline VCU and renal ultrasound showed a normal upper urinary tract. Functional classification was failure to empty. Intermittent catheterization was initially started every 4 hours in efforts to keep residual urines under 20 percent of L.J.'s bladder capacity. The nurse explained the importance of limiting fluids to prevent bladder overdistention and instructed L.J. how to keep input and output records. As stimulated voiding volumes, through valsalva/crede maneuver, increased and residual urines remained consistently under 100ml, per bladder ultrasound, L.J.'s intermittent catheterizations were discontinued. A normal sitting position was encouraged to facilitate voiding, and a program to strengthen abdominal muscles began. In order to maintain a bladder capacity of approximately 350ml, the nurse worked with L.J. to determine her voiding schedule by correlating fluid intake with predicted urinary output. Even though the bladder program was successful in the hospital, L.J. elected to manage her elimination dysfunction with an indwelling catheter. L.J. felt that her hectic work and travel schedule would not afford her the opportunity to adhere to a rigid bladder emptying schedule or intermittent catheterization. The nurse instructed L.J. on insertion and care techniques of an indwelling catheter, as well as proper positioning and taping to reduce urethral damage. Other predischarge instructions included: the risk of catheter-associated ascendng bacteriuria, signs and symptoms of UTI and preventive measures, fluid intake of at least 3000ml per day, daily perineal hygiene and drainage bag care, maintaining the urine pH around 5, and catheter management for sexual activity.

References And Selected Bibliography

Agency for Health Care Policy and Research (AHCPR) (1996). *Urinary incontinence in adults: Acute and chronic management, clinical practice guideline.* AHCPR Publication No. 96-0682. Rockville, MD: U.S. Department of Health and Human Services.

American Association of Spinal Cord Injury Nurses (AASCIN) (1996). *Clinical practice guideline: Autonomic dysreflexia.* Jackson Heights, NY: AASCIN.

Anson, C.A., & Gray, M. (1993). Secondary complications after spinal cord injury. *Urologic Nursing, 13,* 107-112.

Barrett, D.M. & Wein, A.J. (1987). Voiding dysfunction: Diagnosis, classification, and management. In J.Y. Gillenwater, J.T. Grayback, S.S. Howard, & J.W. Duckett (Eds.), *Adult and pediatric urology,* (pp. 863-1099). Chicago: Year Book Medical Publishers.

Berger, R.M., Maizels, M., Moran, G.C., Conway, J.J., (1983). Bladder capacity (onces) equals age (years) plus 2 predicts normal bladder capacity and aids in diagnosis of abnormal voiding patterns. *Journal of Urology, 129*(2), 347-349

Blaivas, J. G., & Oliver, L. (1991). Pathophysiology of urinary incontinence. In D. B. Doughtery (Ed.), *Urinary and fecal incontinence-nursing management* (pp. 23-46). St. Louis, MO: Mosby Year Book.

Booth, A. M., Hisamitsu, T., Kawatani, M., & de Groat, W. C. (1985). Regulation of urinary bladder capacity by endogenous opioid peptides. *Journal of Urology,* 133, 339-342.

Brindley, G. S. (1994). The first 500 patients with sacral anterior root stimulator implants: General description. *Paraplegia,* 32, 795-805.

Coxe, J. (1994). Assessment for biofeedback and behavioral therapy for urinary incontinence. *Urologic Nursing, 14,* 82-84.

Davidoff, G., Schultz, S., Lieb, T., Andrews, K., Wardner, J., Hayes, C., Ward, M., Karunas, R., & Maynard, F. (1990). Rehospitalization after initial rehabilitation for spinal cord injury: Incidence and risk factors. *Archives of Physical Medicine and Rehabilitation, 71,* 121-124.

Devivo, M.J., Black, K.J., & Stover, S.L. (1993). Causes of death during the first 12 years after spinal cord injury. *Archives of Physical Medicine and Rehabilitation, 74,* 248-254.

Dewire, D.M, Owens, R.S., Anderson, G.A., Gottlieb, M.S., & Lepor, H. (1992). A comparison of the urological complications associated with long-term management of quadriplegics with and without chronic indwelling urinary catheters. *Journal of Urology, 147,* 1069-1072.

Dittmar, S.S. (Ed.) (1989). *Rehabilitation nursing process and application.* St. Louis, MO: C.V. Mosby.

Dougherty, D. B. (Ed.) (1991). *Urinary and fecal incontinence - nursing management.* St. Louis, MO: Mosby Year Book.

Emick-Herring, B. (1993). Bladder elimination. In A. E. McCourt (3rd ed.), *The specialty practice of rehabilitation nursing: A core curriculum* (pp. 100-107). Skokie, IL: The Rehabilitation Nursing Foundation of the Association of Rehabilitation Nurses.

Fiers, S. (1994). Indwelling catheters and devices: Avoiding the problems. *Urologic Nursing, 14,* 141-144.

Filmer, R. B. & Spencer, J. R. (1990). Malignancies in bladder augmentations and intestinal conduits. *Journal of Urology, 143*, 671-673.

Finkbeiner, A. E. (1985). Is bethanechol chloride clinically effective in promoting bladder emptying?: A literature review. *Journal of Urology, 134*, 443-449.

Geisler, W.O., Jousse, A.T., Wynne-Jones, M., & Breithaupt, D. (1983). Survival in traumatic spinal cord injury. *Paraplegia, 21*, 364-373.

Ghoneim, G. (1996). Pharmacologic therapy for urinary incontinence. *Urologic Nursing, 16*, 55-58.

Giroux, J. (1988). Alterations in bladder elimination. In P. Holsclaw Mitchell, L. C. Hodges, M. Muwaswes, & C. A. Walleck (Eds.), *AANN's Neuroscience nursing* (pp.431-440). Norwalk: Appleton & Lange.

Gowing-Farhat, C. (1994). The Florida pouch. *Urologic Nursing, 14*, 1-5.

Gray, M. (1991). Assessment of patients with urinary incontinence. In D.B. Doughtery (Ed.), *Urinary and fecal incontinence: Nursing management*, (pp. 47-94). St. Louis: Mosby-Year Book.

Gray, M. (1992). Electrostimulation in management of voiding dysfunction. *Urologic Nursing, 12*, 73-74.

Gray, M. & Dobkin, K. (1993). Genitourinary system. In J.M. Thompson, G.K. McFarland, J.E. Hirsch, & S.M. Tucker (Eds.), *Mosby's clinical nursing* (pp. 957-1028). St. Louis, MO: Mosby.

Gray, M. & King, C. J. (1993). Urodynamic evaluation of the intrinsically incompetent sphincter. *Urologic Nursing, 13*, 67-69.

Hackler, R.H. (1977). A 24-year prospective mortality study in the spinal cord injured patient: Comparison with the long term living paraplegia. *Journal of Urology, 117*, 486-488.

Hampton, B.G. & Bryant, R.A. (Eds.) (1992). *Ostomies and continent diversions - nursing management.* St. Louis, MO: Mosby Year Book.

Hanak, M. (Ed.) (1992). *Rehabilitation nursing for the neurological patient.* New York: Springer.

Hickey, J.V. (Ed.) (1992). *Neurological and neurosurgical nursing* (3rd ed.). Philadelphia: J.B. Lippincott.

Jonas, U. & Truss, M. (1991). Continent urinary reservoir in neurogenic bladder disease. In R. J. Krane & M. B. Siroky (Eds.), *Clinical neuro-urology* (pp. 575-592). Boston: Little, Brown.

Joseph, A. C., Juma, S., & Niku, S. D. (1994). Endourethral prosthesis for treatment of detrusor sphincter dyssynergia: Impact on quality of life for persons with spinal cord injury. *SCI Nursing, 11*, 95-99.

Kaplan, S. A., Chancellor, M. B., & Blaivas, J. C. (1991). Bladder and sphincter behavior in patients with spinal cord lesions. *Journal of Urology, 146*, 113-116.

Karlowicz, K., & Meredith, C. (1995). Adult voiding dysfunction. In K. Karlowicz (Ed.), *Urologic nursing principles and practice* (pp. 377-407). Philadelphia: W.B. Saunders.

Kuemmel, P. & Brook, M. (1988). A rational approach to urinary incontinence in the elderly. *Journal of American Academy Physician Assistants, 1*, 362-364.

Kurtz, M., Van Zandt, D., & Sapp, L. (1996). A new technique in independent intermittent catheterization: The mitrofanoff catheterizable channel. *Rehabilitation Nursing, 21*(6), 311-314.

Lanig, I. (1992). The genitourinary system. In G. G. Whiteneck, S. W. Charlifue, K. A. Gerhart, D. P. Lammertse, S. Manley, R. R. Menter & K. R. Seedroff (Eds.), *Aging with Spinal Cord Injury* pp. 105-115). New York: Demos Publications.

Lindstrom, S., Fall, M., Carlsson, C. A., & Erlandson, B. E. (1983). The neurophysiological basis of bladder inhibition in response to intravaginal electrical stimulation. *Journal of Urology, 129*, 405-408.

Linsenmeyer, T. A. & Stone, J. M. (1993). Neurogenic bladder and bowel dysfunction. In J. A. Delisa & B. M. Gans (Eds.), *Rehabilitation medicine principles and practice* (pp. 733-762). Philadelphia: J.B. Lippincott.

McCourt, A. E. (Ed.). (1993). *The specialty practice of rehabilitation nursing: a core curriculum* (3rd ed.). Skokie, IL: The Rehabilitation Nursing Foundation of the Association of Rehabilitation Nurses.

Muller, S.C., Riedmiller, H., Thuroff, J.W., & Hohenfellner, R. (1991). Bladder augmentation and continent urinary diversion with use of the appendix. In F.F. Marshall (Ed.), *Operative Urology*, (pp. 157-172). Philadelphia: W. B. Saunders Company.

National Institute on Disability and Rehabilitation Research Consensus Statement. (1992). The prevention and management of urinary tract infection among people with spinal cord injuries. *Journal of the American Paraplegia Society, 15*, 194-204.

Newman, D. (1989). The treatment of urinary incontinence in adults. *Nurse Practitioner, 14*, 21-32.

Snow, B. W. & Cartwright, P. C. (1996). Bladder autoaugmentation. *Urologic Clinics of North America, 23*, 323-331.

Snow, J.C., Sideropoulos, H.P., Kripke, B.J., Freed, M.M., Shah, N.K., & Schlesinger, R.M. (1978). Autonomic hyperreflexia during cystoscopy in patients with high spinal cord injuries. *Paraplegia, 1*, 327-332.

Sogal, E.S., Deatrick, J.A., & Hagelgaus, N.A. (1995). The determinants of successful self-catherization program in children with myelomeningocele. *Journal of Pediatric Nursing, 10*(2), 82-88.

Stamm, W.E. (1991). Catheter-associated urinary tract infections: Epidemiology, pathogenesis, and prevention. *American Journal of Medicine, 91*, 655-715.

Steele, D. (1993). Caring for the patient with neurogenic bladder. *Innovations in Urology Nursing, 4*, 1-16.

Steers, W.D., Barrett, D.M., & Wein, A.J. (1996). Voiding dysfunction: Diagnosis, classification, and management. In J.Y. Gillenwater, J.T. Grayhack, S.S. Howards, & J.W. Duckett (Eds.), *Adult and pediatric urology* (pp. 1220-1325). St. Louis, MO: Mosby.

Stover, S.L., Lloyd, L.K., Waites, K.B., & Jackson, A.B. (1989). Urinary tract infection in spinal cord injury. *Archives of Physical Medicine and Rehabilitation, 70*, 47-54.

Tanagho, E.A. (1995). Neuropathic bladder disorders. In E.A. Tanagho & J.W. McAninch (Eds.), *Smith's general urology* (13th ed., pp. 454-472). Norwalk: Appleton & Lange.

Tanagho, E. A. (1995). Urinary incontinence. In E. A. Tanagho & J.W. McAninch (Eds.), *Smith's general urology* (13th ed., pp. 536-551). Norwalk: Appleton & Lange.

Tanagho, E. A., Schmidt, R. A., & Orvis, B. R. (1989). Neural stimulation for control of voiding disorders: A preliminary report in 22 patients with serious neuropathic voiding disorders. *Journal of Urology, 142*, 340-343.

Thomas, D. G., & Lucas, M. G. (1990). The urinary tract following spinal cord injury. In G. D. Chislom & W. R. Fair (Eds.), *Scientific foundations of urology* (pp. 286-299). Chicago: Year Book Medical Publishers.

Vaidyanathan, S, Rao, M. S., Mapa, M. K., Bapna, B. C., Chary, K. S., & Swamy, R. P. (1981). Study of intravesical instillation of 1 A(s)-15 methy prostaglandin F2 in patients with neurogenic bladder dysfunction. *Journal of Urology, 126*, 81-85.

Wallack, C. A. (1994). Central nervous system II: Spinal cord injury. In V. D. Cardona, P. D. Hurn, P. J. Bastnagel Mason, & S. W. Veise-Berry (Eds.), *Trauma nursing from resuscitation through rehabilitation* (pp. 435-465). Philadelphia: W. B. Saunders.

Warren, J.W. (1987). Catheter-associated urinary tract infections. *Infectious Disease Clinics of North America, 1*, 823-854.

Watanabe, T., Rivas, D. A., & Chancellor, M. B. (1996). Urodynamics of spinal cord injury. *Urologic Clinics of North America, 23*, 459-473.

Wein, A.J. (1991). Classification of neurogenic voiding dysfunction. *Journal of Urology, 125*, 605-610.

Wein, A. J. (1992). Neuromuscular dysfunction of the lower urinary tract. In P. C. Walsh, A. B. Retik, T. A. Stamey, & E. D. Vaughan (Eds.), *Campbell's urology 6th ed* (pp. 573-642). Philadelphia: W. B. Saunders.

Wheeler, J. S. & Walter, J. W. (1993). Acute urologic management of the patient with spinal cord injury. *Urologic Clinics of North America*, 20, 403-411.

Zejdlik, C.P. (ED) (1992). *Management of spinal cord injury*. (2nd ed.). Boston: Jones and Bartlett Publishers.

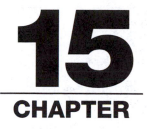

15
CHAPTER

Nutrition

Cynthia Kraft Fine, MSN, RN, CRRN
Audrey Nelson, PhD, RN, FAAN

I. Learning Objectives

A. State four items included in a nursing nutritional assessment.

B. Identify the ideal body weight for individuals with spinal cord impairment (SCI).

C. List two nutritional complications and two preventive nursing interventions.

II. Introduction

This chapter presents the nursing process for the functional alterations in nutritional status in persons with SCI. Metabolic and nutritional responses after SCI indicate that caloric requirements decrease from the moment of injury and remain lower throughout life (Zejdlik, 1992). People with SCI experience a reduction in energy needs proportioned to the amount of muscle that has been denerated. Nutritional requirements for the SCI population must be calculated specifically but generally are 20 percent less than those of the non-injured population.

A. **Demographics:** All persons with SCI have the potential for alterations in nutritional status.

B. **Etiology and Precipitating Factors:**
   1. SCI: Spinal cord trauma affects the organs that are responsible for maintaining nutritional status. Associated internal injuries and malnutritional during the critical phase following SCI frequently compound complications.
   2. Age, neuromuscular process, and structural deficiencies may alter swallowing. The complex innervation to eating and swallowing process can result in multiple variations of impairment. (See to Table 15-1).
   3. Individuals with chronic, progressive diseases, such as cerebral palsy, multiple sclerosis, and amyotrophic lateral sclerosis may develop progressive degeneration of swallowing ability.

Table 15-1 Neuromuscular Diseases Associated With Poor Deglutition

Stages of deglutition	Disease	Characteristics
Oral preparatory	Cerebral palsy	Poor suck reflex. Inappropriate reflexive behaviors.
	Parkinson's disease	Poor mastication
	Multiple sclerosis (when cranial nerve XII is involved)	Foods inadequately chewed.
	Amyotrophic lateral sclerosis Cerebrovascular accident Huntington's disease Head trauma	Poor tongue control on mobility
Lingual	Cerebrovascular accident	Delay in swallow reflex
	Huntington's disease Head trauma Cerebral palsy Parkinson's disease Multiple sclerosis (when cranial nerve IX is involved)	Choking or coughing
	Cerebrovascular accident	Lingual hemiparesis
Pharyngeal	Parkinson's disease Poliomyelitis	Impaired pharyngeal motility and peristalsis
	Cerebrovascular accident Myasthenia gravis	Residue remains in valleculae and pyriform sinuses
	Myotonic dystrophy Head trauma Amyotrophic lateral sclerosis	Aspiration

From Eating and Swallowing, by N.H. Glenn, 1996, in S.P. Hoeman (Ed.), *Rehabilitation Nursing: Process and Application* (2nd Ed.) (p. 350), St. Louis: Mosby. Reprinted with permission.

C. **Anatomy and Physiology of the Digestive System:**
 1. Alimentary canal:
    a. Mouth
    b. Esophagus
    c. Stomach
    d. Small intestine
    e. Large intestine
    f. Anal canal
 2. Neurophysiologic control:
    a. Primarily autonomic control, except for voluntary control of chewing, swallowing, and defecation
    b. Effect of spinal cord injury on motor and secretory functions of digestion is generally temporary.
    c. Functions usually return when spinal shock resolves.
 3. Physiologic functions affected by SCI:
    a. Peristalsis
       (1) Parasympathetic control transmitted by vagus nerve
    b. Secretion of digestive juices

     (1)   Parasympathetic control transmitted by vagus nerve

     (2)   Individuals with tetraplegia may experience hyperchlorhydria: excessive acidic condition due to preservation of the parasympathetic system and interruption of the sympathetic system.

  c. Impairment in oral preparatory phase characterized by poor sensation and perception about the quantity and location of food in the mouth.

  d. Impaired motor control of muscles and tongue movement.

  e. Impaired pharyngeal motility characterized by swallowing problems with increased risk for aspiration.

  f. Impaired head and trunk control, which necessitates special attention to posture and head positioning.

III. Nursing Assessment

A. **Nursing History:**
1. How many meals do you eat each day?
2. Are there any food(s) that you like or dislike?
3. What do your typical meals contain?
4. Do you have any food allergies?
5. Are there any religious or cultural beliefs that influence what you do or do not eat?
6. How much do you drink each day?
7. What types of fluids do you drink?
8. How would you describe your appetite before the SCI?
9. How would you describe your appetite since the SCI?
10. Do you ever experience nausea, vomiting, bloating, diarrhea?
11. Are there any foods that may cause these symptoms?
12. Do you take medications (that may alter nutritional status)?
13. Do you tire easily or become short of breath while eating?
14. Do you sit in any particular position while eating or soon after?
15. Do you have a history of aspiration pneumonia?
16. Do you have pain with swallowing?
17. Do foods get stuck in your throat?
18. Do you have difficulty with swallowing solid or soft foods?
19. Does your food regurgitate nasally?
20. Do you experience choking or coughing when eating?
21. Do you have difficulty with swallowing liquids? (Glenn, 1996)

B. **Physical Assessment:**
1. Observe the person. Are they underweight or overweight? What is the condition of their skin and hair? Assess balance, head control, and facial symmetry.
2. What is their current height and weight? How does this compare with their "Ideal Weight"?
3. Muscle mass and body fat: Upper arm measurements may not be valid in an individual with tetraplegia because of variations associated with disuse atrophy.
4. Inspect the oral cavity, looking for signs of dehydration in mucosa, abnormalities in the teeth, presence of dentures, and ability to move the tongue.
5. Assess chewing and swallowing ability (See Table 15-2)
6. Assess function of lower gastrointestinal tract (See Table 15-3)
7. Assess functional ability related to feeding

C. **Diagnostic Studies:**
1. Lab findings
  a. Hematocrit and hemoglobin low?
  b. Serum Albumin: Elevation is not uncommon, especially early after injury.
  c. Serum Protein
     (1)   After SCI, all body proteins become functional; no storage occurs.
     (2)   Negative nitrogen balance may be induced.

Table 15-2 Assessing Chewing and Swallowing Ability

Purpose
To identify problems associated with malnutrition and to promote safety by preventing choking and aspiration.

Action	Rationale
1. First examine the mouth.	Dental caries, absent teeth, and gum disease may be painful and hamper chewing ability. Young people may have impacted wisdom teeth. Periodontal problems with reddened, swollen, or spongy gums that bleed easily are most common in patients over 40. A major problem in the elderly is ill-fitting dentures due to shrinking gums.
2. Check for any swallowing difficulties.	Although not associated with SCI per se, a patient with a very high cervical cord injury may experience ascending edema, affecting the lower brain stem and subduing the swallowing reflex.
3. To check for gag reflex, brush the eyelash lightly with a piece of soft tissue.	Usually if the blink reflex is present so is an intact gag reflex.
4. Observe the tracheal aspirate for evidence of oral or tube feedings. Routinely add blue food coloring to all tube feeds in the critical care setting. Note if swallowing becomes painful (burning sensation) on a continuing care basis.	To distinguish oral and pulmonary secretions from aspirated tube feedings. A positive result will confirm the connection between the trachea and the esophagus. It may also suggest a rare but more serious complication, tracheoesophageal fistula. Differentiating the two requires radiology or endoscopy, but a fistula takes 2 to 4 weeks to develop, so a positive dye test before then probably indicates swallowing dysfunction. Although this problem usually disappears after the airway is removed, the patient requiring prolonged use may have difficulty meeting nutritional requirements.
5. Closely observe ability to swallow in patients who have just had a halo-thoracic brace applied or who are in cervical traction.	Maintaining the neck in the desired degree of hyperextension may cause swallowing difficulties. However, with very slight adjustment of the bars by the physician this problem can usually be solved. Traction-related problems can be more difficult to solve. Relying on liquid/soft diets is probably the best temporary solution.

From Maintaining Optimal Nutrition, by C.P. Zejdlik, 1992, in C.P. Zejdlik (Ed.), *Management of Spinal Cord Injury* (2nd ed., p. 334), Boston: Jones & Bartlett. Copyright 1992 by Jones & Bartlett. Reprinted with permission.

Table 15-3 Assessing the Function of the Lower Gastrointestinal Tract

Purpose
To determine function of the lower gastrointestinal system, primarily to determine route(s) of nutritional intake possible. Perform an abdominal assessment, observe the consistency and frequency of stool, and look for systemic signs and symptoms of gastric upset.

Action	Rationale
1. Check the abdomen.	Normal bowel sounds are intermittent and vary in intensity but indicate a functional/usable gastrointestinal system. Be alert for absent, occasional, or weak sounds immediately following injury, indicating that the tract is still sluggish and absorption would be impaired. Flatus, stooling, and decreasing amounts of nasogastric returns are better indicators of returning gastrointestinal function.
• First, listen for bowel sounds by auscultating the abdomen in all four quadrants. • Next percuss and palpate the abdomen. • Note flatus, stooling.	The techniques of percussion and palpation should follow auscultation as manual pressure applied to the abdomen may change peristaltic activity. The abdomen should be soft and flat without evidence of distension, swelling, or rigidity related to paralytic ileus.
2. Recognize physical discomfort.	When large portions of the body trunk are without sensation, appreciation of localized pain is not possible.
• In addition to the obvious signs of nausea and vomiting, be alert for generalized tension, malaise, anorexia, shoulder tip pain (the most common referred pain); and, in tetraplegic patients, headache, perspiring, or chills.	These signs and symptoms are indicative of abdominal abnormality.
• Above all, be alert for an increased pulse rate or an elevated systemic temperature and/or white blood count without other apparent cause.	This may signal acute abdominal distress or peritonitis, which may cause death if unrecognized or unchecked.
3. Examine bowel elimination patterns in detail.	Lack of control and bouts of constipation or diarrhea greatly affect the patient's nutritional status.

From Maintaining optimal nutrition by C.P. Zejdlik, 1992, in C.P. Zejdlik (Ed.), *Management of Spinal Cord Injury* (2nd ed., p. 335). Boston: James & Bartlett. Copyright 1992 by Jones & Bartlett. Reprinted with permission.

2. Dysphagia:
   a. Bedside swallow exam
   b. Manometry modified barium swallow with videofluoroscopy
   c. Videoendoscopy

IV. Nursing Process: Acute Spinal Cord Injury

A. **Nursing Diagnosis:** Alteration in nutrition: less than body requirements.

B. **Defining Characteristics:** In the days following injury, it is not uncommon for the spinal cord injured individual to lose a significant amount of weight (10-30 lbs.). Malnutrition is due to the increased caloric needs of the body when dealing with a major physiologic stress and decreased intake ability associated with paralytic ileus and/or associated internal injuries.

C. **Expected Outcomes:**
   1. Maintenance and/or improvement of current nutritional status. The goal is for delivery and absorption of adequate nutrients. This can be demonstrated in a variety of ways:
      a. Body weight acceptance for height and build.
      b. Weight gain of 1-2 lbs. each week.
      c. Positive nitrogen balance.
      d. Blood hematology and chemistry within normal limits.
   2. Appropriate absorption of nutrients without side effect. Able to tolerate the type of nutritional support being given, without experiencing diarrhea or vomiting.
      a. Serum electrolytes are within normal limits.
      b. Other lab studies are within normal limits.
      c. No diarrhea or vomiting experienced with the support being given.
   3. Remain without nutritional complications.

D. **Nursing Interventions:**
   1. Fluid Intake:
      a. Supplement nutritionally as soon as possible; intravenous (IV) solutions have no nutritional value.
      b. Adequate fluid intake is a minimum of 2000 ml/24 hours.
      c. Replace IV's with oral fluid intake as soon as possible.
   2. Caloric and protein intake:
      a. Needs to be monitored closely early on.
      b. Oral intake needs to begin as soon as paralytic ileus has resolved.
      c. Intake may need to be small, frequent meals.
      d. Often high protein, high calorie is needed.
      e. Monitor intake and output (I&O).
      f. Prevent aspiration.
      g. Encourage good nutritional habits. Three balanced meals per day, as well as snacks may be required.
      h. Oral intake may need to be supplemented with either total parenteral nutrition (TPN) or enteral feedings.
      i. Encourage families to bring in food that may help to stimulate the person's appetite.
      j. Increase activity as tolerated and as stability permits.
      k. Begin a bowel program to avoid bowel complications.
      l. Provide health education.
   3. Prevent complications:
      a. Paralytic Ileus:
         (1) Definition: Absence of normal peristalsis in the small bowel, allowing fluid and gas to accumulate.
         (2) Interventions include:
            (a) Nothing by mouth for first 48-72 hours post-injury. Replace fluids via IV.
            (b) Auscultate the abdomen for bowel sounds.

194

(c) Observe for changing abdominal size. Measurements at the umbilicus are helpful.

(d) Do a rectal check and remove any stool gently.

(e) Place a rectal tube for thirty minutes at a time.

(f) Monitor for the passing of the ileus: return of bowel sounds and the passing of stool or flatus.

(g) Insert nasogastric (NG) tube as ordered to decompress stomach and reduce risk of aspiration.

    b. Gastric ulcers (Stress ulcer or acute peptic ulcer):

      (1) Definition: Gastrointestinal hemorrhage associated with a spinal cord injury.

      (2) Interventions include:

(a) Administer histamine-blocking agents as ordered.

(b) Monitor for signs and symptoms of gastric bleeding, including referred shoulder tip pain in individuals with tetraplegia.

(c) May need to insert a nasogastric tube attached to suction and give an iced saline lavage, and/or blood replacement.

(d) Post-op measures to maintain comfort and prevent post-op complications, when surgery is needed.

    c. Post-traumatic malnutrition:

      (1) Definition: Undernourishment of the individual due to inability to meet the caloric needs imposed by the physiologic stress of the injury. Caloric needs generally increase up to 50 percent immediately post-injury.

      (2) Interventions:

(a) Nutritional history and assessment are completed ideally within 24 hours of injury.

(b) Request a consult from a specialized nutritional assessment.

(c) When caloric needs are not being met, may need to institute either enteral feedings or TPN, depending on gastrointestinal function.

(d) Monitor caloric and protein intake.

(e) Monitor weight.

E. Evaluation:

1. Review documentation to determine intake. Utilize this data to determine if any changes need to occur in the manner in which nutritional needs are being met. If nutritional supplements of any type are required, determine which is the best manner for this to occur: oral, enteral or TPN.

    a. If enteral feedings have been instituted already, is the person able to tolerate them?

    b. Is the person experiencing bloating, diarrhea?

    c. Monitor blood chemistry and hematology.

2. Determine if any of the following complications have occurred and if the individual has recovered from them:

    a. Paralytic ileus

    b. Gastrointestinal ulcer

    c. Malnutrition

V. Nursing Process: Long-Term Spinal Cord Injury

A. **Nursing Diagnosis:** Alteration in nutrition: more than body requirements

B. **Defining Characteristics:** In the years after injury, it is not uncommon for the spinal cord injured individual to gain a significant amount of weight (10-30 lbs.), due to lack of regulating intake to amount of energy expended.

C. **Expected Outcomes:**

1. Maintain the ideal body weight.

    a. Ideal weight for individual with paraplegia: 10-15 lbs. below Metropolitan Life Insurance ideal body weight.

    b. Ideal weight for individual with tetraplegia: 15-20 lbs. below Metropolitan Life Insurance ideal body weight.

  2. Maintain a healthy and appropriate nutritional intake.

D. Nursing Interventions:

1. Fluid intake
    a. Remember juices and non-diet sodas have calories.
    b. Replace above fluids with water and diet sodas, as much as possible.
    c. Adequate fluid intake is 2000 ml/24 hours, depending on bladder program.
2. Caloric intake
    a. Needs to be monitored. Caloric needs decrease as the individual ages with a disability and as the individual's activity decreases. May need to keep a logbook.
    b. Intake may need to be small, frequent meals.
    c. Encourage good nutritional habits. Three balanced meals per day, as well as low-calorie snacks, may be required.
    d. Increase activity.
    e. Health education: consult a Registered Dietician as needed.

E. Evaluation:
Review documentation to determine caloric and fluid intake. Utilize this data to determine if any changes need to occur in the manner in which nutritional needs are being met.
1. Is the person losing weight, if that is the goal?
2. Is the person maintaining weight, if that is the goal?

VI. Nursing Process: Spinal Cord Disorders

A. Nursing Diagnoses:
1. High risk for aspiration
2. Fluid volume deficit or risk
3. Knowledge deficit in nutrition or adaptive equipment

B. Defining Characteristics:
1. Weight loss/gain
2. Sensation impairment in mouth or throat
3. Impaired motor control of tongue
4. Impaired pharyngeal motility/difficulty swallowing
5. Impaired motor control of head and trunk

C. Expected Outcomes:
1. Maintain maximal level of independence in eating
2. Adequate nutritional intake
3. Prevent aspiration
4. Maintain adequate body weight
5. Correct use of adaptive equipment

D. Nursing Interventions:
1. Compensatory techniques (Glenn, 1996,pp. 354-355).
    a. Begin by placing the client in an upright sitting position with the head bent slightly forward. The forward tilt of the head is important to prevent food from hitting the posterior pharyngeal wall before the swallow reflex begins.
    b. If the client has poor head control and the head falls forward, hold the head up by placing the palm of your hand on the client's forehead for support.
    c. Sit down when assisting the client to eat. This action communicates time and willingness to help.

d. Initially use small amounts of soft food that are easy to swallow (applesauce, purees).

e. Place a half teaspoonful on the middle to back part of the tongue. However, if the client has tongue or facial paralysis or has had a partial laryngectomy, the correct placement is on the unaffected intact side, not midline.

f. With the spoon, push down on the tongue as you remove the food from the spoon.

g. If swallowing does not occur, remove the spoon from the client's mouth.

h. Instruct the client to move the food around and toward the rear of the mouth.

i. If the swallow comes slowly, press on the tip of the client's head with the palm of your hand. This action will decrease laryngeal tension and facilitate swallowing.

j. Check to see that the client's lips are sealed or the swallowing reflex will not begin. Manually seal the lips together or use a jaw control manuever to pull the jaws together.

k. If swallowing does not occur, try placing your thumb on the client's chin, moving the chin downward toward the sternum to facilitate the swallow.

2. Adequate fluid intake:
   a. Collaborate with rehab team to plan interventions based on diagnostic test results.
   b. Liquids may be thickened.
   c. Assure safety if individual chokes.

3. Health education:
   a. Diet
   b. Nutrition
   c. Assistive devices for feeding
   d. Activities and exercise

VII. Health Education

The following topics need to be covered when teaching nutrition:

A. Anatomy and Physiology of Digestion
1. Digestion
2. Peristalsis
3. Bowel function

B. Food and Fluids
1. Basic Food Groups: Food Guide Pyramid (US Department of Agriculture, 1997)
   a. Fats, oils, sweets
   b. Milk, yogurt and cheese
   c. Meat, poultry, fish, dried beans, eggs and nuts
   d. Vegetables
   e. Fruits
   f. Bread, cereal, rice and pasta
2. Discuss the importance of each food group:
   a. How much should you eat of each?
   b. Caloric and fat content
   c. Fiber requirements
3. Types of Fluids
   a. Juices
   b. Water
   c. Soda
   d. Caffeinated hot beverages (coffee, tea, hot chocolate)
4. Discuss the importance of fluids:
   a. How much of each should you drink?
   b. Caloric content?
   c. Fluid regulation for bladder management met?

   C. **How to eat a "Balanced" diet:**
      1. Three meals versus six smaller meals.
      2. How to incorporate each food group into your diet.

VII. Special Issues Related to Pediatric Care

   A. **Goal:** The goal of nutritional management is to support normal growth based on a child's growth curve.

   B. **Caloric needs for normal growth (Heller, Bujold, Baer, & Harris, 1996)**
      1. Infants need 120 kilocalories/kg/day.
      2. Older child needs 60 to 80 kilocalories/kg/day.
      3. With an acute SCI basal needs are increased to account for ongoing catabolic state.
         a. Protein requirements to achieve an anabolic state may be twice as high as the recommended daily allowance. Nutritional support must be started early and within 48 hours because protein catabolism starts within several hours of injury.
         b. Calcium requirements (65 mg/kg/day depending on child's age) need to be closely monitored in an acute SCI or during early rehabilitation because of risk of hypercalcemia (serum calcium greater than 11 mg/dl). This usually resolves within 18 months following injury.
            (1) Symptoms include irritability, headache, polydypsia, malaise. Small children may be unable to relate symptoms.
            (2) Treatment consists of calcium-limited diet, mobilization, and weight bearing when possible.
      4. To meet appropriate caloric needs, children with cervical injuries may be considered for percutaneous endoscopic or surgical gastrostomy. Oral feedings are given if airway is protected and oral motor function is adequate.
      5. The child with an associated head injury or cognitive dysfunction will need close supervision and/or calorie restriction because of a potential impairment of hunger, satiety cues, or regulation.
      6. Maintaining an appropriate weight is important regardless of the type of spinal cord impairment. Increased weight or obesity decreases level and type of activity and limits the child's ability to participate in activities of daily living (ADL) and normal childhood activities.
      7. Attention must be given to crossover allergies (especially avocados, bananas, and tropical fruits) with latex allergies in children with spina bifida, SCI, and congenital urinary defects.
      8. Long-term caloric needs must be balanced between intake of calories and expenditure of energy. Caloric needs for the child with spina bifida and SCI are usually under the norm following the acute phase.

   C. **Suggested Maintenance Fluid Needs (Heller et al, 1996):**
      1. 100 cc/kg/day for first 10 kg.
      2. 50 cc/kg/day for next 10 kg.
      3. 25 cc/kg/day for every additional 10kg.
      4. Fluid needs increase with fevers, sweating, illness.
      5. Appropriate or adequate fluid intake may be difficult to obtain and maintain, especially in the child with myelomeningocele and SCI. The sense of hunger and thirst may be altered (especially in the children under 5 years) and the ability to obtain fluids independently may make the goal of adequate fluid intake difficult to achieve. A minimal fluid goal, a schedule, and fluid delivery method (cup, sport bottle, chair cup holder, etc.) need to be established to promote the intake of adequate fluids.

   D. **Gastrointestinal Complications:**
      1. Children may not represent with classic signs and symptoms of an acute abdomen, so children with acute SCI should be suspected of having and intra-abdominal injury.

2. Paralytic ileus is common in children and may lead to abdominal distention resulting in emesis and impaired respiratory function, due to compression of the diaphragm.

3. Stress ulcer prophylaxis should be considered in all children who experience an acute injury or surgical intervention. A histamine-blocking agent is usually effective in preventing this complication. Potential adverse reactions of these drugs should be considered when the child has an associated head injury. Children with a tracheostomy or gastrostomy tube should be treated with a histamine-blocking agent even after the acute period.

4. Gastroesophageal reflux should be suspected in all children with acute SCI, and duodenal feedings should be considered. Reflux precautions should be taken with the head of bed elevated for 30 minutes after feeding.

Practical Application #1

J.H. is a 22-year-old male who was injured 20 days earlier in a motorcycle crash and sustained C5 tetraplegia, necessitating halo placement and a tracheotomy. Prior to his injury, J.H. was in good health, 6'2" tall and weighed 180 lbs. He was very active and reported that he did not necessarily eat three meals a day. His most common pattern was to eat lunch and dinner (most of the time at a restaurant), and snack throughout the day. He disliked few foods and would "eat just about anything." Since sustained his injury, J.H. reported loss of appetite and discomfort with swallowing. He lost 25 lbs and now weighed 155 pounds. His family offered to bring in food from home, but even that did not piqued his appetite.

Upon reviewing his prior eating patterns, the nurse discovered that fruits and vegetables (including fruit juices) were almost non-existent in J.H.'s diet. He did eat quite a bit of meat and cheese, and he drank soda. The nurse reviewed J.H.'s nutritional assessment and found that he had no food allergies and did not subscribe to any cultural food habits. Although J.H. had a good appetite prior to his injury, he told his nurse he did not feel like eating nor did he now have any energy. J.H. appeared to be undernourished, his skin was ashen in color, hair dull, and he was thin. Review of the lab values indicated that his serum albumin was elevated and that he was in negative nitrogen balance.

Education included a discussion on the four food groups and the meaning of J.H.'s lab values. The nurse discussed with J.H. and his family ways to make food more appealing; for example, smaller meals served more frequently. J.H. agreed to try the six-meal plan and promised to try to incorporate all food groups into his daily food choices. He started a food diary and set a goal not to lose any more weight within the next two weeks.

Two weeks later, review of his food diary showed those days that J.H. accomplished incorporating the four food groups into his meals, as well as those days in which he did not accomplish the goal. The nurse reviewed with him what could have been done differently on those days that he did not succeed. He lost less than a pound in the time frame monitored and in fact, that occurred in the first week.

The next goal jointly set was that J.H. would keep track of his intake only on those days when he had questions about his diet and he would continue to maintain his weight. The amount of weight to be gained was the next goal.

Practical Application #2

J.M., a 40-year-old female, was injured 20 years earlier in a fall resulting in T6 paraplegia. At the time of injury, J.M. weighed 110 pounds and was 5'4" in height. Over the years, she gained some weight, which she wants to lose. She related that after she was injured, she lost approximately 20 lbs and had difficulty at that time gaining some of the weight she had lost. She started eating several small meals, and found that she was able to gain back the weight. Her goal then was to weigh approximately what she had weighed at the time of injury. Over the years, she steadily added weight, to the point that she now weighed 175 pounds. She is no longer independent in transfers or dressing, needs assistance with picking things up from the floor, and generally, does not feel good about herself. She has had some skin issues lately, which she believed were weight-related.

A review of her eating habits revealed that the four food groups were not represented daily and that although J.M. reported she only ate three meals a day, she snacked frequently. She added that she felt as though she did not eat much. J.M. has a sedentary job and her physical activity is limited to pushing her wheelchair. The plan was for J.M. to keep an activity and diet log including what she eats, when she eats and her daily activity for one week. Although J.M. thought she didn't eat much, a review of her log showed that her caloric and fat intake were high. The four food groups were not represented throughout the week, and she indeed led a sedentary lifestyle.

The plan was for J.M. to gradually lose the weight that she put on over the years. She sets a goal to lose 40 pounds over a period of 18 months. The first part of the program was to give J.M. some alternatives to the high-caloric foods that she ate, which would also satisfy her appetite. She agreed to incorporate more vegetables and fruits into her diet and to cut down on snacking and portion size. She also agreed that after she saw her physician, she would increase her activity, either by joining a gym or by simply beginning to push her wheelchair more.

Three months later, J.M. returned for follow-up. She had lost twelve pounds and stated that she was feeling better about herself. Her eating habits were more appropriate for her activity level and age. She planned to continue on the course set three months earlier; however, believed that her goal of 40 pounds over 18 months may be a little low, and she may need to eventually readjust it.

References and Selected Bibliography

Bayley, E.W. & Turcke, S. (1992). *A comprehensive curriculum for trauma nursing.* Boston: Jones & Bartlett.

Blissitt, P.A. (1990). Nutrition in acute spinal cord injury. *Critical Care Nursing Clinics of North America, 2*(3), 375-384.

Chin, D.E. & Kearns, P. (1991). Nutrition in the spinal injured patient. *Nutrition in Clinical Practice, 6,* 213-222.

Glenn, N.H. (1996). Eating and swallowing. In S.P. Hoeman (Ed.), *Rehabilitation nursing: Process and application* (2nd Ed.). (pp. 347-360). St. Louis, MO: Mosby.

Heller, L., Bujold, C., Baer, M., & Harris, A. (1996). Nutrition for children with special health care needs. *Nutrition Focus, 11*(3), 1-9.

Lagger, L. (1983). Spinal cord injury: Nutritional management. *Journal of Neuroscience Nursing, 15*(5), 310-312.

Reed, M.A. (1987). Nursing considerations in acute spinal cord injury. *Critical Care Clinics, 3*(3), 679-691.

Rice, H. B., Ponichtera-Mulcare, J. A., & Glaser, R. M. (1995). Nutrition and the spinal cord injured individual. *Clinical Kinesiology, 49,* 21-27.

U.S. Department of Agriculture. (1997). *Food guide pyramid: A guide to daily food choices.* Washington, DC: U.S. Department of Health and Human Services.

Worthington, P., Crowe, M. A., & Armenti, V. T. (1993). Nutritional support for patients with spinal cord injury. *Trauma, 9*(2), 82-92.

Zejdlik, C.P. (Ed.) (1992). *Management of spinal cord injury.* (2nd ed.). Boston: Jones & Bartlett.

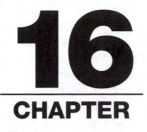

CHAPTER

Bowel Elimination and Continence
Audrey Nelson, PhD, RN, FAAN
Cynthia Kraft Fine, MSN, RN, CRRN

I. Learning Objectives

A. Identify the common pathophysiology of upper motor neuron (UMN) bowel, lower motor neuron (LMN) bowel, uninhibited neurogenic bowel, and motor paralytic bowel, as seen in spinal cord impairment (SCI).

B. Identify goals for establishing bowel control after SCI.

C. List the common nursing interventions utilized in managing a neurogenic bowel.

D. Describe a comprehensive assessment, management, and education plan for gastrointestinal (GI) complications.

E. Discuss the long-term implications of neurogenic bowel dysfunction.

II. Introduction

Altered bowel function may occur whenever the central nervous system (CNS) has been impaired. When disease or disability results in loss of bowel control, incontinence may become as devastating a problem as the SCI itself. This chapter presents the nursing process for the functional alterations of elimination in bowel in persons with multiple sclerosis, tumor, myelomeningocele, intervertebral disk disease, and traumatic injury to the spinal cord. Control of incontinence and prevention of constipation and diarrhea are possible through an effective bowel program. The development of an effective program requires knowledge of normal and altered bowel physiology as well as an in-depth assessment of bowel function.

A. **Demographics**
   1. All persons living with SCI have the potential for alteration in bowel elimination.
   2. As many as 23 percent of persons with long-term SCI have required hospitalization for

neurogenic bowel complications (Kirk, King, Temple, Bourjalais, & Thomas, 1997; Stone, Nino-Murcia, Wolfe, & Perkash, 1990a).

3. Bowel dysfunction affects life activities or life style in 41 percent of the SCI population (Kirk, et. al., 1997) including depression, sexuality, and social discomfort.

4. Many individuals with SCI rank bowel and bladder dysfunction as one of their major (54 percent) life-limiting problems (Stone et al., 1990a). Levi, Hultling, Nash, & Seiger (1995) noted that 41 percent of the Stockholm spinal cord injury study rated bowel care management as a moderate to severe life problem.

5. Unidentified gastrointestinal complications may account for 5 to 10 percent of deaths associated with SCI (Charney, Juler & Comarr, 1975; Miller, Staas & Herbison, 1975; Juler & Eltorai, 1985; Whiteneck et al., 1992). Gore, Mintzer & Calenoff (1981) found that 11 percent of persons with SCI had serious gastrointestinal complications, excluding nausea, vomiting, diarrhea, constipation and transient abdominal pain. These complications were more frequent among individuals with cervical and upper thoracic injuries (14 percent and 11 percent, respectively) than among individuals with more caudal injuries (5 to 6 percent). Complications observed during the first month post-injury included reflex ileus (4.6 percent), peptic ulcers (1.4 percent), and pancreatitis (2.2 percent). Fecal impaction was the most common complication during the chronic period, followed by peptic ulcers.

B. **Etiology:** Damage to the central nervous system and subsequent dysfunction of the sensory, motor, or autonomic nervous systems may leave the individual unable to feel the urge to defecate, perceive gastrointestinal symptoms, or evacuate the bowel voluntarily and completely.

1. Etiology of UMN bowel includes:
   a. Spinal cord trauma, tumor, vascular disease, syringomyelia, and multiple sclerosis.
   b. Level of spinal cord lesion above T12 to L1.
   c. Resultant pattern of incontinence: Infrequent, sudden, unexpected.

2. Etiology of LMN bowel includes:
   a. Spinal cord trauma, tumor, spina bifida, and intervertebral disk disease.
   b. Level of spinal lesion at or below T12 to L1.
   c. Resultant pattern of incontinence: May be continuous or induced by exercise or stress.

3. Uninhibited neurogenic bowel:
   a. Results from damage to upper motor neurons; typically seen after stroke, traumatic brain injury, multiple sclerosis, and trauma.
   b. Internal and external sphincters are intact or hypertonic.
   c. Saddle sensation usually is preserved.
   d. Bulbocavernosus (BC) reflex is varied or increased.
   e. Sacral reflex is intact.
   f. Defecation is involuntary and sudden.

4. Motor paralytic bowel:
   a. Results from damage to the anterior horn cells or S2, S3, and S4 ventral roots, such as with poliomyelitis, intervertebral disk disease, trauma, or tumor.
   b. Saddle sensation is intact.
   c. Bulbocavernosus reflex and anal reflex are absent.
   d. Incontinence is rare except in widespread disease.

C. **Anatomy of the Lower Gastrointestinal (GI) Tract**
1. Large intestine:
   a. Ascending colon
   b. Transverse colon
   c. Descending colon
   d. Sigmoid colon

2. Two sphincters control the anal canal (rectum):
   a. Internal Sphincter: a thickened portion of smooth circular muscle surrounding the canal just inside the anus.
      (1) Smooth muscle innervated by the sympathetic nerves.
      (2) Maintains continence of liquids and gas.

       (3)   High pressure in this area leads to evacuation.

       (4)   Under involuntary control.

       (5)   Major contributor to the resting pressure of closed anal canal thus maintaining continence.

  b. External Sphincter: a circular band of striated muscle that is continuous with the pelvic floor; visible portion of anus.

       (1)   Under voluntary motor control that is mediated by the pudendal and inferior rectal nerves.

       (2)   Maintains continence of solid feces.

D. Neural Control of Bowel Function

1. Intrinsic control is achieved through nerve fibers in the large bowel that respond to local stimulation. When the bowel becomes overdistended, peristalsis is stimulated.

2. The autonomic nervous system provides both parasympathetic and sympathetic stimulation to the bowel. Parasympathetic fibers emerge from the vagus nerve and sacral (S2-S4) outflow to terminate in the colon, rectum, and internal and external anal sphincters. Sympathetic fibers emerge from the lower thoracolumbar (T6-L3) outflow to innervate the same areas. Parasympathetic stimulation increases motility and peristalsis, maintains tone, stimulates secretions, and usually relaxes sphincter activity; sympathetic stimulation provides antagonistic control and thus decreases motility, slows peristalsis, inhibits secretions, and generally contracts sphincters (Zejdlik, 1992).

3. Defecation is controlled by communications from the brain, via the sacral spinal cord (S3-S4), to the external anal sphincter. As stool enters the rectum, the urge to defecate is felt, and voluntary relaxation of the external anal sphincter allows stool to be passed. If the external anal sphincter is kept tonically contracted, the defecation reflex is suppressed and disappears for several hours (Zejdlik, 1992).

4. Actual elimination of stool may be aided through the Valsalva maneuver, unless contraindicated. The person takes a deep breath and attempts to exhale against a closed glottis while at the same time tightening the abdominal muscles, which requires intact innervation to the lower thoracic cord (T6-T12). The actual increase in intra-abdominal pressure forces stool into the rectum (Zejdlik, 1992).

E. Reflexes Utilized

1. Present after the cessation of spinal shock in individuals with an upper motor neuron injury.

2. Reflex contractions of external sphincter (S2-S4)

  a. The most important reflex in maintaining bowel continence in spinal cord injured individuals.

  b. Present in UMN injuries, absent in LMN injuries.

  c. Increase in fecal volume leads to an increase in rectal tone.

3. Rectocolic reflex (S2-S4)

  a. Mediated by the pelvic splanchnic nerves.

  b. Described as the feeling that you have when a fecal mass or high volume of fluid is present in the rectum, leading to gastric rush. You control this by squeezing the external sphincter.

4. Gastrocolic reflex (Myenteric and Mesoteric Plexus): Peristalsis which occurs following the entrance of food into the stomach.

5. Bulbocavernosus reflex

  a. A positive bulbocavernosus reflex indicates that the reflex activity of the sacral cord is intact. This reflex causes a palpable and visible contracture of the anal sphincter when pressure is applied to the glans penis or clitoris. The bulbocavernosus reflex is usually present very soon after injury, before spinal shock fully subsides. It indicates an UMN bowel dysfunction.

  b. Presence indicates that S2-S4 intact.

6. Anocutaneous wink (S2-S4)

  a. The anal reflex, or anal wink, if present, also indicates an UMN bowel dysfunction. This reflex causes a visible contraction of the external anal sphincter in response to a pinprick.

  b. Indicates whether S2-S4 is intact bilaterally.

F. **Physiology**
1. The ileum, cecum, and colon promote active absorption of water and sodium and trigger secretion of mucus, potassium, and bicarbonate essential to stool formation.
2. Functions of the colon
   a. Secretion.
   b. Absorption.
   c. Movement of stool towards the rectum. Rectal compliance and capacity are critical factors in maintaining bowel continence.

G. **Defecation Process**
1. The gastrocolic response or "reflex" is initiated by eating, which increases propulsive small intestine and colonic motility. With distention of colon, rectal stretch receptors stimulate inferior hypogastric plexus and inferior mesenteric plexus; impulses enter spinal cord, ascend to cortex, and initiate awareness of colonic and rectal distention.
2. Peristalsis of colon propels feces to rectum, which initiates a reflex rectal contraction mediated by pelvic splanchnic nerves originating from S2, S3, and S4.
3. Rectal reflexes relax internal sphincter and contract external sphincter so that stool can be expelled.
4. Voluntary defecation begins with closure of the glottis, followed by descent of diaphragm and contraction of abdominal muscles; this provides increased intra-abdominal pressure, which promotes movement of stool.
5. Pelvic musculature relaxes simultaneously with internal and external anal sphincters until complete emptying occurs.
6. Following rectal emptying, pelvic floor rises and anal sphincters return to their tonic state of contraction (Zejdlik, 1992).

III. Initial Assessment

The findings of the history and examination, considered together with the individual's overall capabilities, resources, and lifestyle, provide information for planning, managing, and evaluating a bowel program.

A. **Nursing History:**
1. Describe bowel function before SCI.
2. Did anything in particular trigger bowel movements (e.g., warm beverage, breakfast)?
3. What was the stool consistency and amount?
4. Was there a history of bowel disease (e.g., Crohn's, Colitis, Diverticulitis)?
5. Describe typical diet. Did any food cause constipation or diarrhea?
6. Describe typical activity pattern, including exercise routine.
7. Describe typical fluid intake.
8. Describe how the injury (disease) has affected bowel function.
9. Describe problems with bowel elimination, such as abdominal distention, difficulty of evacuation, respiratory embarrassment, early satiety, nausea, rectal bleeding, constipation, diarrhea, or pain.
10. Describe lifestyle, e.g., schedule for work or school; availability of assistance, if needed; amount of time needed to complete bowel care regime.
11. Describe current bowel program:
    a. Frequency.
    b. Time of day.
    c. Method of management.
    d. Position (bed, commode chair).
12. Explore use of medications that influence bowel activity, including:
    a. Diuretics.
    b. Antacids.
    c. Nonsteroidal and anti-inflammatory agents.
    d. Anticholinergics.

    e. Antidepressants.

    f. Antibiotics.

    g. Antispasmotics.

    h. Laxatives and enemas.

13. Use of alcohol and/or drugs.

B. Examination:
1. Examine height and weight, hydration status, skin.
2. Auscultate for bowel sounds. This is especially important early after injury (within the first seven to fifteen days). Absent or present? Normal or hyperactive? Where did you hear them?
3. Inspect the abdomen for distention. If present, measure abdominal girth at level of umbilicus on a daily basis (at the same time each day).
4. Palpate the abdomen to determine if it is soft, hard, or tender.
5. Percuss the abdomen to determine distention and presence/absence of stool.
6. Examination of stool: A normal stool is softly formed and has a characteristic odor caused by the bacteria present in the large bowel to aid digestion. A normal stool is composed of 75 percent water and 25 percent solid materials, such as undigested roughage and other digestive wastes. Note any hard, dry stools that are difficult to pass or any loose, watery stools. During the first four weeks after injury, when gastric ulceration is most frequent, be alert for dark, tarry stools (melena) (Zejdlik, 1992).
7. Rectal exam:
    a. Fecal impaction.
    b. Guaiac stool.
    c. Internal and external sphincter tone.
    d. Internal and external hemorrhoids.
    e. Rectal prolapse.
8. Functional ability:
    a. Ability to use bathroom, toilet, chair, or assistive devices.
    b. Toileting ability: Ability to remove clothing and perform necessary hygiene.
    c. Transfer ability: Ability to transfer onto a commode or shower chair.
    d. Sitting tolerance, trunk balance.
    e. Ability to use arms; hand function; presence of wrist flexion.
    f. Ability to bend laterally and return to upright position.

C. Diagnostic Studies
1. Flat plate of the abdomen.
2. Sigmoidoscopy.
3. Colonoscopy.
4. Colonic transit times.

IV. Neurogenic Bowel

A. Nursing Diagnosis:
1. Alteration in bowel elimination secondary to upper motor neuron (UMN) damage (also known as reflex neurogenic bowel or spastic bowel).
2. Alteration in bowel elimination secondary to lower motor neuron (LMN) damage (also known as areflexic neurogenic bowel, flaccid bowel, or autonomous neurogenic bowel).
3. Alteration in bowel elimination secondary to uninhibited neurogenic bowel.
4. Alteration in bowel elimination secondary to motor paralytic bowel.

B. Defining Characteristics:
1. UMN
    a. Defecation is involuntary; there is sudden, mass emptying when rectal vault becomes full (due to sacral reflex).
    b. Partial or total sensory loss in perineum and/or rectum.
    c. Partial or total loss of external sphincter control.

2. LMN
   a. Hard, formed stool requiring disimpaction.
   b. Stool leakage with activity and/or stress.
   c. Partial or total sensory loss in rectum and perineum.
   d. Partial or total loss of external sphincter control.
3. Uninhibited neurogenic bowel:
   a. Internal and external sphincters are intact or hypertonic.
   b. Saddle sensation usually is preserved.
   c. Defecation is involuntary and sudden.
4. Motor paralytic bowel:
   a. Saddle sensation is intact.
   b. Incontinence is rare except in widespread disease.

C. **Expected Outcomes:**
   1. Effectiveness: Design a bowel management program that provides predictable and effective elimination and that minimizes GI complaints and evacuation problems and is compatible with individual lifestyle and developmental needs. The ultimate goal is that the individual's bowel routine prevents unplanned bowel movements. The individual is aware of the importance of completing bowel care on a regular basis to provide the predictability of evacuation and continence.
   2. Acceptability to the patient and significant other(s): The bowel routine must be one that the patient, caregiver, and significant other(s) find acceptable and workable. For example, will the primary caregiver be able to transfer the spinal cord injured individual on and off the commode chair? Is this expectation realistic?
   3. Cost effective: Is the bowel routine cost effective? Are the least costly medications being utilized? Can the individual afford the medications if they are not covered by insurance?
   4. Health maintenance: Is the bowel program effective in preventing complications? Are the results from the program appropriate, given food intake?

D. **Interventions:**
   1. Factors to consider when establishing a bowel care regime:
      a. Cognition: Are there any cognitive problems that would interfere with learning?
      b. Systemic and local factors: Viruses, any acute illness. Is an impaction present?
      c. Hormonal factors: Any change in hormonal balance (e.g. menstrual cycle) can lead to loose stool.
      d. Metabolic changes: Changes in serum potassium level can lead to loose stool.
      e. Polypharmacology: What medications is the patient on? Diuretics can lead to constipation; antacids (depending on the contents) can lead to either diarrhea or constipation; antibiotics can lead to diarrhea.
      f. Current health status: Did the patient have any abdominal trauma associated with the spinal cord injury? Acute abdomen?
      g. Psychosocial: How is the patient dealing with the loss of bowel control? How effective is the support system?
   2. Guidelines prior to setting up a program:
      a. Establish a baseline: Determine if an impaction is present. If so, eliminate prior to starting a routine.
      b. Data collection: If necessary, keep a daily log of fluid and food intake and the impact on the bowel program.
      c. The routine MUST be done on a consistent basis, even if incontinence has occurred.
      d. Bowel routines should be started as soon as consistent bowel sounds are heard. Determine if ileus is present if decreased sounds heard.
      e. Think about discharge plans early after the injury: If possible, determine with the patient and family the following:
         (1) What was the evacuation pattern prior to injury? Was it morning or evening? Daily? Every other day?
         (2) Is the patient and/or family able to anticipate when the best time for doing the routine may be, given other commitments?

    f. Bowel routines are most effective when done in the upright position. However, a side-lying position in bed is a legitimate alternative if the individual is unable to tolerate sitting upright, cannot sit due to skin problems, or will be unable to utilize this position when discharged.

    g. If a routine is ineffective, change only one element at a time. Allow time after the change to evaluate the effectiveness of the new routine.

    h. Once a pattern has been established, bowel programs may be advanced to less frequency or decreasing medication. Remember that if the changes lead to incontinence, you may need to go back to what was previously successful.

3. Estabilishing a bowel program: (See Figure 16-1)

    a. Program is set up on an every day to every other day schedule, utilizing data collected from nursing assessment. The scheduled time of the routine should take into account patterns prior to SCI as well as discharge plans.

    b. Oral medications most commonly used include a stool softener and a mild colonic stimulant. Remember to administer the medications at the time that will provide the best medication effect.

    c. For UMN (spastic bowel):

      (1) Determine which type of suppository will provide the maximum effect with the minimum amount of medication.

      (2) Advise the patient of the benefit of drinking 6-8 ounces of warm liquid, or eating a meal thirty minutes prior to bowel care to take advantage of gastrocolic reflex.

      (3) Insert a gloved, lubricated finger into rectum and remove any stool present.

      (4) Stimulate the bowel, using proper procedure for digital stimulation, for approximately one minute. Repeat stimulation every ten minutes, three or four times.

      (5) If there is no response to digital stimulation, then mechanical stimulation, such as a suppository, stimulates the intestinal mucosa by an irritant action, causing stool to move down into the rectum.

      (6) Fifteen to thirty minutes after the suppository has been inserted, if appropriate, transfer the patient to the toilet or commode chair. Encourage the patient to try to bear down (if possible) or to try abdominal massage. Have the patient lean forward, if able. If no results within thirty minutes, gently insert a gloved well-lubricated finger into the rectum and try digital stimulation.

      (7) Individuals who have experienced autonomic dysreflexia when passing stool or during digital stimulation should have a prophylactic topical anesthetic ointment inserted into the rectum five minutes prior to digital stimulation as per physician's order.

    d. For LMN (flaccid bowel):

      (1) Daily manual removal of stool with a gloved well-lubricated finger is performed in cases of flaccid bowel, which results in a relaxed anal sphincter.

      (2) Transfer the patient to the commode or toilet, if possible.

      (3) Encourage the patient to try to bear down (if possible) or try abdominal massage.

      (4) Have the patient lean forward, if able to tolerate.

      (5) If all of the above interventions do not provide results, stool should be gently, manually removed from the rectum.

      (6) Once the stool has been removed, insert a solid suppository up in the rectum as high up as possible.

    e. Upon completion of bowel care, the buttock and perineal areas should be cleaned with soap and water and blotted dry.

4. Use of medications in treating neurogenic bowel:

    a. Medication guidelines:

      (1) Medications usually require more time to take effect with a neurogenic bowel than a non-neurogenic bowel.

      (2) Utilize the minimum dosage, increasing slowly.

      (3) Medications should be timed with colonic motility.

(4) The long term goal is to have a regulated bowel routine with utilization of a minimum amount of medications.

(5) The use of laxatives over a long period of time is strongly discouraged.

b. Commonly used medications:

(1) Stool softeners:

(a) Usually given 2-3 times a day.

(b) Eight ounces of fluid with each dose.

(2) Colonic Stimulants:

(a) Chemically irritate the bowel to increase motility.

(b) Give 8-10 hours before the scheduled bowel routine.

(3) Bulk formers:

(a) Increase bolus of stool and increase consistency.

(b) Eight ounces of fluid should be taken with each dose.

(c) Can cause constipation if fluids are inadequate.

(4) Suppositories:

(a) Irritate the wall of the colon (chemically and mechanically) to increase peristalsis and evacuation.

(b) Rectum should be empty prior to giving suppository.

(c) May need to use digital stimulation and/or manual evacuation.

(5) Liquid suppositories (for UMN):

(a) Irritate the wall of the colon (chemically and mechanically) to increase peristalsis and evacuation.

(b) May need to use digital stimulation and/or manual evacuation.

(c) Advantageous over a solid suppository because the medication is already dispersed in a liquid form, leading to quicker absorption and evacuation.

5. Other modalities:

a. Digital stimulation (for UMN):

(1) Insert a gloved and lubricated finger into the rectum.

(2) Utilize a gentle, circular motion, for approximately one minute or until stool begins to evacuate. Be careful not to damage the mucosal wall.

(3) Stimulation may need to be repeated every 5-10 minutes, 3-4 times.

b. Manual removal:

(1) Insert a gloved and lubricated finger into the rectum.

(2) Gently remove stool from the rectum, being careful not to damage the mucosal wall.

c. Abdominal massage, push-ups, Valsalva maneuver, and leaning forward.

d. Deep breathing.

e. Large-volume enemas are not used for routine bowel care due to potential for bowel overdistention.

f. High tech modalities (for UMN):

(1) Functional Electrical Stimulation (FES):

(a) Looks similar to a vibrator. Provides low-voltage stimulation to the rectum.

(b) The goal is to increase rectal tone, leading to increased sphincter control and continence.

(c) Is most successful in individuals with complete tetraplegia or high-level paraplegia.

(2) Biofeedback:

(a) Utilizes biofeedback to strengthen the accessory rectal muscles and rectum.

(b) The goal is to increase rectal tone leading to increased sphincter control and continence.

(c) Is most successful in individuals with incomplete tetraplegia or high paraplegia.

(d) Biofeedback is not likely to be an effective treatment modality in most persons with spinal cord injury.

Figure 16-1: Designing a Neurogenic Bowel Management Program for Spinal Cord Injury Individuals

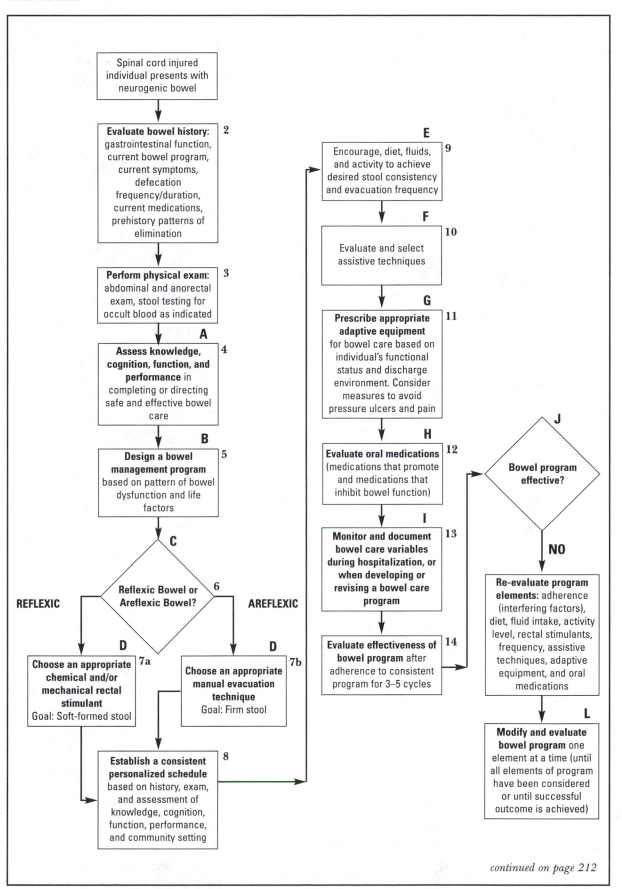

continued on page 212

Figure 16-1: Continued

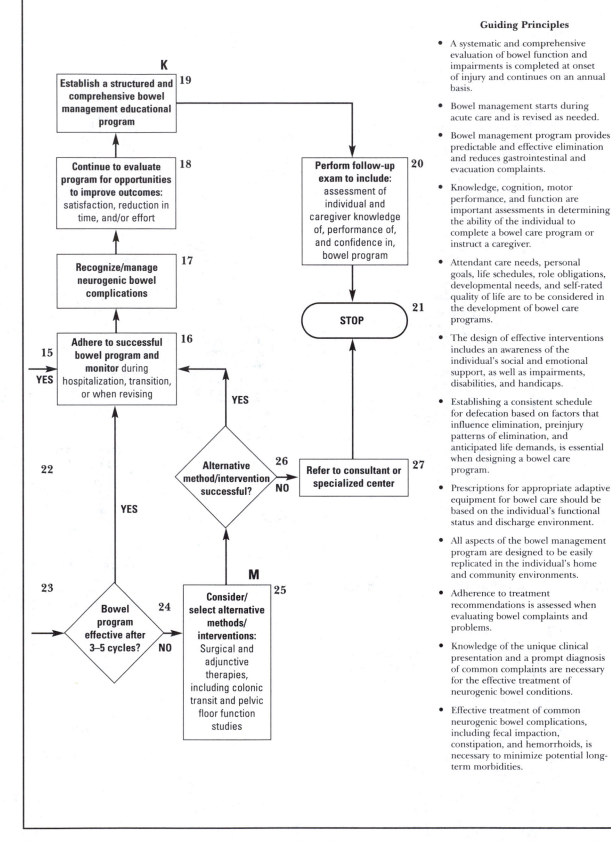

Guiding Principles

- A systematic and comprehensive evaluation of bowel function and impairments is completed at onset of injury and continues on an annual basis.

- Bowel management starts during acute care and is revised as needed.

- Bowel management program provides predictable and effective elimination and reduces gastrointestinal and evacuation complaints.

- Knowledge, cognition, motor performance, and function are important assessments in determining the ability of the individual to complete a bowel care program or instruct a caregiver.

- Attendant care needs, personal goals, life schedules, role obligations, developmental needs, and self-rated quality of life are to be considered in the development of bowel care programs.

- The design of effective interventions includes an awareness of the individual's social and emotional support, as well as impairments, disabilities, and handicaps.

- Establishing a consistent schedule for defecation based on factors that influence elimination, preinjury patterns of elimination, and anticipated life demands, is essential when designing a bowel care program.

- Prescriptions for appropriate adaptive equipment for bowel care should be based on the individual's functional status and discharge environment.

- All aspects of the bowel management program are designed to be easily replicated in the individual's home and community environments.

- Adherence to treatment recommendations is assessed when evaluating bowel complaints and problems.

- Knowledge of the unique clinical presentation and a prompt diagnosis of common complaints are necessary for the effective treatment of neurogenic bowel conditions.

- Effective treatment of common neurogenic bowel complications, including fecal impaction, constipation, and hemorrhoids, is necessary to minimize potential long-term morbidities.

From *Neurogenic bowel management in adults with spinal cord injury,* by Consortium for Spinal Cord Medicine (1998, March). Washington, DC: Paralyzed Veterans of America. Reprinted with permission.

V. Constipation

A. **Nursing Diagnosis:** Colonic Constipation.

B. **Defining Characteristics:** Pattern of elimination characterized by hard, dry stool resulting from delay in passage of food residue.
1. Decreased frequency.
2. Hard, dry stool.
3. Straining, bleeding.
4. Painful defecation.
5. Abdominal distention, pain, cramping.
6. Headache (may be a sign of autonomic dysreflexia—Refer to Chapter 13).
7. Decreased appetite, nausea.
8. Increased spasticity in individuals with neurogenic impairments.
9. Rectal pressure, pain.
10. Related factors/etiologies (Zejdlik, 1992):
    a. Change in or less than adequate physical activity; impaired mobility.
    b. Change in or less than adequate intake of fluids or dietary fiber.
    c. Sensorimotor disorders.
    d. Postoperative complications.
    e. Side effects of medication regimen.
    f. Slowed peristalsis from disorder of central nervous system or autonomic nervous system.

C. **Expected Outcomes:**
1. Regular, routine bowel evacuation.
2. Avoidance of factors that contribute to development of constipation.
3. Knowledgeable regarding relationship among diet, activity, and constipation.

D. **Interventions:**
1. Increase fluid intake as tolerated and monitor intake and output.
2. Increase bulk and fiber in diet.
3. Provide for colonic and rectal emptying through use of stimulants or irritant cathartics, bulk-forming agents (to be taken at least 6 to 8 hours prior to expected and/or desired emptying); use low-volume enemas or suppositories alone or in conjunction with oral medications for complete emptying.
4. Promote use of stool softeners and/or bulk formers.
5. Promote habitual toilet routine.
6. Use seated position to maximize effect of gravity on evacuation.
7. Instruct client and family about symptoms of developing impaction and about the risks associated with it.
8. Reinforce need to limit routine use of laxatives and enemas.

VI. Monitoring Bowel Function/Evaluating Program Effectiveness

A. **Monitoring:** The following variables are monitored after every bowel care procedure:
1. Date.
2. Total time (time from rectal stimulation to end of stool flow).
3. Stimulating agent(s).
4. Position.
5. Color, consistency, and amount of stool.
6. Adverse reactions (e.g., dysreflexia, abdominal cramping, pressure ulcers, bleeding).
7. Unplanned spontaneous evacuations.

B. **Mondifying a Bowel Program:** A bowel program can take months to establish and requires careful management to maintain. Reassess the client's bowel program and modify as needed. Consider the following when modifying a bowel care regime:

1. In the absence of adverse reactions and indicators for potential medical complications, the bowel program management should be evaluated after 3-5 bowel care cycles before considering possible modifications.
2. Indications for changing the bowel care regime include:
   a. Evacuation problems
   b. Adverse reactions
   c. Consumer and caregiver dissatisfaction
   d. Resource availability
3. When modifying a bowel management program, change only one element at a time.

C. **Consumer/caregiver knowledge/skills:** Evaluation of teaching programs should include knowledge of prescribed bowel care program; factors that promote successful bowel management; role of regularity, timing, and positioning in successful bowel management; safe and effective use of assistive devices/equipment; techniques for manual evacuation, digital stimulation and suppository insertion; prescribed bowel medications. Competency and confidence in performing each of the techniques applicable to the prescribed bowel care program should be assessed for the person who will be responsible for performing the regime. Furthermore, problem solving skills for common bowel problems (constipation, impactions, diarrhea, hemorrhoids, incontinence, and autonomic hyperreflexia) should be evident, and the individual and/or caregiver should be able to verbalize when and how to make changes in medications and schedules.

VII. Potential Problems/Complications

A. **Delayed Evacuation:** The time it takes to complete bowel care will vary from one individual to another. Typically, a bowel movement should occur within 1 hour of planned time. It often takes a newly-injured person with a SCI longer to evacuate the bowel. A goal for many persons with a spinal cord injury is to complete a bowel care program in less than one hour (Zejdlik, 1992). Carefully assess contributing factors and consider modifying bowel care regime.

B. **Unplanned Bowel Movements:** Predictive and effective bowel evacuation can be restored and maintained (Gender, 1996). With a well-planned bowel management program, the goal for many persons with a spinal cord injury is to avoid unexpected bowel movements at unplanned times. Initiate early corrective treatment for incontinence, to prevent skin breakdown of perineal area, and to evaluate and adjust bowel program to prevent recurrence (Zejdlik, 1992). Carefully assess contributing factors before deciding to alter bowel care regime.

C. **Consumer/caregiver dissatisfaction:** Individuals should be satisfied and actively involved in monitoring their bowel care program, and possess a preventative focus and problem-solving skills to manage changes or problems (Zejdlik, 1992). Decision making related to changes in a bowel program should reflect the input and preferences of the patient and family. Furthermore, the program should be safe, reliable, convenient, effective, and individualized based on lifestyle and emotional, cultural, and family needs.

D. **Potential Bowel Complications:** Effective management of complications of the neurogenic bowel begins with prevention, and prompt recognition and management of commonly associated complications.
   1. Diarrhea.
   2. Constipation.
   3. Impaction.
   4. Hemorrhoids.
   5. Exacerbation of pain, spasticity, or autonomic dysreflexia.
   6. Falls during transport, transfer, or while reaching to complete bowel care procedure (Malassigne, Nelson, Amerson, Salzstein, & Binard, 1993; Nelson, Malassigne, Murray, 1994).
   7. Pressure ulcers as a result of trauma or positioning during bowel care procedures (Malassigne, Nelson, Amerson, Salzstein, & Binard, 1993; Nelson et al, 1994).

8. Urinary tract infections (Gender, 1996; Zejdlik, 1992).
9. The most common GI complications during the first month following spinal cord injury include ileus, gastric stress ulcers, and gastric dilatation (Gore et al 1981).
10. The most common complaint in SCI patients with abdominal pathology is anorexia. VIII.

VIII. Reassessment

A. Review documentation to determine if and when incontinence has occurred. Utilize this data to determine if any changes need to be made to the program, such as a change in medication or a change in the time of day the program is done, e.g., if the individual is incontinent every morning, a morning program may be more appropriate.
1. Is there a specific time that the individual has a bowel movement? Is it daily; every other day?
2. What is the current bowel routine? Is it reliable? Effective? How long does it take? With what aspects of the program does the individual need assistance? Does the caregiver perceive the bowel routine to be reliable and effective?
3. What is the consistency of the stool? How much stool is evacuated with each movement?
4. Are there episodes of incontinence? Is there any one thing that triggers incontinence?
5. Is there a history of bowel disease (e.g., Crohn's, Colitis, Diverticulitis)?
6. What types of foods are routinely eaten? Did any food increase constipation or diarrhea?
7. What is the typical level of activity, including exercise routine?
8. What is the typical fluid intake?
9. How has the SCI affected the bowel program?
10. If spasticity is present, has there been any change in the level of spasticity recently?

B. Determine if the following complications have occurred:
1. Diarrhea
   a. Assess:
      (1) Recent illness.
      (2) Change in diet.
      (3) Effect of medications.
      (4) Stress level.
      (5) Change in caregiver.
      (6) Sign of possible impaction.
   b. Identify the cause, and treat
2. Constipation
   a. Assess:
      (1) Change in diet.
      (2) Change in fluid intake.
      (3) Possibly dehydrated.
      (4) Change in weather.
      (5) Effect of medications.
      (6) Change in caregiver.
      (7) Change in activity level.
      (8) Consistency in completing bowel care.
      (9) Change in bowel management routine.
   b. Identify the cause and treat.
3. Impaction
   a. Assess for reason that the individual has been constipated:
      (1) Medications.
      (2) Diet.
      (3) Fluids.
      (4) Skipping routine.
   b. Relieve impaction according to institution protocol.
   c. Prevent future impactions.
4. Hemorrhoids/rectal bleeding:
   a. May be secondary to long-term suppository use.

    b. Assess if stool removal is too aggressive; use adequate lubrication.

    c. Assess for constipation.

    d. Treat hemorrhoids.

    e. Rule out other causes of rectal bleeding.

5. Proctitis:

    a. May be secondary to long-term suppository use.

    b. If suppository use cannot be decreased or eliminated, medication may be needed prior to bowel routine to decrease pain.

6. Incontinence:

    a. Assess what has changed in the person's life:

      (1) Medications.

      (2) Diet.

      (3) Type and amount of fluids.

      (4) Recent illness.

      (5) Activity Level.

      (6) Consistency in completing bowel care routine.

    b. Identify the cause, and treat.

IX. Education

A. **Content of education programs:** Educational programs for bowel management in SCI should be structured, organized, and comprehensive, and should be directed at all levels of health care providers, patients, and family or caregivers. An educational program for bowel management should include:

1. Anatomy.

2. Process of defecation.

3. How bowel function is affected by SCI.

4. Goals, description, and rationale for successful bowel program management.

5. Factors that promote successful bowel management.

6. Role of regularity, timing, and positioning in successful bowel management.

7. Safe and effective use of assistive devices/equipment.

8. Manual evacuation or digital stimulation and suppository insertion techniques.

9. Prescribed bowel medications.

10. Prevention and problem solving skills for common bowel problems (constipation, impactions, diarrhea, hemorrhoids, incontinence, and autonomic hyperreflexia).

11. When and how to make changes in medications and schedules.

12. Long-term implications associated with neurogenic bowel dysfunction.

B. **Evaluating adherence and effectiveness:** Patient and caregiver knowledge of and adherence to the recommended bowel management program or to the program as adjusted by patient and family should be assessed at each follow-up evaluation. Educational assessments should not only include mastery of knowledge related to bowel care practices, technique, physiology, and related conditions/skills, but should also carefully address confidence and performance. Attempts to evaluate bowel care program changes in effectiveness should also address the generalized ability of training across settings (inpatient to outpatient, etc.). Careful elucidation of factors related to increasing adherence, while accommodating creative approaches to problem solving, should be encouraged.

X. Special Issues Related to Pediatric Care

A. **Neurogenic Bowel in Children:** Management of neurogenic bowel dysfunction in children is similar to adult management and includes age-appropriate considerations and social implications. Bowel programs may need to be more frequent and bowel medications may be somewhat different.

B. **Special Considerations** (Edwards-Beckett & King, 1996; Leibold, Braun, Cole, & Peterson, 1995).

1. Bowel programs need to be daily due to increased normal stooling patterns in children, and then decreased to every other day, if appropriate. The infant and toddler may even require a bowel program twice each day.
2. For the child with SCI, the bowel program should be based on preinjury status.
3. Children with congenital disorders such as spina bifida may have functionally altered GI tracts which may or may not be physiologically altered. Because these children have never had normal bowel function, the routine bowel continence program for neurogenic bowel may need to be adjusted to obtain and maintain continence. Refer to the Spina Bifida Association Management Guidelines (Rauen & Aubert, 1995).
4. The child's and family's schedule, the child's cognitive and functional level, additional activities, and the length of time needed to complete the bowel program should be considered when determining the time of day the bowel program will be done. Early morning school needs usually make the evening a more acceptable time.
5. Children may be placed on the commode for bowel program. Young children with poor sitting balance may be placed on the commode backwards (facing wall) to gain a sense of security.

C. **Medications for Neurogenic Bowel**: Bowel program medications differ somewhat in children. It is important when considering these medications that over-use does not lead to medication induced incontinence.
1. Stool softener (Colace is recommended).
2. Stimulants: Senna/Senokot, Pericolace (combination softener and stimulant), and bisacodyl (Dulcolax) recommended. Senna or Pericolace should be given 8-10 hours before planned evacuation. Therevac (mini-enema) is as effective as Dulcolax, but less irritating. The faster acting "Magic Bullet" may be the suppository of choice for the older or active child or when time is an issue for compliance or convenience.
3. Saline products (fleet enema and Milk of Magnesia recommended).
4. Bulk products are not commonly used in children.
5. Lubricants (mineral oil enema recommended).
6. Osmotics (glycerin suppository should be tried in the infant and young child before the stronger, more stimulating bisacodyl suppository. Lactulose may be used in children.)
7. Some parents prefer the use of homeopathic medication over the traditional prescribed medications.
8. High fiber diet recommended.

Practical Application #1

B.J., a 34 year old female, who was injured in a motor vehicle accident three weeks previously, resulting in a C8, ASIA A spinal cord injury. Her spine was stabilized and she is now using a wheelchair and active in therapies. Her diet is poor to fair, with many of meals consisting of fluids and dessert. Fluid intake is approximately two liters per day. She is incontinent of bowel approximately every other morning.

Her discharge plans are to return home to her family (husband and two children, ages 4 and 6), eventually returning to her part-time job, three days per week. Attendant care will be primarily in the evening.

Prior to her injury B.J. was very active, engaging in running 3-4 miles several times a week and playing tennis twice a week. Her diet was well balanced. She moved her bowels, usually daily after breakfast when she had a cup of coffee.

B.J. started a bowel regimen of a stool softener and bulk former daily. Her bowel program included rectal digital stimulation every other evening on a commode chair. Stool results were moderate in size and soft in consistency. Incontinency frequently occurred in the morning. She often refused her bowel program if she was incontinent that morning.

B.J. and her husband attended a family educational session that included: neurogenic bowel function, medications, diet and fluid intake, and the importance of activity and of maintaining a consistent bowel management routine. After talking with her nurse, B.J. agreed to try eat a more balanced diet, incorporating all four food groups. She would drink a minimum of 2 liters of fluids each day, but would not exceed 3 liters, and she would follow an evening bowel program, even if incontinent. At this point, evening still seemed to be the best time for the program given her discharge plan. The agreed upon timeframe for re-evaluation was two weeks.

At the end of the two week period, B.J. noted that her incontinencies had decreased to one time that week and that her program was working much more reliably. Over the next month, her incidence of incontinence was zero. She was able to do the routine in fifty minutes from start to finish and believed that this time would continue to decrease. With the cessation of incontinencies B.J. was able to attend therapies on a consistent basis and felt better about herself.

Practical Application #2

J.H. is a 20 year old male L2 paraplegia secondary to a gunshot wound which occurred during a robbery attempt at the store where he was employed. He was admitted to rehab seven days after his injury. His dietary intake is variable, "doesn't like hospital food" and depend upon his family and friends to bring him food that he liked. Fluid intake was inconsistent, less than a liter a day to three liters per day. He just started therapy.

Prior to his injury, J.H. was an active young man who went to school full time and worked part time. He lived at home with his parents and fourteen year-old-sister. He engaged in intramural sports and enjoyed being physically active.

J.H. was unable to report any bowel elimination pattern and denies any gastrointestinal problems prior to his injury. Discharge plans are to return home with his parents and sister. He plans to return to work and school within the next year.

J.H. started a bowel routine of a stool softener twice daily and manual removal of stool in the evening on a commode chair. Stool results were small and hard. When J.H. started therapy, he progressed quickly. He was able to transfer himself independently from wheelchair to mat and became independent in push-up pressure reliefs.

However, he frequently passed small amounts of stool whenever he engaged in these activities and announced "I will never go out of the house again. I'd be too embarrassed that I would have a bowel accident."

Patient teaching included: neurogenic bowel, diet, fluids, activity, and medications. J.H. agreed that his diet was at best "minimal in incorporating all four food groups routinely" and that his fluid intake was inconsistent. His activity level, however was increasing, as he began to have more endurance and feel better.

J.H.'s new plan included the previous medication regime, a healthier and consistent diet including all four food groups and increased fiber intake and fluid intake of 2 liters per day. In two weeks, this plan would be evaluated.

At the end of the two-week timeframe, J.H. was independent in performing his bowel routine and he followed a more consistent diet, incorporating the four food groups and adequate fiber. His fluid intake was consistently 2 liters. Stool incontinency has dramatically decreased, and J.H. is beginning to believe that he will be able to return to work and school.

References and Selected Bibliography

Banwell, J.G., Creasey, G.H., Aggarwal, A.M., & Mortimer, J.T. (1993). Management of the neurogenic bowel in patients with spinal cord injury. *Urologic Clinics of North America, 20*(3), 517-526.

Behm, R. (1985). A special recipe to banish constipation. *Geriatric Nursing, 6,* 216-217.

Boss, B. J., Pecanty, L., McFarland, S. M., & Sasser, L. (1995). Self-care competence among persons with spinal cord injury. *Spinal Cord Injury Nursing, 12,* 48-53.

Brocklehurst, J.C. (1980). Disorders of the lower bowel in old age. *Geriatrics, 35,* 47-54.

Brown, M.K., & Everett, I. (1990). Gentler bowel fitness with fiber: A recipe for bowel regularity and cost savings too. *Geriatric Nursing, 11,* 26-27.

Cameron, K. J., Nyulasi, I. B., Collier, G. R., & Brown, D. J. (1996). Assessment of the effect of increased dietary fiber intake on bowel function in patients with spinal cord injury. *Spinal Cord, 34,*(5), 277-83.

Chang, K.J., Erickson, R.A., Schnadler, S., Caye, T. & Moody, C. (1991). Per-rectal pulsed irrigation versus per-oral colonic lavage for colonoscopy preparation: A randomized, controlled trial. *Gastrointestinal Endoscopy, 37*(4), 444-8.

Charney K, Juler G, & Comarr, A. (1975). General surgery problems in patients with spinal cord injuries. *Archives of Surgery, 110,* 1083-1088.

Chin, D. E., & Kearns, P. (1991). Nutrition in the spinal injured patient. *Nutrition in Clinical Practice, 6,* 213-222.

Coffman, S. (1986). Description of a nursing diagnosis: alteration in bowel elimination related to neurogenic bowel in children with myelomeningocele. *Issues in Comprehensive Pediatric Nursing, 8,* 179-199.

Consortium for Spinal Cord Medicine (1998, March). *Neurogenic bowel management in adults with spinal cord injury.* Washington, DC: Paralyzed Veterans of America.

Cornell, S. A., Campion, L., Bacero, S., Frazier, J., Kjellstrom, M., & Purdy, S. (1973). Comparison of three bowel management programs during rehabilitation of spinal cord injured patients. *Nursing Research, 22*(4), 321-8.

Dunn, K. L. & Galka, M.L. (1994). A comparison of the effectiveness of Therevac SB and bisacodyl suppositories in SCI patients' bowel programs. *Rehabilitation Nursing, 19*(6), 334-8.

Edwards-Beckett, J. & King, H. (1996). The impact of spinal pathology on bowel control in children. *Rehabilitation Nursing, 21*(6), 292-297.

Ellickson, E.B. (1988). Bowel management plan for the homebound elderly. *Journal of Gerontological Nursing, 14,* 16019, 40-42.

Friedman, G. (1989). Nutritional therapy of irritable bowel syndrome. *Gastroenterology Clinics of North America, 18,* 513-524.

Frisbie, J. H., Tun, C. G., & Nguyen, C. H. (1986). Effect of enterostomy on quality of life in spinal cord injury patients. *Journal of the American Paraplegia Society, 9*(1-2), 3-5.

Gender, A. (1996). Bowel regulation and elimination. In Hoeman, S. (Ed.), *Rehabilitation Nursing Process and Application* (2nd ed). (pp. 452-475). St. Louis, MO: Mosby.

Gleeson, R.M. (1990). Bowel continence for the child with a neurogenic bowel. *Rehabilitation Nursing, 15,* 319-321.

Glick, M., Meshinpour, H., Haldeman, S., Hoehler, F., Downey, N., & Bradley, W. (1984). Colonic dysfunction in patients with thoracic spinal cord injury. *Gastroenterology, 86,* 287-294.

Glickman, S., & Kamm, M.A. (1994). Bowel dysfunction in spinal-cord-injury patients. *Lancet, 347,* 1651-53.

Gore, R.M., Mintzer, R.A., & Calenoff, L. (1981). Gastrointestinal complications of spinal cord injury. *Spine, 6*(6), 538-44.

Halm, M.A. (1990). Elimination concerns with acute spinal cord trauma: Assessment and interventions. *Critical Care Nursing Clinics of North America, 2*(3), 385-398.

Hanak, M. (ED) (1990). Bowel management—Spinal cord injury: Patient/family teaching plan. In *Educational guide for spinal cord injury nurses: A manual for teaching patients, families and caregivers* (pp. 63-75). Jackson Heights, NY: American Association of Spinal Cord Injury Nurses.

Hanak, M. & Phillips, B. (Eds). (1986). Bowel management—Spinal cord injury: Patient/family teaching plan. *Patient family education guide for spinal cord injury nurses* (pp. 141-189). Jackson Heights: American Association of Spinal Cord Injury Nurses.

Hogstel, M.O., & Nelson, M. (1992). Anticipation and early detection can reduce bowel elimination complications. *Geriatric Nursing, 13,* 28-33.

Holliday, J. (1967). Bowel programs of patients with spinal cord injury: A clinical study. *Nursing Research; 16*(1), 4-15.

Kannisto, M., & Rintala, R. (1995). Bowel function in adults who have sustained spinal cord injury in childhood. *Paraplegia, 33*(12), 701-3.

Kirk, P.M., King, R.B., Temple, R., Bourjalais, J., & Thomas, P. (1997). Long term follow-up of bowel management after spinal cord injury. *SCI Nursing.* 14, 56-63.

Kokozca, J., Nelson, R., Falconio, M., & Abcarian, H. (1994). Treatment of fecal impaction with pulsed irrigation enhanced evacuation. *Diseases of Colon and Rectum, 37*(2), 161-4.

Laven, G.T., Huang, C.T., DeVivo, M.J., Stover, S.L., Kuhlemieier, K.V., & Fine, P.R. (1989). Nutritional status during the acute stage of spinal cord injury. *Archives of Physical Medicine and Rehabilitation, 70,* 277-282.

Leibold, S., Braun, P., Cole, J., & Peterson, P. (1995). *Bowel continence and spina bifida.* Washington, D.C.: Spina Bifida Association of America.

Levi, R., Hultling, C., Nash, M. S., & Seiger, A. (1995). The Stockholm spinal cord injury study: 1. Medical problems in a regional SCI population. *Paraplegia, 33*(6), 308-15.

Malassigne, P., Nelson, A., Amerson, T., Saltzstein, R., & Binard, J. (1993). Toward the design of a new bowel care chair for the spinal cord injured: a pilot study. *SCI Nursing, 10,* 84-90.

Markman, L.J. (1988). Bladder and bowel management of the spinal cord injured patient. *Plastic Surgical Nursing, 8*(4), 141-145.

Matthews, P. & Carlson, C. (eds.) (1987). Spinal cord injury: A guide to rehabilitation nursing, elimination (pp. 99-120). Gaithersburg, MD: Aspen.

McCourt, A. (1993). Elimination pattern. In A. McCourt. (Ed.), *The specialty practice of rehabilitation nursing: A core curriculum* (3rd ed) (pp. 94-107). Skokie, IL: Rehabilitation Nursing Foundation.

Menardo, G., Baujano, G., & Corazziari, E. (1987). Large bowel transit in paraplegic patients. *Diseases of Colon and Rectum, 30,* 924-928.

Miller, L.S., Staas, W.E., & Herbison, G.J. (1975). Abdominal problems in patients with spinal cord injuries. *Archives of Physical Medicine and Rehabilitation, 56,* 405-8.

Munchiando, J.F., & Kendall, K. (1993). Comparison of the effectiveness of two bowel programs for CVA patients. *Rehabilitation Nursing, 18,* 168-172.

Nelson, A., Malassigne, P., Amerson, T., Saltzstein, R., & Binard, J. (1993). Descriptive study of bowel care practices and equipment in spinal cord injury. *SCI Nursing, 10*(2), 65-67.

Nelson, A., Malassigne, P., & Murray, J. (1994). Comparison of seat pressures on three bowel care/shower chairs in spinal cord injury. *SCI Nursing, 11,* 105-107.

Nino-Murcia, M., Stone, J., Chang, P., & Perkash, I. (1990). Colonic transit in spinal cord-injured patients. *Investigative Radiology, 25,* 109-112.

Rauen, K.K., & Aubert, E.J. (1992). A brighter future for adults who have myelomeningocele—one form of spina bifida: A comprehensive overview of this complex disease. *Orthopaedic Nursing, 11,* 16-27.

Richardson, K., Campbell, M.A., Brown, M.R., Masiulis, B., & Liptak, G.S. (1985). Biofeedback therapy for managing bowel incontinence caused by meningomyelocele. *American Journal of Maternal Child Nursing, 10,* 388-392.

Saltzstein, R. J. & Romano, J. (1990). The efficacy of colostomy as a bowel management alternative in selected spinal cord injury patients. *Journal of the American Paraplegia Society, 13,* 9-13.

Saltzstein, R., Mustin, E., & Koch, T. (1995). Gut hormone release in patients after spinal cord injury. *American Journal of Physical Medicine and Rehabilitation, 74,* 339-344.

Smith, K.A. (1990). Bowel and bladder management of the child with myelomeningocele in the school setting. *Journal of Pediatric Healthcare, 4*(40), 175-180.

Staas, W., & Cioschi, H. (1989). Neurogenic bowel dysfunction. *Critical Reviews in Physical and Rehabilitation Medicine, 1*(1), 11-21

Stevick, C. P., Cassells, E. P., & Hicks, F. (1977). An improved rectal suppository for spinal cord injury patients. *Military Medicine, 142*(11), 882-4.

Stiens, S., Bierner-Bergman, S., & Goetz, L. (1997). Neurogenic bowel dysfunction after spinal cord injury: Clinical evaluation and rehabilitative management. *Archives of Physical Medicine and Rehabilitation;78,* S86-S102.

Stiens, S. A. (1995). Reduction in bowel program duration with polyethylene glycol based bisacodyl suppositories. *Archives of Physical Medicine and Rehabilitation, 76,* 674-676.

Stiens, S., Bergman, S., & Goetz, L. (1997). Neurogenic bowel dysfunction after spinal cord injury: Clinical evaluation and rehabilitative management. *Archives of Physical Medicine and Rehabilitation, 78,* S86-S102.

Stone, J.M., Nino-Murcia, M., Wolfe, V.A., & Perkash, I. (1990a). Chronic gastrointestinal problems in spinal cord injury patient: A prospective analysis. *American Journal of Gastroenterology, 85*(9), 1114-1119.

Stone, J. M., Wolfe, V. A., Nino-Murcia, M., & Perkash, I. (1990b). Colostomy as treatment for complications of spinal cord injury. *Archives of Physical Medicine and Rehabilitation, 71*(7), 514-8.

Venn, M.R., Taft, L., Carpentier, I.B., & Applebaugh, A. (1992). The influence of timing and suppository use on efficiency and effectiveness of bowel training after a stroke. *Rehabilitation Nursing, 17,* 116-121.

Wald, A. (1981). Biofeedback therapy for fecal incontinence. *Annals of Internal Medicine, 95,* 145-149.

White, M., & Williams, J. (1992). A good start to a full life: Managing continence in children with spina bifida and hydrocephalus. *Professional Nurse, 7,* 474, 476-477.

Whiteneck, G.G., Charlifue, S.W., Frankel, H.L., Fraser, M.H., Gardner, B.P., Gerhart, K.A., Krishnan, K.R., Menter, R.R., Nuseibeh, I., & Silver, J.R. (1992). Mortality, morbidity, and psychosocial outcomes of persons spinal cord injured more than 20 years ago. *Paraplegia, 30,* 617-30.

Zejdlik, C.P. (1992). Reestablishing Bowel Control. In Zejdlik, C.P. (Ed.), *Management of spinal cord injury 2nd Ed.* (pp. 397-416). Boston: Jones and Bartlett.

CHAPTER

Skin

Susan S. Thomason, MN, RN, CS, CETN

I. Learning Objectives

A. Describe the physical, psychosocial, and financial impact of skin impairments for individuals with spinal cord impairment (SCI).

B. Relate the demographics, etiology, anatomy, and physiology of skin impairments as a complication of SCI.

C. Plan and implement a program to prevent skin impairments.

D. Assess wounds using staging criteria and/or other assessment parameters.

E. Teach the individual with a SCI, family, and/or caregiver the prevention and treatment of skin impairments.

F. Participate in interdisciplinary discharge planning for the prevention and management of skin impairments.

II. Introduction

The skin is the largest organ of the body, essential in maintaining homeostasis, providing a barrier to infection, and serving multiple other functions. In individuals with SCI, the skin is vulnerable to damage due to immobility, decreased sensation, diminished circulation, and other factors. Preventing alterations in skin integrity, such as pressure ulcers and moisture excoriations, should be underscored in the plan of care for all persons with SCI. This chapter reviews the broad spectrum of normal integument and skin impairment as a complication of individuals with SCI. The framework is based on the clinical practice guidelines published by the Agency for Health Care Policy and Research (Agency for Health Care Policy and Research [AHCPR], 1992, l994) and the clinical practice guidelines of the Consortium for Spinal Cord Medicine (2000).

A. **Demographics**
1. General costs:
   a. Costs associated with wounds are physical, psychosocial, and financial.
   b. According to the International Committee on Wound Management, cost-effectiveness in wound care can be calculated by adding direct and indirect costs (Phillips, 1996; Plackett, 1995).
2. Pressure ulcer prevalence:
   a. In a study of 148 hospitals, Meehan (1990) determined prevalence to be 9.2 percent. Pressure ulcer prevalence for individuals with tetraplegia was 60 percent (Richardson & Meyer, 1981), and 25 percent for individuals with SCI in rehabilitation settings (Langemo et al, 1989).
   b. Individuals with tetraplegia are more prone than those with paraplegia to develop pressure ulcers (Richardson & Meyer, 1981).
   c. Persons with complete injuries are more likely to develop pressure ulcers.
3. Length of stay due to pressure ulcers:
   a. The Department of Veterans Affairs long-term and acute-care facilities reported the median length of stay was 27 days (Thomason, Hawley, & Wurzel, 1993).
4. Location of pressure ulcers:
   a. The most common site of a single pressure ulcer is the sacrum (Richardson & Meyer, 1981).
   b. Eighty percent of ulcers develop over the coccyx, trochanter, ischium, or heels (Smith, 1995).

B. **Etiology/Precipitating Factors for Pressure Ulcers**
1. Pressure is the principal etiology of pressure ulcers. A capillary pressure of 17 mm Hg is required to maintain a functional capillary system. Tissue anoxia may occur if capillary pressure exceeds 32 mm Hg (Bryant, Shannon, Pieper, Braden, & Morris, 1992).
   a. Pressure of low intensity over a long period of time may result in tissue necrosis. High intensity pressures over a short period of time may also result in tissue damage (Braden & Bergstrom, 1987).
   b. Tissue tolerance is the ability of skin to redistribute the applied pressure.
2. Friction is the movement of the skin against the support surface, e.g., "sheet burn" from being pulled up in bed. Friction causes damage to the epidermis and/or dermis.
3. Shear is the synergistic effect of friction combined with pressure, e.g., gravitational pull of the individual towards the foot of the bed when in Fowler's position. Shear occurs when the blood vessels in the deeper tissue layers are stretched and angulated. Shear can create undermining due to opposing parallel forces (Bryant et al, 1992; Conner, & Clack, 1993).

C. **Anatomy/Physiology**
1. Normal skin:
   a. The skin is capable of self-regeneration. Regeneration time for the complete cycle of cell mitosis, differentiation, and migration of cells from the stratum basale to the top of the epidermis is about 35 days (Thibodeau & Patton, 1993).
   b. The dermis does not shed and regenerate like the epidermis. If the dermis is impaired, fibroblasts make connective tissue to form a scar.
   c. The integumentary system consists of skin and accessory structures, e.g., hair, nails, glands (Wysocki & Bryant, 1992). Skin layers consist of:
      (1) Epidermis: Top layer of skin, composed of dead cells (protein) and melanocytes (skin pigmentation).
      (2) Basement Membrane Zone (BMZ): Protein that provides support for the epidermis.
      (3) Dermis: Connective tissue that contains fibroblasts that secrete collagen (tensile strength) and elastin (elastic recoil). Contains hair follicles, sweat and sebaceous glands, and blood vessels.
      (4) Subcutaneous: Loose connective tissue that contains fat deposits, blood vessels, lymphatics, and nerves.
      (5) Muscle: Contractile cells that facilitate movement.

Table 17-1: Phases of Wound Healing

	Partial Thickness		Full Thickness	
	Epidermal	Deep Dermal	Subcutaneous	Muscle
Processes:				
Regeneration same cells	X	X		
Repair with different cells		X	X	X
Inflammation	X	X	X	X
Matrix formation with granulation tissue		X	X	X
Contraction by fibroblasts		X	X	X
Remodeling		X	X	X

    d. Functions of the skin include:
      (1) Protection from mechanical forces and ultraviolet radiation.
      (2) Thermoregulation by circulation and sweat glands.
      (3) Sensation via nerve receptors.
      (4) Absorption of medications and fat-soluble vitamins (A,D,E,K).
      (5) Metabolism of vitamin D.
2. Wound healing (See Table 17-1)
    a. The phases of wound healing overlap. Matrix formation begins simultaneously with the formation of granulation tissue. Matrix is first deposited toward the wound periphery, and then centrally (Clark, 1985).
    b. Wounds may be classified as acute or chronic (Lazarus et al., 1994).
      (1) Acute Wounds: Repair in an orderly and timely manner, resulting in functional and anatomical integrity of skin and tissue.
      (2) Chronic Wounds: Repair in a disorderly and untimely manner, resulting in poor functional and anatomical integrity of skin and tissue.
    c. Partial thickness wounds, i.e., those involving the epidermis and/or superficial dermis, heal by epithelialization from the lateral migration at the wound margins and bases of hair follicles (Bates-Jensen, 1995).
    d. Full thickness wounds, i.e., those involving the deep dermis, subcutaneous, and muscle tissue, heal by contraction, granulation, and matrix formation.
    e. No consensus exists regarding terminology used for pressure ulcers filling with granulation (Maklebust & Margolis, 1995). Consider the following examples of terms used to denote healing lesions: Resolving Stage IV pressure ulcer; granulation tissue 100 percent of wound base; wound reduced from 2.5 cm depth to 1.5 cm. depth.
3. Wound healing variables
    a. Lack of cutaneous sensation, neuropathy, and central nervous system lesions cause a diminished perception or response to discomfort, lack of "cues" for position shifts, and compromises the individual with SCI in mounting an effective inflammatory response to wound bacterial growth (Cooper, 1995).
    b. Changes that occur to skin in mature adulthood include: Decreased dermis by 20 percent, increased epidermis turnover time (21 days in young adult vs. double that in

35-year-old), and increased vulnerability to tearing. As aging occurs, there is decreased sensory perception, vitamin D production, sweat gland function, inflammatory response, vascularity, and subcutaneous fat. Additionally, co-existing illnesses impair healing in aging individuals with SCI (Allman, 1989; Loescher, 1995; Stotts & Wipke-Tevis, 1996).

   c. Diminished mobility in individuals with SCI adversely affects wound healing. Individuals who are bed- or chair-bound are at risk for pressure ulcers (Allman, Goode, Patrick, Burst & Bartolucci, 1995).

   d. Healing wounds are dependent upon localized microcirculation for oxygen and nutrients (Hagisawa, Ferguson-Pell, Cardi, & Miller, 1994); hypoxemia and hypovolemia decrease oxygen required for collagen synthesis (Stotts & Wipke-Tevis, 1996).

   e. Nutritional factors adversely affecting wound healing include: Kwashiorkor (deficient protein stores), marasmus (deficient fat stores), and kwashiorkor/marasmus mix (deficient protein and fat stores). Hypoalbuminemia (less than 3.5 mg/dL) results in interstitial edema causing impaired nutrition and oxygen exchange at the cellular level (Brylinsky, 1995). Calories, protein, carbohydrates, fats, vitamin and mineral deficiencies may adversely affect wound healing. (Pinchcofsky-Davis & Kaminski 1986). Vitamin A, Vitamin C, and Zinc may be positively correlated with wound healing, and supplements may be required if the individual is receiving steroids (Hunt, 1986).

   f. Smokers are 2.9 times as likely than non-smokers to develop pressure ulcers (Guralnik, Harris, White, & Cornoni-Huntley, 1988). Nicotine is a potent vasoconstrictor and increases the risk of microvascular thrombosis. Carbon monoxide binds with hemoglobin, lowering oxygen saturation (Stotts & Wipke-Tevis, 1996; Viehbeck, McGlynn, & Harris, 1995).

   g. Individuals with hemoglobin <12 g/100 mL at baseline are more than twice as likely to develop pressure ulcers as those with hemoglobin >12 g/100mL (Guralnik et al, 1988).

   h. Bacterial burden also affects wound healing. Bacteria compete with normal cells for oxygen and nutrients; bacterial byproducts are toxic to cells (Stotts & Wipke-Tevis, 1996).

   i. Additional variables related to high risk individuals with SCI in the acute setting include: Hypotension and length of time on backboards, x-ray tables, and operating room tables.

   j. Other factors adversely affecting wound healing in individuals with SCI include: Altered level of consciousness, leukopenia, decreased body weight, stress, edema, interval of direct patient care, psychosocial factors, and others (Consortium for Spinal Cord Medicine, 2000).

III. Initial Assessment

A. **Nursing History**:
   1. History of present skin impairment, e.g., date of onset, course, pathology, and treatment.
   2. Individual/caregivers' knowledge of wound prevention/treatment.
   3. Previous surgical interventions.
   4. Functional abilities, e.g., functional orthoses.
   5. Bed and wheelchair support surfaces, e.g., cushion, mattress.
   6. Concomitant illness/conditions, e.g., bladder/bowel incontinence.
   7. Allergies to foods/medications.
   8. Frequency and method of skin inspection, e.g., mirror.
   9. Substance abuse, e.g., smoking, non-prescribed drugs, alcohol.
   10. Increased fluid losses, e.g., fluid drainage.
   11. Increased metabolic needs, e.g., infection.
   12. Nutritional history: Usual body weight vs. ideal body weight, food preferences/ intolerances, chewing/swallowing difficulties, social history, income, food purchaser, meal preparer, adaptive utensils, ability to feed self.

B. **Physical Exam** (Refer to Table 17-2)
   1. Perform a risk assessment for pressure ulcers using a quantitative scale:
      a. Braden Scale variables include sensory perception, moisture, activity, mobility, nutrition, and friction/shear (Bergstrom, Braden, Laguzza, & Holman, 1987) (Refer to Table 17-3).

Table 17-2: Wound Assessment Parameters

Location	Tissue	Undermining
Size	• Granulation	Tunnelling/sinuses
Depth	• Necrotic	Erythema
Stage	• Slough	Induration
Volume	• Eschar	Innervation
Pain	Wound Margins	Lymphangitis
Odor	Edema	Hair distribution
Color	Drainage	Capillary refill
Exposed structures	• Serous	Varicosities
• Tendons/Muscles	• Sanguinous	Joint Involvement
• Bones	• Purulent	Epithelialization

    b. Norton Scale variables include physical condition, mental condition, mobility, and incontinence (Norton, 1989)

    c. Other scales and models include Knoll Assessment Scale (Aronovitch, Millenbach, Kelman, & Wing, 1992), Gosnell Scale (Gosnell, 1989), Sessing Scale (Ferrell, Artinian, & Sessing, 1995), and Sparks Risk Assessment Model (Sparks, 1992, 1993).

2. Systematically assess the skin daily with special attention to bony prominences (AHCPR, 1992). Insure that the individual with a SCI has a hand-held mirror, with extension handle, if necessary, to perform self-inspection of the trunk and lower extremities (Thomason, 1990; Zejdlik, 1992).

3. Linear measurements, using the metric system, may be obtained by the following:

    a. Measure longest dimension (length); measure the longest dimension perpendicular to the length (width) (Cutler, et al., 1993). Wound tracings over a thin plastic sheet may be helpful (Etris, Pribble, & LaBrecque, 1994).

    b. Measure depth by placing a Q-tip into the deepest part of the ulcer and measure the Q-tip with a ruler (Bates-Jensen, 1995; Etris, 1995; Cutler, et al., 1993). The depth may increase with further debridement.

    c. Photography may be used with linear measurement in the photo field (Etris et al., 1994).

4. Stage wound based upon the depth of the lesion. If eschar is present, the ulcer may not be staged (AHCPR, 1994). Indicators of a Stage I ulcer include: non-blanchable erythema, induration, and edema (Lyder, 1991). In individuals with darkly pigmented skin, Stage I may present as a purplish/bluish, or eggplant-like color, with taunt, shiny skin (Bennett, 1995) (Refer to Table 17-4).

5. Volume may be determined by measuring the amount of normal saline, dental alginate, or other material used to fill the wound (Plassmann, Melhuish, & Harding, 1994).

6. Scales may be used to track healing parameters and quantify clinical observations: Sessing Scale (Ferrell et al., 1995) or Pressure Sore Status Tool (Bates-Jensen, 1995).

7. Assess wound margins, noting definition and migration of epithelial cells.

8. Describe type of tissue in the wound: Granulation tissue is "beefy red", denoting fibroblast activity and formation of new blood vessels; the color of granulation tissue may reflect the individual's hemoglobin level (Etris, 1995). Necrotic tissue may be composed of slough (stringy whitish, greyish tissue) or eschar (blackish, leathery tissue). Documentation should include the estimated percent age of granulation or necrotic tissue in relationship to the entire wound bed, e.g., 40 percent granulation and 60 percent slough.

9. Differentiate between infected and colonized wounds. Signs of infection may include purulent drainage, temperature elevation, odor, induration, cellulitis, septicemia, and a bacterial colony count >100,000. There is an absence of local and systemic signs of infection when the wound is colonized.

Table 17-3

BRADEN SCALE FOR PREDICTING PRESSURE SORE RISK

Patient's Name _____

Evaluator's Name _____ Date of Assessment _____

SENSORY PERCEPTION Ability to respond meaningfully to pressure-related discomfort	1. Completely Limited: Unresponsive (does not moan, flinch) to painful stimuli, due to diminished level of consciousness or sedation. OR limited ability to feel pain over most of body surface.	2. Very Limited: Responds only to painful stimuli. Cannot communicate discomfort except by moaning or restlessness. OR Has a sensory impairment that limits the ability to feel pain or discomfort over 1/2 of body.	3. Slightly Limited: Responds to verbal commands, but cannot always communicate discomfort or need to be turned. OR has some sensory impairment which limits ability to feel pain or discomfort in 1 or 2 extremities	4. No Impairment: Responds to verbal commands. Has no sensory deficit which would limit ability to feel or voice pain or discomfort.
MOISTURE Degree to which skin is exposed to moisture	1. Constantly Moist: Skin is kept moist almost constantly by perspiration, urine, etc. Dampness is detected every time patient is moved or turned.	2. Very Moist: Skin is often, but not always moist. Linen must be changed approximately once a shift.	3. Occasionally Moist: Skin is occasionally moist, requiring an extra linen change approximately once a day.	4. Rarely Moist: Skin is usually dry, linen only requires changing at routine intervals.
ACTIVITY Degree of physical activity	1. Bedfast: Confined to bed	2. Chairfast: Ability to walk severely limited or non-existent. Cannot bear own weight and/or must be assisted into chair or wheelchair.	3. Walks Occasionally: Walks occasionally during day, but for very short distances, with or without assistance. Spends majority of each shift in bed or chair.	4. Walks Frequently: Walks outside the room at least twice a day and inside room at least once every 2 hours during waking hours.
MOBILITY Ability to change and control body position	1. Completely Immobile: Does not make even slight changes in body or extremity position without assistance.	2. Very Limited: Makes occasional slight changes in body or extremity position but unable to make frequent or significant changes independently.	3. Slightly Limited: Makes frequent though slight changes in body or extremity position independently.	4. No Limitation: Makes major and frequent changes in position without assistance.
NUTRITION Usual food intake pattern	1. Very Poor: Never eats a complete meal. Rarely eats more than 1/3 of any food offered. Eats 2 servings or less of protein (meat or dairy products) per day. Takes fluids poorly. Does not take a liquid dietary supplement. OR Is NPO and/or maintained on clear liquids or IV's for more than 5 days.	2. Probably Inadequate: Rarely eats a complete meal and generally eats only about 1/2 of any food offered. Protein intake includes only 3 servings of meat or dairy products per day. Occasionally will take a dietary supplement. OR Receives less than optimum amount of liquid diet or tube feeding.	3. Adequate: Eats over half of most meals. Eats a total of 4 servings of protein (meat, dairy products) each day. Occasionally will refuse a meal, but will usually take a supplement if offered. OR Is on a tube feeding or TPN regimen, which probably meets most of nutritional needs.	4. Excellent: Eats most of every meal. Never refuses a meal. Usually eats a total of 4 or more servings of meat and dairy products. Occasionally eats between meals. Does not require supplementation.
FRICTION AND SHEAR	1. Problem: Requires moderate to maximum assistance in moving. Complete lifting without sliding against sheets is impossible. Frequently slides down in bed or chair, requiring frequent repositioning with maximum assistance. Spasticity, contractures or agitation leads to almost constant friction.	2. Potential Problem: Moves freely or requires minimum assistance. During a move skin probably slides to some extent against sheets, chair, restraints, or other devices. Maintains relatively good position in chair or bed most of the time but occasionally slides down.	3. No Apparent Problem: Moves in bed and in chair independently and has sufficient muscle strength to lift up completely during move. Maintains good position in bed or chair at all times.	
			Total Score	

From "Clinical Utility of the Braden Scale for Predicting Pressure Sore Risk," by B.J. Braden & N. Bergstrom, 1988, *DECUBITIS*, 2 (3), p. 45. Copyright 1988 by B.J. Braden & N. Bergstrom.

Table 17-4: Pressure Ulcer Staging

STAGE I:	Nonblanchable erythema of intact skin Heralding lesion of skin ulceration In persons with darker skin, discoloration, warmth, induration, edema, or hardness may be indicators.
STAGE II:	Partial thickness skin loss involving epidermis, dermis, or both. Ulcer is superficial and presents as an abrasion, blister, or shallow crater.
STAGE III:	Full thickness skin loss involving damage to or necrosis of subcutaneous tissue that may extend to, but not through, underlying fascia Ulcer presents as deep crater with or without undermining of adjacent tissue
STAGE IV:	Full thickness skin loss with extensive destruction, tissue necrosis, or damage to muscle, bone, or supporting structures, e.g., tendon, joint capsule. Undermining and sinus tracts may be associated.

From Pressure Ulcers in Adults: Prediction and Prevention, by AHCPR, 1992, Rockville, MD: U.S. Government Printing Office.

Table 17-5: Wound Diagnostic Studies

Assessment Parameter	Noninvasive Studies	Invasive Studies
Wound Size	Direct Measurement Wound Tracings Photography Saline installation Computer assisted planimetry Stereophotogrammetry Impression material Structured Light System High Frequency Ultrasound Scanner	
Blood Flow	Ankle-Brachial Index Thermography Doppler Plethysmography	Arteriogram Venogram Fluoroscopy
Oxygenation	Transcutaneous Oxygen	
Infection	X-ray Bone Scan Magnetic Resonance Imaging (MRI) Computerized Tomography (CT) Indium Scan	Tissue Biopsy Bone Biopsy
Innervation	Semmes-Weinstein filaments Pin testing Vibration	Nerve Conduction Electromyography

C. **Diagnostic Studies**
1. Wound assessment parameters include wound size, blood flow, oxygenation, infection, and innervation (Refer to Table 17-5).
2. Nutrition
   a. Somatic protein stores: Evidenced by weight and height, total body fat, and body muscle stores considering disuse atrophy in individuals with SCI, and creatinine height index.
   b. Visceral protein stores:
      (1) Serum Albumin: Normal 3.5-5.0 gm/dL. Major protein synthesized in the liver; main plasma protein; half-life approximately 20 days. Slow to decrease with malnutrition.
      (2) Transferrin: Normal 180-260 mg/dL. Synthesized in the liver; transports iron in the plasma; half-life 7 days; more reflective of current protein status than albumin.
      (3) Total Lymphocyte Count (TLC): Normal >1,800 mm3. Reflects cell-mediated immunity; TLC = White Blood Cells x percent lymphocytes divided by 100.
      (4) Total Protein: Normal 6.6 - 7.9 gm/dL. Determined by serum albumin and globulin; affects colloid osmotic pressure.

IV. Nursing Process Applied to Stage I and II Pressure Ulcers

A. **Nursing Diagnosis**: Impaired skin integrity.

B. **Defining Characteristics**: Pressure, friction, and shear.

C. **Expected Outcomes**:
1. Individual /caregiver verbalizes knowledge of pressure ulcer prevention and treatment of Stage I and II ulcers.
2. Pressure ulcer prevented.
3. Pressure ulcer healing or reduction in surface area of Stage I and II ulcers (specify date).
4. Epithelialization (Stage II).
5. Granulation (deep Stage II).
6. Absence of necrotic tissue.
7. No signs/symptoms of infection.
8. Mobility maintained at pre-ulcer level.
9. Moisture controlled.
10. Nutritional status adequate.
11. Pain/discomfort relieved.

D. **Interventions**:
1. Prevent pressure ulcers (AHCPR, 1992).
   a. Maintain and improve tissue tolerance.
      (1) Maintain skin hygiene.
      (2) Control humidity.
      (3) Avoid temperature extremes.
      (4) Apply moisturizers to dry skin.
      (5) Avoid massage of reddened areas and/or bony prominences.
      (6) Control moisture.
         (a) Institute bowel and bladder management programs.
         (b) Use absorbent underpads, if indicated.
         (c) Apply moisture barrier cream, if indicated.
      (7) Manage nutritional needs via oral diet, supplements, or parenteral or enteral feedings.
      (8) Establish/maintain mobility program.
         (a) Use assistive devices to promote independence, e.g., hand orthoses, handrails.
         (b) Implement physical and occupational therapy programs to enhance/maintain strength, coordination, flexibility, and muscle tone.
         (c) Facilitate independent living activities.

b. Protect against adverse effects of external mechanical forces, e.g., pressure, friction, shear (AHCPR, 1992).
   (1) Reduce pressure.
       (a) Reposition every two hours in bed. Use turning schedule.
       (b) Prone while in bed, if tolerated.
       (c) Have individual shift weight in wheelchair every 15 minutes. If unable to perform pressure releases, caregiver must perform.
       (d) Avoid plantar flexion, i.e., foot drop, by using a footboard, high-topped tennis shoes, or other device.
       (e) Ambulate, if possible, e.g., individual with central cord syndrome.
       (f) Recline in wheelchair to redistribute pressure.
       (g) If skin is reddened, position individual off ulcer 1-3 days (Sather, Weber, Jr., & George, 1977).
       (h) Provide pressure relief for approximately 2 weeks, if necessary, to completely heal an area of induration with abnormal reactive hyperemia (Pires & Muller, 1991).
   (2) Position with devices.
       (a) Use devices to position between bony prominences, e.g., pillows or wedges between knees and behind back (Smith, 1995).
       (b) Use side position at 30 degree oblique angle, not positioning directly on trochanter.
       (c) Flex upper hip and knee at 30 degrees when side-lying (Garber, Campion, & Krouskop, 1982).
       (d) Position heels off the bed (AHCPR, 1992, 1994).
   (3) Control shear.
       (a) Maintain head of bed no higher than 30 degrees.
       (b) If spasms prohibit heel elevation, use thick, synthetic socks.
       (c) Use lift sheet to move individual up in bed.
       (d) Gatch the foot of the bed slightly to avoid sliding down in bed.
       (e) Use elbow pads, particularly if the patient uses a prone litter.
   (4) Lift individual.
       (a) Use two persons to move individual to head of bed.
       (b) Use lifting device, e.g., hydraulic lift, to transfer.
   (5) Select appropriate wheelchair.
       (a) Use properly sized wheelchair seat, foot pedals, armrests, and back.
       (b) Insure correct postural alignment, weight distribution, and balance.
   (6) Wear appropriate clothing.
       (a) Dress in loose clothing with minimal seams.
       (b) Have individual wear shoes one size larger than normal, with rigid soles (Noble, 1981).

V. Nursing Process Applied to Stage III and IV Pressure Ulcers

A. **Nursing Diagnoses**: Impaired tissue integrity and associated alterations in nutritional status, mobility, comfort, and elimination, as well as knowledge deficits.

B. **Defining Characteristics**: Ulcers that heal by granulation, epithelialization, and contraction.

C. **Expected Outcomes**:
1. Individual/caregiver verbalizes knowledge of pressure ulcer prevention and treatment of Stage III and IV ulcers.
2. Pressure ulcers are prevented.
3. Pressure ulcer healing, reduction in surface area, or reduction in volume of Stage III and IV ulcers (specify date).
4. Granulation, matrix formation, and contraction of Stage III and IV ulcers.
5. Absence of necrotic tissue.
6. No signs/symptoms of infection.

7. Mobility maintained at pre-ulcer level.
8. Moisture controlled.
9. Nutritional status adequate.
10. Pain/discomfort relieved.

D. **Interventions**
1. Prevent pressure ulcers (AHCPR, 1992). **See IV. Nursing Process Applied to Stage I and II Pressure Ulcers**. Cleanse ulcer(s) prior to dressing application.
    a. Avoid antiseptic cleansers (e.g., povidone-iodine, Dakin's solution, acetic acid) due to potential damage to fibroblasts (AHCPR, 1994).
    b. Use 0.9 percent sodium chloride (normal saline) for irrigation or biocompatible wound cleanser.
    c. Apply minimal force with gauze: Avoid scrubbing the wound (Baranoski, 1995).
    d. Irrigate with device to provide 15 p.s.i. force, (e.g., 35 cc. syringe with 19g. needle/angiocath) if hospital infection guidelines permit (Barr, 1995).
2. Debride wound of necrotic tissue (e.g., slough, eschar).
    a. Mechanical, non-selective debridement methods (e.g., wet-to-dry dressings, whirlpool therapy) may damage fibroblasts (Moncada, 1992).
    b. Sharp, selective debridement may be done using scissors and scalpel (Fowler & van Rijswijk, 1995; Thomaselli, 1994).
        (1) Cross-hatch eschar prior to enzymatic therapy.
        (2) Avoid sharp debridement of heel ulcer with dry eschar, unless it exhibits edema, erythema, fluctuance, or drainage (AHCPR, 1994).
        (3) Pre-medicate with analgesic, if necessary; obtain informed consent per facility policy.
        (4) If wound is undermined, consider removing the "over-hang" to allow wound margin to adhere to wound bed (Himel, 1995).
        (5) Use a dry gauze dressing 24 hours following sharp debridement.
    c. Enzymatic debridement should be accomplished by applying 1/8" enzyme confined to wound base. Cleanse with Normal Saline prior to applying.
    d. Autolytic debridement may be indicated if wound does not exhibit signs of infection, e.g., purulent drainage, induration, erythema. Use an occlusive or semi-occlusive dressing (e.g., hydrocolloid) for autolytic debridement.
3. Dress wound maintaining a moist wound bed and insure surrounding skin is dry. Provide gentle care, avoid substances that impede the healing process, and maintain a healthy wound environment (Refer to Table 17-6).
    a. Dressings should protect the wound, provide flexibility and comfort, control exudate, and prevent contamination.
    b. Manage hypergranulation tissue, i.e., "proud flesh," using silver nitrate, petrolatum dressing, or other non-occlusive dressing (Kerstein, 1995).
    c. Avoid occlusive and semi-occlusive dressings if there are clinical signs of infection.
    d. Use absorptive dressings to control exudate that dilutes nutrients, macerates the tissue or skin, or accumulates toxins.
    e. Eliminate wound "dead space," i.e., space between the wound bed and cover dressing, by loosely filling or packing cavity (Doughty, 1990).
    f. Use Standard Precautions to protect against exposure to bloodborne pathogens (Refer to Table 17-7).
    g. Consider caregiver time when selecting a dressing.
    h. Use continuous piece of gauze if packing the dressing; use packing strips if tunneling.
4. Use support surface, e.g., mattresses, beds, overlays, to reduce tissue loads by pressure relief or pressure reduction (Ceccio, 1990; Krouskop & van Rijswijk, 1995).
    a. There is no standardization of pressure/shear gradations; direct comparison of these devices must be more qualitative than quantitative (Department of Veterans Affairs, 1992; Tallon, 1996)
    b. Transducers are common devices to measure interface pressures, between body and support surface.

Table 17-6: Wound Dressing Considerations

Gauze Packing	Unlayer into a single thickness to cover a greater surface area. Use wide mesh gauze to debride and entrap exudate (Hess & Miller, 1990) Use fine mesh gauze when wound begins to epithelialize (Sklar, 1985) Use packing strips for fistulas/tunnels; pack loosely to avoid placing pressure on the capillary buds. Avoid packing above the skin surface. Moisten with normal saline to insure wound healing. Change every 4-6 hours to insure wound does not desiccate.
Hydrocolloid	Occlusive dressing for non-infected wounds Contraindicated in heavily exudating wounds, although fillers may be used to enhance absorption Use filler paste/granules to avoid "dead" space between wound bed and wafer. "Picture frame" with tape around wafer to increase wearability and protect dressing while in shower. Wounds may appear larger due to autolytic debridement Gently irrigate gel (normal) from wound when removing. Avoid stretching wafer when applying. Change every 5 days and as needed if seal is broken. Decreases the number of pericapillary fibrin cuffs (Kerstein, 1995) Barrier to bacteria (Shannon & Miller, 1988)
Absorption Agents	Indicated for moderate to heavy exudating wounds. Will desiccate tissue if wound bed dry. Monitor serum K+ for elevations. Rehydrate gel with normal saline before removing. Avoiding packing fistulas with agent due to difficulty cleansing.
Antibiotics	Use systemic antibiotics if cellulitis or systemic signs of infection. Topical and systemic antibiotics may incur resistance or drug reaction. May not penetrate the wound enough to reduce bacterial count.
Enzymes	Some may impair healthy granulation tissue. Used to debride necrotic wound. Apply in thin layer to wound bed. Avoid wound cleansers with heavy metals. Wound may be cross-hatched to facilitate debridement.
Normal	**Saline** Isotonic solution (0.9% NaCl) Used as irrigant or primary dressing solution. Preserves health granulation issue.
Antimicrobial	May be absorbed systemically; observe for hepatic/renal function. Contraindicated if Sulfa allergy, e.g., Silver Sulfadiazine 1%
Transparent	Moisture vapor-permeable dressing Moist healing environment. Contraindicated in infected wounds or copious drainage. Use wet gauze to loosen dressing. Allow 2" margin around wound. Change every 5 days
Hydrogel	Available as sheets, wafers, impregnated gauze, or spray. Indicated for minimal to moderately exudating wounds; Contraindicated in heavily exudating wounds. Wound may increase in size due to autolysis.

Table 17-7: Wound Dressing Guidelines

Impairment	Non-Infected Wound	Infected Wound
Partial Thickness Wounds		
Skin Tear	Hydrocolloid	Silver Sulfadiazine 1 percent
Stage II Pressure Ulcer	Impregnated non-adherent	Mupirocin 2 percent (gram +)
Abrasion	Hydrogel	
	Gel	
	Foam	
	Synthetic barrier	
	Collagen	
	Composite	
	Transparent	
Partial Thickness Wounds		
Pressure Ulcer	Hydrocolloid with filler paste	Silver Sulfadiazine 1 percent
• Deep Stage II	Gauze with Normal Saline (NS)	Antimicrobial Dressings
• Stage III	• Continuous piece of gauze,	Gauze with NS
• Stage IV	if packing	
	• Packing strips, if tunneling	Absorption Dressing
	Alginate	• Calcium Alginate
	Hydrogel	• Copolymer Starch
	Gel	• Beads
	Composite	Hydrogel
	Collagen	Gel
	Contact layers	Composite
	Enzyme	Contact layers
	Foam	
	Growth Factors	
	Skin Substitute	
	Biosynthetic	
	Impregnated Gauze	
Moisture Excoriations	Moisture barrier cream (MBC)	Antifungal, if yeast
	Wound gel/MBC combination	

c. Selection should be made on the basis of the most cost-effective device to accomplish the desired outcomes.

d. Support surfaces may be categorized based upon whether these provide pressure reduction or pressure relief.
    (1) Pressure reduction surfaces decrease capillary arterial pressure between the body and support surface to about 32 mm Hg. These devices, usually composed of foam, gel, or water, are primarily used for prevention of ulcers, or if the individual with a trunk ulcer can remain off the affected site while in bed.
    (2) Pressure relief surfaces decrease capillary arterial pressure to less than 32 mm Hg. These devices, usually comproed of air or ceramic beads, are primarily used for treatment of ulcers affecting more than one trunk surface, post-operatively for flaps or grafts to the trunk, if the individual is hemodynamically unstable and may not be turned, or if he/she has severe moisture excoriations.

e. Limit the use of pads, sheets, etc. between support surface and body; have loose top sheet.

f. Turn every two hours to optimize pressure reduction/relief, maximize ventilation, and provide adequate urinary drainage; keep heels off surface (Refer to Figure 17-1).

g. Keep patient off ulcer, unless unable.

h. Wheelchair cushions are indicated for all individuals with SCI who are wheelchair users. Consider the following when selecting a cushion: Pressure reduction, maintenance requirements, ease of transfer, adaptability, user's ability to perform activities of daily living, functional needs, balance, shear, and pressure distribution (Garber, 1985).

Figure 17-1: Support Surface Guidelines

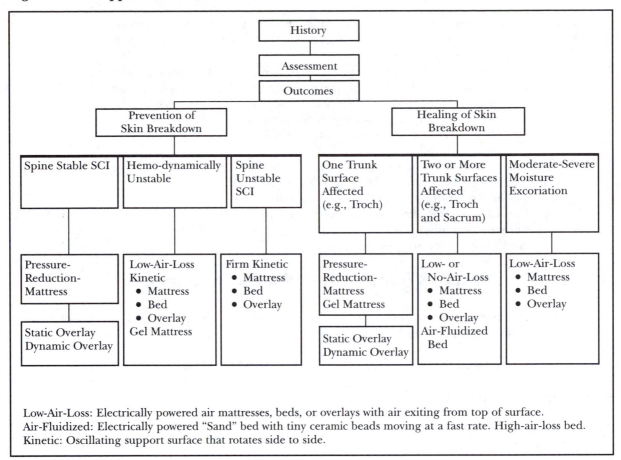

Low-Air-Loss: Electrically powered air mattresses, beds, or overlays with air exiting from top of surface.
Air-Fluidized: Electrically powered "Sand" bed with tiny ceramic beads moving at a fast rate. High-air-loss bed.
Kinetic: Oscillating support surface that rotates side to side.

5. Manage infection that can delay wound healing.
   a. Avoid inappropriate use of antibiotics that may result in an individual with SCI developing an allergy, sensitivity, or resistance to organisms (Leaper, 1994; Thomson & Smith, 1994).
   b. Avoid using occlusive dressings if wounds are infected. However, occlusive dressings have the following infection control advantages when compared to gauze dressings: Reduction in airborne bacteria, effective barrier to infection, decreased aerobic bacteria, and increased number of polymorphonuclear cells in wound fluid to reduce bacterial burden (Hutchinson, 1994; Lawrence, 1994).
   c. Two major complications from pressure ulcers are sepsis and osteomyelitis.
      (1) The incidence of bone infection for persons with Stage IV pressure ulcers is as high as 81 percent (Deloach, DiBenedetto, Womble, & Gilley, 1992).
      (2) Individuals with ulcers that do not heal with appropriate local wound debridement should be evaluated for osteomyelitis.
      (3) The gold standard for diagnosis of osteomyelitis is bone biopsy with evidence of necrosis, or inflammatory cells such as polymorphonuclear leukocytes and lymphocytes, increased white blood cell count (WBC), and increased erythrosedimentation rate (ESR) (AHCPR, 1994).
      (4) Treatment includes surgical debridement to remove devitalized tissue, and antibiotic therapy for 2-8 weeks.
6. Treat surgically with flaps or grafts to protect the wound, prevent desiccation, revascularize previously ischemic areas, and allow for normal physiological response (Deloach et al., 1992; Goldberg, 1995).

237

   a. Common muscle flaps include gluteus maximus flap of the sacrum or ischium, and tensor fascia lata flap of the trochanter.
   b. Pre-operative interventions include: Bowel preparation to prevent infection and contamination, control of muscle spasms, correction of muscle or joint contractures, and improving nutrition.
   c. Post-operative interventions include: Dressing intact for 24 hours, wound drains to low suction, suture care, gradual progression to sitting in appropriate wheelchair, and observation for hematoma, infection, dehiscence, and necrosis.
7. Provide discharge planning with the interdisciplinary team.
   a. Provide comprehensive education to individual with SCI and caregiver to interrupt the pressure ulcer cycle.
   b. Initiate consultation as appropriate, e.g., social worker, therapist, enterostomal therapy nurse, dietitian, pharmacist, and psychologist.
   c. Initiate community referrals, as appropriate.
   d. Consider mental and physical capabilities of individual with a SCI and caregiver, (e.g., difficulty in manipulating transparent dressings with poor hand function) when determining an appropriate dressing.

VI. Nursing Process Applied to Moisture Excoriations

A. **Nursing Diagnoses**: Impaired skin integrity and associated alterations in mobility, comfort, and elimination, as well as knowledge deficits.

B. **Defining Characteristics**: Maceration, excoriation, and bowel/bladder incontinence.

C. **Expected Outcomes**:
   1. Intact skin.
   2. Bowel management with < 1 accident/week.
   3. Bladder management with continence/containment.
   4. Skin hygiene.

D. **Interventions**
   1. Use incontinent cleanser or mild soap after incontinent episode. Rinse well; pat dry.
   2. Consider low air loss specialty support surface if moderate to severe excoriations.
   3. Implement/maintain bladder management program based on urodynamic studies: Intermittent catheterization (IC), external urinary device (EUD), Foley catheter (F/C), or suprapubic catheter (SC).
   4. If penis excoriated with EUD, remove for 48 hours and manage continence with voiding, IC, or F/C.
   5. If yeast infection, apply moisture barrier cream over antifungal cream.
   6. If excoriation due to moisture, apply moisture barrier cream (may combine with wound gel), lift scrotum, and avoid occlusive dressings.
   7. Use "penis pocket" insert device in male underwear, if urine dribbling occurs and no catheter.

VII. Reassessment

A. **Nursing History**
   1. Reassess knowledge demonstrated by individual/caregiver of the prevention and treatment of ulcer/excoriation.
   2. Evaluate ulcer/excoriation recurrence.
   3. Re-evaluate individual's "at-risk" status.

B. **Examination**
   1. Assess weekly or when assessment indicates deterioration in wound status (AHCPR, 1994; van Rijswijk, 1995).

2. If no progress toward healing within 2-4 weeks of therapy initiation, re-evaluate treatment plan (Margolis, 1994).

3. Determine wound healing rate by: Wound perimeter measurement, absolute change in area volume, or percentage change in area or volume (Margolis, 1994).

4. Avoid reverse staging to denote healing progression, as full thickness ulcers are replaced with granulation, and not muscle or subcutaneous tissue (National Pressure Ulcer Advisory Panel (NPUAP), 1995). Therefore, a Stage IV pressure ulcer does not heal to a Stage III ulcer, etc.

5. See **Section III, B** to initiate or re-initiate physical exam parameters.

C. **Diagnostic Studies**: See **Section III, C** to initiate or re-initiate diagnostic tests.

VIII. Health Tips

A. The interdisciplinary team, including nurse, physician, physical and occupational therapists, social worker, dietitian, and others are of critical importance in skin management.

B. Education in the prevention and treatment of pressure ulcers and excoriations must be provided the individual with SCI and the caregiver.

C. Identifying risk factors prompts the nurse to target assessment and treatment of impairments in skin and tissue integrity.

D. Daily skin inspection is imperative; direct observation is essential, as many individuals with SCI are insensate.

E. Pressure ulcer prevention is paramount, as healed tissue has only 80 percent of its original strength, and individuals with SCI are extremely vulnerable to recurrence.

F. Therapy is directed toward doing no harm to the individual (e.g., avoiding antiseptics), while facilitating the wound healing process (e.g., moist dressings to promote epithelization).

G. Less obvious variables (e.g., substance abuse, caregiver issues), must be explored to obtain a thorough assessment of the individual's needs.

H. Skin management should be based upon research findings, not unfounded principles.

I. Every wound "belongs" to a person; the need to address the person with SCI as an individual cannot be overemphasized.

IX. Special Issues Related to Pediatric Care

A. **Risk in Children**: Children may have fewer skin problems due to the distribution and the large amount of subcutaneous tissue. Fat pads are prominent in infants but will disappear over bony prominences as the toddler grows. Older children and adolescents have risks similar to those of adults.

B. **Educational Considerations:**
1. Children with loss of sensation need to gain a respect for their body with the understanding that their body, although they may not feel it, is a part of their total self. This may be accomplished with the help of a mirror, which enables visualization of the entire body. It is difficult for children to develop respect and care for a part of their body that they do not feel.
2. Young children should be taught the names of body parts they do not feel, so they gain an awareness of their bodies. A 15-month-old can learn body parts. A doll is frequently used to teach body parts.

3. Parents need to be taught the risk of pressure ulcers and the need for good skin care habits.

4. The child should be taught the mechanics of skin inspection and to participate in skin checks as soon as possible (by age 5 years) and to gain an understanding of what they must do to prevent skin breakdown or prevent new skin breakdown. Establishing a skin check routine is important for early and effective education of the child and family.

5. Care must be taken to prevent skin breakdown if the child wears an orthotic device, especially over bony prominences, as they grow (Zejdlik, 1992).

6. Seating devices (cushions, size of wheelchair) must be re-evaluated on a scheduled basis because of change in weight and growth spurts.

7. The child and family need to be educated about thermal (hot, cold) and traumatic (shearing, rubbing, friction) injuries. Young children need to be taught the difference between hot and cold and the effect it will have on their skin (frostbite, sunburns, high temperature burns). Care needs to be taken in the home to protect the young child from hot surfaces. Simple things such as hot metal on a wheelchair or seat belt latch can cause an unexpected burn. Older children, while more aware of the effects of hot and cold, will still need reminders to avoid skin injury (e.g., teens with curling irons).

8. The older child and adolescent may for a time show a disregard for their skin and the prevention of skin breakdown. Restricted activities and repeated education and participation may bring an awareness of the necessity of good skin care.

9. Pressure relief (every 15 minutes) reminders such as an alarm watch, commercial breaks on TV, are taught and encouraged. Rest periods at school, standing devices, changes in the position of the chair (reclining or tilt in space chair) and weight shifts aid in the maintenance of good skin.

10. Children who ambulate but have impaired sensation may be at the highest risk for pressure ulcers over the ischial tuberosites, due to the lack of a prevention system. Children may sit in hard chairs in school and not realize the need for pressure releases.

Practical Application

W.S., a 25-year-old professional with C-5 tetraplegia, is admitted to the rehabilitation unit with ulcers on his sacrum and right trochanter. W.S. works as an accountant nine hours per day. He was injured four years ago in a motor vehicle accident, and his brother, who also works full-time, is his primary caregiver. W.S. has a 20 pack-year smoking history, uses a standard mattress at home, and has a pillow for a wheelchair support surface.

On the right trochanter, the W.S. has a 4 x 3 cm. ulcer with 60 percent slough and 40 percent eschar. It is malodorous, with a moderate amount of purulent drainage. On his sacrum, he has a 4 cm., warm, indurated, Stage I ulcer with non-blanchable erythema. He is febrile and diaphoretic. Laboratory values indicate he has an elevated WBC and ESR. A bone x-ray is ordered to rule out osteomyelitis, a tissue biopsy is sent for culture and sensitivity, and blood cultures are drawn.

W.S. is placed on a low-air loss mattress and is on a regular turning schedule to minimize pressure. Consults are initiated to the following disciplines:

Dietitian - Nutritional evaluation and increase calorie/supplemental feedings.
Physical Therapist - Wheelchair and wheelchair cushion evaluation.
Surgery - Debridement of slough and eschar and possible muscle flap.
Substance Abuse Coordinator - Smoking cessation evaluation.

Intravenous antibiotic therapy is initiated for systemic signs and symptoms of infection. Topical treatment of the trochanteric ulcer includes cleansing with a commercial wound cleanser, and application of silver sulfadiazine 1 percent every 6 hours with lightly packed gauze. Education is implemented which includes skin inspection, pressure reduction, positioning, avoiding shear, transferring, wheelchair and clothing considerations, job hour modifications, and other aspects of prevention.

A pressure reduction mattress will be considered at a future time, based upon W.S.'s interdisciplinary discharge plan.

References and Selected Bibliography

Agency for Health Care Policy and Research (AHCPR). (1992). *Pressure ulcers in adults: Prediction and prevention.* Clinical Guideline Number 3. (AHCPR Publication No. 92-00047) Rockville, MD: U.S. Government Printing Office.

Agency for Health Care Policy and Research (AHCPR). (1994). *Treatment of pressure ulcers.* Clinical Practice Guideline Number 15. (AHCPR Publication No. 95-0652). Rockville, MD: U.S. Government Printing Office.

Allman, R.M. (1989). Epidemiology of pressure sores in different populations. *DECUBITUS, 2(2)*,30-33.

Allman, R.M., Goode, P.S., Patrick, M.M., Burst, N., & Bartolucci, A.A. (1995). Pressure ulcer risk factors among hospitalized patients with activity limitation. *Journal of the American Medical Association, 273 (11)*, 865-870.

Aronovitch, S., Millenbach, L., Kelman, G.B., & Wing, P. (1992). Investigation of the Knoll assessment scale in a tertiary care facility. *DECUBITUS, 5(3)*, 70-76.

Baranoski, S. (1995). Wound assessment and dressing selection. *Ostomy/Wound Management, 41*(Suppl. 7A), 7S-12S.

Barr, J.E. (1995). Principles of wound cleansing. *Ostomy/Wound Management, 41*(Suppl. 7A), 14S-22S.

Bates-Jensen, B.M. (1995). Indices to include in wound healing assessment. *Advances in Wound Care, 8(4)*, 25-33.

Bennett, M.A. (1995). Report of the task force on the implications for darkly pigmented intact skin in the prediction and prevention of pressure ulcers. *Advances in Wound Care, 8(6)*, 34-35.

Bergstrom, N., Braden, B.J., Laguzza, A., & Holman, V. (1987). The Braden scale for predicting pressure sore risk. *Nursing Research, 36(4)*, 205-210.

Berlowitz, D.R., & Wilking, S.V.B. (1989). Risk factors for pressure sores. A comparison of cross-sectional and cohort-derived data. *Journal of the American Geriatrics Society, 37(11)*, 1043-1050.

Braden, B., & Bergstrom, N. (1987). A conceptual schema for the study of the etiology of pressure sores. *Rehabilitation Nursing, 12(1)*, 8-12.

Bryant, R.A., Shannon, M.L., Pieper, B., Braden, B.J., & Morris, D.J. (1992). Pressure ulcers. In R.A. Bryant (Ed.). *Acute and chronic wounds: Nursing management* (pp. 105-163). St. Louis, MO: Mosby Year Book.

Brylinsky, C.M. (1995). Nutrition and wound healing: An overview. *Ostomy/Wound Management, 41(10)*, 14-24.

Ceccio, C.M. (1990). Understanding therapeutic beds. *Orthopaedic Nursing, 9(3)*, 57-70.

Clark, R.A.F. (1985). Cutaneous tissue repair: Basic biologic considerations. *Journal of the American Academy of Dermatology, 13(5 Pt 1)*, 701-725.

Conner, L.M., & Clack, J.W. (1993). In vivo (CT scan) comparison of vertical shear in human tissue caused by various support surfaces. *DECUBITUS, 6(2)*, 20-28.

Consortium for Spinal Cord Medicine. (2000). *Pressure ulcer prevention and treatment following spinal cord injury: clinical practice guidelines for health care professionals*. Washington, DC: Author.

Cooper, D.M. (1995). Indices to include in wound assessment. *Advances in Wound Care, 8(4):suppl.,* 15-18.

Cutler, N.R., George, R., Siefert, R.D., Brunelle, R., Sramek, J.J., McNeill, K., & Boyd, W.M. (1993). Comparison of qualitative methodologies to define chronic pressure ulcer measurements. *DECUBITUS, 6(6),* 22-30.

Deloach, E.D., DiBenedetto, R.J., Womble, L., & Gilley, J.D. (1992). The treatment of osteomyelitis underlying pressure ulcers. *DECUBITUS, 5(6),* 32-41.

Department of Veterans Affairs. (1992). *National specialized bed study*. Milwaukee, WI: National Centers for Cost Containment.

Doughty, D. (1990). The process of wound healing: A nursing perspective. *Progressions, 2(1),* 3-12.

Etris, M. (1995). Measuring healing in wounds. *Advances in Wound Care, 8(4):suppl.,* 53-58.

Etris, M., Pribble, J., & LaBrecque, J. (1994). Evaluation of two wound measurement methods in a multi-center, controlled study. *Ostomy/Wound Management, 40(7),* 44-48.

Ferrell, B.A., Artinian, B.M., & Sessing, D. (1995). The Sessing scale for assessment of pressure ulcer healing. *Journal of the American Geriatrics Society, 43(1),* 37-40.

Fowler, E., & van Rijswijk, L. (1995). Using wound debridement to help achieve the goals of care. *Ostomy/Wound Management, 41*(Suppl. 7A), 23S-34S.

Garber, S.L. (1985). Wheelchair cushions for spinal-cord injured individuals. *American Journal of Occupational Therapy, 39(11),* 722-725.

Garber, S.L., Campion, L.J., & Krouskop, T.A. (1982). Trochanteric pressure in spinal cord injury. *Archives of Physical Medicine and Rehabilitation, 63(11),* 549-552.

Goldberg, N.H. (1995). Outcomes in surgical interventions. *Advances in Wound Care, 8(4):Suppl.,* 28-69.

Gosnell, D.J. (1989). Pressure sore risk assessment: A critique. Part I. The Gosnell scale. *DECUBITUS, 2(3),* 32-38.

Guralnik, J. M., Harris, T.B., White, L.R., & Cornoni-Huntley, J.C. (1988). Occurrence and predictors of pressure sores in the national health and nutrition examination survey follow-up. *Journal of the American Geriatrics Society, 36(9),* 807-812.

Hagisawa, S., Ferguson-Pell, M., Cardi, M., & Miller, D. (1994). Assessment of skin blood content and oxygenation in spinal cord injured subjects during reactive hyperemia. *Journal of Rehabilitation Research, 31,* 1-14(1).

Himel, H.N. (1995). Wound healing: Focus on the chronic wound. *WOUNDS, 7*(Suppl. A), 70A-76A.

Hunt, T.K. (1986). Vitamin A and wound healing. *Journal of the American Academy of Dermatology, 15(4 Pt 2),* 817-821.

Hutchinson, J.J. (1994). Infection under occlusion. *Ostomy/Wound Management, 40(30),* 28-33.

Kerstein, M.D. (1995). Moist wound healing: The clinical perspective. *Ostomy/Wound Management,* *41*(Suppl. 7A), 37S-44S.

Krouskop, T., & van Rijswijk, L. (1995). Standardizing performance-based criteria for support surfaces. *Ostomy/Wound Management, 41(1),* 34-45.

Langemo, D.K., Olson, B., Hunter, S., Burd, C., Hansen, D., & Cathcart-Silberberg, T.C. (1989). Incidence of pressure sores in acute care, rehabilitation, extended care, home health, and hospice in one locale. *DECUBITUS, 2(2),* 42.

Lawrence, J.C. (1994). Dressings and wound infection. *The American Journal of Surgery, 167*(Suppl. 1A), 215-245.

Lazarus, G.S., Cooper, D.M., Knighton, D.R., Margolis, D.J., Pecoraro, R.E., Rodeheaver, G., & Robson, M.C. (1994). Definitions and guidelines for assessment of wounds and evaluation of healing. *Archives of Dermatology, 130(4),* 489-493.

Leaper, M.E. (1994). Prophylactic and therapeutic role of antibiotics in wound care. *The American Journal of Surgery, 167*(Suppl. 1A), 155-205.

Loescher, L.J. (1995). The dynamics of skin aging. *Progressions, 7(2),* 3-13.

Lyder, C.H. (1991). Conceptualization of the stage I pressure ulcer. *Journal of ET Nursing, 18(5),* 162-165.

Maklebust, J., & Margolis, D. (1995). Session I: Pressure ulcers: Definition and assessment parameters. *Advances in Wound Care, 8(4):Suppl.,* 6-10.

Margolis, D.J. (1994). Wound healing assessment: The clinical utility of wound healing rates. *Ostomy/Wound Management, 40(8),* 20-27.

Meehan, M. (1990). Multisite pressure ulcer prevalence survey. *DECUBITUS, 3(4),* 14-17.

Moncada, G.A. (l992). The healing wound: Clinical management. *Plastic Surgical Nursing, 12(2),* 56-60.

Noble, P.C. (1981). The prevention of pressure sores in persons with spinal cord injuries. *International Exchange of Information in Rehabilitation.* Monograph Number 11. New York: World Rehabilitation Fund.

Norton, D. (1989). Calculating the risk: Reflections on the Norton scale. *DECUBITUS, 2(3),* 24-31.

National Pressure Ulcer Advisory Panel (NPUAP) (1995). Position on reverse staging of pressure ulcers. *NPUAP Report, 4,* l.

Phillips, T.J. (1996). Cost effectiveness in wound care. *Ostomy/Wound Management, 42(1),* 56-59.

Pinchcofsky-Davis, G.D., & Kaminski, M.V., Jr. (1986). Correlation of pressure sores and nutritional status. *Journal of the American Geriatric Society, 34(6),* 435-440.

Pires, M., & Muller, A. (1991). Detection and management of early tissue pressure indicators: A pictorial essay. *Progressions, 3(3),* 3-11.

Plackett, G. (1995). Proceedings of the international wound management meeting. *Advances in Wound Care, 8(5),* 42-61.

Plassmann, P., Melhuish, J.M., & Harding, K.G. (1994). Methods of measuring wound size. A comparative study. *WOUNDS, 6(7)*, 54-61.

Reichel, S.M. (1958). Shearing force as a factor in decubitus ulcers in paraplegic. *Journal of the American Medical Association, 166(7)*, 762-763.

Richardson, R.R., & Meyer, P.R., Jr. (1981). Prevalence and incidence of pressure sores in acute spinal cord injuries. *Paraplegia, 19(4)*, 235-247.

Sather, M.R., Weber, C.E., Jr., & George, J. (1977). Pressure sores and the spinal cord injury patient. *Drug Intelligence and the Clinical Pharmacist*, 11, 154-169.

Shannon, M.L., & Miller, B. (1988). Evaluation of hydrocolloid dressings on healing pressure ulcers in spinal cord injury patients. *DECUBITUS, 1(1)*, 42-46.

Sklar, C.G. (1985). Pressure ulcer management in the neurologically impaired patient. *Journal of Neurosurgical Nursing, 17(1)*, 30-36.

Smith, D.M. (1995). Pressure ulcers in the nursing home. *Annuals of Internal Medicine, 123(6)*, 433-442.

Sparks, S.M. (1992). Nurse validation of pressure ulcer risk factors for a nursing diagnosis. *DECUBITUS, 5(1)*, 26-28, 32-35.

Sparks, S.M. (1993). Clinical validation of pressure ulcer risk factors. *Ostomy/Wound Management, 39(4)*, 40-41.

Stotts, N.A., & Wipke-Tevis, D. (1996). Co-factors in impaired wound healing. *Ostomy/Wound Management, 42(2)*, 44-56.

Tallon, R. (1996). Support surfaces—A technology review. *Nursing Management, 27(2)*, 58-62.

Thibodeau, G.A., & Patton, K.T. (1993). *Anatomy and physiology* (2nd Ed.). St. Louis, MO: Mosby.

Thomaselli, N. (1994). *WOCN position statement for conservative sharp wound debridement for registered nurses* (pp. 1-2). Wound, Ostomy and Continence Nursing Society.

Thomason, S.S. (1990). Preventing and detecting unique complications in the spinal cord injured. *Home Healthcare Nurse, 8(5)*, 16-21.

Thomason, S.S., Hawley, G.G., & Wurzel, J. (1993). Specialty support surfaces: A cost containment perspective. *DECUBITUS, 6(6)*, 32-40.

Thomson, P.D., & Smith, O.J., Jr. (1994). What is infection? *The American Journal of Surgery, 167 (1A Suppl)*, 7S-11S, Review.

van Rijswijk, L. (1995). Frequency of reassessment of pressure ulcers. *Advances in Wound Care, 8(4)*, Suppl. 19-24.

Viehbeck, M., McGlynn, J., & Harris, S. (1995). Pressure ulcers and wound healing: Educating the spinal cord injured individual on the effects of cigarette smoking. *SCI Nursing, 12(3)*, 73-76.

Wysocki, A.B. & Bryant, R.A. (1992). Skin. In R.A. Bryant (Ed.), *Acute and chronic wounds: Nursing management* (pp. 1-30). St. Louis, MO: Mosby Year Book.

Zejdlik, C.P. (Ed.) (1992). *Management of spinal cord injury*. (2nd Ed.). Boston: Jones & Bartlett.

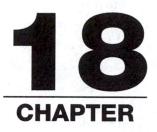

CHAPTER

Musculoskeletal

Joan Stelling, MSN, RN, CRRN
Audrey Nelson, Ph.D., RN, FAAN

I. Objectives

A. Describe general techniques for musculoskeletal management in spinal cord impairment (SCI)

B. Identify the etiology, clinical manifestations, and treatment modalities of the musculoskeletal system following SCI.

C. Discuss health education as it relates to the musculoskeletal system after SCI.

D. Describe common complications of the musculoskeletal system following SCI.

II. Introduction

This chapter describes nursing assessments, general management, and long term implications of functional deficits related to impaired physical mobility and body alignment. In addition to SCI, the chapter includes information on demyelimation disorders affecting the spine (Guillain-Barré, multiple sclerosis, and amyotrophic lateral sclerosis), and congenital spinal disorders (spina bifida, scoliosis, lordosis, and kyphosis).

Refer to Chapter 17 for information on skin, Chapter 19 related to sensation, Chapter 20 related to spasticity, and Chapter 25 related to activity and exercise.

A. **Anatomy/Physiology** (Refer also to Chapter 7)
1. Muscle:
    a. Constitutes 40-50 percent of total body weight (Borgman-Gainer, 1996).
    b. Characterized by irritability, contractility, extensibility, and elasticity.
    c. Functions to produce motion, maintain posture, and produce heat through contraction.
    d. Movement is a result of either conscious, deliberate choice, or involuntary, reflex process.

Table 18-1: Classification of Joints and Movements

Name	Type	Movements
Atlantoaxial	Pivot	Pivoting or partial rotation of head
Shoulder	Ball and socket	Flexion, extension, abduction, adduction, rotation, circumduction
Elbow	Hinge	Flexion, extension
Radioulnar	Pivot	Supination, pronation
Wrist	Condyloid	Flexion, extension, abduction (ulnar deviation), adduction (radial deviation)
Carpal	Gliding	Gliding
Hand		
Metacarpals	Hinge	Flexion, extension, abduction, adduction
Thumb	Saddle	Flexion, extension, abduction, adduction, rotation, circumduction, opposition
Hip	Ball and socket	Flexion, extension, abduction, adduction, rotation, circumduction
Knee	Hinge	Flexion, extension Ankle Hinge Dorsiflexion, plantar flexion
Ankle	Hinge	Dorsiflexion, plantar flexion
Foot		
Between tarsals	Gliding	Inversion, eversion
Between metatarsals, phalanges	Hinge	Flexion, extension, adduction, abduction

From Independent Function: Movement and Mobility, by M. Borgman-Gainer, 1996, in S.P. Hoeman (Ed.), *Rehabilitation Nursing: Process and Application* (2nd ed., p. 229), St. Louis: Mosby. Reprinted with permission.

2. Nervous system:
   a. Voluntary movement involves the:
      (1) Cerebral cortex
      (2) Descending pathways of the spinal cord
      (3) Anterior horn of the spinal cord
   b. Loss of function of the lower motor neuron (LMN) pathway through SCI results in flaccid paralysis or loss of both reflex and voluntary movement.
   c. Loss of function of the upper motor neuron (UMN) pathway through SCI results in continued muscle contraction, evidenced by spastic tone and exaggerated reflexes.
   d. Dysfunction of the cerebellum or in the extra pyramidal tracts can result in loss of coordinated, controlled voluntary movement, as found in multiple sclerosis.
3. Skeletal:
   a. The skeletal structure serves to:
      (1) Protect vital organs, such as the brain, heart, and lungs.
      (2) Act as hemoregulatory system by producing red blood cells in marrow of long bones.
      (3) Facilitate movement.
      (4) Store salts and minerals.
   b. There are 206 bones in the skeletal structure. (Refer to Table 18-1 for a classification of joints and movements).

III. Nursing Assessment of the Musculoskeletal System

The following assessment variables should be considered (Refer to Table 18-2).

A. **General Impression and Health History.**

B. **Range of Motion (ROM)**: Note pain with movement, tenderness or swelling, and abnormalities such as contractures.

C. **Muscle Tone, Strength, Hypertrophy/atrophy.**

D. **Deep tendon reflexes.**

E. **Proprioception and position sense.**

F. **Balance and coordination.**

G. **Gait assessment.**

H. **Posture and body alignment.**

IV. Nursing Process Applied to Musculoskeletal System Management

A. **Nursing Diagnoses**:
1. Impaired physical mobility of the upper extremities.
2. Impaired physical mobility of the lower extremities.
3. Impaired balance and coordination.
4. Dysfunctional gait pattern.
5. Impaired skeletal alignment.
6. At risk due to immobilization.
7. Impaired spinal stability.

B. **Defining Characteristics**:
1. Impaired ability to move purposefully within environment; impaired balance.
2. Medical or mechanical restriction of movement:
   a. Skeletal immobilization.
   b. Bed rest.
3. Decreased muscle tone, strength, range of motion.
4. Impaired sensation, pain.
5. Musculoskeletal impairment:
   a. Heterotopic bone formation: abnormal bone deposits in paralyzed joints
   b. Osteoporosis: disease process, reduction of bone density; fracture is usually first clinical sign. There are three types (Rehabilitation Nursing Foundation, 1993):
      (1) Type I: postmenopausal, related to decreased estrogen.
      (2) Type II: senile.
      (3) Type III: disuse, seen in individuals with disability
   c. Contractures: loss of muscle tone and range.
   d. Pathologic fractures: fractures caused by an increase in porosity and softness of bones related to disuse.
   e. Spasticity: exaggerated muscle tone with increased tendon reflexes associated with UMN lesion.
   f. Ankylosis: joint immobility which can lead to severe loss of function.
   g. Flaccidity: damage to LMN pathways causing destruction of reflex arc.
6. Musculoskeletal Malalignment
   a. Scoliosis.
   b. Kyphosis.
   c. Lordosis.

Table 18-2: Nursing Assessment of Movement

I. General impression:
   A. During interview assess client's external appearance.
   B. Observe client for posture, especially for stooped shoulders; asymmetry; unevenness of length of extremities; absent digits and abnormalities of hands, feet, arms or legs; extremity edema; asymmetry of facial expression and involuntary movement; extremity weakness during activities of daily living such as walking, sitting, rising, writing or dressing; movements that precipitate pain.

II. General range of motion (ROM):
   A. Note
      1. Any deviation of limitation
      2. Joint instability (dislocation or subluxation).
      3. Joint stiffness or fixation (ankylosis).
      4. Joint swelling, heat, or tenderness.
      5. Bogginess and bone enlargement.
      6. Muscle tone and strength, skin condition, subcutaneous tissue, muscle size and shape.
      7. Palpate for crepitus or a grating sensation.

III. Specific ROM (head to toe assessment)
   A. Head and neck
      1. Palpate jaw or temporomandibular joint for tenderness or swelling; check ROM as client opens mouth.
      2. Inspect neck for symmetry and form and size.
      3. Palpate cervical spine muscle and tapezius for tenderness.
      4. Assess neck ROM: the following degree guide is for formal ROM; make adjustments for clients with arthritis or fracture and elderly persons:
         a. Flexion (45 degrees): ask client to touch chin to chest.
         b. Extension (55 degrees): ask client to put head back.
         c. Lateral flexion (40 degrees): ask client to touch ear to corresponding shoulder.
         d. Rotation (70 degrees): ask client to turn head to left, then to right.
   B. Trunk (client stands, if possible):
      1. Inspect posterior for exaggerated C- or S-shaped lateral curvature (scoliosis), exaggerated curvature of thoracic spine (kyphosis), and exaggerated curvature of lumbar spine (lordosis).
      2. Observe differences in height of shoulders or iliac crest.
      3. Palpate paravertebral muscles for tenderness.
      4. Assess spine ROM:
         a. Forward flexion (75-90 degrees): ask client to touch toes while bending from the waist and note rounding of lumbar concavity.
         b. Extension (30 degrees): ask client to lean back from pelvis.
         c. Lateral flexion (35 degrees): ask client to lean to each side.
         d. Rotation (30 degrees): ask client to turn shoulders to the right and then to the left.
      5. Inspect anterior and posterior aspects of trunk:
         a. Compare right side to left.
         b. Compare proximal to distal for symmetry and weakness.
   C. Shoulder girdle and arms:
      1. Observe for swelling; atrophy; altered shape, size, or form.
      2. Palpate sternoclavicular joint, the acromioclavicular joint, and the shoulder joint for tenderness.
      3. Assess ROM:
         a. Extension (50 degrees): ask client to swing both arms back as if reaching back for something.
         b. Forward flexion (180 degrees): ask client to raise arms above head.
         c. Internal and external rotation (90 degrees):
            (1) Internal: ask client to place hands behind in the small of the back.
            (2) External: ask client to place hands behind the neck with elbows out to the side.
         d. Adduction (50 degrees): ask client to reach the right hand to the left hand while crossing extended arms in front of the body; reverse the process for the shoulder.
         e. Abduction (180 degrees): ask the client to bring the arms away from the body as far as possible.
      4. Inspect elbow while flexed at 70 degrees; palpate the olecranon process and grooves with the lateral epicondyle for tenderness, swelling, or nodules.
      5. Assess elbow ROM (0 degrees extension to 160 degrees flexion): ask client to bend and straighten the arms at the elbow.
      6. Inspect the radioulnar joint.
      7. Assess supination (palms up) and pronation (palms down and ROM 90 degrees).
   D. Hands and wrists:
      1. Inspect for swelling, redness, nodules, deformity, atrophy or fasciculations (involuntary twitchings of isolated bundles of muscle fibers).
      2. Palpate joints for tenderness, swelling, bogginess, or enlargement.
      3. Assess ROM of hands and digits: ask client to spread the fingers of each hand and make a fist with the thumb across the knuckles.
         a. Extension (70 degrees).
         b. Flexion (0 degrees).
         c. Radial deviation (20 degrees).
         d. Ulnar deviation (55 degrees).
         e. Metacarpophalangeal joint: hyperextension (30 degrees), flexion (90 degrees).
         f. Proximal interphalangeal joint: hypertenson (0 degrees/neutral), flexion (120 degrees).
   E. Hips: Ask client to stand, if possible:
      1. Observe form and asymmetry of iliac crest.
      2. Palpate for crepitus, nodules, or atrophy.
      3. Assess ROM of hip: client is supine flexion (90

continued on page 251

Table 18-2: Continued

degrees) with knees straight — ask client to raise each leg separately with knee straight, then with knee bent:
- a. Flexion (120 degrees) with knee flexed.
- b. Hyperextension (15 degrees): have client prone and ask client to lift each leg separately off surface.
- c. Adduction (30 degrees): ask client to cross the right leg over the left leg and vice versa.
- d. Abduction (45 degrees): ask client to slide the leg toward the outer edge of bed.
- e. Internal rotation (40 degrees): ask client to bend the knee and hip and gently pull the knee laterally and the hip will rotate externally.
- f. External rotation (45 degrees): ask client to bend the knee and hip and gently push the knee medially and the hip will rotate internally.

F. Knees:
1. Observe for changes in form, shape, or size; atrophy of quadriceps or loss of usual hollows around the patella.
2. Palpate the suprapatellar pouch and over the tibiofemoral joint for thickening, bogginess, tenderness, or fluid.
3. Palpate the popliteal space.
4. Test for bulge sign using fluid and ballottement of a floating patella.
    - a. Bulge sign test:
        - (1) Use the ball of the hand to milk the medial aspect of the knee firmly upward two or three times and displace any fluid.
        - (2) Tap the knee just behind the lateral margin of the patella and watch for a bulge of returning fluid in the hollow medial area of the patella.
        - (3) Grasp the thigh above the patella with one hand, forcing fluid out of the suprapatellarspace; with fingers of the other hand, push the patella sharply against the femur.
5. Assess ROM:
    - a. Hyperextension (15 degrees): ask client to straighten knee.
    - b. Flexion (130 degrees): ask client to flex the hip and lift the lower leg off the bed.

G. Legs and calf:
1. Measure thigh and calf for baseline recording.
2. Observe for any changes in size; Record in centimeters as measured at the same location on the leg.
3. Test circulation in feet and ankles; assess popliteal and femoral pulses; if compression stockings are used, assess proper application and fit.
4. Note whether client is receiving anticoagulant drugs.

H. Ankle and feet:
1. Observe for altered shape, size or form; for swelling, nodules, corns, calluses, or bunions.
2. Palpate Achilles tendon, anterior ankle surface, and the metatarsophalangeal joint.
3. Assess ROM:
    - a. Dorsiflexion (20 degrees): ask client to point toes up.
    - b. Plantar flexion (45 degrees): ask client to point toes down.
    - c. Inversion (30 degrees): client turns sole inward while nurse stabilizes the ankle.
    - d. Eversion (20 degrees): client turns sole outward while nurse stabilizes the ankle.
    - e. Metatarsophalangeal joints: ask client to ball up toes and release them.

I. Muscle tone and strength:
1. Observe tone, flaccidity, spasticity (increased tone), rigidity (inability to relax either flexor or extensor muscles).
2. Note equal or unequal strength on both sides of the body and in proximal and distal positions.
3. Assess relative strength by applying resistance to client's movement attempts during ROM.
4. Assess the upper extremities by asking client to grasp and squeeze the nurse's hands; note differences or sameness on the right and left side; scales for grading muscle strength often used.

J. Deep tendon reflexes:
1. Position client comfortably so that the muscle to be tested is mildly stretched.
2. Use a reflex hammer to strike the tendon briskly – which, in turn, produces a sudden tendon stretch.
3. Major reflexes include the following:
    - a. Biceps: reflects cervical functions between C5-C6.
    - b. Triceps: reflects cervical segments C6-C8.
    - c. Brachioradial: reflects cervical cord functions C5-C6.
    - d. Patellar: reflects L2-L4 functioning.
    - e. Achilles: reflects S1-S2 functioning.
4. Grade reflex from 0-4 +; compare right and left side and upper and lower extremities; hyperactive reflexes are associated with spastic muscle tone and hypoactive reflexes are associated with flaccid muscle tone.

K. Proprioceptive and position sense:
1. Upper extremity: hold client's thumb between the nurse's thumb and index finger; move thumb up and down and ask client to correctly identify the position of the thumb with eyes closed; if unable to identify the thumb position, other joints of the upper extremity such as the wrist, elbow, and shoulder may be tested.
2. Lower extremity: repeat procedure as with toe; if impairment is noted, proceed to the ankle, knee and hip.

continued on page 252

Table 18-2: Continued

<table>
<tr><td>

L. Balance coordination: use appropriate safety precautions:
1. Observe independent and assisted movements in and out of bed, during transfer, and during ambulation.
2. Observe sitting balance while in bed or wheelchair: note whether client slumps or sways to either side.
3. Observe standing balance: note swaying, reeling, or taking backward steps.
4. Perform Romberg test: ask client to stand with feet together, arms stretched in front, and eyes closed; with cerebellar disease, a person falls to the affected side.
5. Perform finger to nose test and heel to shin test.
6. Perform various types of rapidly alternating movements, such as touching the thumb rapidly to each finger or pronating and supinating hands rapidly.

M. Gait:
1. Observe balance, arm sways, inability to negotiate turns, and actual gait patterns; typical gait patterns associated with conditions are:

</td><td>

a. Hemiplegia: a stiff gait; knee flexion is diminished on the affected side; hip circumscribes floor with toes scraping the floor; the affected arm does not swing forward as the opposite foot is advanced.
b. Parkinson's disease: a festinating gait; rhythmic arm swinging is diminished; there is hesitation on initiation of ambulation and steps are small, shifting, and shuffling; client may have difficulty initiating gait manifested as marching in place, or with halting once in motion.
c. Cerebellar problems or posterior column problems; ataxic gaits with broad-base stance and staggering, unsteady gait; difficulty with turns.
d. Multiple sclerosis: a scissors gait; bilateral spastic paralysis of the legs, typified by slow steps.
e. Alpha motor neuron (lower motor problem): a steppage gait making clients appear to be walking up stairs.
f. Progressive neuromuscular disease: a waddling gait may appear.

</td></tr>
</table>

From *Independent Function: Movement and Mobility*, by M. Borgman-Gainer, 1996, in S.P. Hoeman (Ed.), *Rehabilitation Nursing: Process and Application* (2nd ed., p. 233-236), St. Louis: Mosby. Reprinted with permission.

C. **Expected Outcomes**:
1. Achieve optimal independence in activities requiring motor performance.
2. Use assistive devices correctly and consistently. Equipment is tailored to individual based on height, weight, posture, and physical limitations.
3. Maintain physical activity and participate in social and occupational activities.
4. Prevent injury during motor performance.
5. Maintain correct body alignment and prevent complications associated with decreased or absent movement.
6. Maintain range of motion and fitness level.
7. Prevent further neurologic damage and/or facilitate functional return.

D. **Interventions**:
1. Support the body in anatomically correct and functional positions to increase comfort, enhance respiration, promote circulation, prevent gravitational edema, preserve muscle function by preventing contractures, and prevent pressure ulcers.
   a. Side-lying (lateral) position:
      (1) Used to minimize risk of aspiration during mealtime, mobilize secretions, relieve pressure from the sacral area, and decrease spasticity (Zejdlik, 1992).
      (2) Position individual on side, supporting the head and neck with a firm pillow. The lower arm is positioned at the side with the uppermost arm supported by a pillow. The upper leg is flexed at the hip and knee, positioned on a pillow in front of the lower leg. The bottom shoulder is positioned slightly ahead of the rest of the body. Another pillow can be placed behind the back to maintain the position (Borgman-Gainer, 1996).
      (3) Refer to Table 18-3 for potential problems and supportive measures associated with side-lying position.
   b. Supine position:

Table 18-3: Side-Lying (Lateral) Position

Potential Problems	Supportive Measures for Patients with Cervical Injuries	Supportive Measures for Patients with Thoracic or Lumbar Injuries
Excessive lateral neck flexion; fatigue of sterncleidomastoid muscles (which aid respiration)	One-inch foam pad or small, flat pillow placed under head of newly injured patients	Regular pillow under head (high thoracic injured patients may be more comfortable with a small pillow)
Pressure area on ear	Soft protective padding surrounding ears	
Pressure on and pain in dependent shoulder	Grasp scapula and move shoulder through to avoid pressure on nerve plexus	
Loss of correct position; subsequent malalignment of spine and limbs contributing to discomfort and extremity spasticity	Rolled pillow positioned securely behind back	Rolled pillow positioned securely behind back
Skin excoriation under arms; limited chest expansion; compromised circulation to and gravitational edema in paralyzed arms; and internal rotation and adduction of the shoulder with contractures of arm musculature	Pillow under top arm and bottom forearm to support them in good alignment*	Pillow under arms to support in position of comfort
Hip internally rotated and adducted; loss of correct positioning contributing to back discomfort and extremity spasms	Pillows placed lengthwise between legs to maintain good alignment, balance, and comfort	Pillows placed lengthwise between legs to maintain good alignment, balance, and comfort
Foot drop, which complicates sitting in wheelchair, is universal	Support feet in 90 degree position	Support feet in 90 degree position
Pressure areas developing over bony prominences	Padding to separate ankles	Padding to separate ankles

* For most tetraplegic patients position arms in extension to avoid flexion contractures of the elbow. If the patient has a high-level cervical injury with no arm movement, alternate flexion and extension positions to avoid contractures.

From Maintaining Skeletal System Integrity, by C.P. Zejdlik, 1992, in C.P. Zejdlik (Ed.), *Management of Spinal Cord Injury* (2nd ed., p. 423), Boston: Jones & Bartlett. Reprinted with permission.

(1) Used to complete activities of daily living and many general nursing functions, such as bathing (Zejdlik, 1992).

(2) Position individual on the back, with a small, flat pillow supporting the head, neck, and upper shoulders. Position the arms along the side in a neutral position, extending elbows with palms facing downward. Avoid placing pressure on the back of the legs, knees can be slightly flexed. The feet are positioned at a 90 degree angle with the legs, using specialized devices, tightly rolled towels or pillows, or high-top sneakers (Borgman-Gainer, 1996).

(3) Refer to Table 18-4 for potential problems and supportive measures associated with supine position.

c. Sitting position:

(1) Position individual with feet flat on the floor, hips well back in the seat, with weight

Table 18-4: Supine Position

Potential Problems	Supportive Measures for Patients with Cervical Injuries	Supportive Measures for Patients with Thoracic or Lumbar Injuries
Excessive flexion or extension of the head and neck exerting undesirable pressure on injury site	One-inch foam pad or small flat pillow placed under head of newly injured patient	Pillow of suitable thickness placed under head
Flexion of lumbar curvature with undue pressure contributing to back pain and possibly increased neurological deficit		Hyperextension padding (as ordered) to support lumbar curvature and promote reduction of injured spine
Compromises of circulation; gravitational edema of forearms and hands; and elbow contractures	Pillows elevating forearms and hands*	Support not required except as comfort measure
Hyperextension of knees; impaired circulation; and tension on the lower spine	Small pillow or padding under lower thigh to flex legs slightly (optional if full-length padding is used on bed)	Small pillow or padding under lower thigh to flex legs slightly (optional if full-length padding is used on bed)
Foot drop	Pillows or padding and footboard to flex feet at a 90 degree angle	Pillows or padding and footboard to flex feet at a 90 degree angle

* Position most quadriplegic patients with arms extended to avoid flexion contractures of the elbow. If the patient has high-level cervical injury and no arm movement, alternate flexion and extension positions to avoid contractures in either direction.

From Maintaining Skeletal System Integrity, by C.P. Zejdlik, 1992, in C.P Zejdlik (Ed.), *Management of Spinal Cord Injury* (2nd ed., p. 424), Boston: Jones & Bartlett. Reprinted with permission.

Table 18-5: Sitting Position in Bed

Potential Problems	Supportive Measures for Patients with Cervical Injuries	Supportive Measures for Patients with Thoracic or Lumbar Injuries
Loss of neck immobilization with interrupted healing of the bone and possible decrease in function	Position neck orthosis before attempting to sit up	
Loss of position; possibility of falling	Pillows placed at patient's sides to maintain balance	
Shoulder pain; impaired circulation; gravitational edema of forearms and hands	Pillows placed under arms for support	
Strain on fracture site of lower spine	Padding under knees not necessary	Pillow placed under knees to relieve pull on lower spine; eventually long sitting (without supports) allowed
Pressure area on sacrum and heels; foot drop	Padding under ankles to relieve pressure on heels; footboard to maintain plantar flexion	Padding under ankles to relieve pressure on heels; footboard to maintain plantar flexion

* Limit initial time periods in this position, check pressure points frequently.

From Maintaining Skeletal System Integrity, by C.P. Zejdlik, 1992, in C.P Zejdlik (Ed.), *Management of Spinal Cord Injury* (2nd ed., p. 425), Boston: Jones & Bartlett. Reprinted with permission.

distributed evenly over the hips. Avoid positions that aggravate spasticity (Borgman-Gainer, 1996).

(2) During periods of prolonged bed rest, or during the acute phase of SCI, gradual mobilization is needed to prevent postural hypotension.

(3) Refer to Table 18-5 for potential problems and supportive measures with sitting position in bed, and Table 18-6 for proper wheelchair positioning.

   d. Prone position:

(1) Used to counteract prolonged periods of hip and knee flexion, provide pressure relief for ischial tuberosities following prolonged sitting, and provide a position for sleep that minimizes the need for turns.

(2) The prone position is contraindicated for individuals with respiratory deficits, increased intracranial pressure, or cardiovascular deficits.

(3) Refer to Table 18-7 for potential problems and supportive measures with prone position.

2. Use mechanical or positioning devices properly:

   a. Mechanical aids include specialty beds, lifting devices, and transfer aids.

   b. Positioning devices include pillows, trochanter rolls, foot/ankle supports, hand rolls, splints, braces, lap tables, abductor wedges, and wheelchair footrests.

3. Turn according to a regularly set schedule:

   a. Immediately after a SCI, the position should be changed every 2 hours. Minor position changes are required more frequently for comfort.

   b. An individualized turning schedule is developed and adjusted based on individual needs and tolerance.

   c. Persons with impaired sensation and mobility limitations (e.g. persons with SCI, Guillain-Barré, multiple sclerosis, or amyotrophic lateral sclerosis) will need assistance with turning. Depending on strength and mobility, self-turns can be taught.

   d. The prone position can be used, as tolerated, to provide a position for sleep that minimizes the need for turns at night.

4. Prevent complications associated with immobilization:

   a. Individuals who are unable to move part or all of the body, due to SCI or treatment method, can incur a number of complications in a short time. After only three days of bed rest, plasma and calcium are lost, less gastric juice is secreted, less blood flows through the calves, and glucose tolerance is impaired (Borgman-Gainer, 1996, p. 241).

   b. Observe for quality and depth of movement, moisture, effort, and any other cognitive or neurological signs, such as restlessness or forgetfulness, since prolonged bedrest results in decreased respiratory movement, decreased movement of secretions, and disturbed oxygen-carbon dioxide balance. Turning, coughing, and deep breathing, combined with postural drainage and percussion, will enhance respiratory functioning.

   c. Immobilization hypercalcemia can occur in SCI when dehydration and prolonged periods of bed rest are experienced. During this time, bone formation is decreased while the rate of calcium absorption remains elevated. Nursing interventions include vigorous hydration, administration of calatonin, and steroids (Zejdlik, 1992).

   d. Prevention of orthostatic hypotension, increased workload of the heart, and thrombus formation is achieved through active and passive ROM exercises, and self-care activities. Gradual mobilization is also a strategy to minimize the effects of bedrest.

   e. Nutrition is also important for persons on bedrest, due to the resulting negative nitrogen balance. Supplemental protein may be required.

   f. Measures to ensure correct alignment are needed to prevent osteoporosis, contractures, and pressure ulcers.

   g. Nursing interventions for immobilization secondary to spinal instability include proper positioning, use of orthotics, traction devices, and post operative care.

(1) Principles related to orthotic use may include:

(a) The appearance, function, and fit of orthoses.

(b) The method of application (or donning) and removal.

(c) Specific safety precautions and procedures (e.g., wrench is taped to halo brace for quick removal during cardiac arrest).

Table 18-6: Proper Wheelchair Positioning

Body Part	Indications of Improper Seating	Complications	Possible Solutions
PELVIS Neutral*	———		
Oblique	• One hip higher than the other • One shoulder higher than the other	• Increase risk of pressure area on ischial tuberosities • Leads to scoliosis	• Reposition • Solid seat • Custom cushion • Proper seat belt
Rotation	• One knee sticking out farther than the other • One shoulder in front of the other	• Leads to scoliosis • Decrease efficiency in propelling manual wheelchair	• Proper seat belt • Reposition • Rigid pelvic stabilizer
Posterior pelvic tilt	• More than 3 or 4 finger spaces between the front of seat and the back of the knee • Increase kyphosis	• Increase risk of sacral pressure area • Increase risk of pressure area on spinous process • Leads to structural deformity in spine • Respiratory compromise • Decrease in functional activities	• Seat belt • Wedge cushion • Tilt seat • Lumbar support
TRUNK Midline*	———	———	———
Scoliosis	• One shoulder higher than the other	• Structural deformity • Increase pressure on ischial tuberosities that increase pressure areas	• Trunk supports
Leaning	• Person keeps falling to one side	• Jeopardize safety • Decrease in stability • Decrease in functional activities	• Chest strap • Trunk support
Kyphosis	• Forward head • Absence of lumbar lordosis	• Neck pain • Respiratory compromise	• Tilt seat • Lumbar support • Back support
ARMS Shoulder level*	———	———	———
Too much support	• Shrugged shoulders	• Neck pain • Pressure sore development	• Lower armrests • Increase cushion height
Inadequate support	• Dropped shoulders • Subluxation at glenohumeral joint	• Subluxation of glenohumeral joint • Pain • Leads to kyphosis	• Raise armrest height • Lower seat • Add arm troughs
HEAD Midline*	———	———	———
Inadequate support	• Head falling backward, forward, or to one side	• Pain • Compromise airway • Leads to deformity	• Head support

continued on page 257

Table 18-6: Continued

Body Part	Indications of Improper Seating	Complications	Possible Solutions
HIPS 90 degrees*	———	———	———
Greater than 90 degrees	• Thighs overly abducted • Space between the sitting surface and the thighs • Knees hitting under table	• Increase risk of pressure area over bony prominences	• Lower footrests
Less than 90 Degrees	• Thighs abducted with legs internally rotated • Kyphosis • Pelvis tilted back	• Increased risk of pressure sore on great trochanter • Kyphosis	• Raise footrests • Solid seat • Abductor pommel support
THIGHS Even support*	———	———	———
Inadequate Support	• Large space between seat upholstery and back of knees	• Increased risk of pressure area on bony prominences	• Increase seat depth • Reposition • Seat belt (to hold back in chair) must be weighed against inhibiting pressure reliefs
Excessive support	• No space between seat upholstery and back of knee	• Decrease circulation to lower extremities • Increase risk of pressure area on back of knee • Unable to twist in chair to reposition self	• Decrease seat depth • Add back cushion
FEET Midline*	———	———	———
External rotation	• Toes pointing outwardly	• Contributes to improper leg position • Leads to structural deformities	• Change tilt of footrest • Lower footrest • Alter heels on shoes
Internal rotation	• Toes pointing inwardly	• Contributes to improper leg position • Leads to structural deformities	• Straps to secure feet • Raise footrests

* Proper position

From Resuming Physical Activity and Daily Living Skills, by C.P. Zejdlik, 1992, in C.P Zejdlik (Ed.), *Management of Spinal Cord Injury* (2nd ed., p. 488-489), Boston: Jones & Bartlett. Reprinted with permission.

Table 18-7: Prone Position

Potential Problems	Supportive Measures for Patients with Cervical Injuries	Supportive Measures for Patients with Thoracic or Lumbar Injuries
Rotation, flexion, or extension of an unstable neck fracture site with subsequent interruption of bony healing and possible loss of function	Padding to support the chin and forehead and allow a "breathing space".	
Loosening of brace with loss of immobilization resulting in interrupted bony healing and possible loss of function	One or two pillows to support chest and relieve pressure on bars of the halo brace	
Hyperextension of lumbar curve; undue pressure on iliac crests and male genitalia; pressure on female breasts; and difficulty breathing	Pillow placed under abdomen	Pillow placed under abdomen
Hyperextension of knees, undue pressure on knees and toes, and foot drop	Pillow placed under lower legs to flex legs slightly, relieve pressure on knees, and promote plantar flexion	Pillow placed under lower legs to flex legs slightly, relieve pressure on knees, and promote plantar flexion
Brachial plexus damage and impaired circulation	Place arms in comfortable position alleviating pressure on shoulders	Place arms in comfortable position alleviating pressure on shoulders
Undue pressure on toes; foot drop	Position feet between mattress and footboard	Position feet between mattress and footboard

* Turning the patient prone can be simplified with the following techniques. Move the patient to the side of the bed in the supine position, and arrange pillows in the desired position beside the patient. Prepare the patient for turning prone by placing the opposite arm and leg across the body; if turning the patient toward the left, position the right arm and right leg. Tuck the left arm down by the patient's side or place above the head. Finally, logroll the patient toward the pillows.

From Maintaining Skeletal System Integrity, by C.P. Zejdlik, 1992, in C.P Zejdlik (Ed.), *Management of Spinal Cord Injury* (2nd ed., p. 424), Boston: Jones & Bartlett. Reprinted with permission.

      (d) Skin integrity; the contact points on the body where the brace exerts the greatest pressure.
      (e) The degree of physical activity allowed.
      (f) Hygiene.
      (g) Comfort.
    (2) Log rolling techniques are indicated for individuals with unstable neck/spine.
    (3) Interventions are targeted to prevent complications related to neck/spine instability, spinal curvature, chronic pain, or progressive loss of function.
  h. Nursing interventions related to long-term complications associated with muscloskeletal system:
    (1) Heterotopic bone formation is an abnormal deposit of new bone formation around joints of paralyzed limbs, often involving the hip, elbow, or shoulder joints. Etiology is unknown. Signs include localized redness, swelling, or stiffness of the joints, swelling, temperature elevation, and discomfort or referred pain. Nursing interventions include mobilization as soon as possible and gentle ROM at frequent intervals.
    (2) Ankylosis or joint immobility resulting in significant loss of function; surgical removal may be necessary, however, reoccurrence does happen.
    (3) Pathological fractures of the long bones are associated with osteoporotic changes

accompanying paralysis. Deep vein thrombosis is often associated with these fractures. Preventive education includes mobilizing and positioning of affected limb as indicated, managing edema, monitoring skin and pulses.

5. Promote function of upper extremities by maintaining functional position of the hand and arm.
   a. Correct positioning of hands, elbows, and shoulders.
   b. Adequate ROM.
   c. Hand splints may be indicated to prevent contractures and deformities.
   d. Promote self-care.
   e. Prevent degenerative shoulder injuries associated with over-use. Interventions include:
      (1) Shoulder exercise program.
      (2) Prevention of activities that aggravate shoulder problems, particularly overhead activities, such as use of a trapeze for repositioning in bed.
      (3) Correct techniques for transfers and pressure relief activities.
   f. Upper extremity tendon transfer surgery can promote function. Nurses work with therapists and plastic surgeons/orthopedic physicians to optimize outcomes.

6. Participate in the application of technology:
   a. Environmental control units, robotic workstations, voice-activated computer systems, and other technological advancements facilitate independence for persons with mobility deficits.
   b. Lightweight, flexible, durable construction materials enhance functional, vocational, and recreational pursuits.
   c. Functional electrical stimulation (FES) has been used to restore purposeful movement to muscles paralyzed by upper motor neuron lesions. Documented functional uses of FES for persons with SCI include ambulation (Cybulski, Penn, & Jaeger, 1994; Kralji, Bajd, & Turk, 1983; Marsolais & Kobetic, 1987); grasp/release of hand (Peckham, Bajd, & Turk, 1988), sensation, activation of diaphragm for respiratory pacing, control of urinary bladder, and fitness through an FES exercise cycle (Ragnarsson, Pollack, O'Daniel, Edgar, Perofsky, & Nash, 1988). Documented therapeutic use of FES for persons with SCI include muscle strengthening, relief of spasticity, reversal of joint contractures, reversal of muscle adhesions, and correction of spinal curvature (Peckham, 1988). While still in the experimental stage, this technology offers possible solutions to functional deficits.

V. Health Education Tips

A. **Remain mobile and active** to the maximum level possible throughout life.

B. **Prevent complications and injury** by practicing safety, minimizing injury, and exercising regularly.

C. **Schedule medical follow-ups** on a regular basis so that complications such as contractures, pathologic fractures, osteoporosis, spasticity, arthritis, heterotopic ossification, and scoliosis can be identified and treated early.

D. **Maintain proper positioning** in bed and wheelchair to promote optimal musculoskeletal alignment.

E. **Maintain equipment** and have follow-up appointments with rehabilitation professionals for individualized equipment needs.

F. **Follow a therapeutic exercise program** to maintain joint mobility and muscle tone.

VI. Ambulation/Gait Training

The nurse collaborates with physical therapists and reinforces instruction related to the plan for functional independence in ambulation.

A. **Pre-ambulation activities** include exercises in bed to prepare muscles for standing and walking.

B. **Sitting balance** is initiated in bed; the nurse monitors for safety and cardiovascular response.

C. **Standing balance** is initiated once sitting balance has been achieved. Persons require varying levels of assistance to achieve a standing position. Assistive equipment may be used to compensate for plegia or disability. Fall prevention is an important nursing intervention.

D. **Passive standing** minimizes the effects of postural hypotension.
   1. Tilt tables are used for passive standing, generally in a therapy department.
   2. Standing frames allow persons with SCI to benefit from the physiological and psychological rewards of standing.

E. **Assistive devices for ambulation**
   1. Crutches/canes: Requires full use and sufficient strength of upper extremities (UE), with limited lower extremity (LE) function.
   2. Walker: Suitable when there is weakness in both UE and LE.
   3. LE Bracing: Functional ambulation can be accomplished for some persons with paraplegia using a combination of long leg orthotics and crutches/walker.
   4. Wheelchair

VII. Special Issues Related to Pediatric Care

A. **SCI**

The immature spine is prone to developing complex spinal deformities. Children with SCI require varied therapies and equipment to maximize functional abilities and prevent complications. For example, an infant with a myelomeningocele should begin a program at birth to prevent loss of function due to contractures and maximize motor functions.

B. **Scoliosis**
   1. Scoliosis, the most common spinal deformity, usually involves a primary lateral curve with a compensatory secondary curve. Spinal rotation causing rib asymmetry and thoracic involvement occurs. Scoliosis may occur alone or be associated with SCI (Whaley & Wong, 1991). Scoliosis can be congenital or develop during childhood, but most commonly occurs during the growth spurt of adolescence.
   2. Management of scoliosis includes (Dearolf et al, 1990):
      a. Observation, exercise, bracing or surgery may be indicated depending on the specific diagnosis and the extent of deformity.
      b. Exercise and bracing will not correct a curve but may slow progression and help the spine remain flexible and supple during growth periods and treatment.
      c. Depending on the diagnosis, a spine fusion should be delayed as long as possible to enable maximum growth.
      d. Braces are used more often in children than in adults.
      e. Surgical rods, if done for stabilization or fusion, may need to be removed as child grows.
   3. Scoliosis following SCI:
      a. High risk of scoliosis in preadolescent children.
         (1) Rate of curve progression is known to be twice as high in preadolescent children as in adults.
         (2) The development of the scoliosis depends more on the person's age at time of injury than their level of injury.
      b. Treatment may include bracing and spine fusion:
         (1) Body jacket is used to prevent rapid progression of scoliosis until growth is complete. A spine fusion may be necessary to prevent deformity or pulmonary compromise.
         (2) Regardless of when an orthotic device is worn, whether prior to or following surgery, care must be taken to avoid decreased pulmonary function as a result of the brace.

(3) Other treatment measures include proper positioning, wheelchair inserts, and exercise.

(4) Curvature progression should be monitored with x-rays every 6 - 12 months, depending on age.

(5) Surgical rods may need to be removed as child grows.

C. Kyphosis

Kyphosis is an abnormal increase in convex angulation in the curvature of the thoracic spine, causing a "hump back" appearance.

1. Congenital kyphosis:
   a. Severe deformities are recognized at birth and progress rapidly. Lesser deformities may appear as the child grows.
   b. A progressive deformity may result in paraplegia.
   c. Treatment is operative; orthoses are ineffective.
2. Postural kyphosis:
   a. Results from poor posture.
   b. Orthopedic treatment is not generally indicated.
3. Idiopathic kyphosis (Scheuermann disease):
   a. Common (second only to idiopathic scoliosis) as a cause of spinal deformity. There is a rounded back appearance, with or without pain. Cord compression is extremely rare. Treatment is dependent on age, the degree of deformity, and the presence or absence of pain in the apical area.

D. Lordosis

Lordosis is an accentuation/exaggeration of the lumbar curvature.

1. May be idiopathic or the result of a secondary disease process or trauma. Is associated with hip flexion contracture, obesity, congenital hip dislocation, or slipped femoral capital epiphysis. May occur in girls during adolescent growth spurt.
2. Severe lordosis is accompanied by pain.
3. Treatment consists of managing predisposing cause, postural exercises, and/or support garments to relieve discomfort.
4. Congenital lordosis is less common than scoliosis or kyphosis. The major danger with this curve is the reduction of vital capacity. This causes a posterior element synostosis or defect of segmentation while the anterior growth plates continuing to grow. Surgical intervention is usually necessary.

E. Spondylolysis and Spondylolisthesis (Harvel & Hanley, 1995)

1. Spondylolysis is a spinal defect without forward slippage of one vertebra on another.
   a. Most common cause of adolescent low back pain.
   b. It infrequently occurs in children before age five and more commonly between ages seven and ten.
   c. Higher incidence in children involved in sports such as gymnastics because of repetitive stresses.
   d. Treatment is seldom required, but may range from conservative orthopedic management to surgical intervention (posterior spine fusion) if pain is not alleviated.
2. Spondylolisthesis is a forward slippage or displacement of one vertebra in relation to another, usually L5 and S1.
   a. Attributed to hereditary factors, age, skeletal maturity, potential growth, biochemical factors, and trauma. Progression of slippage may be graded.
   b. Occurs in 5 percent of general population and is the most common type.
   c. Defect is present at birth but manifests itself in 5 percent of affected children by age 6.
   d. Usually treated non-surgically
3. Classification system may range from congenital to traumatic or pathological.

F. Heterotopic Ossification (HO)

1. Occurs less frequently in children than in adults.

2. The use of etidronate sodium is not recommended in growing children because it prevents mineralization.

3. Indomethacin has not been studied in the SCI population. The risk of exacerbating a stress ulcer may be too high a risk for it to be used in the pediatric SCI population when the pediatric incidence of HO is so small.

Practical Application

J.C. is a 20 year old female, injured in a motor vehicle accident one month earlier. She presented to the rehabilitation unit with a T6 complete spinal cord injury, wearing a body jacket, and with an external fixator on the left leg due to shattering of the tibia and fibula in the accident. J.C. had a complicated course including pneumonia secondary to a pneumothorax noted on arrival to the emergency department. She had surgery to her thoracic spine with Harrington rods placed at levels T3-T9, as well as orthopedic surgery to repair the shattered left tibia/fibula. J.C. had limited mobility due to her postsurgical course. She was depressed but ready to start rehabilitation so she could return home.

The musculoskeletal plan of care for J.C. included use of a body Jacket when above 30 degrees in bed or out of bed; logroll when flat; diligent inspection for pressure areas and skin care under body jacket. She required attention during transfers with careful positioning of external fixator to prevent damage or dislodging and pin site care to fixator to prevent infection. Harrington rod precautions were followed to prevent flexion of thoracolumbar area and no high level wheelchair activities such as floor to chair transfers were done. She had ongoing spine films to check for alignment and rod position. Patient and family education stressed independence in wheelchair mobility, ADLs, and hygiene. High-level wheelchair skills were delayed until the jacket was removed, surgery healed, and external device removed.

References and Selected Bibliography

Betz, R. (1989). *Children with spinal cord injuries*. Unpublished study, Shriners Hospital for Crippled Children. Philadelphia, PA.

Borgman-Gainer, M. (1996). Independent function: Movement and mobility. In S.P. Hoeman (ed.), *Rehabilitation nursing: Process and application* (2nd Ed.) (pp. 225-269). St. Louis, MO: Mosby.

Cybulski, G., Penn, R., & Jaeger, R. (1994). Lower extremity functional neuromuscular stimulation in cases of spinal cord injury. *Neurosurgery, 15*, 132-146.

Dearolf, WW, Betz, R.R., Vogel, L.C., Levine, J., Clancy, M., Steel, H.H. (1990). Scoliosis in pediatric spinal cord injured patients. *Journal of Pediatric Orthopedics, 10(2)*, 214-218.

Harvel, J. Jr. & Hanley, E., Jr. (1995). Spondylolysis and spondylolisthesis. In D. Pang (Ed.), *Disorders of the pediatric spine*, (pp. 561-574). New York: Raven Press.

Hinck, S. M. (1994). Heterotopic ossification: A review of symptoms and treatment. *Rehabilitation Nursing, 19(3)*, 169-173.

Hoeman, S. P. (1996). *Rehabilitation Nursing: Process and Application (2nd ed.)*. St. Louis, MO: Mosby

Johnson, K. & Persaud, D. (1993). *Spinal cord injury: Education content for professional nursing practice* (2nd ed.) Jackson Heights, NY: American Association of Spinal Cord Injury Nurses.

Kralji, A., Bajd, T., & Turk, R. (1983). Gait restoration in paraplegic patients: A feasibility demonstration using multichannel surface electrode FES. *Journal of Rehabilitation Research and Development, 20* (BPR10-38), 3-20.

Marasolais, E. & Kobetic, R. (1983). Functional walking in paralyzed patients by means of electrical stimulation. *Clinical Orthopaedics, 175*, 30-36.

Marsolais, E. & Kobetic, R. (1987). Implantation techniques and experience with percutaneous intramuscular electrodes in the lower extremities. *Journal of Rehabilitation Research and Development, 23*(6), 1-8.

Meinecke, F. (1973). Pelvis and limb injuries in patients with recent spinal cord injuries. *Proceedings Veterans Administration Spinal Cord Injury Conference, 19 (Oct.)*, 205-212.

Peckham, P. (1988). Functional electrical stimulation: Current status and future prospects of applications to the neuromuscular system in spinal cord injury. *Paraplegia, 25*(3), 279-288.

Ragnarsson, K., Pollack, S., O'Daniel, W. Jr., Edgar, R., Petrofsky, J., & Nash, M. (1988). Clinical evaluation of computerized functional electrical stimulation after spinal cord injury: A multicenter pilot study. *Archives of Physical Medicine and Rehabilitation, 69*(9), 672-677.

Rehabilitation Nursing Foundation. (1993). *The specialty practice of rehabilitation nursing: A core curriculum* (3rd ed., Chapter 7). Skokie, IL: Rehabilitation Nursing Foundation.

Rehabilitation Nursing Foundation. (1995). *Rehabilitation nursing diagnoses: A guide to interventions and outcomes*. Glenview, IL : Rehabilitation Nursing Foundation.

Whaley, L. & Wong, D. (1991). *Nursing care of infants and children* (4th ed.), St. Louis, MO: Mosby.

Zejdlik, CP (Ed.) (1992). *Management of spinal cord injury*, 2nd Edition. Boston: Jones & Bartlett.

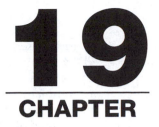

Sensation

Nahid Veit, MSN, RN
Pat Quigley, Ph.D., ARNP, CRRN

I. Learning Objectives

A. Differentiate between acute and chronic pain.

B. Describe pain assessment tools applicable to spinal cord impairment (SCI).

C. Identify four types of pain that occur in SCI.

D. Describe the impact of pain and altered sensation on quality of life.

II. Introduction

A. **Scope of the chapter**: This chapter describes functional alterations of sensation related to acute and chronic pain in persons with SCI. Sensory-perceptual alterations are defined as a state in which the individual experiences, or is at risk for experiencing, a change in the amount, pattern, or interpretation of incoming stimuli (Carpenito, 1995, p.838). The nursing process includes subjective and objective assessment, clinical interventions for treatment of alterations in sensation, and evaluation of patient responses.

B. **Demographics**: All persons with SCI experience alterations in sensation due to trauma or disease of the central and/or peripheral nervous system. The extent of the alteration will vary with the type and extent of disease or injury.

C. **Etiology and Precipitating Factors**: Traumatic injury or pathological disease affects the central and/or peripheral nervous systems. Alterations in sensation result when the sensory neuropathways have been affected. Pain will ensue and may become chronic, depending on its nature.

D. **Anatomy/physiology**: Review of normal anatomy and physiology of the neurological system, pain physiology, and musculoskeletal systems (see Chapters 7 and 18).

III. Initial Assessment

A. **Nursing History**: Loss of sensation or abnormal sensation, especially at the level of injury; paresthesia, unpleasant sensation caused by a stimulus; numbness, a sense of heaviness, weakness, or "deadness" in the affected part of body; location of symptoms; mode of onset and progression of symptoms; course of sensory complaints (intermittent, repetitive or transient); in SCI with incomplete injury, presence of spared sensory functions.
1. Onset and description: Addresses the questions of what precipitated sensation, how it was relieved, and frequency of occurrence.
2. Descriptors of pain:
   a. Pattern
   b. Duration
   c. Location
   d. Severity or intensity of pain based on rating scale 0-10 (Refer to Table 19-1)
   e. Provoking/relieving factors
   f. Associated symptoms
3. Observations
   a. Facial grimacing
   b. Altered muscle tone (decreased; increased) frequency of spasticity
   c. Autonomic responses (diaphoresis, increased blood pressure, increased pulse, pupillary dilation, increased or decreased respiration)
      (1) Abnormal autonomic responses: occur from noxious stimuli below the level of injury, responses include: diaphoresis, increased blood pressure, decreased pulse, pupillary dilation, increased or decreased respiration.
         (a) Noxious stimuli may be full bladder or bowel; pain increases spasticity (See Chapter 20).
         (b) Autonomic dysreflexia/hyperreflexia: a life-threatening event affecting the spinal cord individual with lesion T6 and above (See Chapter 13).
      (2) Clinical manifestations: noxious stimuli below the level of lesion causing disturbances of the reflex mechanisms controlling the autonomic nervous system; manifestations include throbbing, pounding headache, anxiety, visual disturbances, nasal congestion, flushing above the level of injury (Adkins, 1985).
   d. Posture (position of head, trunk, and extremities)
   e. Increase or decrease in activity or physical strength
   f. Changes in level of functional independence
   g. Impact of pain on burden of care and caregiver's burden to provide care
4. Diagnostic studies for alterations in sensation. Invasive and non-invasive tests include: x-rays; CT scan; Magnetic Resonance Imaging (MRI); myelogram; EMG; nerve conduction studies; evoked potentials: Brain (BAER); Visual (VER); Somatosensory (SER)
5. Theories related to pain (Bonica, 1990)
   a. Specificity (Sensory) Theory (formulated by Schiff in 1858 (Bonica, 1990)).
      (1) Pain is a specific sensation, independent of touch and other senses.
      (2) Examined the effects of incisions on sections of the spinal cord to support specificity theory
      (3) Supported later by descriptions of separate spots for warmth, cold, and touch in the skin.
      (4) Further advanced to map pain and touch
   b. Intensive Summation Theory (formulated by Romberg, Henle, & Volkmann, 1840s-1850s (Bonica, 1990))
      (1) Pain resulted from excessive stimulation of the sense of touch
      (2) Every sensory stimulus is capable of producing pain if it reaches sufficient intensity
   c. Central Summation Theory (developed by Livingston, 1943)
      (1) Supports the intensive theory

Table 19-1: Pain Intensity Scales

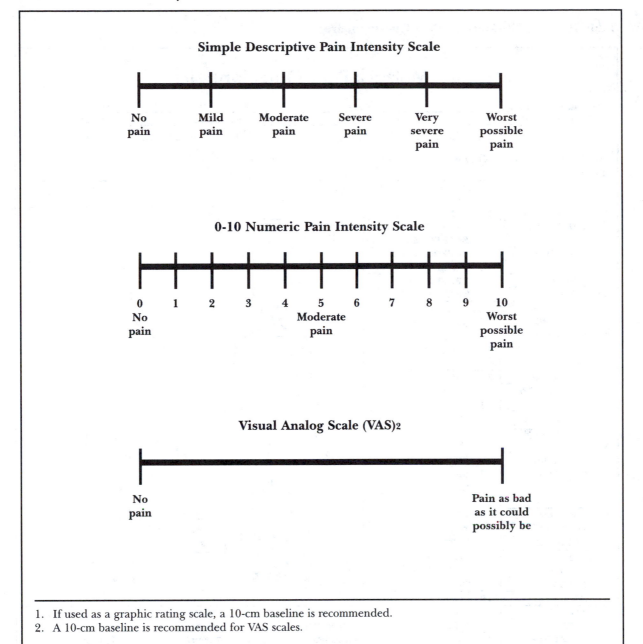

1. If used as a graphic rating scale, a 10-cm baseline is recommended.
2. A 10-cm baseline is recommended for VAS scales.

From *Acute pain management: Operative or medical procedures and trauma* by Agency for Health Care Policy and Research, 1992, Clinical Practice Guideline (AHCPR Publication No. 92-0032). Rockville, MD: U.S. Department of Health and Human Services. Reprinted with permission.

(2) Nerve and tissue damage activates fibers that project to the internuncial neuron pools in the spinal cord, creating abnormal reverbatory activity, which is a closed, self-exciting neural loop.

(3) The abnormal activity spreads to the lateral horn cells and the ventral horn cells of the spinal cord.

(4) The sympathetic nervous system and somatic motor system are activated, producing vasoconstriction.

Table 19-2: McGill-Melzack Pain Questionnaire

McGill - Melzack Pain Questionnaire

Patient's Name_____ Date_____ Time_____ am/pm
Analgesic(s) _____ Dosage _____ Time Given _____ am/pm
_____ Dosage _____ Time Given _____ am/pm

Analgesic Time Difference (hours): +4 +1 +2 +3
PRI: S_____ A_____ E_____ M(S)_____ M(AE)_____ M(T)_____ PRI(T)____
  (1-10)   (11-15)   (16)   (17-19)   (20)   (17-20) (1-20)

1. FLICKERING	11. TIRING
QUIVERING	EXHAUSTING
PULSING	12. SICKENING
THROBBING	SUFFOCATING
BEATING	13. FEARFUL
POUNDING	FRIGHTFUL
2. JUMPING	TERRIFYING
FLASHING	14. PUNISHING
SHOOTING	GRUELLING
3. PRICKING	CRUEL
BORING	VICIOUS
DRILLING	KILLING
STABBING	15. WRETCHED
LANCINATING	BLINDING
4. SHARP	16. ANNOYING
CUTTING	TROUBLESOME
LACERATING	MISERABLE
5. PINCHING	INTENSE
PRESSING	UNBEARABLE
GNAWING	17. SPREADING
CRAMPING	RADIATING
CRUSHING	PENETRATING
6. TUGGING	PIERCING
PULLING	18. TIGHT
WRENCHING	NUMB
7. HOT	DRAWING
BURNING	SQUEEZING
SCALDING	TEARING
SEARING	19. COOL
8. TINGLING	COLD
ITCHY	FREEZING
SMARTING	20. NAGGING
STINGING	NAUSEATING
9. DULL	AGONIZING
SORE	DREADFUL
HURTING	TORTURING
ACHING	PPI
HEAVY	0 No pain
10. TENDER	1 MILD
TAUT	2 DISCOMFORTING
RASPING	3 DISTRESSING
SPLITTING	4 HORRIBLE
	5 EXCRUCIATING

PPI_____   COMMENTS:

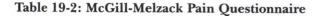

CONSTANT
PERIODIC
BRIEF

ACCOMPANYING SYMPTOMS:	SLEEP:	FOOD INTAKE:
NAUSEA	GOOD	GOOD
HEADACHE	FITFUL	SOME
DIZZINESS	CAN'T SLEEP	LITTLE
DROWSINESS	COMMENTS:	NONE
CONSTIPATION		COMMENTS:
DIARRHEA		
COMMENTS:	ACTIVITY:	COMMENTS:
	GOOD	
	SOME	
	LITTLE	
	NONE	

From The McGill Pain Questionnaire: Appraisal and Current Status, by R. Melzack & J. Katz, 1992, in *Handbook of Pain Assessment*. New York: Guilford Press. Reprinted with permission.

d. Fourth Theory of Pain (formulated by Strong, 1940s (Bonica, 1990)). Pain can be separated into two components:
   (1) Perception of pain based on neural receptive and conductive mechanisms
   (2) Reaction to pain based on physiological, cognitive, and psychological processes
e. Sensory Interaction Theory (formulated by Noordenbos, 1959 (Bonica, 1990)). Two systems are involved in the transmission of pain and other sensory information
   (1) A slow system: involves the unmyelinated and thinly myelinated fibers
   (2) A fast system: involves the myelinated fibers
f. Gate-Control Theory- (formulated by Melzack & Wall, 1950's (Bonica, 1990))
   (1) Transmission of nerve impulses from afferent fibers to the spinal cord T cells is modulated by a spinal gating mechanism in the dorsal horn.
   (2) The spinal gating mechanism is influenced by the relative amount of activity on large diameter and small diameter fibers.
   (3) Spinal gating mechanism is influenced by nerve impulses descending from the brain to the body.
   (4) A specialized system of large diameter rapidly conducting fibers labeled the "central control trigger" activates selective cognitive processes that influence the modulating properties of the spinal gating mechanisms.
   (5) When the output of the spinal cord transmission (T) cells exceeds the critical level, it activates the action system, the neural areas that underlie the complex sequential pattern of behavior and experience characteristics of pain.
g. Psychological/Behavioral Theories (developed by Mersky & Spear, 1970s)
   (1) Chronic pain occurs in the absence of tissue damage or other organic pathology
   (2) Examines relationship between mind and body
   (3) Behavioral conditioning results in chronic pain behaviors (Bonica, 1990)
   (4) Pain Assessment Tools: four common self-report measurement tools useful for assessment of pain intensity and affective distress in adults and children
      (a) Numerical Rating Scale (NRS) (Refer to Table 19-1)
      (b) Visual Analog Scale (VAS) (Refer to Table 19-1)
      (c) Adjective Rating Scale (ARS)
      (d) McGill-Melzack Pain Questionnaire (MMPQ) (Refer to Table 19-2)

B. **Examination**: Physical examination should be conducted symmetrically above and below the level of injury.
1. Central Nervous System: assessment of sensation (pressure, touch and temperature) to determine unilateral and contralateral integrity of spinothalamic tract.
   a. Upper Motor Neuron (UMN) Lesion: interferes with descending pathways, increased muscle tone, increased stretch reflex, varying degrees of weakness, minimal atrophy; pyramidal and extrapyramidal systems, lesions produce hyperactive reflex (facilitate the muscle stretch reflex), bulbocavernosus reflex is positive.
   b. Lower Motor Neuron (LMN) Lesion: anterior horn cells and motor axons; neuromuscular junction and the muscle produce weakness, atrophy, and fasciculations; lesions result in diminished or absent muscle strength, stereognosis
2. Peripheral Nervous System: assessment of dermatomes to determine distribution of abnormality with reference to normal root and peripheral nerve.
   a. Temperature: evaluate by application of cold to skin, using ice packs or ice cubes
   b. Pinprick: evaluate by use of pin by asking the patient to point to stimulated site
   c. Deep pressure: evaluate by applying pressure on tendons using soft, blunt instrument
   d. Vibration: evaluate by using a tuning fork in motion placed over a bony prominence
   e. Joint Position: test by asking the patient to indicate the direction of small passive movement of the fingers and toes while patient's eyes are closed
   f. Romberg's Test: test sway tendency with eyes closed while standing (if appropriate) especially for central cord syndrome
   g. Two-point discrimination: ability to identify two points of sensation on body; examine ability to identify point of touch symmetrically on both sides of body as well as two points on one side of body.

C. **Diagnostic Studies**: Non-invasive vascular studies, Magnetic Resonance Imaging (MRI); laboratory studies, EMG, Nerve conduction studies.

IV. Nursing Process Applied To Sensation

Sensory-perceptual alteration is a state in which the individual experiences or is at risk for experiencing a change in amount, pattern, or interpretation of incoming stimuli (Carpenito, 1995, p. 838). SCI results in altered neurological transmissions of the spinothalamic tract of the afferent horn of the spinal column, affecting pain, temperature, pressure, and touch.

A. **Nursing Diagnoses**: sensory-perceptual alteration — at-risk due to alteration of sensory organs, neurological alteration, metabolic alteration, and/or impaired oxygen for injury related to loss of sensation; sensory alterations — high risk for impaired skin integrity related to lack of protective sensation (Carpenito, 1995). Altered comfort secondary to sensory deficits.

B. **Defining Characteristics**: Affects peripheral receptors, spinal cord and central nervous system — process can alter the experience of sensations to the cortex.
1. Two types of sensory processes
   a. Serial processing: transmission and processing of information
   b. Parallel processing: information-processing operation that produces sensory experience
2. Types of altered sensation
   a. Anesthesia: complete loss of sensation below the level of injury; occurs with complete spinal cord injury
   b. Hyperesthesia: unusual or pathological sensitivity of the skin or a particular sense; occurs in both complete and incomplete spinal cord injury
   c. Dyesthesia: unpleasant sensations, such as burning, stinging, or stabbing sensations, below the level of injury (Davidoff, Roth, Guarracini, Silwa, & Yarkony, 1987); occurs over time, not present immediately after SCI (Beric, Demitrijevic, & Lindblom, 1988).
   d. Phantom sensation: sometimes following total spinal transection, after phase of spinal shock, complaints of phantom sensations of the lower limbs; described as painful, uncomfortable, dreadful, and unpleasant (Pagni, 1969).

C. **Expected Outcomes for Individual**:
1. Understands etiology and possible complications due to sensory deficits
2. Consistently performs compensatory techniques or instructs caregiver in safety techniques
3. Remains safe and free of serious injury
4. Inspects body parts and/or directs caregiver to inspect body correctly
5. Compensates by using another intact sense to compensate for sensory deficit

D. **Interventions**: Safety measures to protect from injury; patient education and adaptive equipment to inspect body parts.

V. Types of Acute Pain

Pain is defined as an unpleasant sensory and emotional experience associated with actual or potential tissue damage. Pain is the most common symptom for which individuals seek help, and can reflect physical or emotional discomfort. Severe pain occurs in five to thirty percent of the SCI population (Chiou-Tan et al., 1996). Presence of spasticity may alter pain perception (Beric et al., 1988; Herman, D'Luzansky, & Ippolito, 1992). The following are types of pain are discussed:

A. **Physical Pain**
1. Result of tissue injury and arises from stimulation of pain endings in somatic and visceral structures.
2. Pain conducting fibers synapse with neurons of the dorsal gray horn of the spinal cord.
3. Pain impulse travels up the contralateral spinothalamic tract to synapses of the midbrain and thalamus, and from the sensory cortex.

B. **Somatic Pain**
1. Tends to be localized
2. Often follows dermatomes or spinal segmental (myotomal) patterns
3. Described in familiar terms
4. Rarely continuous except in certain easily identified acute or subacute tissue-damaging lesions

C. **Visceral Pain**
1. Poorly localized
2. Often spreads from the injured organ to other visceral regions or to somatic dermatomes with a common spinal afferent pathway (referred pain)
3. More difficult to describe
4. More disturbing than somatic pain
5. Precipitated by bladder or rectal distention and is associated with nausea, flushing, headache, and sweating (Pagni, 1969).

D. **Central Pain**
1. Of thalamic origin
2. Characterized as severe and spontaneous or continuous and burning
3. On the contralateral side
4. Greatly accentuated by light touch
5. Painful overreaction to objective stimuli, resulting from lesions confined to the substances of the central nervous system (Pagni, 1969).

E. **Post-traumatic Syringomyelia** (Syrinx formation is discussed in Chapter 9)
1. Pain associated with sensory loss and spasticity
2. Characterized by numbness, weakness, sensory loss (Robinson, 1990).
3. May be unilateral and intermittent initially, and progress to bilateral and continuous (Pagni, 1969).

F. **Reflex-Sympathetic Dystrophy**
1. Continuous pain, central in origin.
2. Includes a complex of sympathetic hyperactivity.
3. Accompanied by disuse (Tasker & Dostrovsky, 1989).

G. **Heterotopic Ossification**
1. Joint pain; in SCI, usually shoulders, hips and elbows.
2. Accompanied by spasticity (Sie, Waters, & Adkins, 1992).

H. **Psychogenic Pain**
1. Pain without pathological or physical cause.
2. Precipitated by stress or crisis situations (emotional or social) (McGrath & Craig, 1989).

I. **Musculoskeletal Pain**
1. Originates from abnormal muscle impulses.
2. May cause involuntary activities, such as spasticity.
3. Long term effects may result in contractures (McGrath & Craig, 1989).

VI. Nursing Process Applied to Acute Pain

Pain is defined as an unpleasant sensory and emotional experience associated with actual or potential tissue damage.

A. **Nursing Diagnosis:** Acute Pain: State in which individual experiences and reports the presence of severe discomfort or an uncomfortable sensation, lasting one second to 6 months (Carpenito, 1995: 217). Acute pain; altered comfort secondary to acute pain.

B. **Defining Characteristics:** unpleasant sensory, perceptual, and emotional experiences; important biological warning; recent onset; symptom — not a disease; self-limiting; transient; brief; situational; occurs under specific circumstances such as trauma or surgery.
   1. Localized
   2. Results from physical or mechanical injury, trauma, or disease state.
   3. May have evidence of peripheral source of involvement affecting the central nervous system, such as neuritis (Balazy, 1992).

C. **Expected Outcomes:**
   1. Decreased pain severity.
   2. Decreased frequency of spasticity.
   3. Increased level of function (low level quadriplegia or paraplegia).
   4. Decreased burden of care to individual and caregiver.

D. **Interventions**
   1. Recognize pain and treat promptly.
   2. Reposition patient.
   3. Provide analgesic medications.
   4. Chart and display pain and relief.
   5. Survey satisfaction with pain treatment.
   6. Inform patient of analgesics and promise alternative analgesic care.
   7. Review the *Patient Family Guide for Acute Pain Management* with individual and family (AHCPR, 1992).
   8. Determine the individual's preferred tool for pain assessment.
   9. Evaluate need for Patient Controlled Analgesia (PCA).
   10. Education/instruction: relaxation, imagery, music distraction, and biofeedback.
   11. Apply physical agents, such as applications of heat or cold, massage, exercise, and immobilization.
   12. Recommend use of transcutaneous electrical nerve stimulation (TENS)
   13. Initiate interdisciplinary involvement in pain management and referrals to pain program, substance abuse program, counseling services.
   14. Pharmacological Management:
      a. Non-steroidal anti-inflammatory drugs (NSAIDs): class of medications, including aspirin, ibuprofen, indomethacin, phenylbutaxone, and a variety of other drugs.
         (1) Have anti-inflammatory and analgesic properties and also prostaglandin inhibitors.
         (2) Therapeutic effect is to decrease pain, and decrease inflammation, while promoting healing.
         (3) For mild to moderate pain (AHCPR, 1994).
      b. Opioid analgesics - analgesics commonly given for moderate to severe persistent pain.
         (1) Should be added to (not substituted for) NSAIDs.
         (2) Produce analgesia by binding to specific receptors both inside and outside the central nervous system.
         (3) For short-term acute pain (AHCPR, 1994).

VII. Nursing Process Applied To Chronic Pain

Defined as pain that persists beyond the usual course; results from pathophysiological effects, psychopathology or environmental factors. Estimates of prevalence of severe/disabling chronic pain in SCI patients range from 18% to 63% (Mariano, 1992). Sie et al. (1992) found 64 percent of persons with paraplegia and 51 percent of those with quadriplegia reported chronic upper extremity pain. Complaints related to carpal tunnel syndrome are the most common, followed by shoulder pain.

A. **Nursing Diagnosis**: Chronic Pain: impaired mobility related to musculoskeletal degeneration; decreased range of motion and loss of muscle strength; self-care deficit related to pain; lack of range of motion and weakness; pain related to disruption of nerve fibers or muscle spasms; altered comfort secondary to chronic pain.

B. **Defining Characteristics**:
1. Persists long after healing has occurred.
2. Unpleasant sensation caused by noxious stimulation of the sensory nerve ending.
3. Lasting longer than 6 months.
4. Expressed verbally or nonverbally.

C. **Expected Outcomes**:
1. Patient is knowledgeable of psychosocial impact of chronic pain.
2. Patient is knowledgeable of adaptive living techniques, posture, nutrition, and exercise.

D. **Interventions**:
1. Institute comfort measures.
2. Identify triggering factors.
3. Initiate interdisciplinary involvement in pain management and patient teaching.
4. Promote rest and relaxation.
5. Introduce visual imagery.
6. Use distraction.
7. Provide self-management strategies (Umlauf, 1992).

VIII. Reassessment

A. Evaluate the extent of sensory deficits, pain intensity, frequency, and patient satisfaction with treatment.

B. Assess the degree of superficial and deep sensation.

C. Evaluate changes in response to treatments.

D. Reassess at least every two weeks during spinal shock.

E. Re-evaluate response to nursing and interdisciplinary interventions:
1. Ability to perform and/or verbalize etiology of sensory deficits, potential complications, and interventions to promote compensation and safety.
2. Reports of increased comfort.
3. Decrease in pain based on patient's rating of pain severity, using one or more pain measurement scales:
   a. McGill-Melzack Pain Questionnaire
   b. Visual Analog Scale
   c. Pain Drawing

IX. Special Issues Related to Pediatric Care

A. **Sensation**
1. As with adults, the degree of sensation will be determined by the level and extent of the SCI.
2. Cognition, age, and developmental level will determine the child's ability to identify and express the type of sensation.
   a. The infant and young child will be unable to specifically identify the areas of sensation or the type of sensation. Staff must be aware of the types of altered sensation (decreased, normal, increased/hypersensitivity) and manage the child appropriately. The infant and young child may scream or cry when touched but be unable to explain why.
   b. The older child, without cognitive impairment, will be able to identify the level and type of sensation.
   c. Increased sensitivity/hypersensitivity and parethesias will interfere with recovery and level of cooperation unless effectively treated with medication and desensitizing techniques.

B. **Acute and Chronic Pain** (AHCPR, 1992).
1. Historically the existence and degree of pain are underestimated in children.
2. Identification of pain by the child is based on the developmental and cognitive level.
3. Caregivers must be educated in pain assessment (verbal, nonverbal, and changes in vital signs) and management and the types of pain associated with SCI.
    a. The infant may exhibit discomfort and pain by their level of irritability, degree of restlessness, or pulling and rubbing a body part.
    b. The young child may use words other than "pain" to describe the degree and location of pain.
    c. The older child will generally verbalize the degree and type of pain.
    d. The parent or caregiver is frequently the best assessor of the amount and type of pain the child is experiencing.
4. A child may deny pain, for several reasons, such as:
    a. Fear of injections.
    b. Belief that pain is a form of punishment for bad behavior.
    c. Child may deny pain to a stranger but admit it to a parent.
5. Pain should not be seen as attention-seeking behavior.
6. A variety of pain rating scales are available for children.
    a. Faces Scales (Wong & Baker, 1988) consists of a series of expressive faces ranging from very happy to very sad. Appropriate for children as young as 3 years.
    b. Numeric Scale: Uses a straight line with numbered markers to determine the degree of pain. Appropriate for children as young as 5 years if they can count and have concept of numbers.
    c. Color Tool (Eland, 1985): Child uses colored crayons or markers to develop own pain scale. Appropriate for children as young as 4 years if they know colors.
    d. Simple Descriptive Scale: Uses a straight line with descriptive words to determine the degree of pain. Appropriate for children as young as 5.
    e. Visual Analog Scale: Uses a straight line without markers and is appropriate for young school-aged children.
7. Pain management may be both nonpharmacologic and pharmacologic.
8. The use of medication is based on its acceptance for use in children, and the child's age and weight.
9. Successful delivery of medication will depend on the route of administration (intraveneous (IV) preferred over intramuscular (IM) or nasogastric (N/G)), the form of medication (tablet or liquid, depending on age), the ability to swallow a pill (chewable form available in some medications), and the person giving the medication (parent frequently preferred over nurse).
10. Children experience chronic pain. Touch stimulation, transcutaneous electrical nerve stimulation (TENS), biofeedback and psychological interventions can be considered for the management but are not always effective.
11. Children should be referred to a pain management specialist if usual methods of pain management are not effective.
12. Refer to *Acute Pain Management: Operative or Medical Procedures and Trauma*, Clinical Practice Guidelines, published by U.S. Department of Health and Human Services (AHCPR, 1992a).

C. **Comfort**
1. All persons gain a degree of comfort from familiar people, places, and things.
2. Children gain comfort and security from their parents, friends, consistent staff, and favorite personal belongings (blanket, stuffed animal). The child without a family at bedside should have scheduled telephone contact times with parents who are unable to visit frequently.
3. A schedule or routine provides the child with structure and sense of security.
4. Familiar objects and belongings make a new environment friendlier.
5. Wearing street clothes (may need to be adapted) during hospitalization provides the child with a sense of normalcy and wellness.

Practical Application

M.A. is a 49-year-old male who grew up in the family trucking business, hauling logs. He sustained T6 paraplegia in 1984 when a log rolled off a truck and fell on him. Shortly after the accident, M.A.'s wife divorced him, and his two children went to live with their mother. M.A. was bitter and depressed. He also complained of constant chronic pain, which he described as "burning, numb, tingling, and electric shock type" over his buttocks, legs, and feet. In the mid-thoracic area, M.A. complained of stabbing pain, which became worse when supine.

M.A. was treated with many different pain medications with no relief. The medications included analgesics, antidepressants and anticonvulsants. M.A. selected a morphine pump for pain relief. He started to abuse alcohol and took non-prescription narcotics, such as cocaine. M.A. stated that the pain persisted.

In 1988, M.A. admitted himself to a substance abuse program. He was eventually weaned off all drugs, including the morphine pump.

M.A.'s family, including brothers, sisters, and parents, were very supportive, realizing the addiction issues. M.A. wanted to go back to work, hauling logs and driving his big truck. With the family's help, many modifications were made to the truck, in particular installing special wheelchair lift and hand controls.

M.A. copes with his chronic pain by staying active, swimming, fishing, and truck driving. M.A. takes acetaminophen occasionally and believes that staying busy and doing what he enjoys helps him to keep his mind off his pain.

References and Selected Bibliography

Adkins, H. (1985). *Spinal cord injury.* (pp. 172-175). New York: Churchill Livingstone.

Agency for Health Care Policy and Research. (AHCPR) (1992a). *Acute pain management: Operative or medical procedures and trauma.* Clinical Practice Guideline (AHCPR Publication No. 92-0032). *Acute pain management: Operative or medical procedures and trauma clinical practice guidelines, patient and family guide.* Rockville, MD: U.S. Department of Health and Human Services.

Agency for Health Care Policy and Research. (AHCPR) (1992b). *Acute pain management in infants, children, and adolescents: Operative and medical procedures.* Quick reference guide for clinicians. Clinical Practice Guidelines. (AHCPR Publication No. 92-0020) Rockville, ND: U.S. Department of Health and Human Services.

Agency for Health Care Policy and Research. (AHCPR) (1994). *Management of cancer pain: Clinical Practice Guidelines, patient and family guide.* Rockville, MD: U.S. Department of Health and Human Services.

Agency for Health Care Policy and Research. (AHCPR) (1994). *Acute low back problems in adults, clinical practice guidelines, patient and family guide.* Rockville, MD: U.S. Department of Health and Human Services.

Balazy, T. (1992). Clinical management of chronic pain in spinal cord injury. *Clinical Journal of Pain, 8*(2), 102-110.

Barker, E. (1994). *Neuroscience nursing.* St. Louis, MO: Mosby.

Beare, P., & Myers, J. (1994). *Principles and practices of adult health nursing. (2nd ed.)* St. Louis, MO: Mosby.

Beric, A., Demitrijevic, M., & Lindblom, U. (1988). Central dysesthia syndrome in spinal cord injury patients. *Pain: The Journal of the International Association for the Study of Pain, 43,* 109-116.

Bonica, J. (1990). *The management of pain, (2nd ed.).* (pp. 388-390). Boston: Lea & Febiger.

Carpenito, L. (1995). *Nursing diagnosis. Application to nursing diagnosis, 6th Ed.* Philadelphia: J.B. Lippincott.

Chiou-Tan, F., Tuel, S., Johnson, J., Priebe, M., Hirsch, D., & Strayer, J. (1996). Effect of mexiletine on spinal cory injury dysesthetic pain. *American Journal of Physical Medicine and Rehabilitation, 75*(2), 84-87.

Christensen, B., & Kockrow, E. (1995). *Foundations of nursing.* St. Louis, MO: Mosby.

Davidoff, G., Roth, E., Guarracini, M., Silwa, J., & Yarkony, G. (1987). Function-limiting dysesthetic pain syndrome among traumatic spinal cord injury patients: A cross-sectional study. *Pain: The Journal of the International Association for the Study of Pain, 29,* 39-48.

Eland , M. (1985). The child who is hurting. *Seminars in Oncology Nursing, 1*(2), 116-122.

Greenburg, D., Aminoff, M., & Simon, R. (1993). *Clinical neurology 2nd ed.* Norwalk: Appleton & Lange.

Herman, R., D'Luzansky, S., & Ippolito, R. (1992). Intrathecal baclofen suppresses central pain in patients with spinal cord lesions: A pilot study. *Clinical Journal in Pain, 8*(4), 338-345.

Lewis, K. & Mueller, W. (1993). Intrathecal baclofen for severe spasticity secondary to spinal cord injury. *Annuals of Pharmacotherapy, 27*(6), 767-774.

McGrath, P. & Craig, K. (1989). Development and psychological factors in children's pain. *Pediatric Clinics of North America, 36*(4), 823-836.

Mariano, A. (1992). Chronic pain and spinal cord injury. *Clinical Journal of Pain, 8*(2), 87-92.

Maynard, F., Karunas, R., & Maring, W. (1990). Epidemiology of spasticity following traumatic spinal cord injury. *Archives of Physical Medicine and Rehabilitation, 71,* 566-569.

Melzack, R., & Katz, J. (1992). The McGill pain questionnaire: Appraisal and current status. In R. Melzack & J. Katz (Eds). *Handbook of Pain Assessment.* New York: Guilford Press.

Pagni, C. (1989). Central pain due to spinal cord and brain stem damage. In R. Melzack & J. Katz (Eds). *Textbook of pain,* (2nd ed.). (pp. 634-637). New York: Churchill Livingstone.

Richards, J. (1992). Chronic pain and spinal cord injury: Review and comment. *Clinical Journal of Pain, 8*(2), 119-22.

Robinson, L. (1990). Motor evoked potentials reflect spinal function in posttraumatic syringomyelia. *American Journal of Rehabilitation Medicine, 69*(6), 307-310.

Sie, I., Waters, R., Adkins, R. & Gellman, R. (1992). Upper extremity pain in the post rehabilitation spinal cord injured patient. *Archives of Physical Medicine Rehabilitation, 73*(1), 44-48.

Tasker, R., & Dostrovsky, F. (1989). Deafferentiation and central pain. In R. Melzack & J. Katz (Eds). *Textbook of pain, (2nd ed.).* (pp. 154-174). New York: Churchill Livingstone.

Umlauf, R. (1992). Psychological interventions for chronic pain following spinal cord injury. *Clinical Journal of Pain, 8*(2), 111-118.

Wong, D. & Baker, C. (1988). Pain in children: comparison of assessment scales. *Oklahoma Nurse, 33*(1), 8.

Zejdlik, C. (1992). *Management of spinal cord injury (2nd Ed.).* Boston: Jones & Bartlett.

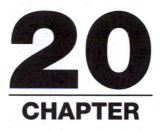

CHAPTER

Spasticity

Nahid Veit, MSN, RN
Pat Quigley, Ph.D., ARNP, CRRN

I. Learning Objectives

A. Differentiate between spasticity and rigidity.

B. Describe a spasticity assessment tool applicable to spinal cord impairment (SCI).

C. Identify treatment interventions for spasticity.

D. Describe the impact of spasticity on quality of life.

II. Introduction

A. **Scope of the Chapter**: This chapter presents functional alterations that occur secondary to spasticity in persons with SCI. The nursing process outlines spasticity assessment, subjective and objective assessment guidelines, clinical interventions for treatment of spasticity, and evaluation of patient responses.

B. **Demographics**: Spasticity is a common complication of persons with SCI. Maynard, Karunas, & Maring (1990) found that 67 percent of persons with SCI exhibit spasticity. The extent of functional alterations varies with the type and/or level of disorder or extent of injury.

C. **Etiology and Precipitating Factors**: Traumatic injury or pathological disease affects the central and/or peripheral nervous systems. Spasticity occurs when descending inhibitory inputs from supraspinal centers do not reach the level of the spinal cord. There is an imbalance between the inhibitory and excitatory impulses. The inhibitory/excitatory imbalance disrupts the inhibition of spinal reflex movements. Disruption of inhibitory functions results in the release of exaggerated reflex movements, which is characterized as spasticity.

D. **Anatomy/Physiology**: Refer to anatomy and physiology of the neurological system and the musculoskeletal systems, Chapters 7 and 18 respectively.

III. Initial Assessment

A. **Nursing History**
1. Onset of injury (during first two years post-injury, individuals with SCI may have increased spasticity)
2. Pattern of spasticity
3. Source of stimulus
4. Functional implications
5. Associated complications resulting in increased spasm (e.g. urinary tract infection (UTI), pressure ulcer)
6. Relationship of spasticity with time of day, activity, posture, or stimuli
7. Determine if pain occurs with spasticity, considering the type of pain

B. **Examination**:
1. Muscle strength, tone, and bulk
2. Degree of spasticity (refer to Table 20-1: Ashworth, Spasm, and Reflex Assessment Scales for Muscle Tone and Frequency of Spasms)
3. Reflex responses to light tap measure degree of spasticity and extent of interference with functional independence
4. Burden of care
5. Neuromuscular examination (include reflexes)
6. Response to touch, pain, and/or passive stretch
7. Presence of clonus
8. Urodynamic studies
9. Bowel function

C. **Diagnostic Studies**: Electromyogram (EMG), x-ray, and laboratory tests.

Table 20-1: Ashworth, Spasm, and Reflex Scale

Ashworth Score	Degree of Muscle Tone
1	No increase in tone
2	Slight increase in tone giving a catch when affected part is moved in flexion or extension
3	More marked increase in tone, but affected part is easily flexed
4	Considerable increase in tone: passive movement is difficult
5	Affected part rigid in flexion or extension

Spasm Score	Frequency of Spasm
0	No spasm
1	No spontaneous spasms: vigorous sensory and motor stimulation results in spasms
2	Occasional spontaneous spasms and easily induced spasms
3	More than 1, but fewer than 10 spontaneous spasms per hour
4	More than 10 spontaneous spasms per hour

Score	Reflexes
0	Absent
1	Hyporeflexive
2	Normoreflexive
3	Mild hyperreflexia
4	3 to 4 beats clonus
5	Clonus

From "Intrathecal Baclofen Infusion: An Innovative Approach for Controlling Spasticity," by S.M. Savoy & J.M. Gianno, 1993, *Rehabilitation Nursing, 18*, pp.105-113. Reprinted with permission.

IV. Nursing Process Applied to Spasticity

Type of hypertonia characterized by gradual increase in tone, causing increased resistance (Barker, 1995); state of exaggerated muscular tone with increased tendon reflexes associated with an upper motor neuron lesion; may be tonic or clonic (intermittent), caused by abnormal increased reflex activity; may interfere with activities of daily living and cause complications such as skin breakdown; and may cause increased pain (Zejdlik, 1992).

A. **Nursing Diagnosis**: impaired physical mobility related to muscle spasms; pain related to muscle spasms; altered comfort secondary to spasticity.

B. **Defining Characteristics**:
1. Gradual increase in muscle tone causing increased resistance; two types of increased muscle tone (hypertonia):
   a. Spasticity: increased tone in arms; flexor tone is greater than extensor tone; resistance tends to be most marked in passive movement; increased tone is velocity dependent; caused by upper motor lesion;
   b. Rigidity: increased resistance to passive movement, independent of the direction of the movement; affects agonist and antagonist muscle groups equally.

C. **Expected Outcomes**:
1. Maintenance optimum joint function and mobility.
2. Increased knowledge of factors contributing to spasticity.
3. Decreased severity of spasm.
4. Decreased pain.
5. Increased functional level and decreased burden of care.

D. **Interventions** (Initiate interdisciplinary involvement in spasticity management)
1. Range of motion (ROM), active and passive.
2. Correct positioning and alignment to inhibit spasticity: prone position, standing position, safety padding, and belt restraints.
3. Cold or heat therapy.
4. Functional or electrical stimulation.
5. Pharmacological management — antispasticity medications:
   a. Baclofen: usually the first drug of choice. Baclofen acts through gamma-aminobutyric acid (GABA) - mediated interference with the release of excitatory neurotransmitters in the spinal cord. Usually administered orally; however intrathecal baclofen is available for management of spasticity when oral drug therapy is ineffective. An implanted pump delivers very small doses of baclofen intrathecally; has the theoretical advantage of focusing the therapy at the site of pathology rather than giving the drug systemically; resulting in fewer complications and central nervous system side effects (Lewis & Mueller, 1993).
   b. Dantrolene: acts directly on muscle itself by interfering with the action potential induced release of calcium ions from the muscle cell; side effect is liver toxicity.
   c. Diazepam (Valium): acts at the spinal cord level by facilitating GABA-mediated presynaptic inhibition; not as effective as dantrolene or baclofen, and has more side effects; is more sedating, and has significant potential for abuse and physical dependence.
6. Surgical treatment: rhizotomy; tendonotomy.
7. Nerve blocks.
8. Ethical Issues: Ensuring patient involvement in goal setting and decision-making for treatment approaches. Consider attitudinal barriers among professionals when treating patient's pain.
9. Incorporate cultural preferences into treatment plan.
10. Health education
    a. Training in positioning and range of motion techniques.
    b. Explanation of possible contributing factors to changes in spasticity.

c. Pharmacological management and possible adverse effects; consequences of abrupt withdrawal of medications.

V. Reassessment

A. Verbalization of decrease in pain severity on scale 0-10.

B. Decreased facial grimacing; relaxed muscle tone; decreased autonomic responses.

C. Decreased frequency of spasticity and severity of spasticity using Ashworth and Spasm Scale (Table 20-1).

D. Increased level of function (low level quadriplegia or paraplegia).

E. Decreased burden of care to individual and caregiver.

F. Changes in functional status due to spasticity.

VI. Evaluation

A. Decrease in spasticity or maintain control of spasticity with minimum intervention to ensure maximal function.

B. Increase or maintain joint ROM and function.

C. Increase safety and comfort.

D. Maintain or increase ability to perform functional activities of daily living.

E. Avoid secondary complications.

VII. Special Issues Related to Pediatric Care

A. **Pharmacological Management** (Medical Economics, 1996):
   1. Diazepam is approved for children 6 months and older. Side effects include sedation and addiction if used long term. Withdrawal is a voided by tapering dose.
   2. Baclofen is recommended in children older than 12 years but also used in younger children. Side effects include sedation, dizziness, and fatigue. Adjust dose for renal compromise. Dose should be tapered when discontinuing drug.
   3. Dantrolene is approved for children 5 years and older. Side effect is hepatic failure. Liver function tests must be done prior to beginning medication and monthly. May worsen overall function because it works on skeletal muscle and does not discriminate muscle that is spastic from that which is normal.
   4. Botox injections may prove to be beneficial in the management of spasticity related to SCI. Although studies have been done on spasticity in multiple sclerosis, this is an emerging treatment in SCI and further investigation is necessary before it can be determined how effective it will be in the SCI population.

Practical Application

D.R. is a 47-year-old male with multiple sclerosis, which was diagnosed 13 years earlier. He was referred to a SCI facility for rehabilitation. D.R. has had three marriages and has one daughter. His third wife left him two years ago. She could not deal with his loss of function and his job. In spite of family problems, D.R. has been able to cope with his situation and maintain a positive, motivated approach toward rehabilitation. He was able to ambulate with a walker, transfer independently, and had bladder and bowel control.

D.R. began having increased spasticity that interfered with his activities. He was treated with baclofen, 5 mg every 8 hours. As his spasticity increased, the baclofen was increased to 120 mg/day, exceeding the recommended daily dose. D.R. began losing independence and could not ambulate. Diazepam was added to the medication regime gradually, to a total dose of 40 mg/day. Clonidine 0.2 mg twice a day was added to control spasticity. As a result of decreased mobility, D.R. became depressed, but continued to participate in rehabilitation. An antidepressant was initiated because of D.R.'s depression. The side effects of the medications became evident. D.R. started feeling sluggish and weak. D.R. became wheelchair dependent and unable to transfer independently.

A year later, D.R. was evaluated for an intrathecal baclofen pump. He received a 50 ug intrathecal bolus test dose, which produced a 2-point decrease in spasticity severity on the Ashworth and Spasm Scale. D.R. underwent a pump implant the following week and started on 100 mg/day. The intrathecal baclofen was gradually increased to 300 mg/day, while the oral baclofen was reduced to 30 mg/day. The diazepam, clonidine and antidepressant were discontinued.

D.R. demonstrated decreased spasticity in his legs and improved physical mobility. Upper extremity spasticity also decreased, and D.R. was able to feed himself independently again. With mild spasticity, D.R. was able to compensate and progress in functional abilities.

References and Selected Bibliography

Adkins, H. (1985). *Spinal cord injury.* (pp. 172-175). New York: Churchill Livingstone.

Agency for Health Care Policy and Research (AHCPR). (1992). *Acute Pain Management: Operative or Medical Procedures and Trauma, Clinical Practice Guidelines, Patient and Family Guide.* Rockville, MD: U.S. Department of Health and Human Services.

Barker, E. (1994). *Neuroscience nursing.* St. Louis, MO: Mosby.

Beare, P. & Myers, J. (1994). *Principles and practices of adult health nursing.* (2nd ed.) St. Louis: Mosby.

Carpenito, L. (1995). Nursing diagnosis. *Application to nursing diagnosis.* (6th ed.) Philadelphia: J.B. Lippincott.

Christensen, B. & Kockrow, E. (1995). *Foundations of nursing.* St. Louis: Mosby.

Craig, K. (1989). *Emotional aspects of pain: Textbook of pain,* (2nd ed.). (pp. 220-228). New York: Churchill Livingstone.

Greenburg, D., Aminoff, M., & Simon, R. (1993). *Clinical neurology.* (2nd ed.) Norwalk: Appleton & Lange.

Lewis, K. & Mueller, W. (1993). Intrathecal baclofen for severe spasticity secondary to spinal cord injury. *Annuals of Pharmacotherapy. 27*(6), 767-774.

Maynard, F., Karunas, R., & Maring, W. (1990). Epidemiology of spasticity following traumatic spinal cord injury. *Archives of Physical Medicine and Rehabilitation, 71,* 566-569.

Medical Economics. (1996). *Physician's desk reference.* Oradell: Medical Economics.

Ricci, M. (1990). Pain and headache: *The management of pain, Vol. I* (2nd ed.). (pp. 613-619). Boston, MA: Lea & Febiger.

Robinson, L.R. (1990). Motor-evoked potential reflect spinal cord function in post-traumatic syringomyelia. *American Journal of Rehabilitation Medicine, 69*(6), 307-310.

Savoy, S.M., & Gianino, J.M. (1993). Intrathecal baclofen infusion: An innovative approach for controlling spasticity. *Rehabilitation Nursing, 18,* 105-113.

Segatore, M. & Miller, M. (1994a). The pharmacotherapy of spinal spasticity: A decade of progress I. Theoretical aspects [Review]. *SCI Nursing, 11* (3), 66-69.

Segatore, M. & Miller, M. (1994b). The pharmacotherapy of spinal spasticity: A decade of progress II. Therapeutics [Review]. *SCI Nursing, 12* (1), 2-7.

Zejdlik, C. (1992). *Management of spinal cord injury* (2nd ed.) Boston: Jones & Bartlett.

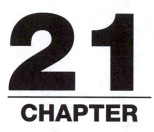

CHAPTER

Sexuality and Reproduction

Kelly Johnson, MSN, RN, CFNP, CRRN

I. Learning Objectives

A. Understand sexual function in individuals with an intact neurologic system.

B. Understand common physical changes that occur in individuals with spinal cord impairment (SCI).

C. Describe sexual health issues including fertility, reproduction, contraception, pregnancy, and obtaining or maintaining erections.

D. Describe physical and psychosocial issues related to comprehensive sexual health care for individuals with SCI.

II. Introduction

Kroll and Klein (1992) eloquently stated that the need for sexual expression is never lost as a result of illness or injury and that every person has the right to sexual expression. It is up to each person to discover the kind of sexual expression that works for him or her and the best way to achieve it.

This chapter provides an overview of sexual function in individuals with an intact neurologic system. Common physical changes that occur in individuals with SCI will be described. Sexual health issues such as fertility, reproduction, contraception, pregnancy, labor, delivery, altered vaginal lubrication, and obtaining or maintaining erections will be discussed. Lastly, physical and psychosocial issues related to comprehensive sexual health care for individuals with SCI are explored.

A. **Demographics**: All individuals experiencing spinal cord injury (SCI) with neurological deficit will experience some change in sexual function and/or sexual health.

B. **Etiology/Precipitating factors related to sexual dysfunction**
1. Altered body structure or function
   a. Paralysis/Paraparesis
   b. Alteration in sensation
   c. Autonomic dysreflexia (AD)
   d. Spasticity
   e. Alteration in elimination pattern
   f. Pain
   g. Positioning difficulties
   h. Mobility deficits
   i. Erectile dysfunction
   j. Alteration in ejaculation
   k. Alteration in vaginal lubrication
   l. Alteration in orgasms
2. Medications
3. Substance use/abuse
4. Alteration in self-esteem
5. Alteration in body image
6. Impaired relationship with significant other
7. Knowledge deficit related to sexuality and SCI and sexual health

C. **Anatomy/ Physiology**
1. Male anatomy and neurophysiology
   a. Male sexual organs (Johnson & Lanig, 1996) (Refer to Figure 21-1)
      (1) Penis: Consists of the shaft or corpora, which is formed by three columns of vascular erectile tissue bound together by elastic connective tissue. The urethra is located in the center of the penis and opens at the tip. The urethra allows passage of semen and urine.
      (2) Scrotum: A loose, wrinkled pouch consisting of skin and subcutaneous tissue, which is separated into two sacs containing the testes.
      (3) Testes: Produce spermatozoa (sperm) and testosterone.
      (4) Epididymis: Located on the posterior surface of the testicles and stores sperm until mature.
      (5) Vas deferens: Cord-like structure that begins at the tail of the epididymis, ascends through the scrotal sac, passes through the external inguinal ring to the abdomen and pelvis, and enters the urethra within the prostate gland. Sperm passes from the testes and epididymis, through the vas deferens, into the urethra. Secretions from the vas deferens, as well as the seminal vesicles and prostate, contribute to the semen.
      (6) Prostate gland: A firm, glandular organ surrounding the proximal (prostatic) urethra. Prostatic secretions empty into the urethra and aid in the motility of sperm.
      (7) Seminal vesicles: The seminal vesicles join the vas deferens behind the bladder; seminal fluid is mixed here.
   b. Neurophysiology of erection and ejaculation
      (1) Erection
         (a) Initiation: Two components of the erection process exist, reflex and psychogenic; in males without SCI, stimulation to elicit both components is needed in order to maintain a firm erection adequate for intercourse (Williams, 1993).
         (b) Filling: The spongy erectile tissue of the corpus cavernosus becomes engorged with blood by arterial dilation.
         (c) Storage: Venous restriction reduces blood flow from penis.
         (d) Neural control (Refer to Figure 21-2) Sympathetic preganglionic fibers from T10 to L2, parasympathetic fibers from S2 to S4. Erections are the result of synergistic activity of the sympathetic and parasympathetic influences (Szasz, 1992).

Figure 21-1: Male Anatomy

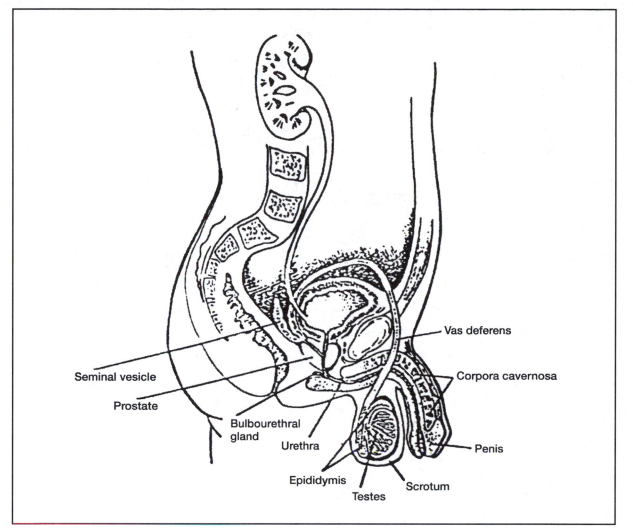

Seminal vesicle

Prostate

Bulbourethral gland

Urethra

Epididymis

Testes

Scrotum

Penis

Corpora cavernosa

Vas deferens

From *Structure and Function of the Human Body* (5th ed.), by R. Memmler, et al., illustration by Anthony Raviella, 1992, Philadelphia: J.B. Lippencott. Copyright 1992. Reprinted with permission.

(2) Emission: The process by which sperm is transported from the epididymis to the prostatic urethra in anticipation of ejaculation.
(a) Peristaltic contractions of the vas deferens, seminal vesicles, and prostate cause the forward movement.
(b) Seminal fluid from the seminal vesicles and prostate mixes with sperm at the level of the prostatic urethra.
(c) Bladder neck partially closes, semen moves beyond the prostatic urethra to the posterior urethra.
(d) Primarily under thoracolumbar sympathetic influence.
(3) Ejaculation: Pulsatile release of semen
(a) Rhythmic contractions of the pelvic floor striated musculature
(b) Semen forced along the urethra and out the urethral meatus
(c) Bladder neck closure complete for antegrade ejaculation
(d) Primarily mediated by parasympathetic sacral impulses and somatic efferents
2. Female anatomy and neurophysiology
a. Female sexual organs (Johnson & Lanig, 1996) (Refer to Figure 21-3).

Figure 21-2: Innervation of Sexual Orgasms

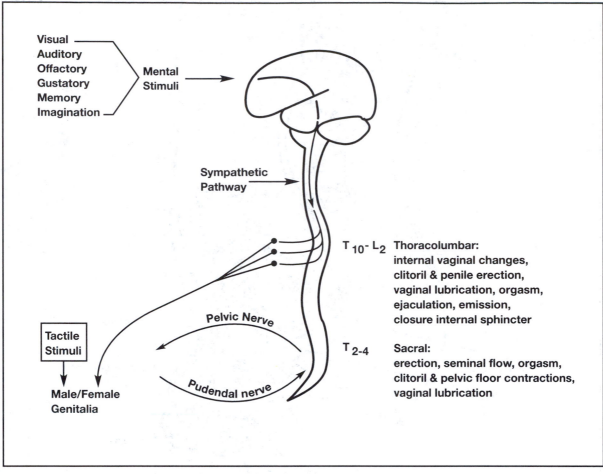

From *Management of Spinal Cord Injury* (2nd ed., p. 180), by C.P. Zejdlik, Ed., 1992, Boston: Jones & Bartlett. Copyright 1992. Reprinted with permission.

(1)   Clitoris: Structure of erectile tissue located anterior to the vaginal opening; extremely sensitive to touch and increases sexual excitement.
(2)   Labia minora and majora: Cover the opening to the vagina
(3)   Vagina: A hollow canal, located between the rectum and urethra, extends from the opening of the labia to the cervix.
(4)   Cervix: The lower, constricted portion of the uterus
(5)   Uterus: A hollow muscular organ, which carries a fetus during pregnancy
(6)   Ovaries: Secrete the hormones estrogen, progesterone, and testosterone and produce ova (eggs). The hormones stimulate pubertal growth and secondary sex characteristics.
(7)   Fallopian tubes: Transport ova

  b. Neurophysiology of sexual response in females: Female sexual response has not been studied as extensively as that of males, although neurologic pathways for female sexual response have been hypothesized as similar to those of males

(1)   Erection: The clitoris becomes engorged. Neural centers at T11 to L1 and S2 to S4 mediate clitoral erection (Szasz, 1992). Vaginal lubrication occurs. Reflexive vaginal lubrication: Probably mediated by sacral parasympathetics. Psychogenic vaginal lubrication: Probably mediated by thoracolumbar sympathetics and sacral parasympathetics.
(2)   Emission: Emission of fluid at the time of orgasm will occur in some women

Figure 21-3: Female Anatomy

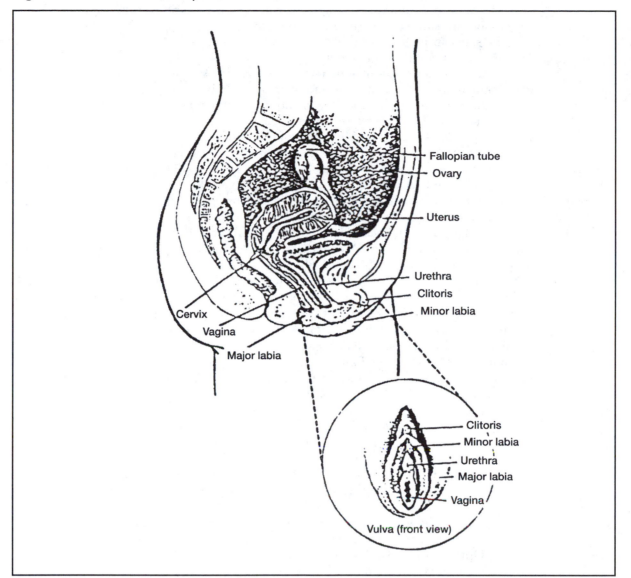

Vulva (front view)

From *Structure and Function of the Human Body* (5th ed.), by R. Memmler et al., illustration by Anthony Raviella, 1992, Philadelphia: J.B. Lippencott. Copyright 1992. Reprinted with permission.

        (3)   Ejaculation: Uterine and pelvic floor contractions mediated by neural centers at T11 to L1 and S2 to S4

  3. Physiologic Sexual Response: Masters and Johnson (1966) outlined four phases of physiologic sexual response

    a. Excitement

      (1)   Males experience penile erection, elevation of the testicles, nipple erection, breast enlargement, beginning of sexual flush, and increased blood pressure, heart rate, and respiration.

      (2)   Females experience vaginal lubrication, enlargement of the clitoris, labial engorgement and separation, nipple erection, breast enlargement, and increased blood pressure, heart rate, and respiration.

    b. Plateau

      (1)   Males continue to experience engorgement of the penis, increased sexual flush, and maximal levels of respiration, blood pressure and heart rate just prior to orgasm.

289

(2) Females experience dilation and elongation of the inner two-thirds of the vagina. The outer one-third of the vagina becomes engorged and constricts (Geiger, 1979). Blood pressure and heart rate continue to increase and blood flow may increase to the skin causing a "sex flush".

c. Orgasm: (Physiological component)

(1) Males experience ejaculation and entire body musculature contractions.

(2) Females in some instances experience an ejaculation. Females will experience entire body musculature contraction, including contractions of the clitoris, uterus, and vagina. Females may experience multiple orgasms.

d. Resolution: This stage is variable in length from person to person

(1) Males experience a refractory period in which further stimulation cannot occur. Detumescence occurs, and there is a gradual resolution of pelvic engorgement. Vital signs return to baseline.

(2) Females experience a gradual reduction of pelvic organ engorgement. Vital signs return to baseline.

4. Common changes in sexual health in men with spinal cord injury

a. Changes in physiologic sexual response are dependent on both level and completeness of SCI (Comarr & Vigue, 1978a, 1978b; Szasz, 1992).

b. Human sexual activity is never a purely physiologic event and is not entirely predictable by level of injury. It is important to encourage individuals with SCI to explore their own bodies, physical capabilities, and physiologic sexual responses (Johnson & Lanig, 1996). It is important, however, for nurses to have knowledge based on how level and degree of injury affect sexual response and orgasm.

c. Common changes in sexual function in males with SCI

(1) Fertility: Severely compromised in SCI for two major reasons; ejaculatory dysfunction and poor semen quality.

(a) Ejaculatory dysfunction
- If the bladder neck fails to close, as in detrussor sphincter dyssynergia, this may result in retrograde ejaculation with sperm being ejaculated into the bladder.
- Fewer than 10 % of men with SCI are able to produce antegrade ejaculation (Bors & Comarr, 1960; Seager & Halstead, 1993), whereby the semen is ejaculated through the end of the urethra.
- A significant number experience retrograde ejaculation (Perkash, Martin, Warner, & Blank, 1985; Sarkarati, Rossier, & Fam, 1987).

(b) Options for sperm retrieval/ejaculation
- Manual stimulation
- Vibratory stimulation: Utilize a vibrator to stimulate ejaculation. Can be done at home. May cause autonomic dysreflexia and skin irritations.
- Electroejaculation: Must be performed by a physician in a clinical setting. Must be monitored for autonomic dysreflexia. May result in retrograde ejaculation. Requires artificial insemination.
- Microaspiration from the epididymis: Surgical procedure to aspirate sperm from the epididymis. Scarring occurs after one or two attempts and will prohibit unlimited attempts at aspiration.
- Subcutaneous physostigmine or intrathecal neostigmine medication: High rate of side effects including nausea, vomiting, headache, autonomic dysreflexia, and death. Not utilized in the United States.

(c) Poor semen quality: Low sperm counts and poor sperm motility (Linsenmeyer, 1988; Linsenmeyer & Perkash, 1991; Phelps et al., 1987; Vervoort, 1987). Poor semen quality is thought to be due to a variety of causes.
- Stasis of seminal fluid
- Recurrent urinary tract infection
- Long-term use of medications such as nitrofurantoin, prostaglandin inhibitors, and alpha blockers.
- Lack of testicular temperature control

(2) Though male fertility may be compromised, contraception should be explored if pregnancy is not desired.

(3) Erectile dysfunction (Courtois, Goulet, Charvier & Leriche, 1999).

  (a) Reflexogenic erection (Refer to Figure 21-4): The result of sensory stimulation and neural transmission via the sacral parasympathetic pathways.
  - Sacral reflex center must be intact
  - Possible in upper motor neuron (UMN) SCI, generally above T11
  - Can be elicited by external tactile stimulation of genitals (e.g., friction from clothing; catheter manipulation; manual or oral stimulation).
  - Can be elicited by internal stimulation (e.g., full bladder).

  (b) Psychogenic erection (Refer to Figure 21-5): Impulses from the hypothalamic area of the brain most likely travel down the lateral columns of the spinal cord to the thoracolumbar sympathetic and sacral parasympathetic pathways to cause psychogenic erections

  (c) (Bennett, Seager, & Vasher, et al, 1988; Linsenmeyer, 1991).
  - May be possible via sympathetic pathways from the brain to thoracolumbar spinal centers.
  - Possible in lower motor neuron (LMN) SCI and UMN SCI if proper pathways are intact.
  - Arise from sights, sounds, smells, or thoughts that are arousing.

Figure 21-4: Reflexogenic Erection

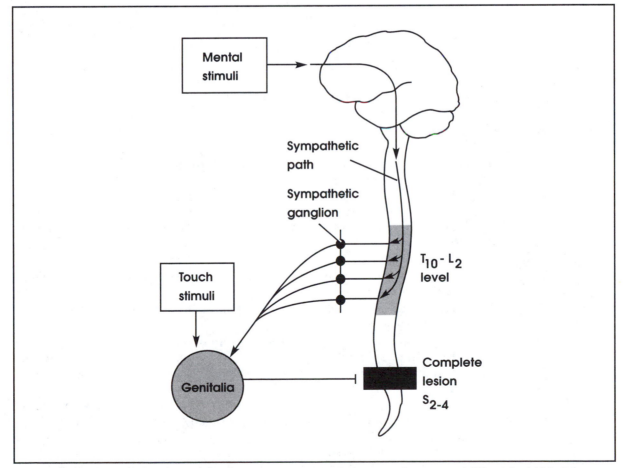

Adapted from *Management of Spinal Cord Injury* (2nd ed., p. 180), by C.P. Zejdlik, Ed., 1992, Boston: Jones & Bartlett. Copyright 1992. Reprinted with permission.

Figure 21-5: Psychogenic Erection

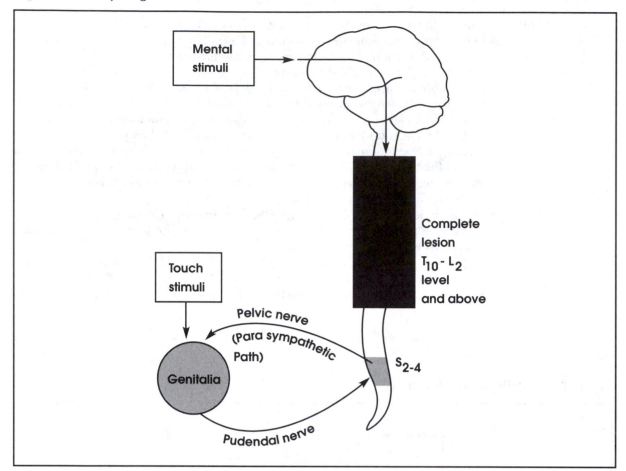

Adapted from *Management of Spinal Cord Injury* (2nd ed., p. 180), by C.P. Zejdlik, Ed., 1992, Boston: Jones & Bartlett. Copyright 1992. Reprinted with permission.

(d) Techniques to restore or compensate erectile function
- Constrictor band
  - Least invasive option
  - Very effective method with strong reflex erection
- Vacuum pump devices or vacuum tumescence devices (Denil, Ohl & Smythe, 1996).
  - Minimally invasive option
  - Avoid/use with caution with perineal skin breakdown, penile implants, anticoagulation therapy.
  - Complications can arise if constriction ring left in place more than 30 minutes or if device used improperly.
  - May require assistance in individuals with limited dexterity.
  - Few complications and high degree of consumer satisfaction if prescribed and used properly (Lloyd, Toth, & Perkash, 1989; Turner, Althof, Levine, & Tobias, 1990).
  - Erection may not be full length and may extend only to base of the penis.
- Intracavernous injection of vasoactive drugs (Yarkony, Chen, Palmer, Roth, Rayner & Lovell, 1995).
  - Non-surgical intervention
  - Papaverine, phentolamine, and prostaglandin E1, either as single drugs or in combination, are the drugs of choice.

- Drugs must be carefully titrated by a qualified health care provider to minimize the risk of complications such as priapism.
- Medication is injected into the cavernosa of the penis.
- Priapism is the most serious complication.
- Individual must be responsible and reliable to utilize this intervention.
  - Transurethral administration of vasoactive drugs.
    - Non-surgical intervention
    - Prostaglandin E1 is available as a suppository, which is administered transurethrally.
    - MUSE (alprostadil) is a prefilled, ready-to-use suppository, inserted with an applicator
    - No need for injection
    - Side effects infrequent but include pain in penis, hypotension, syncope, dizziness, and theoretically priapism (Hellstrom et al, 1996; Padama-Nathan et al, 1997)
  - Oral Sildenifil (Viagra) (Derry, Fraser, Gardner, Gloss, Mayton, Smith, 1998)
    - Non-surgical intervention
    - Effective in men with partial to full reflex erection response
    - Do not use within 48-hours of administration of any nitrate containing medication; may cause severe, life-threatening hypotension
    - Side effects are minimal but may include headache, flushing, dyspepsia, diarrhea, or visual changes such as mild and temporary changes in blue/green colors or increased sensitivity to light
  - Penile prosthesis
    - Inflatable and semi-rigid designs available
    - Operative procedure.
    - Major disadvantage is the cost.
    - Users may be disappointed, as the implants do not typically provide a full-length erection or increase the girth of the penis and this must be discussed prior to implant.
    - Added indication is for maintenance of external catheters.
    - Complications can include rod malfunction, infection, and erosion.
    - Generally an irreversible procedure.
    - Caution should be utilized in recommending for individuals with incomplete injuries early in their recovery.

d. Common changes in sexual health in women with SCI (Jackson & Wadley, 1999)
  (1) Fertility
      (a) Relatively unaffected after SCI
      (b) Temporary amenorrhea for six months to twelve months (50% of women report return of menses after six months, 90% of women report return of menses after 12 months). (Axel, 1982; Charlifue, Gerhart, Menter, Whiteneck, & Manley, 1992; Comarr, 1966; Linsenmeyer, 2000).
  (2) Contraception: options for females should be presented, including known risks and benefits for each method (Refer to Table 21-1).
  (3) Pregnancy: The SCI team and labor and delivery team must work closely together to prevent complications
      (a) Some indication exists that women who are injured while pregnant may experience a higher rate of early labor and low-birth-weight babies (Baker & Cardenas, 1996; Charlifue, et al, 1992; Sipski, 1991; Verduyn, 1986).
      (b) Anemia: Although women with SCI are not more prone to anemia than other women, the effects of anemia can have serious consequences for them:
          - Alteration in skin integrity
          - Decreased energy levels
          - Dietary counseling should be incorporated into prenatal care to avoid or minimize anemia.
          - Iron supplements may be necessary.

Table 21-1: Contraceptive Options

Type	Advantages	Disadvantages
Natural Family Planning (rhythm method or mucous method)	• May be acceptable to couples having religious concerns about other forms of birth control. • No side effects. • Minimal cost. • Can fairly predict start of menstrual periods.	• Taking daily temperature, mucous checks, and record keeping may be a problem. • Temperature and mucous checks may be difficult if hand functions are limited. • Must have a regular cycle to use. • Certain life stresses may alter monthly cycle. • Requires self-control and planning, may limit spontaneity.
Sterilization	• Most definitive method. • After initial surgery, health risks are low.	• Fertility can seldom be restored. • Possibility of swelling, bleeding, autonomic dysreflexia, or infection during postoperative recovery.
Diaphragm	• Can be used only when needed. • Very effective when used correctly. • Minimal side effects. • More effective if used with a condom. • Must be used with a spermicidal jelly or cream.	• Can cause pressure against bladder, leading to infections or unexpected urination. • Can cause irritation to the vagina or cervix. • May become dislodged in women with relaxed vagina. • Must have good hand dexterity to insert and check placement. May require placement by attendant or partner. • Fit must be reexamined every one or two years routinely, after childbirth, and with weight gain or loss. • Must be worn for several hours after intercourse.
Cervical Cap	• Minimal side effects. • Very effective when used correctly. • May be worn longer than a diaphragm. • Less spermicide needed than with a diaphragm. • Can be used with loose vaginal muscles or bladder pressure problems. • More effective if used with a condom.	• Requires full hand function for insertion and removal. May require placement by attendant or partner assistance. • Cannot be used if abnormal pap smear, toxic shock history, vaginitis, or cervicitis. • May cause irritation of the cervix.
Condom	• Protects against sexually transmitted disease. • Improves effectiveness of other methods. • Easy to obtain, no prescription. • Easy to use and dispose of. • Minimal side effects. • Can be used only when needed. • More effective if used with spermicide or barriers.	• May leak or tear, especially if dried out, used with oil-based lubricant, used with no lubricant at all, or not worn properly. • Application necessary, may decrease spontaneity. • May decrease sensation. • Requires cooperation of male. • More effective if used with lubricant. • Failure rate high if used alone.
Spermicides (foam, jelly, cream)	• Easy to obtain, no prescription. • Can be used only as needed. • More effective if used with condom. • Provides vaginal lubrication.	• Must be used at time of intercourse, may decrease spontaneity. • Somewhat messy, may discourage oral sex. Insertion may be difficult if hand function limited. • Chemical may irritate both partners. • Less effective if used in isolation.

continued on page 295

Table 21-1: Continued

Type	Advantages	Disadvantages
Oral Contraceptives	• Regulate menses, reduce cramping. • Shorten menses, decrease flow. • Convenient to use. • Decrease risk of ovarian and endometrial cancer. • Decrease risk of pelvic inflammatory disease. • Very effective in preventing pregnancy. • Decrease risk of benign breast disease. • Can predict start of menstrual periods.	• High risk of blood clots in SCI women who may be unaware because cannot feel the pain of the clot. • Possible interaction with other medications that cause decreased effectiveness of oral contraceptives. • Weight gain possible, which may cause mobility problems. • Potential increased risk of cardiovascular disease, strokes, hypertension, breast cancer. • Must take pill routinely for effectiveness - with even one missed pill, another method must be utilized until back on cycle.
Norplant	• As effective as oral contraceptives. • Easy insertion procedure. • Can be in place for up to five years. • Does not interfere with spontaneity. • No hand function required.	• Side effects may include irregular bleeding. • No long-term studies of use or side effects in SCI women (e.g., blood clots).
Intrauterine Device (IUD)	• Very effective. • Can be in place for up to eight years. • Does not interfere with spontaneity. • No hand function required. • Relatively easy insertion procedure in a health care provider's office.	• Problems such as perforation might go undetected in women with SCI due to inability to feel pain. • More problems with cramping and perforation in women who have never been pregnant. • Increased risk for pelvic inflammatory disease in women with more than one partner. • Increased uterine cramping (which may cause increased dysreflexia in women who experience autonomic dysreflexia with menstrual cramps). • May cause heavier menses.

Adapted from *Spinal Cord Injury Patient Education Manual*, by Craig Hospital, 1992, Englewood, CO. Copyright 1992. Reprinted with permission.

(c) Bladder management issues
- Increased frequency of urinary tract infections due to incomplete bladder emptying. Monitor closely and aggressively prevent and treat. Pyelonephritis may initiate pre-term labor.
- Attempt to eradicate asymptomatic bacteriuria: minimize residual volumes, avoid indwelling catheters if possible, and use antibiotics when needed (Baker& Cardenas, 1996).
- An indwelling catheter may become necessary due to increased frequency of bladder emptying and difficulty with intermittent catheterization because of increased abdominal girth and difficulty with mobility. This intervention should be instituted only after careful consideration of other bladder-emptying techniques.

       (d) Bowel management issues
- Constipation and hemorrhoids: Dietary changes, changes in bowel routines, and changes in medications such as stool softeners, suppositories, and laxatives may be necessary.

       (e) Mobility issues:
- Transfers may require addition of transfer boards or assistance.
- Weight shifts may become more difficult, requiring alterations in equipment, cushions, utilization of assistance, and routines.
- Bed mobility may become difficult, requiring addition of equipment or assistance.

       (f) Thrombophlebitis
- Management of edema is essential.
- May need more frequent elevation of feet or support stockings.

       (g) Pressure ulcers: Risk for development of pressure ulcers increases during pregnancy due to increased weight and size.
- Prevention of anemia is important to prevent pressure ulcer development.
- Adequate weight shifts
- Proper equipment, including wheelchairs and cushions, need to be evaluated and prescribed.

       (h) Medications must be reviewed to determine their safety during pregnancy and breast-feeding.

  (4) Labor

       (a) Women with SCI above the T10 level may not be able to detect the beginning of labor. Women with SCI below T10 should be able to experience labor, although their subjective experience is different than for able-bodied women (Baker & Cardenas, 1996). Pain from the first stage of labor (onset of active labor to complete cervical dilation) is transmitted by sympathetic fibers that enter the spinal cord at T10-T12 and L1. The second stage of labor (from full cervical dilation to delivery) involves pain from pressure and distention of perineal tissues. These signals travel along the pudendal nerve and enter the spinal cord at S2-S4.

       (b) Labor may be detected by appearance of strong abdominal spasms, leg spasms, difficulty breathing, or back pain.

       (c) Close clinical monitoring should begin in weeks 28-32 to detect cervical dilation, which may necessitate bedrest until delivery.

       (d) Labor has been reported to be average or shorter in the first stage, but longer in the second stage, due to the inability to push if the abdominal muscles are affected by SCI.

       (e) Induction of labor can precipitate autonomic dysreflexia and therefore needs careful consideration before it is instituted (Sipski, 1991).

       (f) Autonomic dysreflexia must be managed during labor to prevent further complications.
- Autonomic dysreflexia needs to be differentiated from preeclampsia.
- The hypertension of autonomic dysreflexia generally fluctuates with contractions.
- Bradycardia is usually present.
- The hypertension of preeclampsia does not fluctuate. Tachycardia is usually present. The presence of proteinuria and edema is more consistent with preeclampsia.
- Epidural anesthesia with lidocaine (or its derivitives) or meperidine (Baraka, 1985) can be utilized during labor and delivery to prevent and treat autonomic dysreflexia (Warner, et al, 1987).
- Labor and delivery staff need to be educated regarding care of the woman with SCI, including the risk for pressure ulcer development.

  (5) Delivery

       (a) Women with SCI can carry to term, and deliver normal babies, most often through normal vaginal deliveries (Drench, 1992)

(b) There is a higher incidence of forceps delivery due to a lack of abdominal muscles to push (Sipski, 1991).

(c) Cesarean section is reported in approximately 7 percent of deliveries of women with SCI. It may be indicated in autonomic dysreflexia unresponsive to pharmacological or anesthetic interventions (Baker & Cardenas, 1996).

(d) Regional anesthesia is most widely used to prevent autonomic dysreflexia in labor and delivery (Baker & Cardenas, 1996).

(6) Alterations in vaginal lubrication: There may be changes in a woman's ability to lubricate in preparation for intercourse or other forms of vaginal penetration.

(a) Reflexive vaginal lubrication: Probably mediated by sacral parasympathetics. Most likely occurs in females with upper motor neuron lesions (Sipski, 1991).

(b) Psychogenic vaginal lubrication: Probably mediated by thoracolumbar sympathetics and sacral parasympathetics. May occur in incomplete upper motor neuron lesions, and possible in lower motor neuron lesions (Sipski, 1991).

(7) Orgasm

(a) Overall decrease in ability to achieve orgasm compared to women without SCI (Sipski, Alexander, & Rosen, 1995).

(b) Vagus nerve is a pathway for transmission of non-genital orgasms (DeKoker, 1996).

(c) May take longer time of stimulation to achieve orgasm.

(d) Self-exploration, masturbation, and vibrators may assist women to achieve orgasm.

(e) Degree or type of SCI not related to ability to achieve orgasm (Sipski, 1991).

(f) Knowledge about sexuality has been linked to ability to achieve orgasm and is an important nursing intervention (Sipski et al, 1995).

(g) Sildenifil may improve sexual response/orgasm (Sipski, Rosen, Alexander, Hamer, 2000).

III. Initial Assessment

A. **Nursing sexual health assessment** (Szasz, 1992; Williams, 1993; McBride & Rines, 2000)
1. Determining individual readiness
   a. Determine individual readiness for sexual health assessment.
   b. Secure permission to complete a sexual health assessment.
   c. Provide for privacy and adequate scheduled time for the assessment.
   d. The assessment should be structured to the desires and comfort level of the patient, but ideally should include separate and joint interviews of the patient and the partner (if applicable).
2. Physiological sexual response and activity status/ physical assessment
   a. Presence of genital sensation
   b. Available motor function
   c. Presence of erection, ejaculation, vaginal lubrication, orgasm
   d. Appliances, stomas, and other anatomical considerations for sexual function
3. Sexual knowledge and practices/ psychosocial assessment
   a. Knowledge of sexual function and effects of SCI
   b. Importance of sexual activity
   c. Inventory of personal values: moral and religious concerns pertaining to sexuality, parenting issues.
   d. Pre-injury sexual patterns: to determine areas for exploration with current sexual health status. For example, information on past sexual techniques and practices would help with planning for sexual activity and compensatory methods for techniques for current sexual practice and technique as needed.
   (1) Frequency of sexual activity
   (2) Techniques, practices, and methods of sexual expression
   (3) Erogenous zones

(4) Relationship history
(5) Past difficulties with sexual function
e. Psychological and emotional status.
    (1) Current mental status
    (2) Self-perception and body image
    (3) Fears and concerns
    (4) Prior sexual abuse
f. Current sexual practices: Any sexual experiences since injury
g. Fertility
    (1) Females
        (a) Menstrual and menopausal history
        (b) Knowledge and history of contraception
        (c) Reproductive history
        (d) Previous reproductive difficulties
    (2) Males
        (a) Knowledge and history of contraception
        (b) Reproductive history
        (c) Previous reproductive difficulties
        (d) Erectile difficulties prior to injury and current erectile status
h. Medication and substance use/abuse:
    (1) Many medications can interfere with sexual function or libido; therefore it is important to take a medication history to utilize in sexual health counseling.
    (2) Medications commonly utilized by individuals with SCI can interfere with sexual health
        (a) Alcohol
        (b) Narcotics
        (c) Antispasmodics
        (d) Antihypertensives
        (e) Antidepressants
        (f) Sedatives and tranquilizers

B. **Physical examination**: The physical exam can generally be obtained from the medical history and physical and would not necessarily routinely be obtained by a nurse on initial assessment. The information, however, is critical to a comprehensive sexual health assessment.
1. Motor sensory exam
    a. General motor sensory exam to determine level of injury and motor sensory function.
    b. Motor and sensory exam of the genital area
        (1) Anal contraction.
        (2) Bulbocavernosus Reflex (Szasz, 1992)
            (a) Insert a finger in the rectum, squeeze the tip of the penis or apply pressure to the clitoris to elicit anal contraction.
            (b) If present, the sacral reflex is intact.
            (c) If present, reflex erection is likely in men; significance not determined in women.
2. Genitourinary exam: Physical exam of genito-rectal area

IV. Nursing Process Applied to Promotion and Maintenance of Sexual Health

A. **Nursing Diagnosis**: Actual or potential alteration in sexual health

B. **Defining Characteristics** (Williams, 1993):
1. Reported difficulties in sexual behaviors or activities
2. Limitations in sexual behaviors or activities
3. Changes in sexual behaviors or activities

C. **Expected Outcomes** (Williams, 1993):
1. Demonstrates adequate knowledge of basic sexual function and sexual changes related to spinal cord injury
2. Reports being satisfied with sexuality, sexual activity, and relationships
3. Demonstrates adequate and safe use of contraception.
4. Verbalizes adequate reproductive knowledge, abilities, and resources.
5. Verbalizes knowledge about prevention of sexually transmitted diseases.
6. Verbalizes knowledge about prevention of sexual abuse.

D. **Interventions**: All nursing interventions should be conducted to the level of the patient's knowledge and competence. Nurses should be able to give permission to address the topics involved in sexual health, provide basic level education, and triage individuals with SCI to qualified sexual health practitioners for further information or treatment.
1. Altered body structure or function
   a. Paralysis/Paraparesis: knowledge of level of paralysis or paresis and common physiologic changes by level of injury to provide sexual health education and counseling to the individual with SCI. Health education and counseling may involve suggestions on positioning, adaptive equipment, and suggestions for intimate activity other than intercourse (e.g., caressing, hugging, fondling, kissing, oral sex, self- or mutual masturbation, etc.).
   b. Alteration in sensation: knowledge of level and degree of sensory impairment to provide sexual health education and counseling. Health education and counseling may involve suggestions for self-exploration or exploration with a partner of erogenous zones such as sensate focusing. Health education and counseling may involve suggestions of how to deal with insensate areas or hypersensitive areas during sexual activity (e.g., visualization, fantasy, use or avoidance of hypersensitive areas).
   c. Autonomic dysreflexia (AD): a discussion and anticipatory guidance regarding AD during sexual health education and counseling, including the fact that it may occur during physical sexual activity, orgasm, labor and delivery, etc.
   d. Spasticity: anticipatory guidance and a discussion of suggestions such as positioning and timing of medications.
   e. Altered elimination pattern: health education and counseling regarding bowel and bladder management relative to sexual activity. Individuals with SCI should be educated to plan sexual activity around bowel and bladder care to avoid accidents. Bowel and bladder management should be discussed with the sexual partner. Preparation in the event of an accident should be explored with the patient. The nurse can assist the patient with strategies on how to address these issues. Practical suggestions for how to manage a catheter may include how to manage a catheter tube by removing it or taping it to the abdomen or thigh or keeping a towel handy in case of an accident.
   f. Pain: health education and counseling regarding positioning and other pain management techniques to prevent pain from interfering with sexual activity. The potential effect of pain medications on libido and physical sexual response should be discussed as well.
   g. Positioning difficulties: practical suggestions for positioning in the event the individual with SCI has contractures or respiratory distress that prevent sexual activity in previously utilized positions for that individual.
   h. Mobility deficits: practical suggestions for transfers or other mobility issues that may interfere with an individual's ability to feel sensual in intimate situations. Practical suggestions may also include how to communicate with a partner about turning and positioning, caressing and hugging, or dressing and undressing.
   i. Erectile dysfunction: basic education regarding the effects of SCI on erections by level of injury, thorough evaluation of erectile status, and health education and counseling regarding options for achieving an erection.
   j. Retrograde ejaculation: education and counseling regarding the effect of SCI on ejaculatory function. Options to explore for fertility counseling, including assisted ejaculation, may be discussed with the individual.

k. Alteration in vaginal lubrication: health education regarding vaginal lubrication and the need to use a water-soluble lubricant to prevent tissue trauma during sexual activity.

l. Altered orgasm or anorgasmia: education and counseling regarding the effect of SCI on orgasm. Practical suggestions may include a discussion regarding what orgasm meant before injury and how to focus on those sensations that may occur as orgasm after injury. The psychosocial component of orgasm should be included in this counseling.

2. Medications: Medications need to be reviewed and potential side effects relative to sexual function discussed. Many medications utilized in the management of SCI affect erections, sensations, muscle tone, libido, etc., and thus may interfere with desired sexual function or response.

3. Substance use/abuse: The effects of alcohol, tobacco, and other drugs should be reviewed with individuals with SCI in relation to their effects on sexual function (e.g., the effects of alcohol and marijuana on erections).

4. Alteration in self-esteem: health education and counseling regarding how to establish new or re-establish old relationships, and how to incorporate a discussion of SCI in relation to sexual health. The nurse should foster increased self-esteem by creating an atmosphere of permission and acceptance. Individual counseling and support as well as peer support are helpful interventions.

5. Alteration in body image: sexual health education and counseling regarding personal hygiene or how to dress to feel sexually attractive.

6. Knowledge deficit related to affect of SCI on sexuality and sexual health: sexual health education and anticipatory guidance for the individual with SCI. Partner(s) and family should be provided education and anticipatory guidance as appropriate. Education should include:

a. Basic anatomy and neurophysiology of sexual function.

b. Consequences of SCI on physiologic sexual response and fertility, and options for management.

c. Information regarding sexuality and methods of sexual expression other than intercourse.

d. The impact of SCI on psychosocial sexual response, including sexual self-concept and self-esteem
   (1) Communication and assertiveness training skill building activities.
   (2) Group discussions and peer counseling
   (3) The importance of promoting a positive impression of self to others

e. Safety issues
   (1) Contraception: The need for contraception should be discussed. Risks and benefits of each contraceptive method should be presented.
   (2) Use of sexual aids: Safe use of sexual aids should be covered, to prevent tissue injury and spread of sexually transmitted diseases.
   (3) Sexually transmitted disease: Safer sex practices should be covered with all patients receiving sexual health education.
   (4) Autonomic dysreflexia with sexual activity: Anticipatory guidance should be covered with all patients with T6 injuries and above regarding the potential for AD during intercourse, ejaculation, orgasm, labor and delivery, etc.
   (5) Sexual and physical abuse: The possibility and prevention of physical and sexual abuse, as well as how to report abuse, should be covered during sexual health education.
   (6) Refer to other providers as needed.
      (a) Nurse specialist
      (b) Social worker, psychologist, therapist, or physician
      (c) Fertility or reproduction specialist
      (d) Sex therapist

V. Reassessment

Ideally, individuals with SCI should be reassessed with each preventive or routine entry into the health care system.

A. **Nursing History**:
  1. Identify areas of confusion and misinformation.
  2. Assess changes in the individual's sexual functioning pattern and marital and social relationships over time.
  3. Evaluate readiness to learn additional sexual information such as alternative sexual activities.

B. **Examination**:
  1. Based on specific patient complaints or concerns at the time of re-evaluation.
  2. Motor-sensory exam performed on initial contact, as outlined in initial exam, may have to be repeated.

C. **Diagnostic Studies**:
  1. Based on specific patient complaints or concerns at the time of re-evaluation.
  2. Any or all of the studies outlined in the initial exam may have to be repeated.
  3. Diagnostic studies initiated by a physician or an advanced practice nurse may be utilized for a more comprehensive evaluation of physiologic function for the purpose of diagnosis or to evaluate for more intensive intervention
     a. Erectile studies
       (1) Doppler studies to assess penile blood flow
       (2) Pharmacological erection testing
           (a) Prostaglandin E1
           (b) Papaverine
           (c) Papaverine and phentolamine
     b. Laboratory tests
       (1) Testosterone levels
       (2) Sperm evaluation
       (3) Sperm count
       (4) Sperm motility

VI. Health Education Tips

A. **Sexual health promotion activities** (Johnson & Lanig, 1996).
  1. A comprehensive, interdisciplinary approach to sexual health is most effective.
  2. Patients will approach a variety of members of the health care team for sexual health information as they attemt to secure information pertinent to their sexual selves.
  3. All members of the health care team must be knowledgeable in basic information and available resources.
  4. Training opportunities are often necessary for all staff (including physicians) to enhance their skills in responding professionally and comfortably when confronted with direct or indirect sexual health "information-seeking behaviours" by patients. Training for health professionals is most effective if there is a component of skills development provided through one-on-one practice assessments with one-on-one feedback (Tepper, 1994).
  5. Staff should complete a self-inventory of personal beliefs, values, and comfort levels in regard to sexual health management, know their own knowledge levels and comfort zones, and know when to refer sexual health issues to other members of the team.

B. **Increasing staff comfort with sexuality and SCI** (Herson, Hart, Gordon, Rintala, 1999).
  1. Staff can review and discuss audiovisual and written materials related to sexuality and spinal cord injury.
  2. Role-play question-and-answer sessions regarding questions or specific situations patients or families pose

3. Make a commitment to initiate conversations with patients about sexuality.
4. Sexuality and SCI should be included in nurse orientation and continuing education.

C. **Increasing comfort and knowledge of sexuality for individuals with SCI**
   1. Assess patient readiness before presenting information.
   2. Look for opportunities for patient/family education.
   3. Provide an open and non-judgmental environment.
   4. Address sexuality issues early.
   5. Be aware that differences in verbal styles and skills may have an impact on the ability people have to express their attitudes and needs.
   6. Observe patientís individual learning styles and competency.
   7. Observe the style of communication between that patient and the patientís partner to facilitate a discussion about sexuality concerns.
   8. Focus discussion on the physical and emotional aspects of sexuality.
   9. Consider using gender to gender discussions to promote comfort and open discussions.
   10. Promote peer counseling.

D. **PLISSIT**: defines levels of staff involvement (Annon, 1974).
   1. A widely accepted comprehensive model combines educational strategies with behavioral interventions to integrate human sexuality into the rehabilitation of individuals with SCI (Madorsky & Dixon, 1983).
   2. Allows each member of the health care team to participate at their own level of skill, knowledge, and comfort (Lemon, 1993).
   3. PLISSIT (Refer to Table 21-2)
      a. P = Permission.
         (1) Health professional asks if there are questions or concerns regarding sexuality.
         (2) Lets the individual know that "sex is spoken here" (Szasz, 1992).
         (3) Frequently, this is the only level of intervention required.
         (4) Professionals do not need to be experts on sexual function at this level but do need to be comfortable and have a minimum knowledge base.
         (5) Effective listening skills, interpersonal sensitivity, and a willingness to suspend judgment are important prerequisites (Ducharme & Gill, 1991).
         (6) Example: The nurse may give permission and open the lines for communication by saying to the patient, "Many people who are newly injured have questions about sexuality. If you have any questions or concerns, do not hesitate to ask." Many patients do not ask direct questions but may indicate their need for information

Table 21-2: PLISSIT Model

P =	Permission: Individuals should be assured, through permission giving, that it is permissible, acceptable, and entirely normal to have questions and concerns about their sexuality and to continue to explore and behave in a sexual manner.
LI =	Limited Information: All members of the health care team should be knowledgeable about and comfortable with at least some basic information about sexuality and spinal cord injury and be able to provide limited information to individuals and families with whom they work.
SS =	Specific Suggestions: These should relate to identified areas of concern of an individual and be directed to changing behavior to change those concerns.
IT =	Intensive Therapy: The individual requiring this level of highly individualized intervention should be referred to a professional with the time, experience, and knowledge to address the individual's needs.

From "Sexual Counseling and Spinal Cord Injury" by M. A. Lemon, 1993, *Sexuality and Disability,* *II*(1), pp. 73-96. Copyright 1993. Reprinted with permission.

through indirect questioning during personal care, making statements such as "what good am I to my husband/wife now," or making inappropriate sexual advances. The nurse should reassure the patient that the needs are legitimate and attempt to find out what information they are actually seeking (Lemon, 1993).

    b. LI = Limited information
      (1) Nurses should be knowledgeable in basic information about sexuality and issues after SCI and be able to provide limited information.
      (2) Verbal, written, and/or audiovisual presentations are useful means of delivering information.
      (3) Information dissemination at this level can help correct patient misconceptions or prevent future anxieties.
      (4) Team members must know when to refer an individual for more individual or detailed assistance (Ducharme & Gill, 1991).
      (5) Example: The nurse may provide the patient, and partners if appropriate, information on basic sexual function, effects of SCI on sexual function, and information on bowel and bladder management in relationship to sexual function, based on the patient's desire for these types of information (Lemon, 1993).

    c. SS = Specific suggestions
      (1) Address concerns in greater detail; Generally requires professionals with expertise in SCI and sexual health.
      (2) Specific suggestions on positioning, bowel and bladder management, contraception, reproduction, or options for achieving and maintaining penile erections can be provided (Ducharme & Gill, 1991).
      (3) Example: Nurses may give specific suggestions in regard to planning for intimate activity. If the individual with SCI needs assistance in transferring, undressing, etc., the partner might order out dinner to eliminate an energy-consuming task and reserve more energy and focus on preparing for the intimate events (Lemon, 1993).

    d. IT = Intensive therapy
      (1) Provided by a trained counselor.
      (2) Frequently requires interpersonal relationship counseling or in-depth exploration of sexual identity and psychosocial issues.
      (3) Example: Examples of issues that may require intensive therapy are teaching an individual or a couple social assertion skills

E. **Sexual first aid** (Szasz, 1992)
  1. Although an organized sexual health program is the ideal, it is not always possible in all settings.
  2. Individuals may desire sexual health information at unpredictable moments.
  3. Sexual first aid refers to a form of brief intervention undertaken at the time the need for assistance is perceived (Szasz, 1992).
  4. Four components of sexual first aid.
    a. Acceptance of directly or indirectly expressed sexual concerns
    b. Clarification of concerns
    c. Giving of information
    d. Application of personal knowledge to sexual areas

VII. Special Issues Related to Pediatric Care

A. Issues concerning sexuality naturally surface as children mature and may be particularly difficult for parents to discuss. Concerns such as attractiveness, and being a romantic partner or potential parent can affect body image and esteem, and need to be addressed.

B. **Education**
  1. Child and/or parent may be given information on sexuality regardless of child's age at injury.
  2. Age-appropriate education may be given in different formats based on developmental stage, cognition, and needs of child/parents. Content, with parental consent, may include:

a. Respect for child's body and right to privacy
b. Correct identification of anatomy and use of appropriate terminology, normal physiology, and changes that occur during puberty
c. Physiological function based on level of injury
d. Dating
e. Fertility
f. Safe sex
g. Contraception, including latex allergy concerns
h. Gynecological consultation for adolescent girls

C. **Physical, sexual, emotional abuse**
1. Should be discussed early and with each new developmental stage.
2. Children with disabilities may be at a higher risk for abuse.

Practical Application #1

S.W., a 28-year old female with T4 paraplegia, was preparing for her first weekend visit home. The woman was married three years prior to her injury. She and her husband have no children, but are planning a family next year after he finishes graduate school. S.W. expressed fear about what her first visit home will be like and how her husband will react to her disability. The primary nurse developed a comfortable professional relationship with S.W. and felt comfortable with her basic knowledge of SCI and sexual function. The nurse asked S.W. if she would like to further discuss her concerns. S.W. said she would, but she needed to get to therapy. The nurse made an appointment to meet later that day with S.W. in a private conference room. The nurse prepared for the meeting by gathering appropriate written and audiovisual resources and planned to further explore immediate concerns, fears, and needs that should be addressed prior to her home visit. The nurse also planned to explore if and when S.W. would like her husband brought into the discussion and educational process. The nurse will then determine what she can provide in the form of support, education, and counseling, and what other resources may be needed to continue the support and educational process. One of the most immediate concerns the nurse must address prior to the home visit is the issue of contraception. The nurse should explore what method of contraception was practiced prior to SCI and explore alternatives for current contraceptive use if pregnancy is not desired at this time.

Practical Application #2

B.T., a 25-year old homosexual male with T12 paraplegia asked his primary nurse questions about his sexual function. In particular he was interested in learning if he will ever be able to have erections again. He has no partner, but was sexually active prior to his injury and anticipates being active after he is discharged from the hospital and reintegrates into the community. His primary nurse was somewhat embarrassed to discuss B.T.'s sexual needs and felt she had limited information regarding sexual health and homosexuality to be able to appropriately educate him. The nurse validated B.T.'s need for information and asked his permission to refer his needs to the clinical nurse specialist. B.T. agreed, and also agreed to have the primary nurse participate in the learning experience with him and the clinical nurse specialist so that she could gain knowledge to deal with a similar situation in the future. The clinical nurse specialist covered the potential effects of the SCI on erectile function and explored with B.T. how he could self explore his ability to have erections. The clinical nurse specialist also gave B.T. some written information on options for managing erectile dysfunction should this be a future need. The clinical nurse specialist provided B.T. with information on prevention of sexually transmitted diseases as well as on prevention of sexual abuse. The clinical nurse specialist made a follow-up appointment with B.T. for a later date to further explore sexual health issues. The clinical specialist also planned a meeting with the primary nurse to discuss her learning needs regarding sexual health and SCI.

References and Selected Bibliography

Annon, J. (1974). *The behavioral treatment of sexual problems* (Vol. 1). Honolulu, HI: Kapioniani Health Services.

Axel, S.J. (1982). Spinal cord injured women's concerns: Menstruation and pregnancy. *Rehabilitation Nursing, 7*(5), 10-15.

Baker, E.R., & Cardenas, D.D. (1996). Pregnancy in spinal cord injured women. *Archives of Physical Medicine and Rehabilitation, 77*, 501-7.

Baraka, A. (1985). Epidural meperidine for control of autonomic hyperreflexia in a paraplegic patient. *Anesthesiology, 62*, 688.

Bennett, C.J., Seager, S.W., Vasher, E.A. (1988). Sexual dysfunction and electroejaculation in men with spinal cord injury: A review. *Journal of Urology, 139*(3), 453-457.

Bors, E., & Comarr, E., (1960). Neurological disturbances of sexual function with special reference to 529 patients with spinal cord injury. *Urological Survey, 10*, 191-222.

Charlifue, S.W., Gerhart, K.A., Menter, R.R., Whiteneck, G.G., & Manley, S. (1992). Sexual issues of women with spinal cord injury. *International Medical Society of Paraplegia, 30*, 192-199.

Comarr, A.E. (1966). Observations of menstruation and pregnancy among female spinal cord injury patients. *Paraplegia, 3*, 263-272.

Comarr , A., & Vigue, M. (1978a). Sexual counseling among male and female patients with spinal cord injury and/or quada equina injury: part 1. *American Journal of Physical Medicine, 57*, 107-122.

Comarr, A., & Vigue, M. (1978b).). Sexual counseling among male and female patients with spinal cord injury and/or quada equina injury: part 2. *American Journal of Physical Medicine, 57*, 215-227.

Courtois, F.J., Goulet, M.C., Charvier, K.F. & Lericke, A. (1999). Pasttraumatic erectile potential of spinal cord injured men: how physiologic recordings supplement subjective reports. *Archives of Physical Medicine and Rehabilitation, 80*, 1268-1272.

Craig Hospital. (1992). *Spinal Cord Injury Patient Education Manual*. Englewood, CO: Craig Hospital

DeKoker, B. (1996). Sex and the spinal cord: a new pathway for orgasm. *Scientific American, 275(6)*, 30-32.

Denil, J, Ohl, DL & Smythe, C. (1996). Vacuum erection device in spinal cord injured men: patient and partner satisfaction. *Archives of Physical Medicine and Rehabilitation, 77*, 750-753.

Derry, F.A., Dunsmore, W.W., Fraser, M., Gardner, B.P., Glass, C.A., Mayton, M.C. & Smith, M.D. (1998). Efficacy and safety of oral sildenifil (viagra) in men with erectile dysfunction caused by spinal cord injury. *American Academy of Neurology, 51*, 1629-1633.

Drench, M. (1992). Impact of altered sexual function in spinal cord injury: A review. *Sexuality and Disability, 10*(1), 3-13.

Ducharme, S., & Gill, K.M. (1991). Sexual values, training and professional roles. In R.P. Marinelli & A.E. Dell Orto (Eds.), *The psychological and social impact of disability*, (3rd ed.). New York: Springer.

Greiger, R.C. (1979). Neurophysiology of sexual response in spinal cord injury. *Sexuality and Disability, 2*(4), 257-266.

Hellstrom, W.J.G., Bennett, A.H., Gesundheit, N., Kaiser, F.E., Lue, T.F., Padma-Nathan, H., Peterson, C.A., Tam, P.Y., Todd, L.K., Uarady, J.C., & Place, V.A. (1996). A double-blind, placebo-controlled evaluation of the erectile response to transurethral alprostadil. *Urology, 48*(6), 851-856.

Herson, L., Hart, K.A., Gordon, M.J. & Rintala, D.H.> (1999). Identifying and overcoming barriers to providing sexuality information in the clinical setting. *Rehabilitation Nursing, 24(4)*, 148-151.

Kroll, K., & Klein, E.L. (1992). *Enabling romance: A guide to love, sex, and relationships for the disabled (and the people who care about them)*. New York: Harmony.

Jackson, A.B. & Wadley, V. (1999). A multicenter study of women's self-reported reproductive health after spinal cord injury. *Archives of Physical Medicine and Rehabilitation, 80*, 1420-1428.

Johnson, K.M.M., & Lanig, I.S. (1996). Promotion and maintenance of sexual health in individuals with spinal cord injury. In *A practical guide to health promotion after spinal cord injury*, IS Lanig (Ed.).Gaithersburg, MD: Aspen.

Lemon, M.A. (1993). Sexual counseling and spinal cord injury. *Sexuality and Disability, 11*(1), 73-96.

Linsenmeyer, T.A. (1988). Infertility following spinal cord injury: Where are we and where are we going. *Sexuality Update, 1*, 5.

Linsenmeyer, T.A. (1991). Evaluation and treatment of erectile dysfunction following spinal cord injury: A review. *Journal of the American Paraplegia Society, 14*, 43-51.

Linsenmeyer, T.A., & Perkash, I. (1991). Infertility in men with spinal cord injury. *Archives of Physical Medicine and Rehabilitation, 72*, 747-754.

Linsenmeyer, T.A. (2000). Sexual function and infertility following spinal cord injury. *Physical Medicine and Rehabilitation Clinics of North America, 11(1)*, 141-156.

Lloyd, E.E., Toth, L.L., & Perkash, I. (1989). Vacuum tumescence: An option for spinal cord injured males with erectile dysfunction. *SCI Nursing, 6*, 25.

Madorsky, J.G.B., & Dixon, T.P. (1983). Rehabilitation aspects of human sexuality. *Western Journal of Medicine, 139*, 174-176.

Masters, W.H. & Johnson, V.E. (1966). *Human sexual inadequacy*. Boston: Little Brown.

McBride, K.E. & Rines, B. (2000). Sexuality and spinal cord injury: a road map for nurses. *SCI Nursing, 17(1)*, 8-13.

Memmler, R. , et.al. (1992). *Structure and function of the human body* (5th Edition). Philadelphia, PA: J.B.Lippincott.

Padama-Nathan, H., Hellstrom, W.J.G., Kaiser, F.E., Labashy, R.F., Lue, T.F., Nolten, W.E., Norweeod, P.C., Peterson, C.A., Shaksigh, R., Tam, P.Y., Place, V.A., & Gesundheit, N. (1997). Treatment of men with erectile dysfunction with transurethral alprostadil. *New England Journal of Medicine, 336*, 1-7.

Perkash, I., Martin, D.E., Warner, H., & Blank, M.S. (1985). Reproductive biology of paraplegics: Results of semen collection, testicular biopsy and serum hormone. Journal of Urology, 134, 284-288.

Phelps, G., Brown, M. Chen, J., Dunn, M., Lloyd, E., Stefanick, M.L., Davidson, J.M., & Perkash, I. (1987). Sexual experience and plasma testosterone levels in male veterans after spinal cord injury. *Archives of Physical Medicine and Rehabilitation, 64*, 47-52.

Sarkarati, M., Rossier, A.B., & Fam, B.A. (1987). Experience in vibratory and electroejaculation techniques in spinal cord injury patients: A preliminary report. *Journal of Urology*, 138, 59-62.

Sawin, K. (1994). Women with chronic illness and disability. In E. Youngkin & M. Davis (Eds.), *Women's health: A primary care clinical guide* (pp. 697-719). East Norwalk, CT: Appleton & Lang.

Seager, S.W.J., & Halstead, L.S. (1993). Fertility options and success after spinal cord injury. *Urology Clinics of North America, 20*, 543-548.

Sipski, M.L. (1991). The impact of spinal cord injury on female sexuality, menstruation and pregnancy: A review of the literature. *Journal of the American Paraplegia Society, 14*, 122-126.

Sipski, M.L. (1991). Spinal cord injury: What is the effect on sexual response. *The Journal of the American Paraplegia Society, 14*, 40-43.

Sipski, M.L., Alexander, C.J., & Rosen, R.C. (1995). Orgasm in women with spinal cord injuries: A laboratory-based assessment. *Archives of Physical Medicine and Rehabilitation, 76*, 1097-1102.

Sipski, M.L., Rosen, R.C., Alexander, C.J. & Hamer, R.M. (2000). Sildenifil effects on sexual and cardiovascular responses in women with spinal cord injury. *Urology, 55(6)*, 812-815.

Sloan, S. (1994). *Sexuality and the person with spina bifida*. Washington, DC: Spina Bifida Association of America.

Szasz, G. (1992). Sexual health care. In C.P. Zedjlik (Ed.), *Management of spinal cord injury* (2nd ed., pp. 175-202). Boston: Jones & Bartlett.

Tepper, M.C. (1994). Providing comprehensive sexual health care in SCI rehabilitation. Unpublished manuscript.

Turner, L.A., Althof, S.E., Levine, S.B., & Tobias, T.R. (1990). Treating erectile dysfunction with external vacuum devices: Impact upon sexual, psychological, and marital functioning. *Journal of Urology, 144*, 79-82.

Verduyn, W.H. (1986). Spinal cord injured women, pregnancy and delivery. *Paraplegia, 24*, 231-240.

Vervoort, S.M. (1987). Infertility in the spinal cord injured male. *Urology, 29*, 157-165.

Warner, M.B., Rageth, C.J., & Zach, G.A. (1987). Pregnancy and autonomic hyperreflexia in patients with spinal cord lesions. *Paraplegia, 25*, 482-490.

Williams, L.D. (1993). Sexuality: Reproductive pattern. AE McCourt (Ed.). In *The Specialty Practice of Rehabilitation Nursing: A Core Curriculum* (3rd Edition) Skokie, IL: Rehabilitation Nursing Foundation.

Yarkony, G.M., Chen, D., Palmer, J., Roth, E.J., Rayner, S. & Lovell, L. (1995). Management of impotence due to spinal cord injury using low dose papaverine. *Paraplegia, 33*, 77-79.

Zejdlik, C.P. (ED.) (1992). *Management of spinal cord injury* (2nd ed.). Boston: Jones & Bartlett.

Health Education Resources

Becker, E.F. (1991). *Love - where to find it, how to keep it.* Bloomington: Cheever Publications.

Campion, M.J. (1990). *The baby challenge: A handbook on pregnancy for women with a physical disability.* New York: Routledge, Chapman & Hall.

Fine, M., Asch, A. (Eds.). (1988). *Women with disabilities: Essays in psychology, culture, and politics.* Philadelphia: Temple University Press.

Kroll, K. & Klein, E.L. (1992). *Enabling romance: An illustrated guide to romantic and sexual relationships.* New York: Crown Publishers.

McDonald, S.E., Lloyd, W.M., Murphy, D., Russert, M.G. (1993). *Sexuality and spinal cord injury.* Milwaukee, WI: The Spinal Cord Injury Center.

Mother to be: A guide to pregnancy and birth for women and disabilities. (1991). New York: Demos Publications.

Rabin. B. (1980). Sensuous wheeler, sexual adjustment for the spinal cord injured. *New mobility.* Malibu, CA: Miramar Communication.

Sexual adjustment: A guide for the spinal cord injured. (1993). Bloomington: Cheever Publications.

Sexual reborn. (1993). West Orange, NJ: Kessler Institure for Rehabilitation.

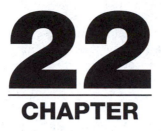

CHAPTER

Body Image and Self-Concept

Laureen Doloresco, MN, RN, CNAA

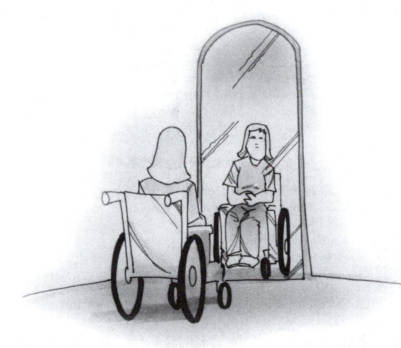

I.   Learning Objectives

A. Describe the relationship among body image, self-concept, and self-esteem.

B. Identify factors that may contribute to disturbances in body image and self-esteem following spinal cord impairment (SCI).

C. Discuss strategies to enhance the image of individuals with SCI.

II. Introduction

A. **Scope of the chapter**
   1. Provides an overview of the concepts of body image, self-concept, and self-esteem.
      a. Body image: the view of the body as a whole, its various parts, functions, and sensations. Body image development is a lifelong process that changes based on life experiences, health, and relationships. Body image represents physical dimensions of the self-concept. Perceptions of others are incorporated into the body image.
      b. Self-concept: consists of body image, self-esteem, and life experiences, which include social and cultural influences. The self-concept is how a person perceives and values self; it guides behavior.
      c. Self-esteem: a measure of self-acceptance and self-approval originating early in life, influenced by interactions with others. Self-esteem is maximal self-love, whether or not one is successful at any point in life.
   2. Discusses factors which may alter body image and self-concept following SCI.
   3. Identifies strategies to enhance the body image and self-concept of individuals with SCI.

B. **Demographics of self-concept and body image disturbance following SCI**
   1. The individual experience of disability makes it difficult to generalize about psychological changes subsequent to SCI. However, many authors have recognized the high incidence and adverse effects of depression among those with physical disabilities and underscore the importance of personal and social factors in the development of depression (Burns, 1980; Dunn & Herman, 1982; Elliott & Frank, 1980; Reidy & Caplan, 1994). Four characteristics describe a depressed self-image: defeated, defective, deserted, and deprived (Beck, 1970).
   2. Low self-concept is a characteristic feature of depression. Illogical, self-defeating, and negative thoughts about disability contribute to low self-concept. Poor body image magnifies physical imperfections into an overwhelming symbol of personal failure. Elliott (1991) emphasized the importance of cultivating interpersonal skills of persons with SCI to contribute to their self-concept and success in social interactions and relationships. Elliott found that depression and psychosocial impairment following SCI were decreased in individuals with self-reported competence in problem solving, assertiveness, and social support. Those with relationships that reaffirmed their sense of self -worth had lower levels of depression.
   3. Individuals with disabilities who demonstrate depressed behavior evoke negative reactions and rejection from others, including rehabilitation staff (Dunn & Herman, 1982; Elliott & Frank, 1980; Nelson, 1990). Conversely, those who demonstrate effective interpersonal skills challenge stereotypes about disability, put others at ease, and elicit positive social reactions.

C. **Etiology/precipitating factors related to alteration in self-concept and body image**
   1. Negative societal perceptions and beliefs: Society generally devalues individuals with disabilities. Multiple social barriers must be surmounted in the process of re-socialization (Dunn & Herman, 1982).
      a. Public attitudes: Typically, able-bodied people are anxious and uncomfortable interacting with people with disabilities. In turn, the person with a disability may reflect this attitude by responding with passivity and discomfort.
      b. Patronizing behaviors of the able-bodied: A cultural norm is to be kind and helpful toward individuals with disabilities. As a result, patronizing behaviors get in the way of appropriate criticisms and negative feedback for the person with SCI. Left unchecked, inappropriate behavior will result in a tendency toward aggression or passivity, and decreased self-esteem. (Refer to Figure 22-1).
      c. Sensitive social situations: Potentially embarrassing situations (e.g., fear of an accidental bowel movement, or of falling out of the wheelchair) may inhibit the person with SCI from taking an active role in public life.
      d. Insufficient assertiveness training: The rehabilitation center often provides insufficient training and experiences to prepare for the stigmatizing consequences of disability. Instead, the person with SCI must learn through trial and error how to resume interpersonal relationships and initiate social contacts. Social isolation may result for

Figure 22-1: Cultural Norms Make it Difficult for a Person with a Disability to Receive Negative Feedback

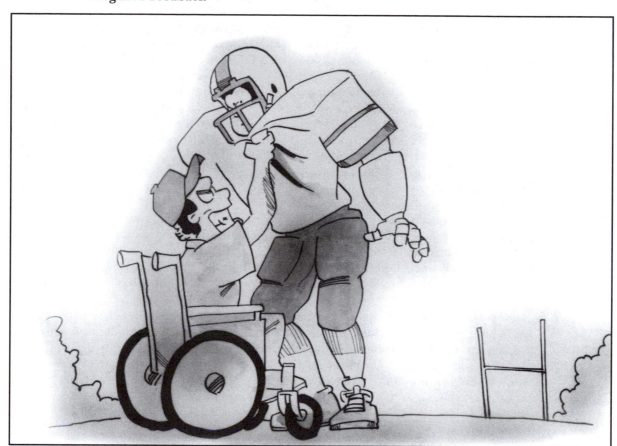

those who do not learn to assert themselves and reduce discomfort in others regarding their disability.

2. Multiple losses may precipitate changes in self-concept.
   a. Significant alterations in body appearance and function affect the entire self-concept. These may include impaired mobility and sensation, altered sexual functioning, loss of bowel and bladder control, and pain and spasticity.
   b. The loss of independence in performing tasks that once were automatic may lead to feelings of helplessness and uselessness.
   c. External sources of self-esteem, such as praise from others, achievements, and possessions may be depleted following SCI. Self-confidence — the ability to cope with life and feel competent in social settings — may decline.
3. Perceptions of femininity, masculinity, physical stamina, and capabilities may be damaged if the individual is unable to value physical and emotional attributes that remain intact. In a society that values youth, beauty, productivity, and relationships, the person with SCI is challenged to rebuild a life with a body that is forever changed. Wheelchairs and other assistive devices become essential tools of life. For those who place great value on physical attributes, the loss of musculature and physique and intrusion of assistive devices are assaults to self-esteem.
4. An important influence on the self-concept of the person who has experienced a spinal cord impairment is the process of rehabilitation (Fitting, Salisbury, Davies, & Mayclin, 1978; Dunn & Herman, 1982; Trieschmann, 1988; Koehler, 1989; Nelson, 1990; Zejdlik, 1992; Hancock, Craig, Tennant & Chang, 1993; Yoshida, 1994). Many rehabilitation programs emphasize physical aspects of rehabilitation at the expense of psychosocial restoration and fall short in providing appropriate experiences to prepare persons with SCI for community

reintegration. Nelson (1990) identifies a series of critical phases that must occur during rehabilitation to preserve the patient's self-worth: buffering, transcending, toughening, and launching.

    a. Buffering occurs when staff and family nurture and protect the patient who is coming to grips with extensive losses. This strategy is appropriate when patients are in situations that decrease their sense of control (e.g., on admission to the unit, first day in therapy, during medical setbacks, first weekend pass, prior to discharge).

    b. Transcending begins in rehabilitation and continues throughout life when individuals with disabilities rise above negative stereotypes and perceptions held by the general public. Staff optimism regarding the client's abilities reinforces a sense of hardiness. Exposure to "older" injuries (persons experienced with living with a SCI) who have developed strategies for transcending attitudinal and physical barriers in the community is essential in this phase. Less-experienced staff may impede transcendence by emphasizing physical aspects of care, which intensifies the client's feelings of dependency.

    c. Toughening concentrates on compensating for physical limitations and acquiring maximal independence while maintaining healthy interpersonal relationships. Many individuals learn to "use" their disabilities and manipulate able-bodied persons to acquire special concessions and attention. This behavior leads to decreased self-esteem, social isolation, and excessive dependency. In the toughening phase, other patients, whose injuries are of longer duration, act as role models by sharing expectations for conduct to reinforce appropriate behavior and discourage antisocial behavior.

    d. Launching exposes the client to the community outside the rehabilitation setting in preparation for the adjustment in lifestyle that results from disability. The rehabilitation facility provides a safe but artificial environment, which does not expose the individual to obstacles in the community. Recreational outings and therapeutic passes provide gradual exposure to the harsh realities of life outside the hospital.

D. Anatomy/physiology

1. SCI alters the body in a variety of ways—some are readily discernible, others less obvious. For the person who requires a wheelchair for mobility, the chair represents a visible symbol of disability. Use of a wheelchair not only reduces physical stature, but also limits accessibility to many environments and social interactions. This may lead to decreased feelings of competence and confidence in social settings. Use of other assistive devices such as hand splints, leg bags, and urinary catheters accentuates the altered body image. (Refer to Figure 22-2).

2. The loss of dependability, predictability, and control may be the harshest elements in the disability experience. Loss of control of bowel and bladder is one of the most sensitive issues surrounding body image for the person with SCI. Early in life, we are taught that control of these body functions is essential for social acceptance.

3. The completeness and level of spinal cord injury affect sexual functioning. Erectile, ejaculatory, and fertility problems are common in males. Fertility in females is not affected by SCI. Sexual activity and intimacy may be inhibited by fear of experimentation and gender/role identity issues. However, sexual expression, intimacy, and satisfaction are attainable following disability. (Refer to Figure 22-3).

4. Visible changes in physique may occur over time to further modify body image.

    a. Loss of muscle mass and tone and contractures result in a distorted appearance of the hands, arms, or legs.

    b. Decreased muscle tone produces a soft, protruding abdomen.

    c. Atrophy of lower body muscles results in a disproportionate body appearance.

Figure 22-2: Use of a Wheelchair Can Limit Accessibility, Socially and in the Environment

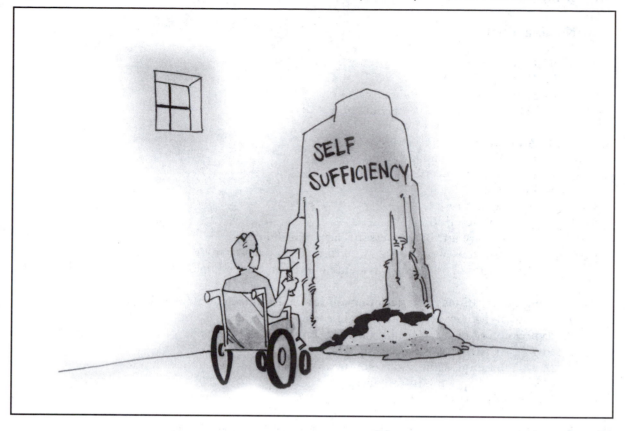

Figure 22-3: A Spinal Cord Injury Affects Sexual Functioning

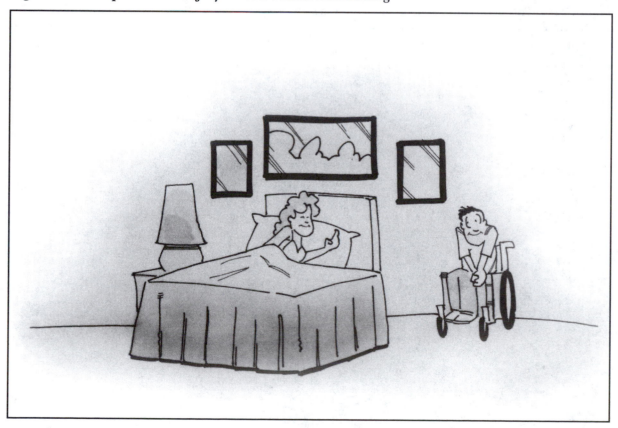

III. Initial Assessment

A. **Nursing history**
1. Patient's perception of SCI
    a. Cause/onset
    b. Feelings about SCI
    c. Expectations of rehabilitation
        (1) Most important rehabilitation goal
        (2) Expectations of staff
    d. Anticipated changes in lifestyle
        (1) Ability to manage at home
        (2) Major concerns and fears about SCI
2. Self-concept
    a. Self-perception
        (1) Self-description
        (2) Positive attributes, personal accomplishments
        (3) Attitudes about people with disabilities prior to injury
    b. Perceptions of others: how patient believes others see him or her self before and after SCI

B. **Nursing observations: Manifestations of low self-esteem and depression**
1. Change in activity level: withdrawal or agitation
2. Expression of negative feelings toward self, e.g., self-blame
3. Regressive wishes: desire to escape, hide, and die
4. Mood alteration: sadness, loneliness, and apathy
5. Sleep and/or appetite disturbances
6. Hypersensitivity to criticism

IV. Nursing Process Applied to Body Image Disturbance

(Refer to Figure 22-4).

Figure 22-4: Potential Body Image Disturbance in SCI

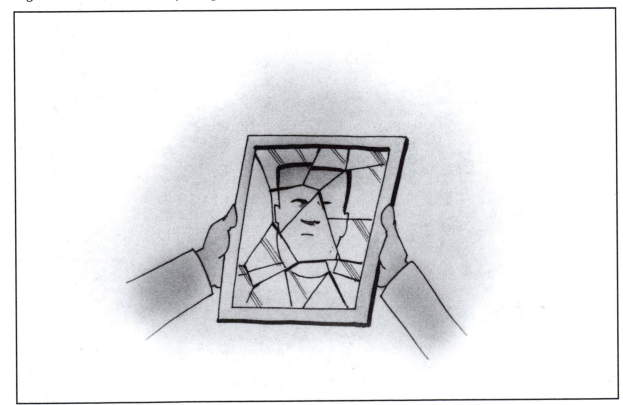

A. **Nursing Diagnosis:** Body image disturbance

B. **Defining characteristics** (Doenges & Moorhouse, 1996)
   1. Verbal response to actual or perceived change in structure and/or function, or
   2. Nonverbal response to actual or perceived change in structure and/or function

C. **Clinical manifestations**
   1. Refusal to look at or touch body part
   2. Unwillingness to discuss disability
   3. Refusal to participate in care
   4. Verbalized negative feelings about body
   5. Social isolation
   6. Fear of rejection or of reaction by others
   7. Focus on past strengths, function, or appearance
   8. Feelings of helplessness, hopelessness, or powerlessness
   9. Preoccupation with change or loss

D. **Expected outcomes** (Doenges & Moorhouse, 1996). (Refer to Figure 22-5).
   1. Communicate acceptance of self post-spinal cord injury
   2. Verbalize relief of anxiety and adaptation to altered body image
   3. Express understanding of body changes
   4. Recognize and incorporate body image change into self-concept in accurate manner without negating self-esteem
   5. Seek information and growth experiences
   6. Acknowledge responsibility for self
   7. Use adaptive devices appropriately

Figure 22-5: An Expected Outcome of Rehabilitation is a Healthy Body Image and Self-Esteem

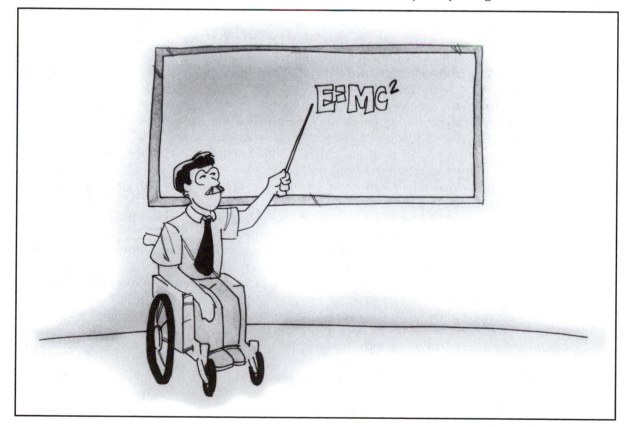

E. Interventions

1. Assess client/family knowledge of body changes secondary to SCI and provide appropriate information based on learning needs.
   a. Encourage identification of personal strengths and limitations and explore how client believes others view self.
   b. Discuss meaning of disability to client (e.g., current and future expectations).
   c. Assess understanding of concepts of independence, masculinity/femininity, self-worth, and help client re-interpret these concepts in light of SCI.
   d. Discuss positive achievements and successes in detail, steering away from negative thinking associated with the trauma of SCI.

2. Establish a therapeutic relationship that communicates and validates the client's competence and worth as a fully functioning human being.
   a. Develop a comfortable nurse/client relationship to create an atmosphere of acceptance and trust and communicate the client is a respected and worthwhile human being (Nelson, 1990). Staff/patient relationships based mutual self-disclosure and friendship demonstrate that disability is not an obstacle the development of healthy interpersonal relationships.
   b. Acknowledge feelings of dependency, grief, and anger. Provide opportunities to express feelings without fear of rejection. Clients may be inhibited to discuss difficulties and problems out of fear they may be criticized for complaining or may be humiliated by admitting to emotional problems.

3. Evaluate coping skills
   a. Assess current level of adaptation
   b. Identify previously used coping strategies and effectiveness
   c. Determine support system/resources
   d. Identify positive coping behaviors
      (1) Talk problems out to reduce tension and get input on how to cope
      (2) Seek comfort from family, friends
      (3) Work off tension through exercise, physical activity
      (4) Step-by-step problem solving (e.g., define problems, generate alternative solutions, evaluate potential outcomes)
      (5) Use humor to alleviate tension

4. Assist client to apply cognitive coping techniques. All moods are created by thoughts, so by changing the way individuals interpret and perceive their disability, self-esteem can be enhanced. Challenging irrational beliefs and negative thinking helps the person with SCI develop a more realistic self-evaluation. Simple "mood elevating" techniques may be applied to increase self-esteem (Burns, 1980).
   a. Recognize and write down self-critical thoughts related to disability.
   b. Self-monitor negative thoughts throughout the day and score at the end of each day.
   c. Refute self-critical thoughts and develop positive coping behaviors to address difficulties.
   d. Visualize success: Break down activities into small manageable tasks to combat overwhelming feelings of not being able to do what is needed.

5. Promote an optimal rehabilitation milieu by assisting clients through the four phases of reintegration (Nelson, 1990).
   a. Buffering: Provide emotional support to allay anxiety, meet critical patient needs, build confidence, and forge a bond with the rehab program
      (1) Assign consistent nursing staff to provide care throughout hospitalization to build rapport and offer continuous support through the myriad of stressful situations that arise during rehabilitation (e.g., stand by to give moral support when client is transferring independently for the first time into bed from wheelchair).
      (2) Provide attention and specific explanations about the client's condition to promote a sense of being understood and confidence in the rehab team. Protect the client from physical or emotional exhaustion to encourage future efforts and successes in rehabilitation.
      (3) Create a unit environment that promotes a sense of belonging and "community."

    (4) Provide maximal privacy during routines to maintain the client's integrity as a sentient human being.

b. Transcending: Strategies to promote a sense of hardiness prepare persons with disabilities to rise above negative stereotypes and social barriers.

    (1) Provide opportunities for patients experienced with living with SCI to help newly injured patients to overcome barriers (e.g., dealing with condescending attitudes, re-establishing sexual activity).

    (2) Create flexibility in treatment approaches to personalize care; minimize structured ward routines that de-emphasize individual identity.

    (3) Establish a daily program and promote self-care activities to mobilize constructive motivations and redirect from self-preoccupation to an interest in external goals and activities.

    (4) Convey a rehabilitation philosophy of optimism, challenge, and goal attainment.

    (5) Use subtle distractions during physical care to minimize dependency (e.g., discussing common interests, joking).

    (6) Promote involvement of family and friends during rehabilitation to reaffirm relationships. Discuss community and family roles and relationships and adjustments to role changes.

    (7) Encourage family involvement in support groups to discuss impact of SCI on the family unit and survival strategies.

c. Toughening: Seasoned staff and patients experienced at living with a SCI are most effective at "toughening up" the newly injured person.

    (1) Provide critical feedback regarding inappropriate behavior and set boundaries to convey their responsibility for their own behavior. Convey the message that disability does not afford them unique rights or excuse inappropriate behavior.

    (2) Confront feigned helplessness. Many individuals capitalize on the dependency aspects of SCI and manipulate social interactions to get others to do things for them that they are capable of doing themselves. This behavior intensifies dependency, reduces self-esteem, and alienates family and friends. Refraining from providing assistance when the person with SCI is capable of completing a task promotes independence. Open confrontation of attempts to "use the disability" conveys confidence in their abilities and increases self-worth. Determining when to "push" and when to assist requires the acumen of an expert rehabilitation nurse.

    (3) Assist client in building social skills in the areas of self-awareness, anger management, and sensitivity.

    (4) Promote healthy competition between clients in therapies to push them toward maximal functional independence.

    (5) Teach appropriate use of adaptive equipment (e.g., wheelchair etiquette, grooming to minimize body changes and enhance appearance). Encourage expression of personal style through appearance and attire. Dispel fashion "myths" and tendency for conformity in dress taught in rehabilitation (e.g., sweatpants, athletic shoes, and warm-up suits).

    (6) Provide praise based on progress in mobility, attitude, energy, and endurance.

    (7) Emphasize positive attributes and unique personal assets to help develop vocational, recreational, and spiritual pursuits.

d. Launching: Full involvement of clients in all aspects of decision making and goal setting about their care and future in the community promotes self-directed behavior and maximal autonomy.

    (1) Facilitate pursuit of pre-injury goals and aspirations to the fullest extent possible.

    (2) Use peer modeling with patients experienced at living with a SCI to share creative approaches for managing embarrassing situations to minimize trauma to self and others (e.g., fall out of wheelchair, external catheter pops off).

    (3) Role play social situations to project an image and attitude that encourage positive social interactions with able-bodied individuals (e.g., how to turn down or ask for help, how to maintain a calm exterior and put others at ease when experiencing muscle spasms).

(4) Gradually expose clients to barriers in the community (e.g., therapeutic passes, recreational outings, and small social gatherings).

(5) Encourage networking among clients with SCI in the community to establish a supportive web of information and friendships.

F. **Evaluation**
   1. Client/family responses to interventions and teaching
   2. Progress toward desired outcomes/goals

V. Reassessment

A. **Nursing history**
   1. Use self-report assessment to evaluate changes in the patient's knowledge and feelings related to body changes, competence and comfort in social situations.
   2. Assess client's involvement in decision making, problem solving.
   3. Solicit objective feedback from staff and family members to evaluate client's behavior and social skills (e.g., mood, assertiveness, and anger management) and evaluate inconsistencies in self-report assessment of social skills.
   4. Determine readiness for community reintegration and availability of support systems (e.g., significant others, friends, groups).

B. **Consultation/referrals:** Refer to appropriate support groups, counseling, or therapy based on specific client complaints or concerns at time of re-evaluation.

VI. Health Education Tips

A. **"Self-efficacy"** — the perceived strength and capabilities to deal with prospective situations — is enhanced by successful performance (Bandura, 1977). Rehabilitation staff can assist clients with SCI to master physical and social skills in the face of multiple obstacles to achieve increased self-confidence. Reinforce self-efficacy by providing incentives to encourage the individual's participation in activities that are perceived as threatening, yet are relatively safe (e.g., self bowel care and catheterizations, recreational travel, participation in wheelchair sports).
   1. Provide gradual experiences to gain feelings of control and mastery.
   2. Structure the environment so individuals with SCI can perform successfully despite physical limitations (e.g., wheelchair accessibility, use of assistive devices).
   3. Promote opportunities to see others with SCI successfully manage the challenges of disability.
   4. Verbally reinforce capabilities and point out improvements and gains.
   5. Demonstrate proficient ways of handling threatening situations (e.g., accidental bowel movement). (Refer to Figure 22-6).
   6. Encourage health-promoting behaviors (e.g., proper diet, rest, and physical exercise) to reduce stress and preserve strength and stamina.

B. **Social Skills training:** Reinforce social skills of clients, families, and rehabilitation staff. Examine staff, family, and client attitudes about independence and achievement. Attitudes and beliefs may perpetuate negative cultural stereotypes about persons with disabilities. Social skills training facilitates comfort in interactions and the full inclusion of persons with disabilities in society. Relevant training includes:
   1. Self-awareness/self-acceptance
   2. Assertiveness training
   3. Anger management
   4. Sensitivity to others (e.g., reading emotional cues, knowing when and where it is more advantageous to use passive or assertive behavior)

C. **Teach "wheelchair etiquette"** (Klemz, 1989); behavioral guidelines for individuals who use wheelchairs and those who interact with them

Figure 22-6: Anticipate Ways to Handle Threatening Situations

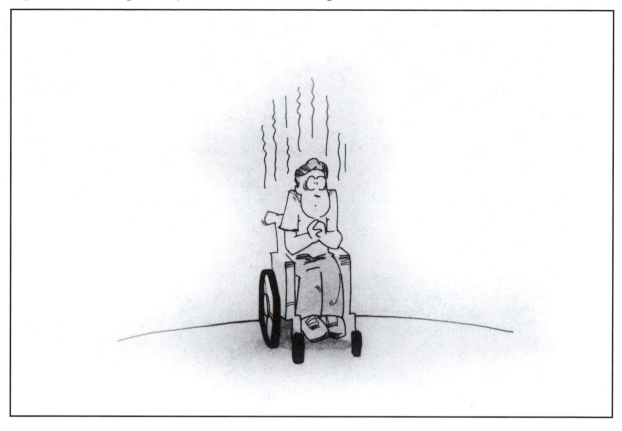

Figure 22-7: Wheelchair Etiquette Can be Taught

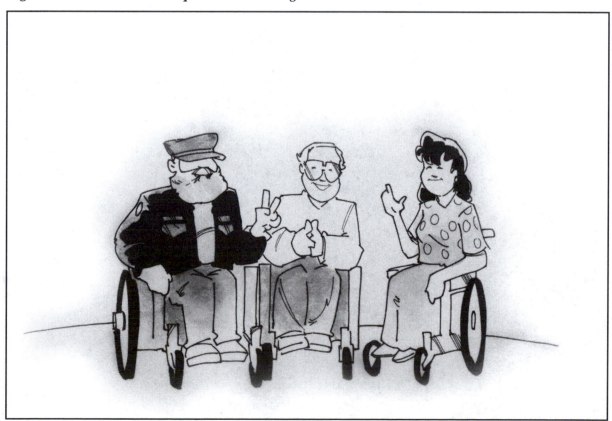

319

1. Illustrate and problem solve situations commonly encountered by people who use wheelchairs.
2. Discuss conversational strategies for minimizing disability. (Refer to Figure 22-7).
   a. Establish eye-level contact.
   b. Avoid descriptions that stereotype people who use wheelchairs as ill (e.g., "crippled," "confined to a wheelchair," or "handicapped").
   c. Refer to person in wheelchair by relationship, not by disability (e.g., "my friend, Bill" instead of "my friend, Bill, who is a paraplegic").
   d. Avoid encroaching on personal space of the person who uses a wheelchair (e.g., leaning on chair, using excessive hand gestures when talking).
   e. Teach "rules of the road" for individuals who use wheelchairs (e.g., avoid sudden stops, travel to the right, and go with the flow of traffic). (Refer to Figure 22-8).

D. **Emphasize projection of a positive image to others.** (Refer to Figure 22-9).
   1. Identify preferences and cultivate ways to express personal style through attire.
   2. Maximize positive physical attributes (e.g., a bright smile, clear voice).
      a. Dress for the occasion
      b. Cosmetics
      c. Hygiene/grooming tips
   3. Discuss inappropriate behavior.
      a. Exposed leg bags, urinals
      b. Pajamas in public
   4. Explore forms of sexual expression and ways to share intimacy.

E. **Facilitate adjustment to role changes**
   1. Discuss previous roles (e.g., mother, teacher, and Girl Scout troop leader). (Refer to Figure 22-10).
   2. Assess how SCI has altered roles and discuss new strategies for providing valuable contributions to family and community.

Figure 22-8: Teach "Rules of the Road" for Individuals Using a Wheelchair

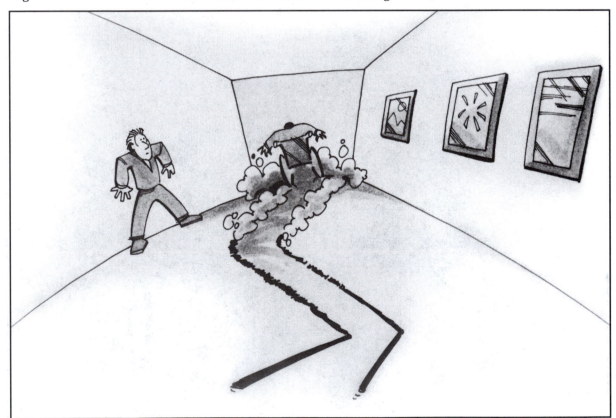

Figure 22-9: Emphasize the Need to Project a Positive Image

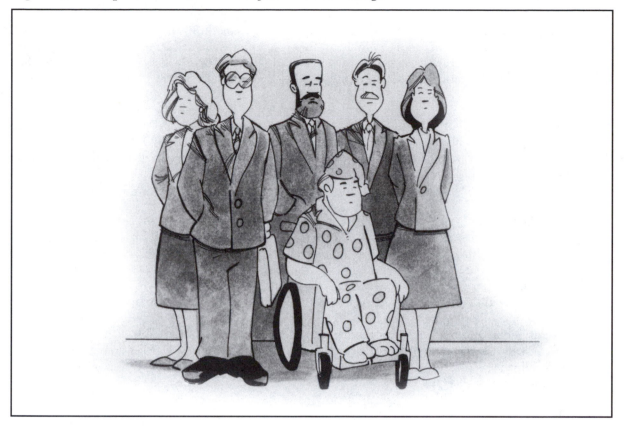

Figure 22-10: Facilitate Adjustment to Role Changes

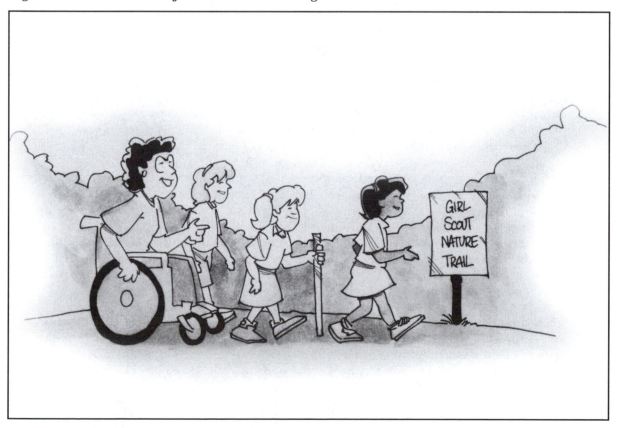

Practical Application # 1

S. K., an 18-year old high school senior, placed great value on his physique, strength and skill as an athlete. He was active in football and hockey, and was elected by teammates as captain of the hockey team. S.K. was very popular and proud of his status as a star athlete. He enjoyed an active dating life and had steady relations with two girlfriends. He viewed himself as very "macho."

During the final football game of the season, S. K. sustained a C 5-6 spinal cord injury that abruptly changed his life. He became totally dependent in all activities of daily living. Following a frightening stay in a critical care unit, he entered rehabilitation. When he looked in the mirror, he was transformed from a tall, strong athlete to a "a sick wimp in a wheelchair." He'd lost 55 lbs.—his muscular physique was a thing of the past.

S.K.'s family and friends were very supportive throughout the arduous process of rehabilitation. His father assumed the role of primary caregiver, doing everything in his power to assist S.K. to a return to health and maximal independence. After six weeks of rehabilitation, S.K. returned home with his parents. He attempted to resume intimate relations with his girlfriends, engaging in sexual experimentation to reaffirm his sexuality. During rehabilitation, staff had not discussed sexual functioning and options with him, and he'd had no contact with older injuries. After repeated attempts and embarrassing failures, including external catheter "blowouts" and urinary incontinence, S. K. decided to give up on sexual relations. He felt extremely frustrated and defeated and eventually broke off relations with his girlfriends. He couldn't accept the pain of recalling the pleasures of past. He was resigned to life alone—with no hopes of ever being intimate again.

Over the next few years, S. K. became more isolated. Fear of rejection caused him to avoid others. In social settings, he avoided interactions and was rude to keep others at a distance. He no longer felt like a man. Though he had the support of a caring family and high school "buddies" to hang out with, he felt his life was empty. At 23 years of age, he longed for his former body and former self. He felt unfulfilled and resentful about the profound losses and physical changes he experienced.

S. K. was angry about the loss of control over his life. He had difficulty asking for assistance and asserting his needs and frequently put his health at risk. He restricted his fluid intake out of fear of not having access to a wheelchair accessible restroom, and became predisposed to urinary tract infections. He had a passion for winter outdoor activities, and hated that he could no longer play hockey or go ice fishing. His stubborn refusal to take sufficient precautions against the cold weather placed him at risk for overexposure. Family and friends were concerned about the effect S. K.'s "devil-may-care" attitude would have on his health.

Eventually, a female acquaintance from high school approached S.K. at a party at the home of one of his close friends. She talked with him about mutual friends and shared high school memories. She seemed to accept S.K. completely and was eager to learn more about him. She asked if they could see each other again, and he agreed. Inwardly, he felt very insecure about seeing her again, but also felt renewed by her presence. She saw through his physical differences and was determined to get to know S. K. better. Her unconditional acceptance of him and matter-of-fact approach to his care provided a major boost to S. K.'s self-esteem and a resurgence of his masculinity and self-confidence.

They continued to date, and developed a relationship based on mutual respect, trust, and love—culminating in a rich and fulfilling marriage. S. K. earned a master's degree in social work to blend a successful career in health care with a rewarding family life. Looking back, he recalls how unprepared he was for the realities of living with SCI after rehabilitation.

Practical Application #2

P. L. is a 64 year old female, with post-polio syndrome, who developed cancer of the rectum which required a permanent colostomy. She had polio as a child and over the years has demonstrated an excellent adjustment to the challenges of living with a disability. She has a solid marriage of 23 years. She and her husband have successful careers in real estate sales, specializing in selling accessible houses for persons with disabilities. P. L. volunteers as a peer counselor at a local rehabilitation center and is considered a role model for other females with physical disabilities. P.L. ambulates with a walker and uses a wheelchair for longer distances.

When P.L. learned she had cancer and would need a colostomy, she became very despondent. It was more than she could bear. First polio, and now cancer and a colostomy. As a successful career woman, she took pride in her dress and appearance, firmly believing in the adage, "Dress for success." The thought of a colostomy was repulsive; however, she agreed to surgery.

Post-operatively, she received an excellent prognosis. Her primary nurse was concerned about P. L.'s refusal to look at her colostomy and assume care for it. She consulted a Certified Enterostomal Therapy Nurse (CETN). The CETN discussed P. L.'s concerns about sexuality, femininity, and resumption of physical activity with a colostomy. She involved P. L.'s husband in teaching and entertained his questions to provide clarification about life with an ostomy. She gradually involved P. L. in care of the colostomy, helping her to see that it could be incorporated into her daily life. She provided simple instruction to teach application and cleansing of appliances, use of pouch covers during sexual activity and deodorant appliances and filters. The CETN taught P. L. how to observe for complications and troubleshoot problems at home. She made provisions for follow-up care to assure a successful transition to home.

Swimming was one of P. L.'s favorite recreational activities. The CETN assured P. L. she would be able to safely resume swimming, work, and all former activities. P. L. gained knowledge and confidence to live with a colostomy and return to an active and fulfilling life.

References and Selected Bibliography

Arnhoff, F. & Mehl, M. (1963). Body image deterioration in paraplegia. *Journal of Nervous and Mental Disease, 137*, 88-92.

Askevold, F. (1975). Measuring body image. *Psychotherapy and Psychosomatics, 26*(2), 71-77.

Bach, C. & McDaniel, R. (1993). Quality of life in quadriplegic adults: a focus group study. *Rehabilitation Nursing, 18*, 364-374.

Bandura, A. (1977). Self-efficacy: Toward a unifying theory of behavior. *Psychological Review, 84*(2), 191-215.

Bandura, A. (1982). Self-efficacy mechanism in human agency. *American Psychologist, 37*, 122-147.

Barry, P. (1989). *Psychosocial nursing: Assessment and intervention—care of the physically ill person* (2nd ed.). Philadelphia: Lippincott.

Beck, A. (1970). *Depression: Causes and treatments*. Philadelphia: University of Pennsylvania Press.

Beeken, J. (1978). Body changes in plegia. *Journal of Neurosurgical Nursing, 10*(1), 20-23.

Bednar, R., Wells, M., & Peterson, S. (1989). *Self-esteem: paradoxes and innovations in clinical theory and practice*. Washington, DC: American Psychological Association.

Berkowitz, M., Harvey, C., Greene, C., & Wilson, S. (1992). *The economic consequences of traumatic spinal cord injury*. New York: Demos.

Bourdon, S. (1986). Psychological impact of neurotrauma in the acute care setting. *Nursing Clinics of North America, 21*, 629-640.

Branden, N. (1987). *How to raise your self-esteem*. Toronto, CAN: Bantam.

Brennan, J. (1994). A vital component of care: The nurse's role in recognizing altered body image. *Professional Nurse, 9*(5), 298-303.

Burns, D. (1980). *Feeling good: The new mood therapy*. New York: Avon Books.

Charmaz, K. (1983). Loss of self: a fundamental form of suffering in the chronically ill. *Sociology of Health and Illness, 5*(2), 168-195.

Chase, B. & King, K (1990). Psychosocial adjustment of persons with spinal cord injury. *International Journal of Rehabilitation Research, 13*(4), 325-327.

Conomy, J. (1973). Disorders of body image after spinal cord injury. *Neurology, 23*(8), 842-850.

Craig, A., Hancock, K., & Chang, E. (1994). The influence of spinal cord injury on coping styles and self-perceptions two years after the injury. *Australian and New Zealand Journal of Psychiatry, 28*(2), 307-312.

Denis, M. (1989). Spinal cord injured adolescents and young adults: The meaning of body changes. *Journal of Advanced Nursing, 14*(5), 389-396.

Doenges, M. & Moorhouse, M. (1996). *Nurse's pocket guide: Nursing diagnoses with interventions* (5th ed.). Philadelphia: F. A. Davis.

Doloresco, L., Simmons, B., Klemz, S., & Brown, J. (1996). *Image enhancement: An educational model for SCI reintegration*. Paper presented at the meeting of the American Association of Spinal Cord Injury Nurses, Las Vegas, NV.

Drench, M. (1994). Changes in body image secondary to disease and injury. *Rehabilitation Nursing, 19*, 31-36.

Dunn, M. & Herman, S. (1982). Social skills and disability. In R. Doleys, D. Meredith, & R. Ciminero (Eds.), *Behavioral psychology in medicine: Assessment and training strategies*. New York: Plenum Press.

Eisenberg, M. (1984). Spinal cord injuries. In H. B. Roback (Ed.), *Helping patients and their families cope with medical problems: A guide to therapeutic group work in clinical settings* (pp. 107-129). San Francisco: Jossey-Bass.

Elliott, R. (1991). Interpersonal behavior and adjustment of persons with spinal cord injury. *SCI Psychosocial Process, 4*(3), 82-87.

Elliott, R., & Frank, R. (1980). Social and interpersonal reactions to depression and disability. *Rehabilitation Psychology, 35*(3), 135-147.

Fisher, S. & Cleveland, S. (1968). *Body image and personality*. New York: Dover.

Fitting, M., Salisbury, S., Davies, N., & Mayclin, D. (1978). Self-concept and sexuality of spinal cord injured women. *Archives of Sexual Behavior, 7*(2), 143-156.

French, J. & Phillips, J. (1991). Shattered images: Recovery for the SCI client. *Rehabilitation Nursing, 16*(3), 134-136.

Frye, B. A. (1986). A model of wellness seeking behavior in traumatic spinal cord injury victims. *Rehabilitation Nursing, 11*(5), 6-7, 14.

Gorman, L., Sultan, D., & Luna-Raines, M. (1989). *Psychosocial nursing handbook for the non-psychiatric nurse*. Baltimore: Williams and Wilkins.

Green, B., Pratt, C., & Grigsby, T. (1985). Self-concept among persons with long-term spinal cord injury. *Archives of Physical Medicine and Rehabilitation, 65*(12), 751-754.

Grunbaum, J. (1985). Helping your patient build a sturdier body image. *RN 48*(10), 51-55.

Hancock, K., Craig, A., Tennant, C., & Change, E. (1993). The influence of spinal cord injury on coping styles and self-perceptions: A controlled study. *Australian and New Zealand Journal of Psychiatry, 27*(3), 450-456.

Helman, C. (1995). The body image in health and disease: Exploring patients' maps of body and self. *Patient Education and Counseling, 26*(1-3),169-175.

Jiwa, T. (1995). Multiple sclerosis and self esteem. *Axon, 16*(4), 87-90.

Kinney, W. & Coyle, C. (1992). Predicting life satisfaction among adults with physical disabilities. *Archives of Physical Medicine and Rehabilitation, 73*, 863-869.

Klemz (1989). *Wheelchair Etiquette*. Tampa, FL: James A. Haley Veterans Hospital.

Koehler, M. (1989). Relationship between self-concept and successful rehabilitation. *Rehabilitation Nursing, 14*(1), 9-12.

Lasfargues, J., Custis, D., Morrone, F., Carswell, J., & Nguyen, T. (1995). A model for estimating spinal cord injury prevalence in the United States. *Paraplegia, 33*(2), 62-68.

Lenhehan, G. (1986). Emotional impact of trauma. *Nursing Clinics of North America, 21*(4), 629-640.

Mattsson, E. (1975). Psychological aspects of severe physical injury and its treatment. *The Journal of Trauma, 15*(3), 217-234.

Mayer, T. & Andrews, H. (1981). Changes in self-concept following a spinal cord injury. *Journal of Applied Rehabilitation and Counselling, 12*, 135-137.

Moore, A., Bombardier, C., Brown, P., & Patterson, D. (1994). Coping and emotional attributions following spinal cord injury. *International Journal of Rehabilitation Research 17*(1), 39-48.

Morse, J. & O'Brien, B. (1995). Preserving self: From victim, to patient, to disabled person. *Journal of Advanced Nursing, 21*(5), 886-896.

Nelson, A. (1990). Patients' perspectives of a spinal cord injury unit. *SCI Nursing, 7*(3), 44-63.

Partridge, C. (1994). Spinal cord injuries: Aspects of psychological care. *British Journal of Nursing, 3*(1), 12-15.

Perry, P. & Sutcliffe, S. (1982). Conceptual frameworks for clinical practice. *The Journal of Neurosurgical Nursing, 14*(6), 318-321.

Piazza, D., Holcombe, J., Fotte, A., Paul, P., Love, S., & Daffin, P. (1991). Hope, social support, and self-esteem of patients with spinal cord injuries. *Journal of Neuroscience Nursing, 23*(4), 224-230.

Piotrowski, M. (1982). Body image after a stroke. *Rehabilitation Nursing, 7*(1), 11-13.

Price, M. (1993). Exploration of body listening: Health and physical self-awareness in chronic illness. *Advances in Nursing Science, 15*(4), 37-52.

Reidy, K. & Caplan, B. (1994). Causal factors in spinal cord injury: Patients' evolving perceptions and association with depression. *Archives of Physical Medicine and Rehabilitation, 75*(8), 837-842.

Richmond, T. & Craig, M. (1986). Family-centered care for the neurotrauma patient. *Nursing Clinics of North America, 21*(4), 641-651.

Rieve, J. (1989). Sexuality and the adult with acquired physical disability. *Nursing Clinics of North America, 24*(1), 265-276.

Shontz, F. (1974). Body image and its disorders. *International Journal of Psychiatry in Medicine, 5*(4), 461-472.

Stein, K. (1995). Schema model of the self-concept. *Image: Journal of Nursing Scholarship, 27*(3), 187-193.

Stensman, R. (1989). Body image among 22 persons with acquired and congenital severe mobility impairment. *Paraplegia, 27*(1), 27-35.

Stubbins, J. (Ed.) (1977). *Social and psychological aspects of disability: A handbook for practitioners.* Baltimore: University Park Press.

Swanson, B., Cronin-Stubbs, D., & Sheldon, J. (1989). The impact of psychosocial factors on adapting to physical disability: A review of the research literature. *Rehabilitation Nursing, 14*(4), 64-68.

Trieschmann, R. (1988). *Spinal cord injuries: psychological, social, and vocational rehabilitation* (2nd ed.). New York: Demos.

Turnbull, A., Patterson, J., Behr MD, S., Murphy, D., Marquis, J., & Blue-Banning, M. (1993). *Cognitive coping, families, and disabilities.* Baltimore MD: Paul H. Brooks.

Ulman, R. & Brother, D. (1988). *The shattered self: A psychoanalytic study of trauma.* Hillsdale, NJ: The Analytic Press.

Vamos, M. (1993). Body image in chronic illness: A re-conceptualization. *International Journal of Psychiatry in Medicine, 23*(2), 163-178.

Vardenbout, J., Van Son-Schoones, N., Schipper, J., & Groffen, C. (1988). Attributional cognition, coping behavior, and self esteem in inpatients with severe spinal cord injuries. *Journal of Clinical Psychology, 44*(10), 17-22.

Weinberg, J. (1982). Human sexuality and spinal cord injury. *Nursing Clinics of North America, 17*(3), 407-419.

Wortman, C. & Cohen Silver, R. (1989). The myths of coping with loss. *Journal of Consulting and Clinical Psychology, 57*(3), 349-357.

Yoshida, K. (1994). Institutional impact on self-concept among persons with spinal cord injury. *International Journal of Rehabilitation Research, 17*(2), 95-107.

Zejdlik, C. (Ed.) (1992). *Management of spinal cord injuries* (2nd Ed.). Boston: Jones & Bartlett.

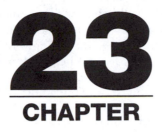

CHAPTER

Family

Constance Captain, Ph.D., RN

I. Learning Objectives

A. Increase nurses' understanding of family nursing practice.

B. Identify family needs and responses across the spinal cord impairment (SCI) care continuum.

C. Enhance nurses' ability to conduct family assessments based on family theoretical models.

D. Expand nurses' knowledge of family nursing interventions using family- focused nursing diagnoses.

II. Introduction

A. Scope

Serious illness or injury dramatically affects not only the individual, but the family as well. This is especially true in health conditions that require on going health maintenance to prevent secondary complications, as in SCI, or diseases with an episodic or downward trajectory, as in multiple sclerosis (MS). Failure of nurses and other health care providers to attend to family needs and to include the family in treatment has the potential for far-reaching negative consequences for the patient and family alike. In this chapter, SCI is discussed from the perspective of what is known about family needs and responses across the continuum of care; acute, rehabilitation, and lifetime health maintenance. Family assessment and interventions are presented within the context of family theoretical models and family nursing diagnoses. The focus is on maintaining and improving family functioning in SCI.

B. Background

For many years, nurses have provided family-centered care— care of individuals within the context of the family. In a family-centered care delivery model, care is directed at the identified patient, and the family is recognized as one, among many, contributors in health/illness outcomes. Much of what is known about the family in SCI derives from this family-centered model. That is, information about the family is presented from the perspective of how family factors affect the care and treatment of the patient, rather than, how SCI affects or alters family functioning and the health and well-being of family members. Nursing reports and research published in the past decade suggest a shift in focus from an emphasis on individuals to interest in the family as the primary unit of care. Increasingly, nurses are expanding the scope of their practice and assuming responsibility for the health care of families. When nurses focus on the family as the "identified patient," this is called family nursing practice rather than family-centered nursing practice. An emphasis on family nursing is expected to continue as health care delivery shifts from an illness orientation to an emphasis on prevention, health promotion, and concerns about maximizing health care resources. The family in SCI is a major resource in the ongoing care of the patient and in the maintenance of the patient's health. Accordingly, this chapter addresses the provision of SCI nursing from a family nursing perspective.

C. **Definitions**
  1. Family: A group of persons with common ancestry, who share a household, have common features or proportions, and are united by certain convictions or a common affiliation. It is the basic biosocial unit in society, having as its nucleus two or more adults living together and cooperating in the care and rearing of offspring (Webster, 1990).
      a. An analysis of the literature by Stuart (1991) identified specific attributes of a family. These include:
          (1) A social system/unit, self-defined by its members, that is ever-changing and developing.
          (2) Members who may or may not be related by birth, adoption, or marriage and may or may not live under one roof.
          (3) A unit that may or may not have dependent children.
          (4) Evidence of commitment and attachment among members that develops over time and demonstrates future obligation.
          (5) Members who carry out specific care-giving functions, such as protection, nourishment, and socialization.
      b. For this chapter, family is defined as: Two or more persons who are emotionally involved with each other, interact, communicate within social roles, assume responsibilities of managing a household, and share a common culture established by its members.
  2. Types of families
      a. Nuclear Family: conjugal unit composed of a husband and wife and their children.
      b. Family of orientation: the family unit into which one is born.
      c. Extended family: a nuclear family and other related (blood/adopted) members joined across generations by emotional ties and a shared sense of commitment.
      d. Diverse family: all forms of family that deviate from the traditional nuclear family structure; term that reflects changing life styles such as single-parent families, same-gender unions, and other communal living arrangements.
  3. Family-centered nursing: health care of individuals within the context of family.
  4. Family nursing: health care of the family as the unit of nursing care.

III. Family Theories

A. **Family Lifecycle Developmental Perspective** (Duvall, 1977) (Refer to Table 23-1).
  1. Description: family as a unit proceeds sequentially through predictable developmental stages over its life span; that is, from its inception through old age and dissolution.
  2. Key concepts
      a. Like individuals, families go through successive stages of development
      b. There are eight stages over the life cycle of a family.
      c. Each stage is characterized by stage-specific developmental tasks that need to be accomplished to proceed intact to the next stage.

Table 23-1: Eight-Stage Family Life Cycle

Stage I	Marriage (beginning of family)
Stage II	Childbearing Family (oldest child under 30 months)
Stage III	Family with Preschoolers (oldest child 30 months to 60 months)
Stage IV	Family with School Children (oldest child 6-13 years)
Stage V	Family with Teenagers (oldest child 13-20 years)
Stage VI	Launching Families (last child leaving home)
Stage VII	Middle Years Families (empty nest through retirement)
Stage VIII	Retirement and Old Age Families (retirement to death of partners)

From *Family Development* (5th ed.), by E. Duvall, 1977, Philadelphia: J.B. Lippincott. Reprinted with permission.

    d. Stages may overlap or be repeated as families assume the complex arrangements often seen in our contemporary lifestyles (e.g. divorce, remarriage, and blended families.) Complexity signals potential problems.
    e. Societal, ethnic, and cultural values as well as expectations alter developmental tasks.
    f. Family tasks should incorporate the stage-specific tasks of its individual members.
    g. The developmental stage of the family guides family dynamics, i.e., how the family functions and deals with internal and external challenges.
    h. Families may arrive at similar developmental outcomes through quite different processes.
3. Assessment areas: Nurse identifies the specific developmental stage of the family and determines the degree to which stage-specific tasks are being accomplished.
    a. Developmental stage; family constellation and age of oldest child. For example, a family with a newborn and a school-aged child would be classified as a Family with School Age Children.
    b. Stage-specific family health status (e.g., 50- year- old wife of SCI spouse has annual papanicolaou (PAP) exams.)
    c. Current status with accomplishing developmental tasks
    d. Developmental stage concerns and issues
    e. Impact of SCI on family stage of development and task accomplishment

B. **Systems Theory**
1. Description: a family system is a goal-directed unit of interacting, interdependent members which endures over a period of time (Freidman, 1981).
2. Key concepts
    a. A change in any part of the system creates change in the entire system. For example, an illness in a family alters routine living activities of every member.
    b. Systems are constantly changing and evolving; failure to do so contributes to family dysfunction.
    c. Once changed, a family does not revert to a former pattern.
    d. Embedded within systems are subsystems. In traditional families, there is a parental subsystem and sibling subsystems. Other alliances are seen and may suggest a need for further inquiries by the nurse to better understand family interaction.
    e. Boundaries differentiate the family from the outside world and maintain the integrity of internal subsystems.
    f. Systems are classified as open or closed, denoting the extent of exchange with external environments.
    g. Systems operate through circular feedback mechanisms that function to maintain a steady state (homeostasis).

     h. Family structure refers to the organization of family members into roles with system-defined responsibilities.

     i. Family function is how a family interacts, adapts, and changes to meet its goals.

  3. Assessment areas: Nurse observes family interactions and asks questions to determine how well members relate to one another.

     a. Family subsystems; the members and how do they relate to each other.

     b. Degree of system openness (family boundaries) and its effect on the family's ability to adapt to changing demands and circumstances.

     c. Communication patters and behaviors (feedback mechanisms) that affect family structure and function.

     d. Strategies used by the family system to maintain equilibrium — which is balance change with stability.

     e. How the family uses other systems to facilitate growth and survival.

C. Role Theory

  1. Description: family unit seen as an interacting, independent set of defined roles assumed by its members to carryout the functions of family life. Role theory is a component of symbolic interaction theory.

  2. Key concepts

     a. A role is an integrated set of socially prescribed expectations about how persons ought to behave in certain situations (Burr, Leigh, Day, & Constantine, 1979).

     b. Role behavior, performance and enactment are terms used to describe how a person carries out role expectations. This is influenced by many factors; individual perceptions, cultural values, exposure to role models, number of roles, member personalities, the environment, and circumstances within which the behavior occurs.

     c. Role strain occurs when a person experiences difficulty in fulfilling role obligations.

     d. Role conflict occurs when incompatibilities exist among roles, i.e., the expected behavior of one role conflicts with the expected behavior of another role.

     e. The quality of role enactment is determined by clarity of role expectations, importance of the role to the person, knowledge and skill in performing the behavior required, and cooperation when reciprocal or complementary roles are needed to accomplish a goal.

     f. Roles are dynamic, changing over time to meet developmental and situational family needs.

     g. Each family member assumes multiple roles; formal (mother, father, employee, student) and informal (caregiver, peacemaker, martyr, others).

     h. Factors that affect role accomplishment include the person's understanding of the socially or culturally sanctioned expectations, and the number of role obligations and responsibilities.

  3. Assessment areas: Nurse observes family members' ability to fulfill expected roles.

     a. Who are the members of the family and what are their roles?

     b. Is there evidence to suggest role conflict, strain, or incompatibilities?

     c. Do family members demonstrate role enactment competency? If not, what are the barriers?

     d. What roles are shared or require reciprocal role enactment to accomplish role obligations?

     e. Are family members assuming new roles or changing the nature of existing roles?

     f. How is SCI affecting role assignments and responsibilities?

D. Family Stress Theory - Double ABCX Model (McCubbin & Patterson, 1983). (Refer to Figure 23-1).

  1. Description: Explains family adaptation following a crisis event by examining how families balance demands and capabilities to achieve positive outcomes. Builds upon Hill's (1958) ABCX Model, which addressed only pre-crisis variables to account for differences in family adaptation to crisis.

  2. Key concepts

     a. Stress in a family becomes a crisis when there is a continual imbalance between

Figure 23-1: Double ABCX Family Stress Model

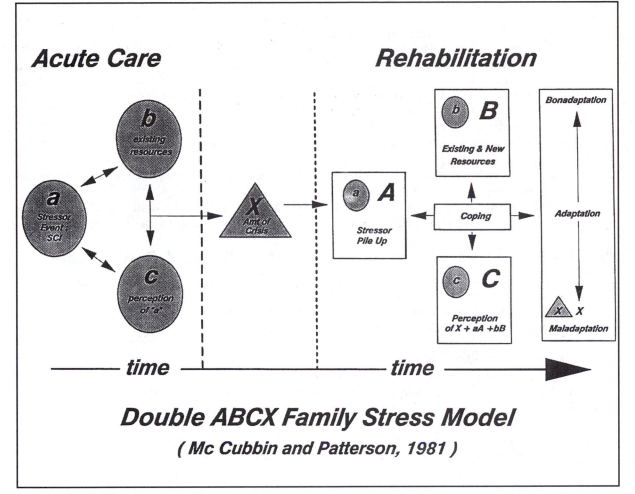

Double ABCX Family Stress Model
(Mc Cubbin and Patterson, 1981)

From *Family Assessment Inventories for Research and Practice* ; by H.I. Thompson (1987), Madison, WI: University of Wisconsin: Madison. Reprinted with permission.

demand-capabilities, so family stability cannot be maintained without making major changes in the way the family functions.

b. The central question guiding family stress assessment is (1) how much and what kinds of stressors; (2) mediated by what personal, family, and community resources and by what family coping responses; and (3) what family processes shape the course and ease of family adjustment and adaptation over time (McCubbin & Patterson, 1983, p 7).

c. Key variables are: Pile-up of System Demands (Aa), Resources (Bb), Perception (Cc), Coping (a bridging concept), and Adaptation.

   (1) Pile-up - cumulative stress from additional demands, residual deficits and added stresses over time.

   (2) Resources - existing and new resources that emerge because of the crisis.

   (3) Perception - family's subjective appraisal of the crisis and their ability to make adjustments.

   (4) Coping - mediating cognitive and behavioral strategies used by the family to restore balance in family life.

   (5) Adaptation - outcome of the situation; occurs on a continuum from maladaptation to bonadaptation.

d. Stress is viewed in this model as the family system members response to change. Interest is on identifying the stress-regulating factors used by the family to mediate change.

e. Families respond to similar situations in very different ways. Family perception of their situation is the critical factor in how change will be managed.

f. Recent research in the stress theory tradition has focused on family strengths and strategies to enhance family strengths.

g. Adaptation to crisis is an ongoing process of adjustments whereby families strive to balance demands and resources to achieve optimal family functioning, given their circumstances.

3. Assessment areas: Nurse assesses the family for strengths and weaknesses.

a. Identify family pile-up of demands, resources, perception of their situation, coping behaviors, and degree of adaptation.

b. Explore how family members view their situation; strengths, weaknesses, and expected outcomes.

c. Determine what the family believes they need to do to stabilize or improve family functioning.

d. Examine strategies aimed at balancing family demands with family capabilities in the context of recommendations that are feasible and acceptable to the specific family.

IV. Family Nursing Care During the Acute/Critical Care Phase

A. **Nursing Diagnoses**
1. Alteration in family processes related to member SCI crisis
2. Potential for family self-care deficits

B. **Desired Family Outcomes**
1. Support family member with SCI and each other.
2. Maintain, and as necessary, redefine hope regarding prognosis of family member with SCI.
3. Develop confidence and trust in healthcare team by establishing a relationship with providers.
4. Minimize family disruption and maintain essential family activities.
5. Communicate needs and concerns to providers and one another.
6. Participate in patient care planning.
7. Balance understanding with information overload; synthesize multiple suggestions and recommendations.
8. Engage in own self-care activities to decrease physical and psychological stress.

C. **Assessment**
1. Family responses
   a. Crisis event; period of major stress
   b. Emotional turmoil; anxiety, fear, grief, hope, uncertainty
   c. Central fear; survival of family member with SCI
   d. Exhaustion; physical and psychological
2. Family needs
   a. Visitation; being in close proximity to the family member with SCI
   b. Information; honest, timely and delivered with concern
   c. Reassurance; patient receiving the best care possible
   d. Support (to patient and among other family members)
   e. Ventilation; expression of concerns and feeling
   f. Environmental amenities
3. Family function: Focus areas in acute SCI phase: What to look for.
   a. Family membership
      (1) Relationship of visitors to patient
      (2) Contact person(s)
      (3) Potential primary caregiver(s)
   b. Adaptive family processes during acute crisis
      (1) Accurate cognitive appraisal of the situation
      (2) Balancing responsibilities of hospital, home, and work

        (3)   Open information exchange among family members and providers

        (4)   Maintaining integrity of family relationships

        (5)   Decision-making and problem-solving skills; who is involved and how decisions are made

        (6)   Assuming new role responsibilities

    c. Resources

        (1)   Prior experience with serious, acute illness

        (2)   Effective coping behaviors

        (3)   Ability to mobilize a support network

        (4)   Ability to express needs to each other and providers

        (5)   Ability to assimilate information

    d. Family health

        (1)   Management of psychological responses

        (2)   Care for their own health

        (3)   Family member sensitivity to one another's emotional needs

        (4)   Ongoing maintenance of family member health needs

        (5)   Ability to assimilate information

D. Interventions Based on Family Needs

  1. General principles to consider when planning nursing care (Leske, 1992)

    a. Family is a critical aspect of patient's environment for recovery.

    b. Interactions among family members and nurses greatly influence perceptions about the quality of care being provided.

    c. Information exchanged among family members and providers is easily distorted and requires constant validation and clarification.

    d. Patient education and rehabilitation begins on admission and needs to include the family. Positive reinforcement goes a long way.

    e. Use every family contact as an opportunity to assess family needs, plan and provide interventions.

    f. There is considerable research based evidence regarding family responses and needs during acute illness and when individual is in an intensive care unit.

    g. There is little research-based evidence regarding the effectiveness of nursing interventions to address family needs at this stage.

  2. Family visitation

    a. Promote physical access and proximity to the patient.

    b. Contract with family for appropriate visitation schedule.

    c. Determine family member's expectations regarding visitation. Do they want time alone with patient, or to assist with caregiving, or to receive instructions about how to relate to the patient?

    d. Encourage family member self-care activities, such as physical needs of rest and nutrition and psychological needs for breaks and maintaining daily living responsibilities.

  3. Information management

    a. Provide timely, current, realistic information regarding patient's condition; validate accuracy of information received.

        (1)   Information decreases uncertainty and may restore a sense of control (Lynn-McHale & Smith, 1991).

        (2)   Ability to assimilate information is altered during crisis.

        (3)   Families need help to maintain a balance between reality and optimism.

    b. Identify contact persons: a family member and a primary care provider, to serve as the major conduit for information exchange.

  4. Reassurance

    a. Develop relationship of trust and confidence with family members through planned interactions and active listening.

    b. Orient family members to hospital routine, care procedures, and need for special equipment to allay concerns and fears of the unfamiliar.

    c. Provide continuity of primary care providers.

5. Support
   a. Strengthen family's ability to provide support to patient and one another.
      (1) Family support has a mediating effect on patient's ability to cope with frightening acute-care hospital environment and painful procedures; desire to recover; psychological distress; and physiological state.
      (2) Staff support to family yields reciprocal support of family members to patient.
      (3) Family members are receptive to staff influence at a time of crisis (Cobb, 1976; Norbeck, 1988).
      (4) Family "peer" support groups are an important resource for families.
   b. Provide staff accessibility to family members; inquire about family needs and well being.
      (1) Investigators found that families perceive staff to be too busy to be concerned about their needs (Artinian, 1989; Hampe, 1975).
      (2) Family contact needs vary; individualize based on family preference.
6. Ventilation
   a. Provide opportunities for family members to express concerns and feelings.
      (1) Families exhibit variations in the need for expressing emotions and in the ability to do so.
      (2) Study findings suggest that encouraging emotional release is not helpful for some families (Lynn-McHale & Bellinger, 1988).
   b. Reassure family members that they are a vital part of the patient's care and recovery process (Lynn-McHale & Smith, 1991).
7. Environmental amenities
   a. Facilitate physical comfort of the family by offering comfort items such as pillows and blankets, providing easy access to a telephone and, orienting to facilities accessible to the hospital, especially available accommodations for out-of-town visitors.
   b. Provide information about available institutional support services (e.g. social worker, psychologist, and chaplain.)
   c. Initiate referrals and coordinate follow-up through the care team.

E. **Health Education Tips**
   1. Factors affecting teaching/learning:
      a. Limited time for teaching; stay in intensive care is usually brief
      b. Ability to learn and comprehend are compromised by personal and environmental factors inherent in a life-threatening, crisis situation (e.g., fear and anxiety, decreased ability to focus attention and process information, and environmental distractions.)
      c. Nurses should assess and validate comprehension with liberal use of repetition and clarification.
   2. Content
      a. Concrete information about diagnosis and condition status
      b. Purpose of procedures, tests, and equipment
      c. Hospital/unit rules, routines, and amenities and services available
      d. Strategies and rationale for family self-care activities

V. Family Needs and Responses in Rehabilitation

A. **Nursing Diagnoses:**
   1. Alterations in family process due to rehabilitation needs
   2. Potential for family self-care deficits
   3. Potential alteration in family members' health maintenance
   4. Impaired home-maintenance management
   5. Grieving related to decreased functional status of a family member
   6. Potential for ineffective family coping
   7. Powerlessness

B. **Desired Family Outcomes**:
   1. Reestablish family stability.
   2. Maintain open communication among members.

3. Reallocate member roles to accommodate restructured responsibilities.
4. Realign relationships among family members.
5. Demonstrate ability to perform SCI rehabilitation requirements.

C. **Assessment**: Nurse observes family efforts to pull together as a unit and respond to the demands of rehabilitation.
1. Family responses
   a. Post-crisis: period of major adjustment
   b. Emotional ups and downs: anxiety, frustration, fear, hope, relief and accomplishment
   c. Central fear: ability to restructure family life to accommodate SCI requirements
   d. Predominant feeling: uncertainty
   e. Magnification of family strengths and weaknesses
2. Family needs
   a. Emotional stability
   b. Information/Instruction
   c. Redefinition of family member relationships, roles, and responsibilities
   d. Development of new networks while maintaining existing ones
   e. Opportunity to grieve for the loss of the family as it was prior to injury
3. Family function - focus areas in rehabilitation phase
   a. Family membership
      (1) Family constellation: who are the members, immediate and extended; subsystems; alliances and barriers.
      (2) Member contributions to family function: strengths and weaknesses.
      (3) Developmental stage and status of stage-specific tasks: family and individual members.
      (4) Potential family member caregiving contributions.
   b. Adaptive family processes during rehabilitation
      (1) Realization of multiple changes
      (2) Reestablishment of family functioning
      (3) Restructuring of family unit: roles and responsibilities
      (4) Realignment of relationships and communication patterns among family members and external systems
      (5) Recognition of the influence of family cultural traditions, values, and behaviors on rehabilitation
   c. Resources
      (1) Ask if family has a social worker to help them obtain essential social services. Does the family know what they need, where to obtain resources and how to access other agencies?
      (2) What is family doing to reestablishing economic stability? Determine need for additional referrals.
      (3) Assist family in obtaining a home environment assessment. Ask family about their plans for accommodating to the changes; talking through their plans often helps clarify concerns.
      (4) Explore coping behaviors of family members; what has worked in the past?
   d. Family health
      (1) Implications of pre-injury lifestyle on rehabilitation requirements
      (2) Ongoing family health care requirements
      (3) Ability to problem solve, make decisions, and prioritize family needs/demands
      (4) Effects of rehabilitation requirements on each family member and family system

D. **Interventions - Based on Family Needs**
1. General principles: Factors associated with better family functioning:
   a. Time since injury is less than 2 years or more than 5 years (McGowan & Roth, 1987).
   b. Communication among family members is clear, direct, and responsive (McGowan & Roth, 1987).
   c. Family members understand and accept role responsibilities (McGowan & Roth, 1987).
   d. Strong marital relationship (Baxter, 1981).
   e. First marriage (El Ghatit & Hanson, 1976).

    f. Marital partners are older (DeVivo & Richards, 1992).

    g. Married after injury (Crewe & Krause, 1988).

    h. Ability to manage conflict (Urey & Henggeler, 1987).

    i. Family communicates sense of worth toward SCI member.

2. Emotional stability

    a. Offer reassurance that fluctuations in emotional responses are normal.

    b. Encourage expression, provide support and assist family to manage feelings.

      (1) Once patient survival is assured, the family experiences decreased anxiety, fear, and other intense emotions. This relief is short-lived, as the realities of the disability generate uncertainty and daily challenges in adjusting to the demands of rehabilitation.

      (2) Progress and setbacks are accompanied by fluctuating psychological responses that may not be readily understood by the patient, family members, or providers.

    c. Psychological adjustment is as important as physical adjustment if the family and patient are to regain control and mastery over their lives and attain rehabilitation goals. Families would benefit from family counseling. A referral and support from the nurse can facilitate that decision.

3. Information/Instruction

    a. Provide timely, accurate, instructive updates on patient's condition and progress with treatment and rehabilitation goals.

    b. Involve patient and family in well-planned comprehensive educational program.

      (1) Early rehabilitation requires the patient and family to assimilate vast amount of information, learn many skills, and develop dexterity with unfamiliar equipment and procedures in order to achieve success.

      (2) Family involvement is a key factor in successful rehabilitation i.e., positive reinforcement by family is related to better performance (Litman, 1964); patients who perceive their family as supportive and responsive show higher levels of self-initiation of activities (McGowan & Roth, 1987).

      (3) See *Educational Guide for Spinal Cord Injury Nurses* (Hanak, 1990) for comprehensive text on meeting educational needs.

4. Redefinition family member relationships, roles, and responsibilities

    a. Interpersonal adjustment is a process that family members need to work through. Assistance from the entire rehabilitation team is required.

    b. Keep the SCI family member in control of the rehabilitation process. Teach family members the benefits derived from active self – care, such as in the decreasing passivity and dependency and preventing the development of unhealthy self - care patterns.

    c. Assist family members to jointly redefine family structure and member contributions in adjusting to SCI.

    d. Functional independence, within the limitations of the disability, is necessary for the identified patient and the family. Failure to achieve this often leads to dysfunction of the family unit and poor rehabilitation outcomes.

5. Development new support networks while maintaining existing ones

    a. Identify family's support network: membership and type of support provided (emotional, instrumental, and/or informational).

      (1) Discuss effectiveness of support and strategies to maintain support (e.g., reciprocity/preventing overload or burden.)

      (2) Social support that offers professional advice and tangible assistance may minimize distress soon after injury, while peer support may be more helpful over time (Elliot, 1991).

    b. Encourage contact with other families who have had positive rehabilitation outcomes.

      (1) Rehabilitation adjustment problems are less intense when family members can talk with others who have "been there" and can provide practical suggestions based upon what worked for them.

      (2) Nelson (1990) notes that SCI individuals have a great influence on one another. Observation suggests that this occurs with families as well.

    c. Make appropriate referrals based on careful assessment of family needs and agency services. Link families with organizations and publications to help them stay abreast of changes in rehabilitation treatment. Local chapters of some organizations, such as Paralyzed Veterans of America (PVA), have social functions and other opportunities to become involved, informed, and to network with others.

    d. Monitor family relationships for areas of tension and potential dysfunction. Provide opportunities to discuss situations. Alert treatment team.

6. Grieve for the loss of the family as it was prior to the injury

    a. Reinforce therapy/consultant recommendations. This assumes that psychologist and social worker interventions were provided.

    b. Recognize emotional responses of grief, loss, and helplessness and provide opportunities for discussion. Keep team members informed. Identify interventions in the plan of care.

    c. Explore family-specific alternatives for accepting and resolving the impact of SCI on adjustment (Miller & Eggerth, 1994). For example, discuss past family activities and explore ways the family could alter activities to accommodate the changes imposed by altered physical abilities.

    d. Discuss benefits of brief family therapy.

E. Health Education Tips

1. Factors affecting teaching/learning:

    a. Learning style, needs, and level of assimilation vary among family members; frequent assessment and adjustment are required.

    b. Psychological factors and emotional responses greatly influence learning and performance. These may need to be addressed prior to proceeding with planned instruction.

2. Content

    a. SCI-specific information and skills to achieve independent living

    b. How to ask for and receive help; applies to both patient and family members.

    c. Communication and problem-solving skills

    d. Time management

    e. Resource acquisition

    f. Strategies for re-entry into the community (e.g., dealing with negative/positive attitudes toward disability.)

VI. Family Needs and Responses in Lifetime Health Maintenance

A. Nursing Diagnoses:

1. Alteration in family process due to:

    a. Disability/chronic illness

    b. Acute illness episode

2. Alterations in family members' health maintenance

3. Impaired home-maintenance management

4. Ineffective family coping

5. Family self-care deficit

6. Alteration in parenting

7. Potential diversional activity deficit

B. Desired Family Outcomes:

1. Maintain family stability

2. Practice health behaviors that prevent secondary complications and impairments

3. Promote stage-specific independent living skills among its members

4. Balance family demands with resources

5. Strive for an acceptable quality of life.

C. Assessment

1. Family responses

    a. Residual sense of vulnerability

    b. Attitude of caution and vigilance; awareness that good health cannot be taken for granted.

     c. General emotional stability

     d. Problem-solving abilities and coping skills based on experience in having worked through difficult situations.

     e. Resilience

2. Family needs

     a. Maintenance of a satisfying, high-quality family life

     b. Involvement in a supportive social network

     c. Absence of medical and psychological complications

     d. Independent lifestyle

     e. Economic stability

3. Family function: focus areas in lifetime health maintenance

     a. Family membership

        (1) Family constellation; the members and their roles and responsibilities?

        (2) Member contributions to family function

        (3) Developmental stage and status of stage-specific tasks

     b. Adaptive family processes

        (1) Strategies used by the family to maintain stability of family life

        (2) Areas of strengths and weaknesses in family functioning.

        (3) Evidence of family goals and plans for achieving them.

     c. Resources

        (1) Knowledge and use of social services; areas of deficits or over dependence

        (2) Evidence of participation in social network and community activities

        (3) Adequate financial support

        (4) Status of family demands and capabilities

        (5) Barriers to work, education, housing, transportation, and other factors necessary to achieve a satisfying family life

     d. Health

        (1) Implications of SCI on "normal" process of aging

        (2) Ongoing developmental stage-specific health care requirements of members.

        (3) Adequacy of illness prevention and health promotion efforts

D. Interventions Based on Family Needs

1. General principles

     a. The literature that evaluates the long-term adjustment of an entire family in which one individual has SCI is relatively sparse. There are few clinical reports and minimal research.

     b. Family coping and adjustment to SCI is a lifelong process.

     c. Studies of parenting and parent-child relationships suggest no negative consequences of parental SCI on children's psychological adjustment or general development (Buck & Hohmann, 1981; 1982).

     d. SCI has a short-term negative impact on marriage and divorce. Studies of divorce rate in SCI within 5 years of injury suggest slightly higher rates seen in couples without injury (DeVivo & Richards, 1992). Marriages that do survive are generally viewed as satisfying (Crewe & Krause, 1988).

     e. Regardless of adaptation outcomes, family life is complex and requires a greater amount of member effort and commitment to attain quality family life.

2. Maintenance of sustain a satisfying, quality family life

     a. Assess family adjustment at each opportunity of contact — annual physical, routine exams, episodic treatment. Allocate additional time to address family needs through inquiry and observation of members who accompany the patient member.

     b. Create opportunities to interact with family members and observe family dynamics (e.g., invite input from family members at routine visits, attend social functions attended by extended family).

     c. Recognize behavioral patterns of inappropriate or destructive family relationships. Consider referral for family therapy when family members evidence signs of difficulty such as chronic complaining, treatment sabotage, extreme over-protectiveness, increasing somatic complaints, overt hostility, unhealthy close relationships, and psychosocial deprivation (Munro, 1985).

    d. Promote and advocate for health care delivery models that address provisions for continuity of care, such as a primary care provider, follow-up (especially home visits). The best way to assess family adjustment in spinal cord dysfunction is by actually observing the environment in which health maintenance occurs.

    e. Be aware that a family may not wish to openly express its feelings and concerns; therefore, close contact over a period of time is needed to establish trust.

    f. Assess for degree of burden on any one family member and determine how this is managed by the family.

    g. Realize that encouragement and empowerment are two strategies that facilitate family adaptation to SCI and increase the ability to attain quality family life.

    h. Explore family expectations and discuss in terms of realistic outcomes.

3. Involvement in a supportive social network

    a. Access adequacy of support available to the family. Who provides support? What is the relationship of the supportive persons to the family? What help is provided? Is the assistance helpful?

    b. Explore options for strengthening supportive relationships. Address issue of reciprocity.

    c. Identify opportunities for peer counseling; consider recommending that the family receive or provide this type of assistance.

4. Absence of medical and psychological complications

    a. Evaluate family members' knowledge and understanding of essential illness prevention and health maintenance regimens to sustain a healthy lifestyle.

    b. Evaluate family members' ability to recognize early symptoms of potential medical and psychological problems.

    c. Assess degree of compliance in managing health maintenance regimens. Identify factors that may interfere, such as; time, comfort, energy, supplies, motivation, expenses, and assistance.

    d. Determine whether family has an organized plan for medical emergency situations, (e.g., ready access to critical telephone numbers, written instructions on what to do).

5. Independent lifestyle

    a. Identify environmental barriers to participation in usual activities of daily living, such as; work, transportation, housing, education, and finances, and accessibility to public and private facilities/events.

    b. Examine family problem-solving abilities and coping strategies.

    c. Assess usual level of participation in social and community activities. For example, "What does your family do for fun?"

    d. Determine sources of stress and what the family does to alleviate stress.

6. Economic stability

    a. Refer to social worker to assess financial status.

    b. Identify deficits and possible sources that could be mobilized to meet these needs.

    c. Consult with, or refer family to, useful social services.

E. **Health Education Tips**

1. Factors affecting teaching/learning

    a. Few SCI Centers offer educational programs for outpatients and families.

    b. Providers need to develop programs and outreach strategies to involve families in illness prevention and health promotion programs.

2. Content

    a. Survival skills, (e.g., prevention of medical complications, promotion of wellness, updates on advances in treatment, managing personal care attendants).

    b. Healthy living and enrichment programs aimed at skill development, expanding leisure and vocational activities, and information/discussion groups for improving family life.

Practical Application

At 3:00 in the morning, Kay received a call from the West General Hospital stating that her husband, R.E. had been in an auto accident and was a patient in the Intensive Care Unit (ICU). He was semi-conscious and had asked for her. Kay immediately called her parents to come stay with the couple's 18-month-old son. Upon arrival in the ICU, Kay's fears escalated to panic. She couldn't speak and felt faint. The nurse had been watching for her arrival and came to her side. She introduced herself and asked Kay if she wanted to sit down a minute. The nurse attempted to normalize Kay's reaction with "This place often frightens people when they first come in." She invited Kay to express her feelings and immediate concerns. She then accompanied Kay to her husband's bedside, offering realistic reassurances and information en route. "We don't know the extent of the injury just yet; his spinal cord was injured here, as she pointed to the T7 area of Kay's back. Your husband has had some medication that should decrease the swelling and pressure, but it takes time to see how well the medication will work, and we need to do more tests to see how much damage there has been. I will keep you informed as we learn more." It's okay to touch him and talk to him. Have a seat here by the bed. I'll be right here with you. Feel free to ask questions." Kay took her husband's hand and slowly looked him over from top to bottom. "Nothing looks broken. What is wrong with him?" The nurse sat down next to Kay and provided a brief but simple explanation about spinal cord trauma, and what the staff would be doing and looking for in the next 24 hours. She frequently checked Kay's understanding of the information and watched for her emotional responses. The nurse viewed Kay as "her patient," knowing that she needed to help Kay maintain optimal functioning during this crisis. Her message to Kay was "We want you to feel comfortable here. You are very important to R.E.'s recovery." Her actions toward Kay communicated care and concern and were motivated by a desire to establish a trusting relationship. As the nurse provided care, she explained what she was doing and why. She began a family assessment by casually inquiring about the couple's son, R.E.'s parents, and others who might be visiting R.E. The nurse used sensitive listening and careful observation to develop an initial understanding of R.E.'s family and the role members might play in the days ahead.

At a break in R.E.'s care, the nurse oriented Kay to the ICU visitation policies, and physical surroundings, and on a walking tour, pointing out the telephones, lounge and rest areas, and snack machines. She gave Kay "Information About the ICU," a unit developed pamphlet with the same information. On the cover, the nurse had written her name, the physician's name, and other key staff with telephone numbers. She explained that she was R.E.'s primary nurse and would be coordinating his care while in the ICU. Before going off duty, she set up a meeting for the physician to talk with Kay and any other family members. As the nurse explained, "It's important for you to have the support of your family or friends at a time like this." The nurse introduced Kay to her replacement and noted she would be back on duty at 3:30 PM. "I'll be working 3:30 to 12:00 AM all week. When I return, I want to hear that you went home for some rest and nourishment. Will you be able to do that?"

The nurse provided family nursing care by addressing both R.E.'s and Kay's needs. During the initial hours in the acute care setting, the nurse accomplished the following: 1) demonstrated that R.E. was receiving excellent care from a knowledgeable nurse, 2) reduced Kay's anxiety, 3) began to develop a relationship with Kay, 4) promoted physical access and proximity to R.E., 5) provided Kay with realistic information about her husband's condition, 6) validated Kay's understanding of information, 7) conducted initial assessment of family structure and function, 8) provided opportunities for Kay to express concerns and ask questions, 9) facilitated Kay's coping, and 10) set up the expectation that Kay needs to take care of herself is she going to be an ally in R.E.'s recovery.

References and Selected Bibliography

Adams, K. (1981). Impact on marriages of adult-onset paraplegia. *Paraplegia, 19*, 253-259.

Alston, R. & McCowan, C. (1995). Perception of family competence and adaptation to illness among African Americans with disabilities. *Journal of Rehabilitation, 61*(1), 27-32.

Artinian, N. (1989). Family member perceptions of a cardiac surgery event. *Focus on Critical Care, 16*, 301-308.

Baxter, R. (1981). Divorce: The second trauma. *Accent, 2*, 47-52.

Brewer, N. & Warren, M. (1994). Altered family processes related to an ill family member: A validation study. *Nursing Diagnosis, 5*(3), 115-120.

Brown, J. & Giesy, B. (1986). Marital status of persons with spinal cord injury. *Social Science Medicine, 23* (3), 313-322.

Buck, F. & Hohmann, G. (1981). Personality, behavior, values, and family relations of children of fathers with a spinal cord injury. *Archives of Physical Medicine and Rehabilitation, 62*(9), 432-438.

Buck, F. & Hohmann, G. (1982). Child adjustment as related to severity of paternal disability. *Archives of Physical Medicine and Rehabilitation, 63*(6), 249-253.

Bucklew, S. & Hanson, S. (1992). Coping and adjustment following spinal cord injury. *SCI Psychosocial Process, 4*(3), 99-103.

Burr, W., Leigh, R., Day, R. & Constantine, J. (1979). Symbolic interaction and the family. In W. Burr, R. Hill, F. Nye, & I. Reiss (Eds.), *Contemporary theories about the family*. New York: The Free Press.

Butcher, L. (1994). A family-focused perspective on chronic illness. *Rehabilitation Nursing, 19* (2), 70-74.

Cleveland, M. (1980). Family adaptation to traumatic spinal cord injury: Response to crisis. *Family Relations, 29*, 558-565.

Cobb, S. (1976). Social support as a moderation of life stress. *Psychosomatic Medicine, 38* (5), 301-313.

Crewe, N., Athelstan, G., & Keumberger, B.A. (1979). Spinal cord injury: A comparison of preinjury and postinjury marriages. *Archives of Physical Medicine and Rehabilitation, 60*(6), 252-266.

Crewe, N. & Krause, J. (1988). Marital relationships and spinal cord injury. *Archives of Physical Medicine and Rehabilitation, 69* (6), 435-438

Decker, S., Schultz, R. & Wood, D. (1989). Determinants of well-being in primary caregivers of spinal cord injured persons. *Rehabilitation Nursing, 14* (1), 6-8.

DeJong, G., Branch, L. & Corcoran, P. (1984). Independent living outcomes in spinal cord injury: Multivariate analysis. *Archives of Physical Medicine and Rehabilitation, 65*(2),66-73.

DeVivo, M. & Fine, P. (1985). Spinal cord injury: Its short-term impact on marital status. *Archives of Physical Medicine and Rehabilitation, 66*(8), 501-504.

DeVivo, M. & Richards, J. (1992). Community reintegration and quality of life following spinal cord injury. *Paraplegia, 30*(2), 108-112.

Duvall, E. (1977). *Family Development* (5th ed.). Philadelphia PA: J.B. Lippincott.

El Ghatit, A. & Hanson, R. (1976). Marriage and divorce after spinal cord injury. *Archives of Physical Medicine and Rehabilitation, 57*(10), 470-472.

Elliot, T. (1991). Interpersonal behavior and adjustment of persons with spinal cord injury. *SCI Psychosocial Process, 4* (3), 82-87.

Friedman, M. (1981). *Family nursing: Theory and assessment.* Norwalk CT: Appleton-Century -Crofts.

Gillies, D. (1988). Role supplementation to overcome interfamilial role insufficiency following physical disability. *Rehabilitation Nursing, 13* (1), 19-23.

Hampe, S. (1975). Needs of the grieving spouse in a hospital setting. *Nursing Research, 24*(2), 113-120.

Hanak, M. (Ed.). (1990). *Educational guide for spinal cord injury nurses.* Jackson Heights, NY: American Association of Spinal Cord Injury Nurses.

Hart, G. (1981). Spinal cord injury: Impact on clients' significant others. *Rehabilitation Nursing, 6*(1), 11-15.

Herbert, J. (1989). Assessing the need for family therapy: A primer for rehabilitation counselors. *Journal of Rehabilitation, 55* (1), 45-51.

Hill, R. (1958). Generic features of families under stress. *Social Casework, 39,* 139-150.

Judd, F., Webber, J., Brown, D., Normand, T., & Burrows, G. (1991). Psychological adjustment following traumatic spinal cord injury: A study using the Psychosocial Adjustment to Illness Scale. *Paraplegia, 29,* 173-179.

Killen, J. (1990). Role stabilization in families after spinal cord injury. *Rehabilitation Nursing, 15*(1), 19-21.

Krause, J. & Crewe, N. (1987). Prediction of long term survival among persons with spinal cord injury: An 11-year prospective study. *Rehabilitation Psychology, 32*(4), 205-213.

Lapham-Randlov, N. (1994). How the family copes with spinal cord injury: A personal perspective. *Rehabilitation Nursing, 19* (2), 80-83.

Leske, J. (1992). Needs of adult family members after critical illness. *Critical Care Nursing of North America, 4* (4), 587-596.

Litman, T. (1964). An analysis of the sociological factors affecting the rehabilitation of physically handicapped patients. *Archives of Physical Medicine and Rehabilitation, 45,* 49-57.

Lynn-McHale, D. & Bellinger, A. (1988). Need satisfaction levels of family members of critical care patients and accuracy of nurses' perceptions. *Heart and Lung, 17*(4), 447-453.

Lynn-McHale, D. & Smith, A. (1991). Comprehensive assessment of families of the critically ill. *Critical Care Nurses, 2* (2), 195-209.

Marlatt, J. (1988). The role of the family in rehabilitation. *Journal of Rehabilitation, 54* (1), 7-8, 77.

McCubbin, H., & Patterson, J. (1983). The family stress process: The double ABCX model of adjustment and adaptation. In H. McCubbin, M. Sussman & J. Patterson (Eds.), *Social stress and the family: Advances and developments in family stress theory and research* (pp. 7-38). New York: Haworth Press.

McCubbin, H & Thompson, AI. (1987). *Family assessment inventories for research and practice.* Madison, WI: University of Wisconsin.

McNett, S.C. (1987). Social support, threat and coping responses and effectiveness in the functional disabled. *Nursing Research, 36*(2), 103.

McGowan, M. & Roth, S. (1987). Family Functioning and functional independence in spinal cord adjustment. *Paraplegia, 25*(4), 357-365.

Miller, T. & Eggerth, D. (1994). Spinal cord as a stressful life event. *SCI Psychosocial Process, 7*(1), 3-7.

Munro, J. (1985). Counseling severely dysfunctional families of mentally and physically disabled persons. *Clinical Social Work, 13* (1), 18-31.

Nelson, A. (1990). Patient's perspectives of a spinal cord injury unit. *SCI Nursing, 7* (3), 14-16.

Norbeck, J. (1988). Social support. *Annual Review of Nursing Research, 6,* 85-109.

Potter, P. (1979). Stress and the intensive care unit-the family's perception. *Missouri Nurse, 48*(4), 5-8.

Richmond, T. (1990). Spinal cord injury. *Nursing Clinics of North America, 25* (1), 57-67.

Rintala, D. & Willems, E. (1987). Behavioral and demographic predictors of post-discharge outcomes in spinal cord injury. *Archives of Physical Medicine and Rehabilitation, 68*(6), 357-362.

Simmons, S. & Bael, S.E. (1984). Marital adjustment and self-actualization in couples married before and after spinal cord injury. *Journal of Marriage and the Family, 46,* 943-945.

Stambrook, M., Psych, C., MacBeath, S., Moore, A., Peters, L., Zubeck, E. & Friesen, I. (1991). Social role functioning following spinal cord injury. *Paraplegia, 29*(5), 318-323.

Stuart, M. (1991). An analysis of the concept of family. In *Family theory development in nursing state of the science and art.* (pp 31-42). Philadelphia PA: F.A. Davis Company.

Trieschmann, R. (1988). *Spinal cord injuries: Psychological, social, and vocational rehabilitation New York, NY:* (2nd ed.). Demos.

Urey, J. & Henggeler, S. (1987). Marital adjustment following spinal cord injury. *Archives of Physical Medicine and Rehabilitation, 68*(2), 74.

Vargo, F. (1984). Adaptation to disability by the wives of spinal cord males - A phenomenological approach. *Journal of Applied Rehabilitation Counseling, 15* (1), 28-32.

Versluys, H. (1980). Physical rehabilitation and family dynamics. *Rehabilitation Literature, 41* (3-4), 58-65.

Webster's new collegiate dictionary. (1990). Springfield MA: G. & C. Merriam.

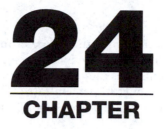

CHAPTER

Stress and Coping

Barbara Simmons, MSN, RN

I. Learning Objectives

A. Describe the concept of coping.

B. Identify the relationship between stress and significant life events.

C. List six symptoms of depression.

D. Describe the progression of substance abuse.

II. Introduction

Spinal cord impairment (SCI) represents one of life's greatest challenges. SCI can result from traumatic injury or from a disease process. Nonetheless, the etiology of SCI does not change its impact on the life of individuals or their family members. Whether sudden in onset or through progressive deterioration, SCI clearly requires the individual to draw upon all psychological, physical, social, spiritual and economic resources to adjust to this major life-changing event. Nurses must be capable of identifying and evaluating effective coping strategies. Equally important, is understanding stress as a response to SCI. Stress occurs when one experiences or perceives an event that threatens or exceeds the ability to cope. When existing coping strategies fail, the person with SCI may experience depression or turn to substance abuse to alleviate their discomfort. This chapter focuses on coping and stress as critical elements affecting success or failure in rehabilitation. When stress exceeds an individual's ability to cope, depression or substance abuse may occur.

A. **Background**

Care of the person with SCI typically emphasizes the physical process, with minimal resources allocated for psychosocial care. Psychological adjustment, as a prediction of successful reintegration and quality of life, has been investigated and reported (Dunnum, 1990; Tate, Forcheimer, & Maynard, 1993; and Trieschmann, 1988). Shorter lengths of stay, decreased recidivism, improved rehabilitation outcomes and greater reintegration have all been positively correlated with successful adjustment to SCI (Tate, Maynard, & Forchheimer, 1993; Trieschmann, 1988).

B. Demographics
Between forty to fifty percent of persons with SCI are estimated to have sustained their injuries while using alcohol or drugs. Reports on the incidence of depression among persons with SCI range broadly from 13-44 percent. This range has been attributed to variations in definitions of depression among studies. However, a 13 percent rate of depression among persons with SCI is more than double the 5.7 percent rate reported among the general population.

III. Theories of Stress

A. **"Fight or Flight" Syndrome** (Cannon, 1932).
1. Description: When faced with imminent threat, the nervous system responds by preparing the individual physiologically to fight or to flee to safety.
2. Key concepts (manifestations)
   a. Epinephrine is released by the adrenal medulla.
   b. Blood supply to the heart, brain, and muscles increases.
   c. Blood supply to visceral organs decreases.
   d. Blood pressure and heart rate increase.
   e. Blood supply to the skin diminishes and blood coagulates more rapidly to prevent blood loss.
   f. Respiration increases.
   g. Digestive processes cease.
   h. Perspiration increases cooling the body.

B. **Stress** (Selye, 1984).
1. Definition of Stress:"Stress is the state manifested by a specific syndrome which consists of all the nonspecifically - induced changes within a biologic system" (Selye, 1984, p.64).
2. Key concepts
   a. Stress is a specific syndrome but has no specific cause.
   b. A stressor is any source of stress.
   c. Stressors may be unpleasant or pleasant.
   d. The bodily response to stress is nonspecific, responding in the same way to both pleasant and unpleasant stressors.
   e. Stressors are specific to the individual and vary in the degree to which they produce stress.

C. **General Adaptation Syndrome** (GAS)
1. Definition: General adaptation syndrome is the whole body's response to stress over time (Selye, 1984).
2. Key concepts: General adaptation is comprised of three stages.
   a. Alarm reaction is the initial phase, when the organism's defenses against stressors are mobilized.
   b. Stage of resistance occurs when the body adapts to survive the sustained exposure to the stressor.
   c. Stage of exhaustion occurs when the body can no longer endure the prolonged exposure to stress.
3. Manifestations of stress
   a. Irritability, depression
   b. Dry mouth and throat
   c. Increased perspiration
   d. Increased heart rate
   e. Inability to concentrate
   f. Tremulousness

g. Substance abuse

h. Accident prone

i. Increase or decrease in appetite

D. **Concept of Stress: The Dynamic Concept** (King, 1981).

1. Definition: "Stress is a dynamic state whereby a human being interacts with the environment to maintain balance for growth, development, and performance, which involves an exchange of information between the person and the environment for regulation and control of stressors" (King, 1981, p.98).

2. Key concepts

a. Stress is dynamic. Life events may be pleasant or unpleasant. As circumstances change, so do levels of stress.

b. Stress is both temporal and spatial. Stressful life events occur at specific times and in particular situations. Stressful events can be predictors of illness or disease.

c. Stress is individual, personal, and subjective. "A person's response to stress is influenced by the stressors, the situation, the time of the event, and the meaning it has for the person" (King, 1981, p.98).

E. **Concepts of Stress: The Descriptive Concept** (Benner & Wrubel, 1989).

1. Definition: "Stress is defined as the description of meanings, understanding, and smooth functioning so that harm, loss, or challenge is experienced, and sorrow, interpretation, or new skill acquisition is required" (Benner & Wrubel, 1989, p.59).

2. Key concepts

a. Stress infers that the individual's perception of smooth functioning has been disrupted.

b. Stress involves the individual, the event, and the individual's understanding of the situation.

c. Stress is inevitable.

d. Stress cannot be cured.

F. **Assessment**

1. SCI as catastrophic life event

2. History of previous or co-existing stressors

3. Availability of support system

4. Behavioral change (e.g., noncompliance with rehabilitation, angry outbursts)

5. Coping strategies

6. Ability to perform activities of daily living (ADL).

7. History of depression

8. History of substance abuse

9. Smoking

G. **Interventions**

1. Interpret life event of SCI

2. Involve the family in care of the patient.

3. Coach and guide toward appropriate behavior.

4. Utilize progressive rehabilitation, visualization, self-hypnosis, and desensitization.

5. Educate patient regarding mastery of or assistance with ADL.

6. Refer to mental health professional.

H. **Expected Outcomes**

1. Realistic goals for reintegration will be established.

2. Relationship with family will remain intact.

3. Feelings regarding SCI will be expressed.

4. Coping strategies will be used.

5. Participation in rehabilitation will be maintained.

IV. Coping Strategies

A. **Copology** (Hughley, 1994)
1. Definition: "Copology is the branch of learning that studies human beings their functioning, and the process of coping with life events and the associated stress" (Hughley, 1994, p.113).
2. Goals:
   a. Assist individuals to understand themselves in relationship to their SCI.
   b. Teach persons with SCI practical strategies to cope with related stress.
3. Key concepts
   a. Coping factors: Human characteristics used for physical, mental, and social functioning.
   b. Life event: A situation that occurs in life. A life event may be either endogenous (from inside the body) or exogenous (from outside the body).
   c. Sensation: A coping factor comprised of five components — optical, auditory, olfactory, coetaneous and gustatory, which collect information and a "sixth sense".
   d. Thoughts: cognitive means for processing information, and are comprised of five components — analyzation, recognition, integration, comprehension, and decision.
   e. Emotions: A coping factor representing feelings related to SCI and comprised of three components- - love, fear, and anger.
   f. Attitudes: Embedded ideas, beliefs, values, and memories of previous life events. Attitudes may be positive, neutral, or negative.
   g. Behaviors: Actions that carry out the functions of emotions, comprised of three components — digression, freeze and aggression.
   h. Copology identifies parameters for assessing the individual's capacity to cope with SCI. It also provides a framework for understanding the impact of life events.

B. **Concepts of Coping** (Benner & Wrubel, 1989).
1. Definition: Coping is what an individual does to restore meaning when smooth functioning is disrupted. Coping does not refer to choosing from a list of alternatives. Coping is unique to each individual and bound by that individual's concerns, situation, temporality, and embodied intelligence.
2. Key concepts
   a. Temporality: The person lives in the present but is influenced by past events and by what is anticipated for the future.
   b. Role of the body: The person's body is not separate from the mind but rather provides the perspective from which the environment is experienced. For example, anxiety may increase awareness of the outer environment while decreasing awareness of the body's internal environment.
   c. Embodied intelligence: The body is adaptive, knows, and interprets. For example, the body responds to the environment based upon innate knowledge, habitual/cultural knowledge, and complex skills.
   d. Role of the situation: The situation is the unique circumstance of the person involving time, space, events and past, present, and anticipated future experience. Situation is more specific than environment.
   e. Role of personal concern: ".....The ability to have people, events, and things matter to the person in a constitutive and motivating way" (Benner & Wrubel, 1989, p.86).

V. Depression

A. **Clinical Features:** Multiple mood disorders with depressive features exist and are delineated by specific criteria in the *Diagnostic and Statistical Manual of Mental Disorders (DSM IV)*, (Fourth Edition) (American association, 1994). It is not within the scope of SCI nursing to differentiate among mood disorders. Recognition of symptoms of depression will assist the nurse to identify when to recommend referral to a mental health professional. The pathognomonic symptom of depression is the pervasive existence of a depressed mood or loss of interest or pleasure in activities. Depression may include any or all of the following symptoms (Klerman, 1988, p.310-311):
1. Depressed mood characterized by sadness and despondency

2. Inability to experience pleasure
3. Fatigue or loss of energy
4. Psychomotor retardation
5. Psychomotor agitation
6. Insomnia or hypersomia
7. Change in appetite with significant weight loss or gain
8. Physical complaints
9. Decreased sexual interest
10. Loss of interest in work or usual activities
11. Feelings of worthlessness or self-reproach
12. Difficulty concentrating
13. Anxiety
14. Feelings of helplessness
15. Decreased self-esteem
16. Pessimism and hopelessness
17. Thoughts of death or suicide attempts

B. **Differential Diagnosis**
   1. Differentiating a psychiatric diagnosis is the domain of medicine and mental health professionals. Several medical conditions may resemble depression. They include, but are not limited to:
      a. Multiple Sclerosis
      b. Trauma
      c. Thyroid disorders
      d. AIDS
      e. Chronic Fatigue Syndrome
      f. Hyponatremia
      g. Cardiovascular disorders
      h. Chronic pain
      i. Renal failure
      j. Hepatic failure
   2. Medication administration or withdrawal from medications or substances may cause depression. Administration of the following medications may cause depression:
      a. Clonidine
      b. Guanethidine
      c. Hydralazine
      d. Digitalis
      e. Prazosin
      f. Procainimide
      g. Reserpine
      h. Glucocorticoid
      i. Anabolic Steroids
      j. Nifedipine
      k. Baclofen
      l. Dantorlene
      m. Cimetidine
      n. Propranalol
      o. Barbiturates
      p. Benzodiazepines
      q. Verapamil
      r. Narcotics
   3. Withdrawal from the following medications or substances may cause depression:
      a. Amphetamines
      b. Cocaine
      c. Benzodiazepines
      d. Narcotics

351

e. Alcohol

f. Nicotine

C. **Implications:** SCI nurses are often the first to recognize symptoms of depression as impediments to rehabilitation.

1. Nursing Diagnosis: Alteration in mood with associated symptoms of depression.

2. Defining characteristics
   a. Sad expression
   b. Weight loss
   c. Minimal participation in therapy
   d. Social isolation
   e. Remaining in bed for extended periods
   f. Helplessness

3. Expected Outcomes
   a. Improved mood
   b. Improved nutritional status
   c. Active participation in therapy
   d. Involvement with family and friends
   e. Participation in planned activities
   f. Setting goals for rehabilitation

4. Interventions
   a. Encourage expression of feelings
   b. Arrange dietary consultation
   c. Include individual in planning therapy
   d. Involve family in planning care
   e. Involve individual in planning unit activities
   f. Arrange mental health consultation

D. **Health Tips**

1. Promote optimal independence and autonomy.

2. Involve individual in groups that provide coping strategies and problem-oriented approach.

3. Encourage development of new or expanded leisure skills.

4. Encourage maintenance of relationships with family and friends.

VI. Substance Abuse

A. **Clinical Features:** Substance abuse is the use of substances in excessive amounts or for other than their intended purpose, and despite resulting adverse consequences. The DSM IV describes substance abuse as a maladaptive pattern resulting in impairment, as evidenced by continued use despite 1) problems at school, work or home, hazardous circumstances, legal problems, and social and interpersonal problems. Eleven categories of substances were identified (American Psychiatric Association, 1994):

1. Alcohol

2. Amphetamines

3. Caffeine

4. Cannabis

5. Cocaine

6. Hallucinogens

7. Inhalants

8. Nicotine

9. Opioids

10. Phencyclidine (PCP)

11. Sedatives/anxiolytics/hypnotics

Figure 24-1: Pattern of Progression with Implications for Persons with SCI

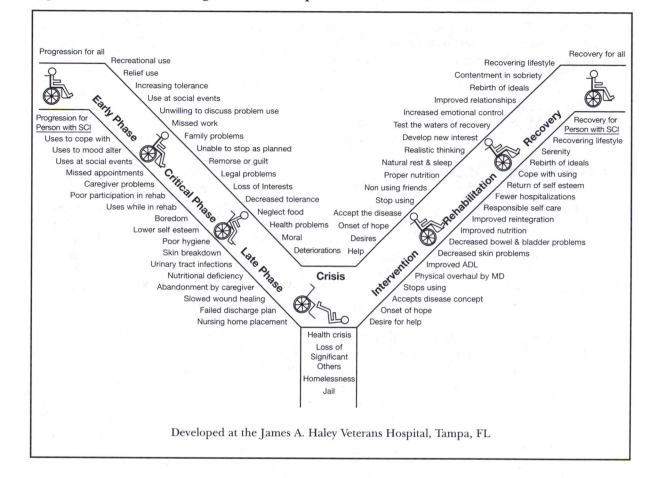

Developed at the James A. Haley Veterans Hospital, Tampa, FL

B. **Key Elements**

1. Substance abuse is a progressive disorder ending in crisis if use continues. See Figure 24-1 for pattern of progression with implications for persons with SCI (Simmons & Judd, 1994).

2. Denial is "the refusal to admit the reality or disavowal of the truth, refusal to acknowledge the presence or existence of. Known also as negation, denial is a primitive defense— an attempt to disavow the existence of unpleasant reality" (Campbell, 1989, p. 90).

3. Enabling is the process by which others collude with the addict or alcoholic in denial that the substance abuse is a problem, thereby providing consciously or unconsciously, the support, needed by the addict or alcoholic to continue to use.

C. **Nursing Diagnosis**: Ineffective coping secondary to substance abuse.

D. **Defining Characteristics**

1. Denial that substance use is a problem
2. Frequent altercations with family
3. Recurrent skin breakdown
4. Second citation for driving under the influence (DUI) in 3 months

E. **Expected Outcomes**

1. Acknowledgment of substance use as a problem
2. Abstinence from substance use
3. Restoration of relationship with family
4. Restoration of skin integrity

F. **Interventions**
1. Refer to substance abuse program
2. Provide information about Alcoholics Anonymous (AA)
3. Refer family to Alcoholics Anonymous
4. Provide education about substance abuse
5. Reinforce education on skin care

G. **Health Tips**
1. Identify leisure activities to fill time and replace abusive behaviors.
2. Develop a realistic exercise program to restore health.

Practical Application

J.H. is a 32-year-old single male admitted to the rehabilitation unit with the diagnosis of C5-C6 incomplete quadriplegia. He sustained a spinal cord injury in a motorcycle accident while on his way to work. Prior to his injury, J.H. worked as a bricklayer and foreman in a successful family-owned contracting business. He is the second of five siblings with an older brother, one younger brother, and two younger sisters. Both parents are alive. J.H. is of Nordic descent. His father believed that hard work was the measure of personal worth. J.H. and his siblings all began work at age 16 and were never without employment.

During visits, the family talked about work and how well the business was doing. On the unit, J.H. was observed as quiet and even sullen. He rarely initiated interaction except to seek assistance with a specific function. Upon admission, he had reported that he had continuous pain but rarely asked for anything to relieve the pain. He was frequently observed listening to his CD player. He attended therapy but was frequently late and was less than enthusiastic in his participation. With the exception of his limited participation in therapy, J.H.'s quiet, stoic behavior was typical for his culture and family. J.H. did admit that since he was paralyzed he thought he had little to gain from therapy. As a result of his injury, his embodied intelligence was disrupted and he perceived his body as unresponsive. His personal concern for hard work was also disrupted, since he could no longer work as a foreman or bricklayer. His role in the situation had dramatically changed.

His primary nurse assured him that even though his life had changed, he could achieve greater independence. He attended an SCI group where he met a person with C4-C5 complete quadriplegia, who had put himself through college and was married after being injured. J.H. was referred to vocational rehabilitation for evaluation for future employment. He realized that he would probably not lay bricks again; however, he could perform several functions as a foreman. He was also exploring other work options. J.H. was provided education regarding SCI, and the importance of therapy. He became an active participant in planning and implementing his care. Twelve weeks later, J.H. was discharged home and continued to work in the family business.

References and Selected Bibliography

American Psychiatric Association. (1994). *Diagnostic and statistical manual of mental disorders (DSM IV)* (4th ed.) Washington, DC: Author.

Benner, P., & Wrubel, J. (1989). *The primacy of caring: Stress and coping in health and illness.* New York: Addison Wesley.

Bozzocco, V. (1990). Vulnerability and alcohol and substance abuse in spinal cord injury. *Rehabilitation Nursing, 15*(2), 70-72.

Bulman, J.R., & Wortman, C.B. (1977). Attributions of blame and coping in the "real world": Severe accident victims react to their lot. *Journal of Personality and Social Psychology, 35*(3), 351-363.

Campbell, R.J. (1989). *Psychiatric dictionary* (6th ed.). New York: Oxford University Press.

Cannon, W.B. (1932). *The wisdom of the body.* New York: Norton.

Clay, D.L., Hagglund, K.J., Frank, R.G., Elliot, T.R., & Chaney, J.M. (1995). Enhancing the accuracy of depression diagnosis in patients with spinal cord injury using Bayesian Analyses. *Rehabilitation Psychology, 40*(3), 171-180.

Cook, D.W. (1979). Psychological adjustment to spinal cord injury: Incidence of denial, depression and anxiety. *Rehabilitation Psychology, 26*(3), 97-104.

Craig, A.R., Hancock, K.M., & Dickson, H.G. (1994). Spinal cord injury: A search for determinants of depression two years after the event. *British Journal of Clinical Psychology, 33*, 221-230.

Craig, A.R., Hancock, K.M., Dickson, H., Martin, J., & Chang, E. (1990). Psychological consequences of spinal injury: A review of the literature. *Australian and New Zealand Journal of Psychiatry, 24*, 418-425.

Crewe, N.M., & Krause, J.S. (1991). Marital status adjustment to spinal cord injury. *Journal of the American Paraplegia Society, 15*(1), 14-18.

Crisp, R. (1992). The long term adjustment of 60 persons with spinal cord injury. *Australian Psychological, 27*(1), 43-47.

Culpepper-Morgan, J.A., Twist, D.J., Petrillo, C.R., Soda, K.M., & Kreek, J.M. (1992). B-Endorphin and cortisol abnormalities in spinal cord individuals. *Metabolism, 41*(6). 578-81.

Cushman, L.A., & Dykers, M. (1991). Depressed mood during rehabilitation of persons with spinal injury. *Journal of Rehabilitation, 57*(2), 35-38.

Davies, H. (1993). Hope as a coping strategy for the spinal cord injured individual. *AXONE, 15*(2), 40-46.

de Miranda, J., Young, M., & Casmer, C.A. (1993). Developing alcohol and drug abuse services in a spinal cord injury program. *SCI Psychosocial Process, 6*(2), 64-68.

Dunnum, L. (1990). Life satisfaction and spinal cord injury: The patient perspective. *Journal of Neuroscience Nursing, 22*(1), 43-47.

Elliott, T.R., & Frank, R.G. (1996). Depression following spinal cord injury. *Archives of Physical Medicine and Rehabilitation, 77*(8), 813-823.

Elliott, T.R., & Harkins, S.W. (1991). Psychosocial concomitants of persistent pain among persons with spinal cord injuries. *Neuro Rehabilitation, 1*(4), 7-16.

Elliot, T.R., Hirrick, S.M., Witty, T.E., Godshall, F., & Spriell, M. (1992). Social support and depression following spinal cord injury. *Rehabilitation Psychology, 37*(1), 37-48.

Frank, R.G., Chaney, J.M., Clay, D.L., Shutty, M.S., Beck, N.C., Kay, D.R., Elliott, T.R., & Grambling, S. (1992) Dysphoria: A major symptom factor in persons with disability or chronic illness. *Psychiatry Research, 43*(3), 231-241.

Frank, R.G. Kashani, J.H., Wonderlich, S.A., Lising, A., & Visot, L.R. (1985). Depression and adrenal function in spinal cord injury. *American Journal of Psychiatry, 142*(2), 252-253.

Fuhrer, M.J., Rintala, D.H., Hart, K.A., Clearman, R., & Young, M.E. (1993). Depressive symptomatology in persons with spinal cord injury who reside in the community. *Archives of Physical Medicine and Rehabilitation, 74*(3), 255-260.

Fullerton, D.T., Harvey, R.F., Klein, M.H., & Howell, T. (1981). Psychiatric disorders in patients with spinal cord injuries. *Archives of General Psychiatry, 38*(12), 1369-1371.

Gehart, K.A., Kozisol-McLain, J., Lowenstein, S.R., & Whiteneck, G.G. (1994). Quality of life following spinal cord injury: Knowledge and attitudes of emergency care providers. *Annals of Emergency Medicine, 23*(4), 807-812.

Gordon, S., & Lewis, D. (1993). Psychological challenges of drugs, violence and spinal cord injury among African American inner-city males. *SCI Psychosocial Process, 8*(2), 53-60.

Hammell, K.R. (1992). Psychological and sociological theories concerning adjustment to traumatic spinal cord injury: The implications for rehabilitation. *Paraplegia, 30*(4), 317-326.

Healy, P.C. (1993) Substance abuse in spinal cord injured people. *SCI Psychosocial Process, 6*(2), 73-76.

Heinemann, A.W. (1991). Substance abuse and spinal cord injury. *Paraplegia News, 47*(7), 16-17.

Hughley, E., Jr. (1994). Copology: A contemporary model useful for coping with the stress of spinal cord injury. *SCI Psychosocial Process, 7*(3), 112-116.

Judd, F.K., & Brown, D.J. (1992). Psychiatric consultation in a spinal injuries unit. *Australian and New Zealand Journal of Psychiatry, 26*(2), 218-222.

Kim, S.P., Davis, S.W., & Sell, G.H. (1977). Amitriptyline in severely depressed spinal cord injured patients: Rapidity of response. *Archives of Physical Medicine and Rehabilitation, 58*(4), 157-161.

King, I.M. (1981). *A theory for nursing: Systems, concepts, process.* New York: John Wiley & Sons.

Kishi, Y., Robinson, R.G., & Forrester, A.W. (1994). Prospective longitudinal study of depression following spinal cord injury. *Journal of Neuropsychiatry and Clinical Neurosciences, 6*(3), 237-244.

Klerman, G.L. (1988). Depression and related disorders of mood (affective disorders). In A.M. Nicoli, Jr. (Ed.), *The new Harvard guide to psychiatry* (pp. 309-336). Cambridge,MA: Belknap Press of Harvard University Press.

MacDonald, M.R., Nielson, W.R., & Cameron, M.G.P. (1987). Depression and activity patterns of spinal cord injured persons living in the community. *Archives of Physical Medicine and Rehabilitation, 68*(6), 339-343.

Mask, J. (1993). Attitudes of staff and spinal cord injured persons toward the problem of substance abuse. *SCI Psychosocial Process, 6*(2), 77-82.

Mawson, A.R., Jacobs, K.W., Winchester, Y., & Bundo, Jr., J.J. (1988). Sensation seeking and traumatic spinal cord injury: Case control study. *Archives of Physical Medicine and Rehabilitation, 69*(12), 1039-1043.

McColl, M.A., Lei, H., & Skinner, H. (1995). Structural relationships between social support and coping. *Social Science and Medicine, 41*(3), 395-407.

McColl, M.A., & Skinner, H. (1995). Assessing inter- and intrapersonal resources: Social support and coping among adults with a disability. *Disability and Rehabilitation, 17*(1), 24-34.

Mower, S.A., William, G.H., & Stimac, D.J. (1995). Estimates of mental disorders in new spinal cord injuries: A brief report. *SCI Psychosocial Process, 9*(2/3), 69-72.

Patterson, D.R., Miller-Perrin, C., McCormick, T.R., & Hudson, L.D. (1993). When life support is questioned in the care of patients with cervical level quadriplegia. *The New England Journal of Medicine, 328*(7), 506-509.

Quigley, M.C. (1995). Impact of spinal cord on the life roles of women. *The American Journal of Occupational Therapy, 49*(8), 780-786.

Radnitz, C.L. (1993). A new program for SCI veterans with substance abuse problems. *SCI Psychosocial Process, 6*(2), 85-86.

Reidy, K., & Caplan, B. (1994). Causal factors in spinal cord injury: Patient's evolving perceptions and association with depression. *Archives of Physical Medicine and Rehabilitation, 75*(8), 837-842.

Richards, J.S. (1986). Psychologic adjustment to spinal cord injury during first post-discharge year. *Archives of Physical Medicine and Rehabilitation, 67*(6), 362-365.

Schmelzer, E.J. (1994). Social work interventions related to substance abuse among spinal cord injury patients: A response to rationalizations. *SCI Psychosocial Process, 7*(3), 117-122.

Selye, H. (1984). *The stress of life* (rev. ed.). New York: McGraw-Hill.

Simmons, B., & Judd, J. (1994, September). *Addiction education: Breaking the grip of denial in substance abuse*. Poster session presented at the annual conference for the American Association of Spinal Cord Injury Nurses, Las Vegas, NV.

Sullivan, J. (1990). Individual and family responses to acute spinal cord injury. *Critical Care Nursing Clinics of North America, 2*(3), 407-414.

Sutherland, M.W. (1993). The prevention of violent spinal cord injuries. *SCI Nursing, 10*(3), 91-95.

Tate, D.G., Forchheimer, M., Daugherty, J., & Maynard, F. (1994). Determining differences in post-discharge outcomes among catastrophically and non-catastrophically sponsored outpatients with spinal cord injury. *American Journal of Physical Medicine and Rehabilitation, 73*(2), 89-97.

Tate, D.G., Maynard, F., & Forchheimer, M. (1993). Predictors of psychologic distress one year after spinal cord injury. *American Journal of Physical Medicine and Rehabilitation, 72*(5), 272-275.

Trieschmann, R.B. (1988). *Spinal cord injuries: Psychological, social, and vocational rehabilitation* (2nd ed.). New York: Demos.

Wineman, N.M., Durand, E.J., & McCullock, B.J. (1994). Examination of the factor structure of the ways of coping questionnaire with clinical populations. *Nursing Research, 43*(5), 268-273.

Wineman, N.M., Durand, E.J., & Steiner, R.P. (1994) A comparative analysis of coping behaviors in persons with multiple sclerosis or spinal cord injury. *Nursing Research and Health, 17*(3), 185-194.

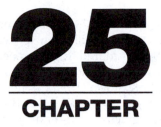

Activity and Exercise

Theresa M. Chase, MA, ND, RN

I. Learning Objectives

A. Identify physical changes caused by spinal cord impairment (SCI) that affect safety and efficacy of fitness training.

B. Identify the fundamentals of exercise within the context of a given individual's age, physical characteristics, previous exercise experience, and functional capacity.

C. Describe the physiological variables according to level of SCI that will affect exercise performance, response, and adaptation.

D. Review safety strategies for injury prevention or reduction during exercise sessions.

E. Discuss adapted equipment for exercise training and identify options that can be utilized in the home or health club.

II. Introduction

The promotion of optimal physical function is a vital component in the rehabilitation and continued development of a person with SCI. Physical disability places additional demands on the body, creating an even greater need for maximal physical function with smaller muscle mass available. For people with SCI, physical fitness plays an especially important role in enhancing functional ability and promoting a better quality of life.

A. **Scope**
   1. The role of fitness in the promotion of optimal physical functioning for adults with SCI is the focus of this chapter. Much of this information is also applicable to children.
   2. Description of the physiological challenges that occur in persons with disability and affect physical fitness activities

3. Description of the components of physical fitness
4. Discussion of physical and psychosocial issues related to a comprehensive fitness plan

B. **Demographics**
1. The long-term survival rate of persons with disabilities continues to increase, as a result of improvements in acute care and rehabilitation services. Indeed, once medically stabilized, persons with SCI need not be considered fragile, in need of protection, or unable to exercise.
2. Respiratory system complications (particularly pneumonia) are the leading cause of death following SCI (DeVivo, Black, & Stover, 1993). Ischemic and non-ischemic heart disease are leading causes of death after paraplegia (DeVivo, Black, & Stover, 1993). Furthermore, the high incidence of obesity, glucose intolerance, altered lipid profile, and impaired cardiovascular function in the SCI population has led clinicians and researchers to hypothesize that physical fitness training and nutritional strategies may overcome negative effects of sedentary lifestyle (Compton, Eisenman, & Henderson, 1989).
3. The cycle of disability illustrates a potential debilitative spiral, in which reduced incentive to exercise leads to deconditioning and a lower capacity for physical work (Figoni, 1991). (Refer to Figure 25-1).

Figure 25-1: Cycle of Disability

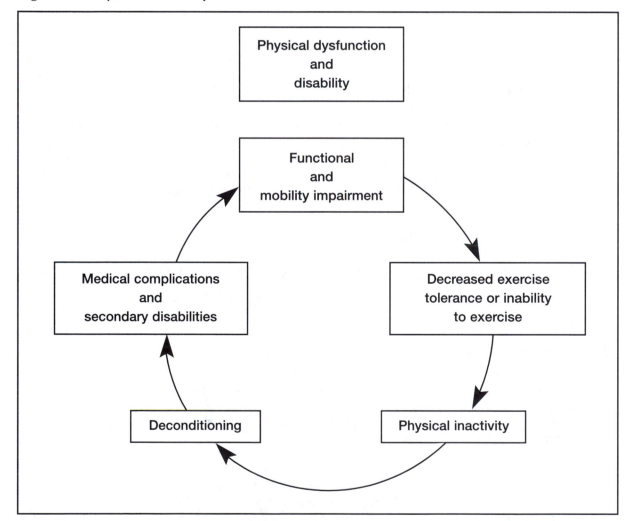

From Physiology of Aerobic Exercise, by S.F. Figoni, 1995, In P. Miller (Ed.), *Fitness Programming and Physical Disability* (p. 52), Champaign, IL: Human Kinetics. Reprinted with permission.

C. **Etiology/Precipitating Factors of Deconditioning**
   1. Altered body structure and function
      a. Paralysis/paraparesis
      b. Alteration in sensation
      c. Autonomic dysreflexia (AD)
      d. Spasticity
      e. Altered elimination
      f. Pain
      g. Mobilization difficulties
   2. Medications
   3. Alterations in self-esteem
   4. Alterations in body-image
   5. Knowledge deficit related to activity and physical exercise

D. **Anatomy/Physiology**
   1. Generally, the higher the level of injury, the greater the loss of voluntary muscle control and cardiovascular capacity, as well as possible disruption of the autonomic nervous system (ANS). Two major exercise-related physiologic consequences can occur and have an impact on the performance of exercise and on the physiological response to exercise:
      a. Progressive loss of skeletal muscle with each incremental level of injury (Claus-Walker & Halstead, 1981).
         (1) Limited muscle mass available for exercise-induced challenges to the heart and lungs
         (2) Limited functional muscle mass
         (3) Blood pooling in the lower extremities due to loss of muscle pump action
         (4) Lower threshold for fatigue in available peripheral muscles
      b. Disruption of sympathetic outflow tract with injury levels above T6 (Claus-Walker & Halstead, 1982).
         (1) Parasympathetic influence unopposed, thus limiting cardiac output and cardio-acceleration properties
         (2) Limited shunting of blood from non-exercising muscles to exercising muscles
         (3) Blunting of heart rate response, often to only approximately 110-120 Beats per minute in those with injuries above T6. With injuries below T6, there is normal regulation of cardiac function, but with lower-extremity venous pooling.
   2. Additional physiological concerns: Alterations in hemodynamic and thermoregulatory response to exercise, and varying degrees of impairment in sensation and trunk/limb control, cause additional physiological concerns (Refer to Chapter 13).
      a. Postural Hypotension
         (1) Persons with SCI at the T6 level and above frequently become hypotensive during activity, due to vasodilatation in exercising upper body muscles without normal compensatory vasoconstriction in non-exercising muscles (Figoni, 1993; Greenhoot & Mauck, 1972).
         (2) Muscle pump action of the lower extremities is absent.
         (3) Pooling of blood in the lower extremities reduces blood supply to the heart and brain, which may cause dizziness, pallor, blurred vision, and sometimes fainting.
         (4) Prevention includes:
            (a) Use abdominal binders and support hose during exercise and activity periods.
            (b) Take frequent rest breaks with gradual increases in exercise time and tolerance.
            (c) Exercising in semi-reclined position may be helpful.
            (d) Timing of blood pressure medication so that drug effectiveness is peaked to coincide with the exercise and activity.
      b. Autonomic Dysreflexia (AD)
         (1) Autonomic dysreflexia is a medical emergency, which must be recognized and treated immediately. AD is discussed in detail in Chapter 13.
         (2) Prevention includes:
            (a) Assess knowledge and previous experience with AD.

(b) Check/empty urinary drainage system.

(c) Check seating position and padding of buttocks, back, and legs.

c. Hyperthermia

   (1) Many individuals with SCI are at a disadvantage during exercise/activity, especially in warm humid environments due to impaired thermoregulatory responses. Impairments of the ANS will interfere with normal heat reduction mechanisms such as sweating and cause core body temperature to rise to dangerous levels if left unchecked.

   (2) Prevention includes:

     (a) Schedule exercise/activity during cool times of the day or in temperature-controlled environments.

     (b) Provide adequate hydration before, during, and after exercise/activity.

     (c) Have patient wearing loose-fitting clothes with some skin exposure, to enhance evaporation.

     (d) Keep a spray or mist bottle on hand for periodic use.

d. Pressure ulcers

   (1) Pressure ulcers are a major concern during exercise/activity for the person with SCI. Pressure ulcers are discussed in detail in Chapter 17 (Skin).

   (2) Prevention includes:

     (a) Ensure proper seating and frequent weight shifts during exercise/activity.

     (b) Remove wet clothing immediately following activity/exercise session.

     (c) Utilize proper padding and specialized cushions during and following an exercise/activity session.

     (d) Have individual wear shoes and other protective clothing during exercise

e. Overuse injury

   (1) Activity/exercise participation can promote stress on upper extremity joints and muscles. This stress of small musculature and joints can result in pain and fatigue, and may lead to more complicated orthopedic problems if not prevented.

   (2) Injuries due to overuse may include blisters, abrasions, or lacerations of the hands and arms, as well as joint pain of the wrists, elbows, and shoulders (Curtis & Dillon, 1985).

   (3) Prevention includes:

     (a) Optimize seating position to prevent overreach and shoulder extension.

     (b) Modify seating position to reduce torque and promote trunk stability during wheelchair propulsion or other seated activities.

     (c) Keep number of transfers to a minimum to reduce stress on shoulders.

     (d) Incorporate strengthening of posterior shoulder and upper back muscles whenever motor function allows.

     (e) Encourage the use of protective equipment (gloves, helmets).

     (f) Instruct in specific joint-sparing techniques during both exercise and routine activity, as well as pacing of activity to conserve energy.

III. Initial Assessment

A. **Nursing History**

1. Obtain adequate information to determine an individual's health status and functional levels, including medical history and risk factors.

  a. Health history

   (1) SCI specific information

   (2) Orthopedic or other medical conditions that would limit exercise participation.

   (3) History of heart disease

   (4) Significant orthostatic hypotension

   (5) Range-of-motion (ROM) limitations due to contracture, fractures, heterotrophic ossification

   (6) Seating / positioning issues

   (7) Upper extremity overuse syndrome complaints

      (8)   Skin status

      (9)   Medications

    (10)   Exercise history

  b. Risk factors for cardiac disease

      (1)   Age

      (2)   Family history

      (3)   Current tobacco use

      (4)   Hypertension

      (5)   Hypercholesterolemia

      (6)   Diabetes mellitus

      (7)   Sedentary lifestyle/ physical inactivity (American College of Sports Medicine (ACSM), 1995)

  c. Physical examination; components of a physical examination specific to exercise include the following:

      (1)   Body weight

      (2)   Pulse rate and regularity

      (3)   Resting blood pressure

      (4)   Auscultation of the lungs

      (5)   Palpation and auscultation of the carotid, abdominal, and femoral arteries

      (6)   Motor control and coordination

      (7)   Balance and trunk stability

      (8)   Spasticity

      (9)   Tests of neurologic function, including reflexes

  d. Psychosocial assessment

      (1)   Understanding of SCI and impact on activity levels and performance of skills

      (2)   Level of motivation

      (3)   Ability to problem solve

      (4)   Ability to articulate needs and ask for help

      (5)   Resources available for transportation, equipment and/or assistance if needed

IV. Nursing Process Applied to Activity and Exercise

A. **Nursing Diagnosis:** Health-Seeking Behavior-Condition in which an individual in stable health actively seeks ways to alter personal habits or the environment in order to move toward optimal health.

B. **Defining Characteristics**

  1. Desire for increased control of health practices

  2. Desire to seek higher levels of wellness

  3. Lack of knowledge about health-promoting behaviors

  4. Concern about effect of environmental conditions or health status

  5. Unfamiliarity with wellness resources

C. **Expected Outcomes**

  1. Expresses understanding of benefits of regular exercise according to functional ability

  2. Understands modified exercise guidelines

  3. Formulates goals for personalized exercise plan

  4. Demonstrates ability to perform exercise properly and/or provide verbal instructions to an assistant

D. **Interventions**

  1. Provide education about:

    a. Benefits of a regular exercise program on overall health with specifics regarding SCI. (Refer to Table 25-1, Table 25-2).

    b. Definition of health-related physical fitness within the context of SCI.

      (1)   Health-related physical fitness is typically defined as including cardiorespiratory

Table 25-1: Physiological Effects of Aerobic Training

System or Organ	Effects of Disuse (Physiological)	Effects of Exercise (Physiological Change, Dependent on SCI Level)	Effects on Performance
Cardiovascular system	Higher resting heart rate. Higher resting blood pressure. Lower cardiac output. Decreased circulation.	Decreased resting heart rate; Decreased resting blood pressure; Greater absolute stroke volume; More efficient cardiac output and pulmonary ventilation. Improved blood redistribution. Increased oxygen extraction and delivery to muscles. Increased blood flow.	Heart is more efficient (pumps same output with fewer beats). Increased endurance. Decreased risk of cardiovascular disease.
Nervous system	Suboptimal coordination. Decreased emotional state, possible depression and lethargy.	Increased activation of motor units in prime movers. Increased EMG responses. Increased appropriate activation of synergists and antagonists.	Increased coordination and skill of movement. Increased accuracy, precision, and balance. Improved self-esteem. Improved mechanical efficiency. Energy reserves.
Muscle	Decreased muscle mass (atrophy) and strength. Early onset of fatigue.	Increased muscle endurance. Increased oxygen utilization by mitochondria; capillary density.	Easier performance of daily activities. Increased ability for wheelchair propulsion on uneven outdoor surfaces.
Connective tissue/bone	Bone demineralization (osteoporosis). Decreased pliability of tendons and ligaments. Contractures. Pressure sores.	Increased bone density and mass. Increased tensile strength in tendons and ligaments. Increased skin elasticity.	Decreased risk of pressure sores. Decreased incidence of injury from overuse activities.
Body composition	Increased percent body fat.	Decreased percent body fat and increase in lean tissue.	Possible decreased risk of cardiovascular disease. Maintenance of healthy weight. Improved body image.

From Conditioning with Physical Disabilities (p. 41), by K. F. Lockette & A. M. Keyes, 1994, Champaign, IL; Human Kinetics. Reprinted with permission.

endurance, muscular strength, and endurance, flexibility, and body composition (ACSM, 1995).

(a) Fitness is associated with lower risk for development of disease and/or functional disability.

(b) Physical fitness for the SCI population embraces modified endurance, strength, and flexibility, as well as conscientious nutritional practices, medical follow-up, and a balance of activities (Chase, 1996).

(2) Basic components of a physical exercise program:

(a) Cardiorespiratory endurance enhances physical work capacity, reduces fatigability, and enhances cardiovascular health.

(b) Cardiorespiratory activities for persons with SCI include:

- Wheelchair pushing
- Swimming

Table 25-2: Physiological Effects of Resistance Training

System or Organ	Effects of Disuse (Physiological)	Effects of Exercise (Physiological Change, Dependent on SCI Level)	Effects on Performance
Nervous system	Suboptimal coordination. Decreased emotional state, possible depression and lethargy.	Increased activation of motor units in prime movers. Increased EMG responses. Increased appropriate activation of synergists and antagonists.	Increased coordination and skill of movement. Increased accuracy, precision, and balance. Smooth, flowing movement. Improved self-esteem.
Muscle	Decreased muscle mass (atrophy) and strength. Early onset of fatigue.	Increased muscle mass (hypertrophy). Increased muscle endurance. Improved ability to generate muscle tension (strength).	Muscle balance. Easier performance of daily activities. Increased ability for wheelchair propulsion on varied surfaces. Improved mechanical efficiency.
Connective tissue/bone	Bone demineralization (osteoporosis). Decreased pliability of tendons and ligaments. Contractures. Pressure sores. Postural changes.	Increased bone density. Increased tensile strength in tendons and ligaments. Increased skin elasticity.	Decrease or elimination of pressure sores. Decreased incidence of injury from overuse activities. Stabilized and protected joints (ligaments).
Body composition	Increased percent body fat.	Increase in lean tissue.	Better mobility; ease of transfer.

From *Conditioning with Physical Disabilities* (p.17), by K. F. Lockette & A. M. Keyes, 1994, Champaign, IL; Human Kinetics. Reprinted with permission.

- Arm-cycle ergometry
- Hand cycling
- Wheelchair aerobics

(c) Modification of training principles for SCI addresses the five factors important in any fitness routine: *Frequency, Intensity, Time, Type, and Enjoyment (FITTE).* The FITTE model is described in Chase (1996). Modifications of the guidelines for each of these factors will depend upon the type of SCI, the functional muscle mass available, and the baseline/current level of activity.

(d) Muscular strength and endurance are the components of fitness most routinely integrated into the rehabilitation and daily activities of persons with SCI. Muscular strength is the ability of a muscle or muscle group to exert maximal force. Muscular endurance is the ability of a muscle or muscle group to perform repeated contractions. Pushing a wheelchair, performing transfers, independent dressing, performing push-up weight shifts, and many other activities require muscular endurance. Floor-to-chair transfers and lifting a wheelchair into a vehicle are activities that require muscular strength.

(e) Resistance training activities that enhance muscular strength and endurance include the following:
- Free weights, dumbbells, cuff weights
- Multi-station weight machines
- Pulley system exercises
- Stretch bands
- Medicine balls

(f) The actual prescription for strength and endurance gains is based on the individual's functional ability and fitness goals. A prescription may include number of repetitions, sets, and frequency of workouts (ACSM, 1995; Lockette & Keyes, 1994).

(g) Flexibility is the ability to move a joint through its full range of motion (ROM) without pain or discomfort. Maintaining flexibility becomes important when counteracting positional strains created by muscle imbalances due to paralysis, spasticity, and sitting in a wheelchair.

- Maintaining flexible joints and supple muscles enhances functional capacity, helps prevent injury, stimulates circulation, and keeps the body in a state of overall preparedness.
- Stretching exercises are useful in maintaining or improving flexibility and can be incorporated into warm-up and cool-down activities or done as part of a daily workout. An excellent resource for suggested stretching activities is *Stretch and Strengthen for Rehabilitation and Development* (Anderson & Bornell, 1987).

(h) Body composition is the proportional relationship among fat tissue, lean or fat-free body mass, and total body mass, expressed as percentages. Calculation of body composition is often used in the able-bodied population to help direct the focus and success of fitness programs. The routine assessment of body composition after SCI however, is limited by lack of effective methods and normative data for this population (Nuhlicek et al., 1988).

2. Encourage activity options that promote fitness goals.
3. Support goals that meet fitness criteria and provide enjoyable activity.
4. Refer to available home-based or community-based exercise program.
5. Encourage sustained participation in prescribed program.
6. Educate individual to notify health care provider of adverse effects experienced during or after an exercise program.
7. Provide patient with literature on exercise guidelines and other resources to reinforce teaching.

V. Re-Assessment

A. **Nursing History**
1. Review patient fitness goals and plans.
2. Assess health status, changes, and concerns.

B. **Examination**
1. Repeat basic physiological measures and compare with baseline levels.
2. Review diagnostic studies as indicated (Lanig, 1996).
3. Address specific complaints or concerns at time of re-assessment.

VI. Health Education Tips: Physical Fitness as a Healthy Choice

A. **Healthy Choice: Why?** Following SCI, some people tend to become sedentary or lead less active lives. It is important to maintain a level of activity sufficient to prevent deconditioning. Getting started is half the battle. Some helpful hints are:
1. Get medical clearance
2. Set reasonable goals
3. Progress slowly
4. Make exercise convenient
5. Pick an enjoyable activity

B. **Healthy Choice: What, How, Where?**
1. Fitness must be defined for each person individually, based on personal goals, extent of SCI,

lifestyle, and motivation. Remember the components of fitness and support the workout plan to improve:

    a. Cardiorespiratory Endurance

    b. Muscular Strength and Endurance

    c. Flexibility

    d. Body Composition

2. General exercise guidelines

    a. Frequency: Make exercise and activity a regular occurrence and try for at least 3 to 5 times per week. Allow for rest days in between to recover.

    b. Intensity: In order for fitness levels to improve, activity must be performed at or above the activity levels encountered in daily life. Intensity can be monitored by heart rate and perceived exertion.

    c. Duration: The appropriate length of exercise will depend on initial level of fitness and conditioning. Working up to a minimum of 15 minutes of continuous vigorous exercise is a good goal, especially if one has not been exercising regularly.

3. Where people exercise is an individual decision, based on time, transportation, and finances.

Practical Application #1

P.R., a 34-year-old female with a T10 paraplegia sustained 5 years earlier, arrived at the out patient clinic for her annual re-evaluation. She had no outstanding medical issues and was in overall good health. She does not smoke and was within 10 pounds of her recommended weight. During her nursing assessment, P.R. expressed a desire to begin an exercise program in her home community. Her stated goals were increasing levels of endurance, weight loss, and a desire to feel better about herself.

The nurse began by reviewing the patent's medical record and diagnostic studies performed during the re-evaluation to rule out any contraindications for exercise. Finding none, the nurse, in conjunction with the rehab team, was then able to gather appropriate information and resources for the patient. Based on P.R.'s stated goal of increased endurance, the nurse recommended activities that would be specific to that goal. Endurance activities such as swimming, wheelchair pushing, arm cycling and a low-weight, high-repetition resistance program were suggested as options. A handout illustrating an upper body stretching routine was also included in the packet of information. The FITTE (frequency, intensity, time, type, enjoyment) factors as well as safety considerations for people with SCI were shared.

The nurse discussed with P.R. the difficulty of losing weight simply by exercise. Additional information was given to P.R. about incorporating low-fat food choices into her daily meals. The nurse also suggested increasing her water intake, as that has also been found to be helpful for some people in losing weight. Adjustments in bladder management were discussed as well.

Since the re-evaluation was only one week long at this particular institution, the nurse suggested components of an individualized exercise plan but could not follow through with implementation. However, P.R. was given enough information to begin a safe, effective exercise plan to continue upon her return home. P.R. will be exercising at a local recreation center and will consult with the fitness leader there for further exercise development.

Practical Application #2

R.M., a 28-year-old male with C7-C8 quadriplegia, contacted the local fitness center with a request to start an exercise program. The fitness director had been in contact with a nurse from the SCI outpatient clinic for some suggestions for this client.

The nurse suggested that the fitness director use the in-house screening and health information forms for initial assessment purposes as well as asking specifics about the SCI history. If the client expressed health issues, such as loss of function or pain in the upper extremities, these should be referred back to the SCI team for evaluation. The nurse assured the fitness director that people with SCI are typically in stable health; however, checking with clients about their health status is not inappropriate.

Exercise options for this particular client might include gravity-reduced exercises on a supporting surface, such as a table, to strengthen triceps. Other exercise options include strap-on weights, the rickshaw, machine exercises with wrist cuffs to access a pulley system, the machine shoulder press, and the upper arm ergometer. If trunk balance is a problem, even with strapping, using an exercise machine is the preferred mode of exercise rather than strap-on weights or free weight exercises. Focus of the program included: back musculature and scapular stabilizers such as the serratus anterior and lower trapezius, to prevent forward posture and shoulder protraction; shoulder depressors (latissimus dorsi), to assist with transfers from the wheelchair; and muscle balance, to strengthen trunk and shoulder muscles.

Safety concerns, prevention, and treatment specific to SCI, were discussed, including autonomic dysreflexia, hypotension, pressure ulcers, overuse injury, and hyperthermia. Additional resources and sources of information were discussed with the fitness director.

References and Selected Bibliography

American Association of Spinal Cord Injury Nurses. (1996). *Clinical practice guideline: Autonomic dysreflexia*. New York: Author.

American College of Sports Medicine (ASCM), (1995). *Guidelines for exercise testing* (5th ed.). Philadelphia: Lea & Febiger.

Anderson, B., & Bornell, D. (1987). *Stretch and strengthen for rehabilitation and development*. Palmer Lake, CO: Stretching.

Borg, G. (1982). Psychosocial bases of perceived exertion. *Medicine and Science in Sports and Exercise, 14*(5), 377-381.

Chase, T. (1996). Physical fitness strategies. In I. S. Lanig (Ed.), *A practical guide to health promotion after spinal cord injury* (pp. 243-306). Gaithersburg, MD: Aspen.

Claus-Walker, J., & Halstead, L. (1981). Metabolic and endocrine changes since spinal cord injury. I) The nervous system before and after transection of the spinal cord. *Archives of Physical Medicine and Rehabilitation, 62*, 595-601.

Claus-Walker, J., & Halstead, L. (1982). Metabolic and endocrine changes since spinal cord injury. II) Consequences of partial decentralization of the autonomic nervous system. *Archives of Physical Medicine and Rehabilitation, 63*, 569-575.

Compton, D., Eisenman, P., & Henderson, H. (1989). Exercise and fitness for persons with disabilities. *Sports Medicine, 7*, 150-162.

Curtis, K., & Dillon, D. (1985). Survey of wheelchair athletic injuries: common patterns and prevention. *Paraplegia, 23*, 170-175.

Davis, G. (1993). Exercise capacity of individuals with paraplegia. *Medicine and Science in Sports and Exercise, 25*(4), 423-432.

DeVivo, M., Black, K., & Stover, S. (1993). Causes of death during the first twelve years after spinal cord injury. *Archives of Physical Medicine and Rehabilitation, 74*(6), 248-254.

Figoni, S. (1991). Physiology of aerobic exercise applications for persons with physical disabilities. In P. Miller (Ed.), *Adapted fitness instructor workbook* (pp. 1-26). Rockville, MD: National Handicapped Sports.

Figoni, S. (1993). Exercise responses and quadriplegia. *Medicine and Science in Sports and Exercise, 21*(4), 433-441.

Glaser, R. (1989). Arm exercise training for wheelchair users. *Medicine and Science in Sports and Exercise, 21*(5Suppl), S149-S157.

Glaser, R. (1992). Cardiovascular problems of the wheelchair disabled. In R. Shephard & H. Miller (Eds.), *Exercise and the heart in health and disease* (pp. 476-499). New York: Marcel Dekkar.

Greenhoot, J., & Mauck, H. (1972). The effect of cervical cord injury on cardiac rhythm and conduction. *American Heart Journal, 83*, 659-662.

Hoffman, M. (1986). Cardiorespiratory fitness and training in quadriplegics and paraplegics. *Sports Medicine, 3*, 312-330.

Lanig, I. (1996). The interdisciplinary assessment of health. In I. Lanig (Ed.), *A practical guide to health promotion after spinal cord injury* (pp. 50-78). Gaithersburg, MD: Aspen.

Lockette, K. F., & Keyes, A. M. (1994). *Conditioning with physical disabilities*. Champaign, IL & Human Kinetics.

Miller, P. (Ed.) (1995). *Fitness programming and physical disability*. Champaign,:IL: Human Kinetics.

Noreau, L., & Shephard, R. (1995). Spinal cord injury, exercise and quality of life. *Sports Medicine, 20*(4), 226-250.

Nuhlicek, D., Spurr, G., Barboriak, J., Rooney, C., El Ghatit, A., & Bongard, R. (1988). Body composition of patients with spinal cord injury. *European Journal of Clinical Nutrition, 42*, 765-773.

Rimmer, J. (1994). *Fitness and rehabilitation programs for special populations*. Champaign, IL & Human Kinetics.

Shephard, R. (1990). *Fitness in special populations*. Champaign, IL & Human Kinetics.

Zejdlik, C. (1992). Maintaining protective functions of the skin. In C. Zejdlik (Ed.), *Management of spinal cord injuries* (2nd ed.). Boston: Jones & Bartlett.

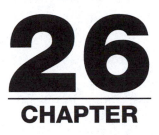

CHAPTER

Spinal Cord Injury Prevention

Mimi Watson Sutherland, MS, BSN, RN, CNRN

I. Learning Objectives

A. Describe the principles of injury prevention.

B. Describe the disease model for controlling injuries.

C. Describe the demographics of injury cost.

D. Identify the characteristics of the at-risk population for spinal cord injury (SCI).

E. Explain why the adolescent and the elderly populations are at risk for SCI.

F. Describe how to identify SCI patterns in your community and compare them to national statistics.

G. Describe the evolution of SCI prevention programs and coalitions.

H. Identify prevention concepts focused on controlling injury and reducing costs.

I. Explain how to develop a strategy to target an appropriate issue for SCI prevention in your community.

J. Define the teaching opportunities for nursing as SCI prevention advocates.

K. Discuss screening of SCI risk by the nurse along the continuum of care.

L. Describe the role of alcohol and other drug abuse in SCI.

M. Identify the scope of the firearm problem in SCI.

      N. Describe the political process role in SCI prevention.

      O. Describe how the nurse can evaluate the effectiveness of an SCI prevention program.

II.   Introduction

A. **History of Injury Prevention:**
Injury prevention has historically been part of the disciplines of epidemiology and public health (Haddon & Baker, 1981). However, other health care disciplines, including medicine and nursing, have become increasingly involved in trauma prevention (Kreis, 1988). Clinicians responded to preventable injuries by developing SCI prevention programs.
1. Federal Government Response: Congress established the Injury Control Program at the Center for Disease Control (CDC) in Atlanta in response to the 1985 landmark report of the Committee on Trauma Research (National Research Council, 1985). The report revealed the magnitude of the problem.
   a. Injuries kill more than 142,000 people in the United States.
   b. More than 62,000,000 people require medical attention, as a result of accidents each year.
   c. Injuries are the single greatest cause of death in individuals from 1 to 44 years of age.
   d. Treatment costs are approximately $133.2 billion each year in the United States.
   e. SCI is one of the most costly of these injuries.
   f. The CDC's research agenda includes:
      (1) Epidemiology
      (2) Prevention
      (3) Biomechanics
      (4) Rehabilitation
      (5) SCI as a mandated reportable health condition
2. Neurosurgical response: The response of America's neurosurgeons to the 12,000 new spinal cord injuries each year (Kennedy, 1986), was to establish a National Head and Spinal Cord Injury Prevention Program in 1986 (Cain & Saxton, 1986). It was designed to:
   a. Document and track incidents.
   b. Identify those at risk for particular injuries.
   c. Determine how to prevent spinal cord injuries.
   d. Establish SCI surveillance as the first step to injury control and to determine the true epidemiology of SCI.
   e. Collaborate with allied health professionals to implement prevention programs.

B. **Epidemiological Variables**
1. Demographics (who gets hurt)
   a. Home address
   b. Age
   c. Gender
   d. Race
   e. Level of injury
   f. Extent of injury (complete or incomplete)
   g. Alcohol
   h. Drugs
   i. Mechanism of injury
   j. Injury site (incident location)
   k. Injury information related to motor vehicle
      (1) Position in or on vehicle
         (a) Driver, passenger
         (b) Front or rear seat
      (2) Protective devices
         (a) Safety belt use (Streff & Geller, 1986)
         (b) Airbag
         (c) Child restraint seat

      (d)   Helmet use
l. Associated injuries
m. Socioeconomic information (occupation, education, insurance)
2. Etiology (how and why individuals sustain SCI)
There are geographic differences in leading causes of SCI from state to state, and among rural, suburban, and urban locations (Crawley et al 1994; Maiman, 1988). Causes include:
  a. Motor vehicle crashes
  b. Pedestrians hit by vehicle
  c. Motorcycles
  d. All terrain vehicles (ATVS)/Mopeds
  e. Bicycles
  f. Diving and water-related injuries
  g. Falls, jumps, and suicide attempts
  h. Penetrating injuries (Sloan, Kellerman, Ready, Ferris, Koepsell, Rivara, Rice, Gray, & LoGerfo, 1988; Sutherland, 1994)
     (1) Gunshot wounds
     (2) Knife wounds
     (3) Screwdrivers
     (4) Spear-diving
     (5) Arrows
     (6) Construction reinforcing rods
  i. Sports
     (1) Football
     (2) Hockey
     (3) Wrestling
     (4) Trampoline
3. Location (where injuries occur)
  a. Highway and other roadways
  b. Home
  c. Pools and other water locations
  d. Work
  e. Playgrounds
  f. Athletic events
4. Incidence (when injuries occur)
  a. Peak incidence by months
     (1) January
     (2) April
     (3) July
     (4) December
  b. Calendar events
     (1) Holidays
     (2) School breaks
  c. Time
     (1) Weekends
     (2) Early evenings
5. Demographic incidence
  a. Male to female ratio 4:1
  b. Most prevalent at ages 16 to 35 and age over 65
6. Cost factors
  a. Average cost of injury computed for
     (1) Acute initial care
     (2) Rehabilitation
     (3) Lifetime care
     (4) Lost productivity
  b. Who pays
     (1) Insurance industry

      (2) Government-funded programs
      (3) Individuals or families
      (4) Society (taxes)
   c. Cost/benefit ratio of preventing injury
7. Critical precipitating factors
   a. Risk-taking behaviors (Rosenberg, 1987)
      (1) Poor judgment
      (2) Alcohol abuse
      (3) Substance abuse
      (4) Carelessness
      (5) Forgetfulness
      (6) Irresponsibility
   b. Associated activities
      (1) Nearby bars
      (2) Secluded areas
      (3) Teen hangouts
      (4) Gangs
      (5) Sporting arenas

C. **Background Information**
  1. Injury definition (Haddon, 1980)
   a. Transfer of energy to body causes tissue damage
   b. It results from inappropriate exposure to energy
   c. SCI cause may be mechanical or kinetic
  2. Trauma is a disease with (Waller, 1985)
   a. Seasonal variations
   b. Epidemic occurrence in certain populations
   c. Environmental causative factors
   d. Identifiable susceptibility factors
   e. Predictable patterns
  3. Injury prevention requires
   a. Changes in basic public attitude
   b. Recognition of most injuries are not accidents
   c. Realization that most injuries are indeed preventable
  4. Injury triangle (Baker, 1985) (Refer to Figure 26-1)

Figure 26-1: Injury Triangle

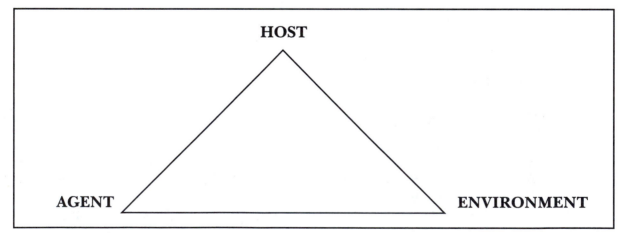

From: "Injury Facts, Risk Groups, and Injury Determinants," by S. Baker, 1985, *Public Health Report,* *100,* pp. 581-582.

a. Host
    (1) At-risk populations
    (2) Susceptibility
    (3) Defenses (protection)
    (4) Exposure (frequency and risk ratio)
       (a) Host characteristics of the young
         - Ages 15-35
         - More males than females
         - Alcohol involved
         - High- risk activity exposure
       (b) Host characteristics of the elderly
         - Over age 65
         - Effects more likely to be permanent
         - High direct cost
         - Lower lifetime cost
         - Risk of death and hospitalization three times higher
         - Osteoarthritis is a predisposing factor

b. Agent
    (1) Identification
    (2) Elimination
    (3) Reduction
    (4) Confinement

c. Environment
    (1) Separation of host from agent
    (2) Modification of environment

III. Aspects of SCI Prevention

A. **Principles of Injury Prevention** (Calonge, 1987; Pottie, 1994)

1. Problem identification
    a. Determine most frequent injuries in each community
    b. Identify population most at risk
    c. Determine most common incident location for each type of injury
    d. Determine the critical precipitating factors for most frequent causes of SCI

2. Data acquisition and analysis: Surveillance systems and research are equally essential to identify high-risk activities in individuals.
    a. Surveillance systems: hospital, county, and state
       (1) State SCI Registry
       (2) Hospital and/or County Trauma Registry
       (3) Uniform Hospital Discharge Data Set
       (4) Hospital Discharge E Codes
       (5) Emergency Department Logs
       (6) Emergency Medical Service records
       (7) Medical Examiner records
       (8) Department of Motor Vehicles records
       (9) Criminal Justice System records
     (10) City/county/state police reports
     (11) School records
     (12) Parks and Recreation Department records
     (13) Vital Statistics records
     (14) Insurance records
     (15) National SCI Database
       (a) Medical insurance
         - Managed Care
         - Health Maintenance Organizations
         - Private Insurance

- Medicaid
- Medicare
- Worker's Compensation
(b) Motor vehicle insurance
(c) Death and disability insurance
(d) Home liability insurance
b. Injury Cause Surveillance Data
(1) Motor Vehicle Crashes
(a) Safety belt use
(b) Excessive speeding
(c) Inexperience
(d) Drivers' education inadequate
(e) Physical limitations
(f) "Showing off"
(g) Unfamiliar roads
(h) Weather
(i) Road conditions
- Grading/curves
- Traffic control signals
- Lighting
- Guardrails
- Roadway markings
- Pavement conditions
(j) Motor vehicle maintenance
(2) Diving and water-related injuries (Eyster & Watts, 1992)
(a) Unknown water depths in swimming pools, lakes, canals, or ocean
(b) Unseen submerged objects
(c) "Showing off", horseplay
(d) Changing water levels: tides, drought, and locks
(e) Lifeguard on duty
(f) Appropriate rescue equipment
(3) Falls
(a) Work-related: roofers, construction workers, window cleaners
(b) Home-related: repairs using ladders
(c) Elderly: unsafe environment, frail or unsteady gait, compromised by medication
(4) Penetrating Injuries
(a) Gunshot wounds
(b) Stab wounds

B. **Components of Injury Control**
1. Epidemiology
2. Biomechanics, mechanism of injury
3. Acute care
4. Rehabilitation
5. Prevention

C. **Plan for Injury Control** (National Academy of Sciences, 1988)
1. Surveillance
a. Define the problem
b. Monitor progress
2. Research
a. Identify risk factors
b. Develop interventions
c. Measure effectiveness

3. Programs
   a. Implement interventions
   b. Measure effectiveness

D. **Injury Prevention Strategies**
   1. Education and awareness
      a. Increases injury visibility and community awareness
      b. Changes knowledge and attitudes
      c. Increases community support
      d. Maybe difficult to evaluate for effectiveness
      e. May lack longevity
      f. May not translate to changes in behavior
      g. Outcome analysis
         (1) Pre-test/post-test
         (2) Self-reported behavior
         (3) Observation
         (4) Rate-based incidence
   2. Legislation and enforcement
      a. Increases awareness
      b. Affects large target groups
      c. Increases compliance
      d. Cannot alone change culture, which must evolve so that society will not accept the unacceptable e.g., (tobacco use)
      e. Can expand from local to state to federal levels
      f. Becomes more acceptable over time
      g. Requires commitments of time and resources
      h. Aims to change behavior
      i. Does not assure compliance
      j. Outcome analysis
         (1) Rate-based incidence
         (2) Injuries
         (3) Citations for non-compliance
   3. Engineering (modification of the environment)
      a. Removes known hazards or design flaws
      b. Reduces risk and exposure, increase safety
      c. Affects large target group
      d. Directly reduces risk
      e. Can be active or passive e.g., (manual or automatic safety belts)
      f. Requires active approach
      g. Legislation may enhance active approach
      h. Maybe costly
      i. Outcome analysis
         (1) Rate-based incidence
         (2) usage
         (3) injuries

E. **Injury Prevention Programs**
   1. Public health approach (Baker, 1985)
      a. Injuries are not accidents (random uncontrollable acts of fate).
      b. Injuries are understandable, predictable and preventable.
      c. Injuries require the same approach as disease epidemics
      d. Detailed study of patterns of injury, working with local data, reveals:
         (1) How the injuries are occurring
         (2) Who in population is most at risk?
         (3) When injuries occur
         (4) Where in community the injuries occur

    (5)   What caused the injuries

    (6)   Cost of injury consider both the financial cost and also the years of potential life lost

2. Haddon Strategies for Injury Prevention (Baker, 1984; Haddon, 1980) (Refer to Figure 26-2)

Figure 26-2: Haddon Matrix - Motor Vehicle Crash Example

	Host	Agent	Environment Physical	Socioeconomic
Pre-Event (Pre-crash)	Driver vision Alcohol use Experience Judgement Driver education	Brakes, tires Speed of travel Car maintenance Ease of control Center of gravity Load characteristics	Visibility Road grade Road surface Divided highway One way streets	Speed limits Alcohol attitudes DUI laws Injury prevention support
Event (Crash)	Safety belt use Osteoarthritis	Vehicle size Speed capability Padded interior Automatic airbags	Guardrails Speed limits Median barriers Recovery areas - shoulders	Safety belt attitudes Safety belt laws Child safety seat laws
Post-Event (Post crash)	Age Physical condition	Fuel system integrity	911 access Distance to and quality of emergency medical services Rehabilitation programs	Training of EMS personnel Support for trauma care systems

From *Haddon Injury Prevention Countermeasures* (Haddon, 1980). Reprinted with permission.

    a. Prevent the creation of the hazard.

    b. Reduce the amount of the hazard.

    c. Prevent the release of a hazard that already exists.

    d. Modify the rate or special distribution of the hazard.

    e. Separate in time or space the hazard from that which is to be protected.

    f. Separate the hazard from that which is to be protected by a material barrier.

    g. Modify relevant basic qualities as a hazard.

    h. Make what is to be protected resistant to damage from the hazard.

    i. Begin to counter the damage already done by the hazard.

    j. Stabilize, repair, and rehabilitate the object of the damage.

3. Precede Model (Green, Kreuter, Deeds, & Partridge, 1980)

    a. Predisposing variables are antecedent to behavior and include relevant knowledge, beliefs, and values.

    b. Enabling variables include availability and accessibility of personnel and community resources required to perform the behavior.

    c. Reinforcing variables are factors subsequent to behavior that provide rewards, incentives, or punishment for continuation of the behavior.

    d. Any injury behavior may be seen as a function of the collective influence of these three factors.

4. Health Belief Model: "Think First Program". The American Association of Neurological Surgeons and the Congress of Neurological Surgeons (Watts & Eyster, 1992) sponsor this spinal cord injury prevention project.

    a. Individual is convinced of seriousness and irreversibility of the potential injury.

    b. Individual is personally susceptible.

    c. Alternatives to risk-taking behavior are accessible, acceptable, and achievable.

    d. Individual is reminded to "Think First. Use your mind to protect your body".

        (1) Program components

            (a)   Basic education

            (b)   Reinforcement activities

            (c)   General public and community awareness

            (d)   Public policy initiatives

        (2) High school program

            (a)   Discussion on definition of SCI and epidemiology by health care professional

            (b)   Showing of film "On The Edge," depicting graphic consequences of risk-taking activities

            (c)   Frank and open discussion between a young person who has sustained an SCI and students (attitudes governed by peers, not adults)

            (d)   Discussion by health care professional of secondary injuries that can occur after incident due to inappropriate handling

        (3) Elementary school program (Think First for Kids)

            (a)   Targets students ages 6-8

            (b)   Adheres to belief that habits developed early continue through adulthood

            (c)   Provides environment for development and reinforcement of safety behaviors

            (d)   Multifaceted program integrated into school curriculum

            (e)   Animated video features "Street Smart" (animated role model who practices safe behaviors), multimedia lesson plans, and reinforcement activities

5. Community Coalitions (Rutledge, 1995)

    a. Identify database specific problem

    b. Define target population

    c. Build a coalition

        (1) Health care providers and organizations

        (2) Third-party payors

        (3) Law enforcement officials

        (4) Fire rescue service providers

        (5) Epidemiologists

        (6) Statisticians

        (7) Patient advocate groups

        (8) Community organizations

    d. Evaluate existing programs

    e. Define time-specific goals and achievement methods

    f. Develop strategy

    g. Identify intervention

    h. Develop budget

        (1) Cost of materials

        (2) Staff time

        (3) Outcome measures and analysis

        (4) Grant funding

    i. Keys to success (Gielen, 1992)

        (1) Start with a reachable goal

        (2) Focus on one goal at a time

        (3) Work collaboratively; build coalition support network

        (4) Identify opposing forces and system to address them

        (5) Be persistent

        (6) Be patient

        (7) Use a multifaceted approach

        (8) Evaluate effectiveness and measurement outcomes

        (9) Share results of program

F. Program Evaluation Methods (Avolio, et al 1993)

    1. Formative evaluation and program development feedback

2. Needs assessment
3. Outcome evaluation, including injury surveillance resources, and mortality and morbidity data
4 Program visibility level, scope of impact
5. Amount and type of legislative action
6. Site visits

IV. Health Education Tips

A. Safety belts save lives and prevent SCI. Buckle up whenever in an automobile, regardless of where you sit, or how far or at what speed you are travelling.

B. Walk carefully into water to check for depths and objects before jumping or diving, even in known waters, since water levels can change.

C. Walk away from arguments before they escalate into violent physical altercations.

D. Keep guns and bullets out of the hands of children.

E. Always wear safety harnesses when working at heights, to prevent falls.

F. To prevent falls in the elderly, provide a safe, well-lighted environment, free of scatter rugs and clutter. Bathrooms should have grab bars in the shower or tub and adjacent to the raised toilet.

G. Wear an approved helmet when engaged in sporting activities or riding a motorcycle or bicycle.

H. When partying with friends, agree to a designated driver who will not drink alcohol.

I. Think first. Use your mind to protect your body.

V. Safety Issues Related to Children

A. **Vehicular Safety Recommendations**
   1. Never place children in a car seat in the front seat of an automobile with airbags. The rear seat is the safest place for a child in a car seat.
   2. Use car seats until age 4 or weight 40 pounds.
   3. Use car seat designed to prevent extreme flexion loads.
   4. Position car seat facing the rear to prevent extreme flexion loads. In cars with air bags, the car seat should be used in the back seat only.
   5. Use appropriate restraint systems after the child graduates from car seat (toddler seat with built-in seat belt, regular seat belt).
   6. Special seats are available for the child with a disability.

B. **All Terrain Vehicles (ATV)**
   1. Teach appropriate management of ATVs.
   2. Children under 15 years of age should be supervised when using ATVs.

C. **Bicycle Safety**
   1. Helmets should be used at all times.
   2. Bicycle safety classes should be encouraged.

D. **Sports**
   1. Proper equipment should be used at all times.
   2. Children with a known risk for SCI should avoid contact sports. For example children with Down Syndrome have an anomaly of the dens.

E. **Swimming/Diving**
   1. Teach how to identify appropriate swimming/diving sites and rules (feet first, first time never swim alone).
   2. Children under 15 years of age should be supervised.

F. **Weapon Safety**
   1. Teach appropriate weapon handling training.
   2. Wear protective equipment, such as orange vests for hunters.
   3. Weapons should be stored, unloaded, in a secured locked place and out of the reach of children.

G. **Alcohol/Drug Abuse**
   1. Encourage use of "designated driver."
   2. A contract between the child and parents, such as "Prom Promise" should be encouraged.
   3. Referrals should be made to drug intervention programs when abuse is suspected or confirmed. A distinction should be made between abuse and experimentation.

References and Selected Bibliography

Agran, P.F., Dunkle, D.E., & Winn, D.G. (1987). Injuries to a sample of seatbelted children evaluated and treated in a hospital emergency room. *Journal of Trauma, 27*, 58-64.

Avolio, A.E., Ramsey, F.L., & Neuwelt, E.A. (1993). Evaluation of a program to prevent head and spinal cord injuries: A comparison between middle school and high school. *Neurosurgery, 31*(3), 557-562.

Baker, S. (1985). Injury facts, risk groups, and injury determinants. *Public Health Report 100*, 581-582

Baker, S.P., O'Neill, B., & Karpf, R.S. (1984). *The injury fact book.* Lexington, MA: Lexington Books.

Bernstein, E., Roth, P.B., Yeh, C., & Lefkowits, D.J. (1988). The emergency physician's role in injury prevention. *Pediatric Emergency Care, 4*, 207-211.

Burns, B. (1994). Think first. Head and spinal cord injuries. *North Carolina Medical Journal, 55*(8), 347-350.

Cain, K., & Saxton, C. (1986). Instruction guide for conducting the National Head and Spinal Cord Injury Prevention Project of the American Association of Neurological Surgeons and the Congress of Neurological Surgeons. *National Head and Spinal Cord Injury Prevention Project.* Park Ridge , IL:

Cales, R., Bietz, D., & Heilig, R. (1985). The trauma registry: A method for providing regional system audit using the microcomputer. *Journal of Trauma, 25*, 181-187.

Calonge, N. (1987). Objectives for injury control intervention: The Department of Public Health and Human Services model. *Public Health Report, 102*, 602-605.

Centers for Disease Control. (1984). Prevention of leading work-related diseases and injuries. *Morbidity and Mortality Weekly Report, 33*, 16.

Crawley, T., Chaloupka, M.M., & Kelker, D.B. (1994). Injury prevention symposium. *Journal of Neuroscience Nursing, 26*(2), 103-106.

Dunn, K.A., Cline, D.M., Grant, T., Masius, B.,Teleki, J.K., Snow, L., & Carroll, E. (1993). Injury prevention instruction in the emergency department. *Annals of Emergency Medicine, 22*(8), 1280-1285.

Eyster, E.F., & Watts, C. (1992). An update of the National Head and Spinal Cord Injury Prevention Program of the American Association of Neurological Surgeons and the Congress of Neurological Surgeons. Think first. *Clinical Neurosurgery, 38*, 252-260.

Gielen, A.C. (1992). Health education and injury control: Integrating approaches. *Health Education Quarterly, 19*, 203-218.

Green, L. W., Kreuter, M.W., Deeds, S.G., & Partridge, K.B. (1980). *Health education planning: A diagnostic approach.* Palo Alto, CA: Mayfield.

Haddon, W. (1980). Advances in the epidemiology of injuries as a basis for public policy. *Public Health Report, 95*, 411-421.

Haddon, W., & Baker, S.P. (1981). Injury control. In D. Clark & B. MacMahon (Eds.), *Preventive and community medicine* (p. 10). Boston: Little, Brown.

Haddon, W., Suchman, E.A., & Klein, D. (1964). *Accident research: Methods and approaches*. New York: Harper & Row.

Kennedy, E.J. (Ed.). (1986). *Spinal cord injury: The facts and figures*. Birmingham, AL: National Spinal Cord Injury Statistical Center, University of Alabama.

Kreis, D.J. Jr. (1988). Trauma systems: An interdisciplinary approach to prevention, treatment and education. *Bulletin NY Academy of Medicine 64*, 835-837.

Loftin, C. (1986). Assaultive violence as a contagious social process. Bulletin NY *Academy of Medicine 62*(5), 551-552.

Maiman, D., (1988). Diving-associated spinal cord injuries during drought conditions: Wisconsin 1988. *Morbidity and Mortality Weekly Report, 37*, 453-454.

Mayhew, M.S. (1991). Strategies for promoting safety and preventing injuries. *Nursing Clinics of North America, 26*(4), 885-893.

National Academy of Sciences. (1988). *Injury control*. Washington, DC: National Academy Press.

National Research Council. (1985). *Injury in America: A continuing public health problem*. Washington, DC: National Academy Press.

Pottie, D. (1994). *The impact of prevention*. Axone, 16(2), 46-49.

Rivara, F.P., Dicker, B.G., Bergman, A.B., Dacey, R., & Herman, C. (1988). The public cost of motorcycle trauma. *Journal of the American Medical Association*, 260, 221-223.

Roberts, M.C., Fanurik, D., & Layfield, D.A. (1987). Behavioral approaches to prevention of childhood injuries. *Journal of Social Issues, 43*, 105-118.

Rosenberg, M.L. (1987). Violence, homicide, assault and suicide. *American Journal of Preventative Medicine, 3*, 164-178.

Rutledge, R. (1995). The goals, development, and use of trauma registries and trauma data sources in decision making in injury. *Surgical Clinics of North America, 75*, 305-326.

Sato, T.B. (1987). Effects of seat belts and injuries resulting from improper use. *Journal of Trauma, 27*, 754-8.

Sloan, J. H., Kellerman, A. L., Reay, D. T., Ferris, J. A., Koepsell, T., Rivara, F. P., Rice, C., Gray, L., & LoGerfo, J. (1988). Handgun regulations, crime, assaults, and homicide: A tale of two cities. *New England Journal of Medicine, 319*(19), 1256-1262.

Streff, F.M., & Geller, E.S. (1986). Strategies for motivating safety belt use: The application of applied behavior analysis. *Health Education Research, Theory and Practice, 1*, 47-59.

Sutherland, M.W. (1994). *The Think First Foundation's violence curriculum*. Park Ridge, IL: Think First Foundation.

Tator, C., & Edmonds, V. (1986). Sports and recreation as a rising cause of spinal cord injury. *Physician Sportsmedicine, 14*, 157-167.

Waller, J.A. (1985). *Injury control: A guide to the causes and prevention of trauma*. Lexington, MA: Lexington Books.

Watts, C., & Eyster, E.F. (1992). National Head and Spinal Cord Injury Prevention Program of the American Association of Neurological Surgeons and the Congress of Neurological Surgeons. *Journal of Neurotrauma, 9*(Suppl. 1), 307-312.

Zuckerman, D., & Zuckerman, B. (1985). Television's impact on children. *Pediatrics, 75*, 233-240.

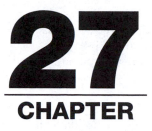

CHAPTER

Trauma Emergency

Holly Watson-Evans, MS, RN
Connie J. Mattera, MS, RN , TNS

I. Learning Objectives

A. Anticipate the possibility of spinal cord injury (SCI) based on type of trauma

B. Identify initial assessment and management strategies completed for SCI

C. Describe methods for immobilizing the vertebral column

D. Prioritize components of initial care

II. Introduction

This chapter discusses the care of the person with traumatic SCI, beginning with the first responder and concluding with the emergency department. Additional information regarding ongoing critical care management of traumatic SCI can be found in Chapter 28.

The ultimate outcome of SCI is greatly influenced by the pre-hospital and emergency room management to prevent or minimize neurological deficit. The difference between permanent paralysis and complete recovery can be affected by the type of care initially administered. "The first person who provides care at the scene of injury begins the rehabilitation process" (Zejdlik, 1992, p. 88).

III. Incidence/Epidemiology of Traumatic SCI

A. **Incidence**
   1. Approximately 8,000-10,000 new SCI cases occur each year. This is about 30-50 per million of population. It is estimated that an additional 20 persons/million sustain SCIs but die prior to hospital admission (Albin, 1987).

2. SCI occurs in 2.6 percent of all severe multiple trauma victims and in 7.5 - 8.9 percent of serious head injuries (Albin, 1987).

B. **Demographics**
1. Common causes of injury include motor vehicle crashes, gunshot wounds, falls, and sporting activities. (Review Chapters 8 and 26).
2. Most frequently occurring levels of trauma in vertebral column (Albin, 1987):
   a. C4, C5, C6 (55 percent).
   b. Thoracic (30 percent).
   c. Lumbar (15 percent).
3. Most frequent times for injuries are holidays and weekends between 12:00 AM and 5:00 AM (Albin, 1987).
4. Sixty-five associated with alcohol or drugs (Albin, 1987).

IV. Initial Assessment/Intervention

A. **Pre-hospital Management**
1. Anticipate the possibility of SCI with any traumatic injury.
   a. Check ABCs and treat accordingly.
   b. Determine if victim is in a dangerous place, requiring mobilization. Wait for trained rescuers if possible.
2. Valuable information can be obtained at the scene. For example the type of incident, whether or not seat restraints were used, and initial neurological status should give clues about the likelihood of SCI.
3. Persons who are unconscious or appear to have impaired judgment due to alcohol or drugs are at risk for overlooked injuries and should be assumed to have SCI until proven otherwise.
4. Be suspicious about the possibility of SCI when one or more of the following are observed:
   a. Injury that suggests violent, sudden movement (deceleration/axial loading/ hyperextension)
   b. Loss of consciousness
   c. Pain at injury site
   d. Paralysis/Paresis
   e. Paresthesia
   f. Priapism (uncontrolled erection in the male)
   g. Parasympathetic/Sympathetic dysfunction
5. Primary survey, and ABCDE approach: The initial assessment of actual or potential SCI includes assuring a patent airway, re-establishing or maintaining adequate breathing and circulation (Zejdlik, 1992).
   a. "A"—Airway: If breathing spontaneously, assess the rate and depth of respirations.
   b. "B"—Breathing:
      (1) LOOK for evidence of breathing difficulty or agitation (a sign of hypoxia).
         (a) Diaphragmatic or paradoxal breathing — the chest does not rise and fall with respiration; abdomen exhibits exaggerated movement just below the rib cage.
         (b) Respiratory rate less than 8 or approaching 35 breaths/minute, consider immediate ventilatory assistance.
         (c) Thoracic SCI often accompanies chest injuries.
      (2) LISTEN for evidence of airway compromise (hoarseness, gurgling).
      (3) FEEL for air exchange, tracheal deformity, and foreign bodies.
      (4) Ensure patent airway with the least amount of manipulation to the neck. Maneuvers to open the airway with cervical SCI are described in Figure 27.1
      (5) In the presence of diminished or absent air movement, an airway should be inserted:
         (a) Oropharyngeal airway — if unconscious
         (b) Nasopharyngeal airway — if responsive
            - Administer supplemental oxygen at 100 percent via non-rebreather mask with gas flow of 12-15 liters/minute.

Figure 27-1: Maneuvers to Open the Airway with Cervical SCI

Purpose:

To avoid hyperextension of the neck, which is the standard maneuver, by minimizing neck movement when opening the upper airway.

Action	Rationale
The Jaw Thrust Maneuver	

1. Be sure that the neck is in the neutral position and the patient is supine.

2. Stand or kneel behind the patient's head if possible; neutral place hands on either side of the patient's head. Work from a stable position. — To maintain the head and neck in a fixed, position without hyperextension or tilting from side to side.

3. Open mouth.

4. Grasp the angles of the patient's lower jaw with fingers, place thumbs carefully on patient's cheekbones. — Positioning of thumbs also provides an opposing point to gain momentum with lifting movement.

5. Using the thumbs to provide a focal point for opposing pressure, thrust (displace) the jaw forward with a lifting movement. — This thrust unlocks the jaw and avoids inadvertent movement of the head.

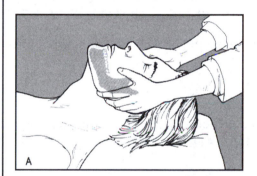 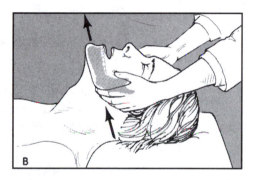

6. If the lips close, quickly move one thumb to retract the lower lip.

7. If this is unsuccessful, tilt the head slightly backward and make another attempt to open the airway or proceed with the chin lift maneuver. — Ensuring an open airway takes priority over treatment of the spinal cord injury.

The Chin Lift Maneuver

1. Using one hand, place your thumb in the patient's mouth with the thumbnail between the patient's teeth; grasp the patient under the chin with your fingers.

2. Lift the patient's chin. — Ensuring an open airway takes priority over treatment of the spinal cord injury.

3. Observe for elevation of the chest to indicate air entry.

From *Management of Spinal Cord Injury* (2nd ed., p.93), by C.P. Zejdlik (Ed.), 1992, Boston: Jones & Bartlett. Reprinted with permission.

        (c) Nasotracheal intubation is the preferred route for SCI, since it can be accomplished with minimal manipulation of the cervical spine.

        (d) The presence of apnea mandates endotrachial intubation and assisted ventilation delivering 12-15 breaths/minute.
- Intubate with neck stabilization.
- Cricothyrotomy

  c. "C"—Circulation

    (1) Assess peripheral and carotid pulses:

        (a) Strong, regular pulses plus good color imply adequate perfusion (circulation).

        (b) Weak, rapid, or absent pulses with pale or ashen color suggest poor perfusion (shock).

        (c) Heart rate may be as slow as 50 or 60 beats per minute (BPM) due to loss of sympathetic innervation to the heart in injuries above T8.

    (2) Blood pressure:

        (a) May be as low as 70/50.

        (b) In the absence of hemorrhage, low blood pressure (BP) is due to associated autonomic nervous impairment.

  d. "D"—Disability: Assess for presence of spinal/neurogenic shock.

  e. "E"—Exposure: Expose the patient to do a secondary survey.

6. Secondary survey: A rapid head-to-toe evaluation performed in an organized and thorough manner. Most of the survey may be done during transport, since those with serious injury should not be kept more than 10 minutes at the scene.

  a. Neurological assessment done at the scene or enroute to the hospital includes general motor and sensory assessments. The initial neurological exam is a key assessment. Subsequent motor and sensory exams will use this as a baseline to determine improvement or deterioration in the sensorimotor status (Refer to Table 27.1).

  b. Examine the entire neck and spine for signs of deformity, hematoma formation, or localized pain.

  c. Chest, abdomen, and long bone exam are done rapidly to determine the presence of injuries to these systems.

7. History

  a. Obtain as much information as possible.

  b. Record the mechanism of injury.

  c. If conscious, ask about neck pain, what is most bothersome, details of the injury (speed of the car, height of the fall, etc.), medical problems, medications, and use of alcohol/drugs.

  d. If unconscious, ask a witness or relative the same questions.

8. Spinal immobilization in the field (Zejdlik, 1992)

  a. Respiratory and cardiovascular stabilization, along with maintaining immobilization, initially remain top priorities.

  b. Cardinal principle in moving person with a suspected SCI is to prevent any further damage to the vertebral column, spinal cord, and nerve roots.

    (1) Use appropriate access techniques to remove stable persons from vehicle with a Kendrick's Extractation Device (KED).

    (2) Fully splint the spine on a long backboard with a lateral head immobilization device.

  c. It is equally important to provide reassurance in an attempt to decrease anxiety and avoid undesirable movement.

  d. Additional hand and body restraints may be necessary to prevent movement during transport.

  e. Refer to Table 27.2 for extrication from the water.

9. Transport: After stabilization in the field, rapid transport to an appropriate medical facility is warranted.

  a. Within 20 minutes of definitive care transfer by ground if traffic permits; otherwise consider helicopter transport.

  b. If the distance is greater than 60 miles (97 km) or terrain makes transport difficult, air evacuation is indicated.

Table 27-1: Secondary Survey: A Focus on Neurological Assessment

Purpose
To detect injury to the spinal cord

Action	Rationale
1. Measure and record vital signs (pulse, respirations, and blood pressure).	Anticipate spinal shock; rule out hypovolemia.
2. Look for lacerations, contusions, or puncture wounds along the spinal column. Deformity is rare.	
3. Assess pain at the injury site. Gently palpate along the spinal column noting tenderness.	
4. Assess motor strength in upper and lower extremities:	SCI must be suspected if the patient has any difficulty in moving extremities on command.
• Ask if there is any paralysis or weakness in arms or legs; note any numbness, tingling, "feeling weird."	If Patient shows any obvious weakness, assume there is injury to the spinal cord. Paralysis is obvious.
• Ask patient to wiggle fingers of both hands. If this is achieved, have patient raise arms, one at a time. Then ask patient to squeeze your fingers with both hands.	Movement of the upper extremity is undertaken if no obvious fractures are present. The strength of patient's grasp should be similar in both hands. If patient cannot move fingers and arms, or
• Ask patient to wiggle toes. If toes of both feet can wiggle, ask patient to raise legs slightly, one at a time.	has obvious weakness, there probably is spinal cord damage in the neck, whereas failure of only the lower extremities to respond indicates injury to the lower back.
5. Perform sensory examination:	The presence of a sensory deficit confirms the suspicion of cord injury. If your touch is felt,
• Ask if there is any numbness in arms or legs.	spinal cord damage is not probable. If your touch is not felt in one or more places, or if there is
• Touch patient's ankles and wrists and ask if your touch is felt.	numbness or tingling, spinal cord damage is likely.
6. Check the condition of the unconscious patient who is a victim of trauma:	The unconscious patient who is a victim of trauma should be suspected of having SCI because the forces necessary to produce a brain
• Observe for *diaphragmatic breathing*.	injury are also in the range of those that cause cervical injuries.
• Prick the fingertips of each hand and soles of the feet or skin of the ankles with a sharp object, such as a pin.	The presence of diaphragmatic breathing in an unconscious patient is the most obvious sign of SCI. If there is no spinal cord damage, the
Note facial grimace without limb movement in response to painful stimuli.	painful stimulus triggers an involuntary muscular reflex and the extremity will move. If the cord is damaged, there will be no reflex reaction. Lack of response to a pinprick in the upper extremities indicates damage to the spinal cord in the neck, whereas failure of only the lower extremities to respond indicates injury in the spinal cord of the back.
7. Note incontinence of urine and possible feces. Urinary retention is also common. Note priapism (a persistent penile erection).	Initial urinary incontinence and involuntary defecation are often followed by retention. Priapism is extremely rare, but if present, is a sure sign of SCI.

From Management of Spinal Cord Injury (2nd ed., p. 98), by C.P. Zejdlik, (Ed.), 1992, Boston: Jones & Bartlett. Reprinted with permission.

    c. Pre-hospital communication with hospital base station includes:

       (1) Age and sex

       (2) Mechanism of injury

       (3) Level of injury (paraplegic or tetraplegic)

       (4) Vital signs and level of consciousness

       (5) Brief history

       (6) Associated injuries that require immediate treatment

       (7) Estimated time of arrival

    d. Complications during transport:

       (1) Impaired respiration results in inadequate air exchange and can lead to hypoxia and hypercapnia (carbon dioxide buildup). Hypoxia can cause additional damage to the oxygen-sensitive spinal cord; hypercapnia can increase brain and spinal cord swelling.

       (2) Spinal shock can cause misleading symptoms.

         (a) Assess for hypotension (BP<80-100/50-60 mm Hg)

         (b) Assess for bradycardia heart rate (HR<60 beats/minute)

         (c) Prehospital management includes conservative fluid replacement to avoid fluid overload.

         (d) Consider careful application of antishock garments or slight elevation at the foot of the spineboard.

         (e) Vasopressors may be indicated.

       (3) Nausea and vomiting can lead to aspiration pneumonia which can be devastating for SCI patients.

         (a) Keep suction equipment nearby.

         (b) Log roll (spineboard and all) onto side if necessary.

         (c) Children are more prone to aspiration (Herzenberg et al, 1989).

Table 27-2: Extrication of a Patient from the Water

Purpose:
To establish an airway and adequate ventilation while immobilizing the spine.

Equipment needed:
Long backboard or substitute, such as a door or any object that provides a rigid, flat surface.

Action:
1. If the patient is found floating face up in the water, maintain in straight position. If the patient is found floating face down in the water, support the head and neck while turning victim over.

First Rescuer:
•   Position yourself at patient's head. Grasp shoulders and stabilize the neck and head between your arms.

Second Rescuer:
•   Start mouth-to-mouth ventilation, if necessary.

2. Position patient on a long backboard (or substitute) before removing victim from water.

First Rescuer:
Hold head, neck, and shoulders firmly in alignment.

Second Rescuer:
Slide long backboard under the patient. Float the board to the edge of the water and gently lift the patient and the board out of the water with additional rescuers.

3. Secure patient to long backboard in preparation for transport.

From *Management of Spinal Cord Injury* (2nd ed., p.103), by C. P. Zejdlik (ED), 1992, Boston: Jones & Bartlett. Reprinted with permission.

(4) Loss of thermoregulation necessitates adequate protection of patient from environmental exposure. Utilize covers or warm fluid replacement, if available.

(5) Pressure areas can develop on bony prominences within hours. Consider carefully padding highly vulnerable areas such as the heels, elbows, back of the head, and sacrum during prolonged transport.

B. **Emergency Department Management:**
1. The environment
   a. Prepare equipment for cardiopulmonary support and skeletal immobilization (traction system, weights, specialized bed).
   b. Obtain preadmission data from transferring personnel.
2. Admission and priorities: evaluation is adjusted to the level of consciousness and performed without any movement to the spine.
   a. Establish level of consciousness, utilizing Glasgow Coma Scale.
   b. Utilize "ABCDE" approach as in pre-hospital care. Be prepared to intubate if needed.
   c. Identify associated injuries.
   d. Continue neck and spine immobilization, utilizing pre-hospital equipment until permanent alternatives are secure.
3. Nursing diagnosis: Ineffective airway clearance
   a. Assessment:
      (1) Inability to talk, gurgling sounds, snorting or grunting noises indicate airway impairment. If unconscious, the oropharynx may be occluded by the tongue. If upper airway obstruction is due to facial fractures, digital clearance of the mouth and suctioning of the oropharynx should be used.
      (2) Retropharyngeal hematoma associated with injury of the upper cervical spine may impinge the airway.
   b. Expected outcome: Upper airway is patent with adequate airflow.
   c. Interventions:
      (1) Manual thrusts, modified jaw thrust, chin lift (Refer to Figure 27.2).
      (2) Artificial airways: depends on presence of gag reflex and absence of facial injuries.
      (3) Assist with intubation as appropriate, minimizing neck movement.
4. Nursing diagnosis: Ineffective breathing pattern related to muscular paralysis and/or gastric distention secondary to ileus.
   a. Assessment: As described in Respiratory Chapter (Chapter 12)
      (1) Assess rate, rhythm, symmetry of chest wall movement, breath sounds, and use of accessory muscles. Retraction of neck muscles is a sign of poor oxygenation and may indicate respiratory decompensation.
      (2) Assess muscular ability with Vital Capacity (VC), Negative Inspiratory Force (NIF), and minute volume on admission. Partial paralysis of the diaphragm can occur in cervical injuries.
      (3) Assess oxygenation with arterial blood gases, pulse oximetry, skin color, and altered level of consciousness.
   b. Expected outcomes:
      (1) Adequate tidal volumes of 10 cc/kg and respiratory rate of 12-20/minute.
      (2) Oxygen saturation within normal limits.
   c. Nursing interventions: initiate interventions early to prevent complications, which tend to escalate rapidly.
5. Nursing diagnosis: Decreased cardiac output related to spinal shock.
   a. Assessment:
      (1) Assess perfusion by noting the rate, quality, and regularity of peripheral pulses. Evaluate skin temperature and moisture. Monitor level of consciousness (LOC) and blood pressure.
      (2) Intractable hypotension in SCI may be due to life-threatening hemorrhage. Neurogenic shock exacerbates hypovolemic shock because the loss of vasoconstrictive reflexes prohibits peripheral shunting of blood to vital organs.
      (3) Monitor cardiac rhythm.

(4) In injuries T6 and above assess for presence of spinal shock (neurological condition occurring immediately following an injury to the spinal cord.) Spinal shock is:

(a) Characterized by hypotension, bradycardia, and hypothermia. (If tachycardia is present, suspect hypovolemic shock.)

(b) Due to a disrupted communication between the sympathetic nervous system and higher centers within the cerebral cortex.

(c) Disappears as spinal neurons gradually regain their excitability several hours to weeks post-injury.

(d) Caused by autonomic nervous system changes that decrease vascular resistance, causing blood to pool in the extremities.

(e) Characterized by flaccid paralysis, loss of motor control, sensory perception, and loss of reflex activity below the level of injury. Absent somatic/visceral sensations below the level of the injury accompanied by bowel distension and loss peristalsis.

(f) Accompanied by marked hemodynamic effects, especially in high cervical injuries.
- Bradycardia and hypotension related to spinal shock are due to absent or impaired autonomic nervous system functioning.
- Blood pools in the enlarged vascular system.
- Venous pooling in the lower extremities causes extreme sensitivity to sudden position changes when moving from a supine to sitting position.
- Occurs in varying degrees.

(5) Critical to differentiate between spinal and hypovolemic shock when estimating the type and amount of fluid replacement therapy. High volumes of fluid given to compensate for hypotension will cause fluid overload.

b. Expected outcomes:
(1) Adequate cardiac output (CO) is maintained.
(2) Heart rate remains regular at 60-100/minute. Blood pressure is adequate to maintain perfusion.
(3) Urine output is 0.5-1.0 ml/kg/hr.
(4) Pulse oximetry is within normal limits.
(5) Skin is warm, dry, and pink; body temperature is normal.
(6) Reflex activity returns below level of injury.
(7) Usually subsides in 4-6 weeks.

c. Nursing interventions:
(1) Monitor vital signs (VS) at least every 15 minutes in acute phase.
(2) Maintain immobilization.
(3) Maintain adequate hydration and volume status through administration of crystalloids as ordered. Management includes establishing intravenous (IV) lines. Neurogenic shock may be treated by increasing CO. Volume resuscitation may be used to increase systemic volume. However, in neurogenic shock not associated with other injuries, parasympathetic blockers and pressor agents may be used.
(4) Carefully monitor response to vasopressors; response may be less than expected since the sympathetic nervous system is compromised.
(5) Consider Swan Ganz catheter insertion if VS do not respond to fluid challenges or medications.

6. Nursing diagnosis: Potential alteration in tissue perfusion related to vasovagal episodes.
a. Assessment:
(1) Re-assess tolerance of vital sign changes by evaluating LOC, signs of hypoxia, feeling of dizziness, shortness of breath, decreased urine output, presence of ectopic beats.
(2) Continuously monitor electrocardiogram (EKG) for severe bradycardia, which may require a pacemaker.
(3) Take measures to prevent deep vein thrombosis. Assess leg color, size, and temperature as a baseline.

   b. Expected outcomes:
- (1) Absence of vasovagal episodes.
- (2) Organs and periphery are adequately perfused.

   c. Nursing interventions:
- (1) Avoid prolonged suctioning, which can precipitate vagal stimulation.
- (2) Hyperoxygenate prior to suctioning.
- (3) Closely monitor heart rate and rhythm.
- (4) Apply sequential compression devices.
- (5) Administer Atropine 0.5 -1.0 mg rapid IV push in symptomatic bradycardia, as ordered.

7. Nursing diagnosis: Alteration in gastrointestinal function (paralytic ileus, stress ulcer).
   a. Assessment:
- (1) Anticipate paralytic ileus for at least the first 48 hours.
- (2) Determine gastric pH; hematest stools and gastric contents.
- (3) Measure abdominal girth, auscultate bowel sounds, and palpate the abdomen in all four quadrants. The patient may be insensitive to pain and not develop a rigid abdomen due to the absence of muscle tone.

   b. Expected outcomes:
- (1) Active bowel sounds.
- (2) Gastric aspiration less than 50ml/ 24 hours without evidence of blood.
- (3) Abdomen flat without distention.

   c. Interventions:
- (1) Insert nasogastric (NG) tube to low suction as ordered to decompress the stomach and assess for blood in upper gastrointestinal tract. Severe gastric distention can impair ventilatory excursion.
- (2) If NG tube is not inserted, utilize vomiting precautions.
- (3) Administer gastric antacids and/or H2 blockers, as ordered to prevent gastric irritation and/or ulcers.

8. Nursing diagnosis: Decreased urine output/retention.
   a. Assessment: Bladder catheterization is important for both drainage and monitoring of fluid status.
   b. Expected outcomes: urine output is 30 cc/hr.
   c. Nursing interventions:
- (1) Insert foley catheter as ordered.
- (2) Anticipate an areflexic bladder associated with spinal shock.
- (3) Assess urine color, clarity, character, and amount.
- (4) Monitor renal function; document intake and output.
- (5) Send urine for urinalysis.
- (6) If blood in urine, prepare patient for further diagnostic tests.

9. Nursing diagnosis: Musculosketal impairment related to pre-existing conditions or associated injuries.
   a. Assessment:
- (1) Extremities: palpate for fractures, abnormal position of the arms or legs.
- (2) Vertebral assessment: consider other pre-existing factors that may compromise the spinal canal and contribute to SCI, such as stenosis, ankylosing spondylitis, or rheumatoid arthritis. Pathologic spine fractures may be associated with degenerative and osteoporotic changes of aging or metastatic lesions at the injury site.
  - (a) Assess for pain, tenderness, and/or deformity at the injury site. Pain occasionally radiates to the arms, the chest and abdomen, or into the lower extremities.
  - (b) Assess the shape, site of injury/fracture for edema, open areas, entry wounds, or deformities.

   b. Expected outcomes: Minimize existing musculoskeletal trauma and prevent secondary complications.
   c. Nursing interventions (Refer to Chapter 18 – Musculoskeletal)

10. Nursing diagnosis: Actual/potential loss of skin integrity related to pressure from immobilization devices, lack of sensation, or voluntary movement, or spinal shock.
    a. Assessment: skin inspection, focusing on areas at risk for pressure ulcer and trauma.
    b. Expected outcomes: skin surfaces remain intact and free of external pressure and infection.
    c. Nursing interventions (Refer to Chapter 17: Skin)
       (1) Protect prominences to prevent pressure ulcers.
       (2) Position patient properly to prevent wrist and foot drop.
11. Nursing diagnosis: Sensory and motor deficits due to SCI and related injuries.
    a. Assessment (Mahon, 1992; Porter, 1994; Restak, 1984):
       (1) Level of Consciousness: consider traumatic brain injury (TBI), chemical impairment, or hypothermia as sources of decreased LOC.
           (a) Mental status exam: awareness, orientation.
           (b) Quantify responses with Glasgow Coma Scale.
       (2) Cranial nerve assessment: especially for high cervical spine injuries and TBI
           (a) In high cervical injuries (C2, C3, C4), traction may affect cranial nerves. Function may be absent or diminished.
           (b) Assess function of Glossopharyngeal (IX), Vagus (X), Accessory (XI) and Hypoglossal (XII) nerves.
           (c) Accessory muscle function may be confused with shoulder shrug ability (CN XI).
       (3) Purpose of spinal neurological exam is to establish baseline neurological level of injury and type of injury (Refer to Chapter 10: Neurological Assessment) (Refer to Figure 27.2).
       (4) Review diagnostic studies as described in Chapter 10 - Neurological Assessment
    b. Expected outcomes: Minimize neurological deficit and facilitate return of motor and sensory function.
    c. Nursing interventions:
       (1) Monitor for changes in sensory level (Refer to Chapter 10: Neurological Assessment).
       (2) Pharmacological interventions (*The Medical Letter*, 1993; Travis, 1992).
           (a) The use of steroids remains controversial. It is believed that steroids stabilize lysosomal membranes and act as free-radical scavengers, thus preventing cell destruction.
               - Methylprednisolone is used because it rapidly crosses cell membranes.
               - Individuals with neurological deficits must begin to receive the drug within 8 hours of injury.
               - Dosage: 30 mg/kg IV bolus over 15 minutes, pause for 45 minutes, 5.4 mg/kg/hr continuous drip over the next 23 hours
           (b) Sygen is an additional drug under investigation. Sygen is generally administered following standard methylprednisolone therapy in non-penetrating injuries with significant neurological deficits.
           (c) 21-aminiosteroids (lazaroids) such as tirilizade mesylate, seem to demonstrate greater antioxidant activity without glucocorticoid action.
           (d) Other drugs used experimentally in the treatment of SCI include Narcan, Thyrotropin, and calcium channel blockers.
       (3) Psychological support.
           (a) During the acute management phase individuals and families are extremely frightened and anxious.
           (b) Honest, frequent communication is a critical element of the treatment protocol.
           (c) Additional information about psychological implications following SCI is found in Chapters 23 and 24.

C. **Reassessment:** Before leaving the emergency room (ER), assure that (Green, 1987):
   1. Airway is cleared and "guaranteed"; suctioning equipment must be available during the transport.
   2. The spine is immobilized in a "neutral" position.

Figure 27-2: Motor Assessment Flow Sheet

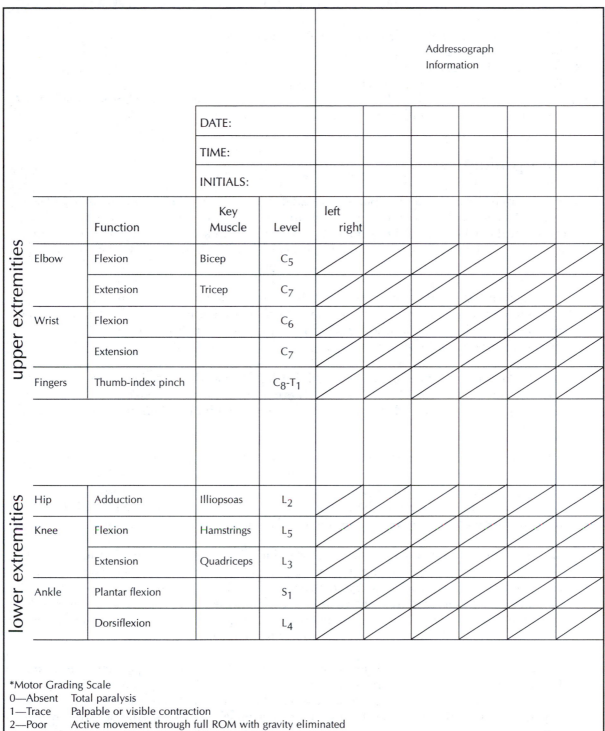

		Function	Key Muscle	Level	left right						
upper extremities	Elbow	Flexion	Bicep	C_5							
		Extension	Tricep	C_7							
	Wrist	Flexion		C_6							
		Extension		C_7							
	Fingers	Thumb-index pinch		C_8-T_1							
lower extremities	Hip	Adduction	Illiopsoas	L_2							
	Knee	Flexion	Hamstrings	L_5							
		Extension	Quadriceps	L_3							
	Ankle	Plantar flexion		S_1							
		Dorsiflexion		L_4							

DATE: / TIME: / INITIALS: / Addressograph Information

*Motor Grading Scale
0—Absent Total paralysis
1—Trace Palpable or visible contraction
2—Poor Active movement through full ROM with gravity eliminated
3—Fair Active movement through full ROM against gravity
4—Good Active movement through full ROM against resistance
5—Normal

Note: ASIA (1989) recommends the use of sensory testing (Procedure 4–2) for levels C_{1-3} (C_4 diaphragm), T_2-L_1, and S_2-S_5.

From Motor Assessment Flow Sheet, by J. Keene, University of Wisconsin Spine Center, in C.P. Zejdlik (Ed.), 1992, *Mangement of Spinal Cord Injury* (2nd ed., p. 74), Boston: Jones & Bartlett. Reprinted with permission.

3. Ventilation is satisfactory with 100 percent oxygen.
4. Pulse/BP are stable and a route (IV site) for further resuscitation has been established.
5. EKG is being monitored.
6. A foley catheter and NG tube to gravity have been passed.
7. Skin is padded under bony prominences.
8. Body warmth is guaranteed.
9. Paralyzed limbs are secured under straps to the backboard.
10. Other unstable injuries have been supported to the best of the referring hospital's ability.
11. A complete medical record and any radiographic studies accompany the patient.

Practical Application

A helicopter crew was paged to respond to a trauma victim in a remote mountain area. M.G., a 64-year-old male, had been riding an all terrain vehicle (ATV) on a dirt road when he was pitched over the handle bars. The victim was not wearing a helmet at the time of the crash. M.G. was said to have landed on his head, forcing his chin into his chest. The local ambulance was on scene.

M.G. was received at the helicopter in full spinal immobilization, with oxygen being administered by non-rebreather mask, and one intravenous line infusing in his left arm. The victim was complaining of neck and back pain and tingling in his arms. The findings on physical exam were as follows:

GENERAL: M.G. was a well-nourished, well-developed male who looked his stated age of 64. He had a medical history of diabetes and hypertension, for which he took oral medications. Initial vital signs were blood pressure 90/50, pulse 66, respirations 28/minute, temperature 96.5 degrees.

NEURO: The victim was awake, alert, and oriented. M.G. had gross motor movement of his arms, fingers, and left toes, but had a fine motor movement deficit in all of his extremities. He had a weak hand grasp and an inability to flex or extend his fingers. He was not able to move his right toes or either leg. The most significant finding was a diaphragmatic breathing pattern. There was no sensation below the nipple line.

HEENT: The victim had obvious facial injuries, including contusions and abrasions of both cheeks, orbits, and forehead, leading to suspected orbital fractures. There was a 3 cm laceration to the bridge of his nose and a laceration of about the same size to the left of his mouth. Blood was leaking from the victim's left ear and nose mixed with a small amount of clear liquid. M.G.'s mandible was painful, swollen, and appeared deformed. In spite of these injuries, M.G .was able to speak and swallow; he denied being nauseated.

CHEST/CV: There were no bruises on the chest or broken ribs palpable on exam. Respirations were shallow, breath sounds were clear and equal, though diminished bilaterally. The heart monitor revealed a regular sinus rhythm without ectopy. Pulse oxygenation was 97 percent on the non-rebreather mask. The victim's blood pressure was initially 90/50 with a pulse rate of 66 and respiratory rate of 28 per minute.

ABD/PELVIS: The abdomen was soft and the pelvis stable to anterior-posterior pressure. There were no bruises or swelling indicating injury. Pain was not elicited below the nipple line due to sensory loss.

ASSESSMENT: Possible spinal cord injury with neurological deficit and potential for spinal shock; possible basilar skull fracture; possible facial fractures to include orbits and mandible; possible internal injuries, potential for ventilatory insufficiency due to diaphragmatic breathing pattern.

TREATMENT:
1)   Maintain an adequate airway and oxygenation level.
2)   Start a second IV line and maintain adequate fluid volume.
3)   Maintain spinal immobilization.
4)   Maintain body temperature with warm blankets and heat.
5)   Observe for signs and symptoms of shock and develop treatment plan as needed.

En route to the trauma center, M.G. had two episodes of hypoxia as measured by pulse oximetry and falling respiratory rate. He received 15 liters of oxygen for about two minutes during each episode. Suction was not needed. Spontaneous respiration and diaphragmatic breathing continued after each hypoxic episode. Pulse oxygenation level was maintained at 93 percent and above throughout the trip.

The trauma team awaited arrival at the trauma center. A complete set of spine X-rays was obtained, as well as chest and pelvis X-rays. Emergency bloodwork showed a normal hematocrit and hemoglobin. CT scans diagnosed a nasal fracture. The spine CT showed a stable fracture of the ring of C-1 with some degeneration of the vertebrae, and swelling indicating a cord contusion and/or hematoma between the areas of C4 and C6. Neurological exam showed fine motor movement impaired, and decreased strength in both hands. There was no antigravity strength of the biceps, triceps, or across the shoulders, and there was some ability to flex and extend the left wrist. Lower extremities were flaccid and there was no sensation in the left lower extremity. The patient did exhibit some minimal sensation and very slight movement of the right ankle and interphalangial joints. Rectal tone was present, though weak. M.G. was maintained in a Philadelphia cervical collar, started on high dose steroids within four hours after the injury, and was admitted to the intensive care unit.

M.G. maintained spontaneous respirations with adequate pulse oxygenation through the night. Normal body temperature was maintained. An NG tube was inserted to keep the stomach empty due to possible development of an ileus. The next day there was improvement in the neuro exam. Improved strength across both shoulders, both biceps, and triceps was noted, indicating some preservation of C-5, C6, and C7. Minimal internal rotation of both hips was demonstrated, left greater than right, with impaired sensation to the pelvic area. Bowel and bladder dysfunction were evident. M.G. was able to withdraw both lower extremities, but not to gravity. There was trace movement of the right lower extremity, but no sensation was noted. M.G. was discharged 16 days after the injury to a rehabilitation hospital.

References and Selected Bibliography

Albin, M.S. (1985). Acute cervical spine injury. *Critical Care Clinics, 1*(2), 267-284.

Albin, M.S. (1987). Epidemiology, pathophysiology, and experimental therapies of acute spinal cord injuries. *Critical Care Clinics, 2*(3), 441-449.

Ball, R. (1990). Don't add insult to injury: Proper handling of head and neck trauma. *Journal of Emergency Medical Services, 10,* 40-54.

Bonegin, L., Hung, T.L., & Chang, G.L. (1987). Biomechanics of spinal cord injury. *Critical Care Clinics, 3*(3), 453-459.

Davis, A.E. (1991). Acute care management of patients with spinal cord injuries. *Critical Care Currents, 9*(1), 1-4.

Errico, T.J., Bauer, R.D., & Wauch, T. (1992). *Spinal trauma.* Philadelphia: Lippincott.

Fontanarosa, P.B. (1991). Avoiding the risks and repercussions of acute spinal cord injury. *Prehospital Care Reports, 15,* 33-42.

Gilbert, M.B. (1987). Critical care management of the patient with an acute spinal cord injury. *Critical Care Clinics, 3*(3), 549-563.

Goldberg, S. (1979). *Neuroanatomy made ridiculously simple.* Miami, FL: Med Master.

Green, B.A. (1987). Spinal cord injury - A systems approach: Prevention, emergency medical services and emergency room management. *Critical Care Clinics, 3*(3), 471-493.

Hanak, M.A., & Scott, A. (1983). *Spinal cord injury: A guide for health professionals.* New York: Springer.

Herzenberg, J., Hensigner, R.E., & Dedrick, D., (1989). Emergency transport and positioning of young children who have an injury of the cervical spine. *Journal of Bone and Joint Surgery, 71A,* 15-22.

Laskowski-Jones, L. (1993). Acute spinal cord injury: How to minimize the damage. *American Journal of Nursing,* 23-30.

Mahon, J.C. (1992). Spinal cord injury. In E.W. Bayley & S.A. Turkle (Eds), *A comprehensive curriculum for trauma nursing* (pp. 285-306). Boston: Jones and Bartlett.

The Medical Letter. (1993). Drugs for acute spinal cord injury. *The Medical Letter, 35*(902), 72-73.

Patterson, D.R., (1993). When life support is questioned early in the care of patients with cervical level quadriplegia. *The New England Journal of Medicine, 328*(7), 506-509.

Porter, D. (1994). New in the field of neurosurgery. *Flight Rounds, Flight For Life, 2*(2), 5.

Przybylski, G.J., & Marion D.W. (1996). Injury to the vertebrae and spinal cord. In Feliciano, Moore, & Mattox (Eds.), *Trauma* (pp. 307-323). Stamford, CT: Appleton & Lange.

Restak, R.M. (1984). *The brain.* Toronto, CAN: Bantam.

Rothman, R.H., & Simeone, F.A. (1992). *The spine* (3rd ed., Vol. 2). Philadelphia: Saunders.

Segatore, M. (1993). Methylprednisolone after spinal cord injury. *SCI Nursing, 10*(1), 8-13.

Sinkinson, C.A. & Egherman W.P. (1991). Cervical spine trauma: On the front lines. *CME-TV Study Guide, University of Arizona: College of Medicine.2*(8), 1-13.

Travis, J. (1992). Spinal cord injuries: New optimism blooms for developing treatments. *Science, 258,* 218-220.

Zejdlik, C.P.(Ed.) (1992). *Management of spinal cord injury,* (2nd ed.). Boston: Jones and Bartlett.

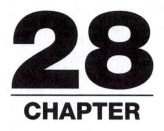

CHAPTER

Critical Care
Holly N. Watson-Evans, MS, RN
Denise Miller Lemke, MSN, RN, CNRN

I. Learning Objectives

A. Prioritize the critical care needs for the individual with a traumatic acute spinal cord injury.

B. Identify key nursing interventions associated with the critical care management of an individual with a traumatic acute SCI.

C. Prioritize the critical care needs of the individual with spinal cord impairment.

D. Identify key nursing interventions associated with the critical care management of an individual with spinal cord impairment.

II. Introduction

This chapter discusses the critical care management of the individual with a traumatic acute spinal cord injury or spinal cord impairment. Traumatic spinal cord injuries are often treated in a critical care setting only until hemodynamic and/or respiratory needs are stabilized. Additional information regarding the initial emergency management of traumatic spinal cord injuries can be found in Chapter 27. Critical care needs for individuals with spinal cord impairment are usually limited to acute respiratory and/or hemodynamic compromise. Determination of location of admission (intensive care unit (ICU) versus acute care unit) is dependent on the clinical status and specific institution admission criteria.

III. General Critical Care

A. **Admission Assessment/History:**
   1. Present injury
   2. Past medical history

    3. Present medications

B. **Review of Systems: Assessment and Management of Complications:**
1. During the first 7-10 days following an acute SCI, priorities revolve around anticipating, preventing, recognizing, and treating complications. Many complications are related to spinal shock and may affect all body systems. Complications are more severe in cervical injuries.
2. Individuals in the critical care area with spinal cord impairment are often admitted for pulmonary and/or hemodynamic instability. Patient care management priorities are directed at optimizing function of these body systems.

C. **Neurologic System:** Specific neurological assessment to define level of injury utilizing American Spinal Injury Association (ASIA) criteria (See Chapter 10).
1. Nursing diagnosis: Neurologic dysfunction related to spinal instability.
2. Expected outcomes:
    a. Maintenance or improvement of neurologic function.
    b. Adequate pain relief.
3. Nursing interventions:
    a. Assess and monitor motor and sensory function as ordered. Be especially aware of ascending paralysis in C5 injuries or above.
    b. Maintain spinal alignment at all times with weights/tongs, halo vest, or other orthotic device.

D. **Cardiovascular System:**
1. Nursing diagnosis: Decreased cardiac output related to spinal shock.
2. Expected outcomes:
    a. Adequate cardiac output/blood pressure is maintained for tissue perfusion.
    b. Heart rate remains regular at 60-100/minute.
    c. Blood pressure is adequate to maintain perfusion.
    d. Urine output is 0.5-1.0 ml/kg/hr.
    e. Pulse oximetry is within normal limits.
    f. Skin is warm, dry, and pink.
    g. Immediate recognition/treatment of autonomic dysreflexia.
    h. Level of Consciousness (LOC) is maintained.
3. Nursing interventions:
    a. Assess heart rate: quality and regularity of peripheral pulses.
    b. Assess blood pressure.
    c. Monitor for vasovagal response, which may result in cardiac arrest due to vagal stimulation and hypoxia.
    d. Stop any activity associated with decrease in heart rate more than 10 percent.
    e. Assess temperature and moisture of skin.
    f. Assess for presence of spinal shock (see Chapter 18).
    g. Take measures to prevent deep vein thrombosis.
        (1) Assess leg color, size, and temperature as a baseline.
        (2) Apply anti embolism stockings, sequential boots, compression sleeves or other devices as ordered.
    h. Maintain adequate hydration and volume status through administration of fluids as ordered.
    i. Monitor poikilothermism. Due to interruption of sympathetic pathway to temperature-regulating centers in hypothalamus individuals will become hypo-or hyper-thermic, depending on room temperature.
        (1) Use warming mattress to prevent hypothermia.
        (2) Maintain cool room temperature (700F) to prevent hyperthermia.
    j. If utilizing inotropics (i.e. dopamine, dobutamine), monitor blood pressure per hospital policy.
    k. Gradually elevate the head of bed. Utilize abdominal binder.

E. **Respiratory System:**
1. Nursing diagnosis: Ineffective breathing patterns related to muscular paralysis and/or gastric distention secondary to ileus.
2. Expected outcomes:
   a. Adequate tidal volumes.
   b. Arterial blood gases (ABGs) within normal limits.
   c. Clear breath sounds.
   d. Effective cough (may require cough assist).
3. Nursing interventions:
   a. Measure respiratory parameters as ordered.
   b. Assess rate, pattern, and depth of respirations.
   c. Assess symmetry of chest wall movements.
   d. Assess use of accessory muscles. Retraction of neck muscles may be a sign of poor oxygenation and may indicate respiratory decompensation.
   e. Apply pulse oximeter.
      (1) Monitor airway patency.
      (2) Monitor chest excursion and diaphragmatic breathing.
      (3) Observe for and report changes in assessment and response to treatment.
   f. If applicable, monitor response to mechanical ventilation.
   g. Suction as necessary. Pre-oxygenate before each suction pass.

F. **Gastrointestinal System:**
1. Nursing diagnosis: Alteration in bowel elimination due to paralytic ileus or altered bowel innervation.
2. Expected outcomes:
   a. Gastric mobility.
   b. Established bowel program without impaction.
3. Nursing interventions:
   a. Anticipate paralytic ileus for at least the first 48 hours.
   b. Insert nasogastric tube to low intermittent suction as ordered to decompress the stomach and assess for blood in the upper gastrointestinal tract.
   c. Be aware that severe gastric distention can impair ventilatory excursion.
   d. Auscultate bowel sounds and monitor for abdominal distention.
   e. Evaluate gastric pH.
   f. Initiate tube feedings with return of peristalsis.
   g. Check for presence of impaction.
   h. Within 72 hours of injury, initiate stool softeners, suppositories, and bowel training program.
   i. Administer gastric antacids and/or H2 blockers to prevent gastric irritation and/or ulcers.
   j. Initiate total parenteral nutrition (TPN) within several days if tube feedings are contraindicated.

G. **Genitourinary System:**
1. Nursing diagnosis: Alteration in urinary elimination related to loss of bladder innervation.
2. Expected outcomes:
   a. Establishment of bladder elimination program.
   b. Absence of urinary tract infection or incontinence.
3. Nursing interventions:
   a. Insert foley catheter as ordered.
   b. Palpate bladder for distention.
   c. Anticipate areflexic bladder.
   d. Monitor renal function; document intake and output (I & 0).
   e. When hemodynamically stable, initiate intermittent catheterization every 4-6 hours to maintain bladder volume of 500 cc or less.
   f. Monitor for signs and symptoms of infection.
      (1) Color and character of urine.

   (2) Odor.

   (3) Elevated temperature.

H. **Integument:**

 1. Nursing diagnosis: High potential for impairment of skin integrity and related loss of sensation.

 2. Expected outcome: Intact skin.

 3. Nursing interventions:

  a. At least every eight hours inspect all skin surfaces for signs of redness.

   (1) Under Halo vest.

   (2) Back of the head.

  b. Turn every 1-2 hours.

  c. Utilize Kinetic Treatment Table (Rotorest Bed) as ordered.

  d. Monitor and protect pressure points every eight hours.

  e. Protect from injury.

I. **Nutrition:**

 1. Nursing diagnosis: Potential for inadequate nutrition related to impaired gastric motility.

 2. Expected outcomes:

  a. Adequate caloric intake.

  b. Adequate fluid intake

 3. Nursing interventions:

  a. Initiate tube feedings with return of peristalsis.

  b. Utilize calorie count if appropriate.

  c. Initiate TPN within several days if tube feedings are contraindicated.

J. **Pharmacotherapy:**

 1. The use of steroids remains controversial. It is believed that steroids stabilize lysosomal membranes and act as free-radical scavengers, thus preventing cell destruction.

  a. Methylprednisolone is used because it rapidly crosses cell membranes.

  b. Individuals with neurological deficits must begin to receive the drug within 8 hours of injury.

 2. Sygen is an additional drug under investigation in clinical trials at 26 U.S. sites. Sygen, a GM-1 Ganglioside is a neurotrophic agent that promotes neuronal growth. Sygen is administered following standard methylprednisolone therapy in non-penetrating injuries with significant neurological deficits.

 3. 21-aminosteroids (lazaroids) such as Tirilizade mesylate, seem to demonstrate greater antioxidant activity without glucocorticoid action.

 4. Nursing interventions with pharmacotherapy include:.

  a. Provide education regarding medication.

  b. Monitor response/side effects to medication.

  c. Report and document response/side effects.

K. **Diagnostic Evaluation** (Refer to Chapter 10):

 1. Magnetic Resonance Imaging (MRI)

 2. Magnetic Resonance Spectroscopy (MRS)

 3. Somatosensory Evoked Potentials (SSEPs)

L. **Surgical Management:**

 1. Timing: dependent on

  a. Type of injury

  b. Extent of injury

  c. Medical stability

 2. Surgical procedures:

  a. Laminectomy

  b. Bony fusion

   c. Spinal instrumentation
   d. Stabilization of associated injuries
3. Post-operative bracing (orthotics):
   a. Cervical Spine
     (1) Halo Brace
     (2) SOMI (Sterno-occipital-mandibular-immobilizer)
     (3) Minerva brace
     (4) Extended cervical collar
     (5) Short cervical collar
   b. Thoracic Spine
     (1) Modified Minerva
     (2) Fabricated orthosis
   c. Lumbar Spine
     (1) Fabricated orthosis

M. Psychological Support:

1. Nursing diagnosis: Ineffectual coping
2. Expected outcome:
   a. Verbalization of concerns
   b. Management of stress and ability to rest
   c. Stabilization of physical functions
3. Nursing interventions:
   a. During the critical care phase following spinal cord trauma, individuals and their families are extremely frightened and anxious.
   b. Individuals with spinal cord impairment who are in critical care areas are also anxious and unsure of what to expect.
   c. Consistent, concise, honest communication is a critical component of nursing care provided to these individuals.
   d. Additional information about psychological implications can be found in Chapters 23 and 24.

References and Selected Bibliography

Albin, M.S. (1985). Acute cervical spine injury. *Critical Care Clinics, 1*(2), 267-284.

Albin, M.S. (1987). Epidemiology, pathophysiology, and experimental therapies of acute spinal cord injuries. *Critical Care Clinics, 2*(3), 441-449.

Ball, R. (1990). Don't add insult to injury: Proper handling of head and neck trauma. *Journal of Emergency Medical Services* (10), 40-54.

Bonegin, L., Hung, T.L., & Chang, G.L. (1987). Biomechanics of spinal cord injury. *Critical Care Clinics 3*(3), 453-459.

Davis, A.E. (1991). Acute care management of patients with spinal cord injuries. *Critical Care Currents, 9*(1), 1-4.

Davis, A.E. (1991). Acute care management of patients with spinal cord injuries. *Critical Care Currents, 9*(2), 1-4.

Errico, T.J., Bauer, R.D., & Wauch, T. (1992). *Spinal trauma*. Philadelphia: Lippincott.

Fontanarosa, P.B. (1991). Avoiding the risks and repercussions of acute spinal cord injury. *Prehospital Care Reports, 15*, 33-42.

Gilbert, M.B. (1987). Critical care management of the patient with an acute spinal cord injury. *Critical Care Clinics, 3*(3), 549-563.

Green, B.A. (1987). Spinal cord injury - A systems approach: Prevention, emergency medical services and emergency room management. *Critical Care Clinics, 3*(3), 471-493.

Goldberg, S. (1979). *Neuroanatomy made ridiculously simple*. Miami, FL: Med Master.

Hanak, M.A., & Scott, A. (1983). *Spinal cord injury: A guide for health professionals*. New York: Springer.

Laskowski-Jones, L. (1993). Acute spinal cord injury: How to minimize the damage. *American Journal of Nursing, 93*,(12), 22-31.

Mahon, J.C. (1992). Spinal cord injury. In E.W. Bayley & S.A. Turkle(Eds), *A comprehensive curriculum for trauma nursing* (pp. 285-306). Boston: Jones & Bartlett.

The Medical Letter (1993). Drugs for acute spinal cord injury. *The Medical Letter, 35*(902), 72.

Patterson, D. R., Everett, J. J., Bombardier, C. H., Questad, K. A., Lee, V. K., Marvin, J. A. (1993). When life support is questioned early in the care of patients with cervical level quadriplegia. *The New England Journal of Medicine, 328*(7), 506-509.

Porter, D. (1994). New in the field of neurosurgery. *Flight Rounds, Flight for Life*, (2) 2, 5.

Przybylski, G.J., & Marion D.W. (1996). Injury to the vertebrae and spinal cord. In Feliciano, Moore & Mattox (Eds.), *Trauma (3rd ed.)*, (pp. 307-323). Stamford, CT: Appleton & Lange.

Restak, R.M. (1984). *The brain*. Toronto, CAN: Bantam.

Rothman, R.H., & Simeone, F.A. (1992). *The spine 6th ed., Vol 2*. Philadelphia: Saunders.

Segatore, M. (1993). Methylprednisolone after spinal cord injury. SCI Nursing, 10(1), 8-13.

Sinkinson, C.A., & Egherman W.P. (1991). Cervical spine trauma: On the front lines. *CME-TV Study Guide, University of Arizona College of Medicine, 2(8)*, 1-13.

Travis, J. (1992). Spinal cord injuries: New optimism blooms for developing treatments. *Science*, 258, 218-220.

Zejdlik, C.P. (Ed.)(1992). *Management of spinal cord injury* (2 ed.) Boston: Jones & Bartlett.

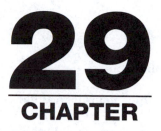

Rehabilitation

Audrey Nelson, PhD, RN, FAAN

I. Learning Objectives

A. Define the concept of rehabilitation.

B. Describe the process of rehabilitation as it relates to persons with spinal cord impairment (SCI).

C. Identify nursing interventions to facilitate rehabilitation in SCI.

II. Introduction

This chapter presents an overview of rehabilitation as it relates to persons with SCI. Rehabilitation begins at the moment of injury or when a disorder is diagnosed. In this documented trajectory of SCI nursing care, rehabilitation follows trauma emergency care (Chapter 27), and critical care (Chapter 28). This chapter complements information found in Chapter 3, "Philosophy, Goals, and Process of SCI Nursing Practice."

III. Definitions of Rehabilitation

A. **Definition #1:** Rehabilitation is a restorative and learning process that seeks to hasten and maximize recovery from SCI by treating the resultant impairments, disabilities, and handicaps (World Health Organization, 1980).
  1. Impairment focuses on how a condition affects the normal structure and function of the body.
  2. Disability focuses on the individual's inability to perform a task in the usual manner.
  3. Handicap focuses on the individual's inability to fulfill usual roles.

B. **Definition #2:** Rehabilitation is a constant process of learning or behavior change, during which an individual with a disability adjusts initially, but must also continually adapt (Trieschmann, 1980).

C. **Definition #3**: Rehabilitation is a creative and individualized process of preparing an individual with a disability to successfully adapt to physical limitations, architectural barriers, and societal prejudices (Nelson, 1990).

IV. Goals of Rehabilitation

A. **Prevention of secondary complications**

B. **Remediation or treatment to reduce neurological deficits**

C. **Compensation to offset and adapt to residual disabilities**

D. **Maintenance of function and promotion of health throughout the life span**

V. Expected Outcomes of Rehabilitation

A. **Markers of Success in rehabilitation** are measured not only by the physical functions regained by the individual, but also by the individual's attitude, motivation, cooperation, and participation in rehabilitation (Albrecht & Higgins, 1977). Failures in rehabilitation are viewed as rehabilitation stalemates—success that has not yet occurred.

B. **Learning to Compensate Without Using the Disability:** The individual learns to compensate for the physical limitations of the injury in a way that promotes safety, comfort, and personal worth. The individual with a newly diagnosed SCI learns effective social skills without having to "use the disability" to get his/her needs met. Persons with SCI "use their disability" when they exploit the guilt, social discomfort, and ignorance of functional abilities many able-bodied persons have about persons with disabilities. Using one's disability is likely to lead to diminished social support system and further isolation in the community(Nelson, 1990).

C. **Housing and Transportation Resources:** Wheelchair-accessible housing is obtained and transportation is available.

D. **Links to Community:** The individual returns to a viable occupation; feels physically attractive; participates in a rich, full social life; and maintains family ties.

E. **Creating New Ways of Achieving Goals:** "Acceptance of disability" has been an ultimate outcome that staff has set for persons with SCI (Kerr & Thompson, 1972). Persons with SCI, on the other hand, may view acceptance as "giving up" or "passive resignation." To them, the ultimate goal of rehabilitation is to create new ways of achieving old goals and life dreams. Optimal rehabilitation programs facilitate the ability to "transcend" cultural stereotypes about disabilities, rather than accept them (Nelson, 1990).

VI. Setting Goals and Measuring Progress in Rehabilitation

A. **Involvement in Goal Setting:** Goal setting is a cultural norm in our society since achievement is so highly valued. Persons with SCI enter the SCI rehabilitation program with varying levels of life experience in goal setting and goal attainment. However, even those most adept at goal-setting strategies find their limited knowledge about SCI impedes their ability to set realistic and appropriate goals. For this reason, staff involvement in the early stages of rehabilitation is intense. Later, staff involvement in setting goals tends to wane as the individual becomes more knowledgeable about SCI and is subsequently encouraged to take more initiative in setting individualized goals (Nelson, 1990).

B. **Purpose of Goal Setting:** Goal setting in SCI rehabilitation serves two major purposes.
1. Goals provide markers for determining progress. These markers provide the stimulus for

ongoing positive feedback to the individual and, in a sense, motivate the patient to continue to work hard.

2. The process of goal setting gives the person with SCI critical cues about the extent of the disability, as well as what can be expected from the staff, the rehabilitation program, and what the prospects are for the future (Gubrium & Buckholdt, 1982).

C. **Progress in Meeting Goals:**

1. As individuals move through the rehabilitation program, more attention is paid to progress and goal attainment. Staff members give patients cues as to the progress they see. For example, a nurse might say, "Well, I think you ought to start going to the dining room for your meals," or "Have you thought about going out on pass for the weekend?" Staff members provide cues to keep patients on course and provide markers for noting when progress has been made.

2 Gubrium and Buckholdt (1982) describe three ways to view progress in rehabilitation; each allows for regression.

   a. The linear model characterizes progress as steps; small changes occur on each day of therapy.

   b. The incremental model views progress as stages; little or no change occurs for a period of time and then at some critical points, the patient leaps to a new level of recovery or gains, which must be consolidated before further progress can occur.

   c. The spontaneous model is sudden; patients go from little or no progress to a remarkable gain, perhaps approaching recovery almost overnight.

3. Persons with disabilities gauge progress as a dichotomy of being dependent or independent in completing tasks, as in the statement, "I couldn't do this and now I can." From a the patient's perspective, the following milestones indicate progress: getting up in the chair for the first time, independent transfers, doing bowel care and catheterizations independently, feeding self, dressing oneself, going on a recreation trip for the first time, first overnight pass, and setting a discharge date.

4. Staff members have a more complex system of gauging progress. For example, muscle strength is graded on a scale from 1-5. Staff also evaluate the level of assistance required, such as dependent, partial assist, stand-by assist, and independent. In addition, staff monitor quality of movement, self-confidence, speed, amount of effort expended to complete a task, ability to solve problems that arise, and the amount of equipment/assistive devices used. Staff also place a heavy emphasis on attitude and cooperation.

5. Often, the progress made in rehabilitation is invisible to the layman, who lacks the necessary knowledge and experience with SCI to see subtle improvements. Furthermore, the person with a newly diagnosed SCI is often preoccupied by comparisons to the pre-injury state.

D. **Information Assimilation:** There are four levels at which a patient assimilates information during rehabilitation.

1. Receipt: The first level of reintegration is characterized by passive receipt of information and casual observation of staff and other persons with SCI on the rehabilitation unit. Generally, patients do not feel that much of what they see or hear about disabilities pertains to them as individuals, since most feel their disability is temporary. Boredom and curiosity lead patients to listen, watch, and experience the essence of rehabilitation in SCI.

2. Response and Imitation: At some point, individuals begin to respond to information and may even imitate others. As individuals are socialized to the unit, they go through the motions of what is expected of them. During this phase, peer counseling is effective, and is meaningful to both the sender and the receiver.

3. Internalization: Individuals start to internalize some of the values and practices and feel a sense of "belonging" and comfort. Frequently, individuals are discharged from the rehabilitation unit during this stage.

4. Accommodation: After discharge, persons with SCI learn to adapt the knowledge and skills learned in rehabilitation to make it fit with their own lifestyle. Furthermore, individuals are able to make lifestyle alterations to accommodate the disability. Individuals show skill in adapting to various environments and situations without undue distress or anxiety.

VII. Teaching and Learning in Rehabilitation

Teaching and learning are central critical factors of the rehabilitation process, determining the eventual degree of success in re-entering the community and living a healthy life.

A. **Format of Educational Programs:** Educational programs in SCI should be structured, organized, comprehensive, and directed to the individual, family, and caregivers.

B. **Timing of Education:** Health education may occur throughout the continuum of care, and should be provided to the individual and caregiver, according to their specific assessed needs. Content and timing of education are dependent on such factors as readiness to learn, importance of the information, medical stability, and safety. Individual and caregiver knowledge of and adherence to treatment regimes should be assessed at follow-up evaluations. Educational assessments should not only include mastery of knowledge, technique, physiology, and related conditions/skills, but should also carefully address confidence and performance.

C. **Readiness for Learning:** Though readiness for learning is acknowledged as important (Hamric, 1981), there are few indicators that let us know when the time is right for teaching the person with SCI. Several factors interfere with readiness to learn: pain, fear, sensory and perceptual disturbances, sleep disruption, and drugs.

D. **Learning Environment:** Providing a good learning environment is critical. A comfortable environment with provisions for privacy is critical especially when presenting skills that could be awkward or embarrassing during the preliminary learning period.

VIII. Phases of Rehabilitation

SCI rehabilitation nursing practice can be characterized by four distinct approaches: buffering, transcending, toughening, and launching (Nelson, 1990).

A. **Buffering:** Individuals must necessarily cope with the multitude of losses associated with SCI as well as the indignities and problems resulting from extended hospitalization. Buffering, is the nurturing and protective process of helping patients to gather the physical and emotional strength necessary for a strenuous rehabilitation program.
   1. Expected outcomes of buffering:
      a. Garnering physical and emotional strength to fully participate in the strenuous rehabilitation program.
      b. Easing the transition between the intensive care unit and the unique environment of the rehabilitation unit
      c. Establishing trusting, comfortable relationship with the staff
      d. Establishing effective coping skills
   2. When buffering is most needed
      a. When the individual is first admitted to the rehabilitation unit
      b. In crisis situations, where resources are quickly depleted
      c. When the individual is experiencing something for the first time
   3. Components necessary for buffering
      a. Effective relationships
      b. Competent staff who recognize and tend to critical needs
      c. Continuity of personnel
      d. Creation of a caring environment
      e. Peer support program
      f. Focus on short-term goals
      g. Instillation of a sense of hope

B. **Transcending:** Accepting the cultural stereotypes of how a person with a disability should act severely limits life options and choices related to vocation, social relationships, intimacy, and

412

recreation. Transcending, is the process of rising above these negative, stereotypical beliefs (Vash, 1978).

1. Expected outcomes of transcending:
   a. Coming to terms with the negative stereotypes and then developing strategies to overcome them.
   b. Learning not to "use the disability" to secure special favors or attention.
   c. Acquiring techniques for handling strangers and for developing relationships where the disability will cease to be a crucial factor.

2. Conditions for transcending:
   a. Persons with disabilities will face new challenges and barriers, which require transcending throughout life.
   b. Peer counselors can promote transcending behaviors.
   c. Staff attitudes and beliefs are readily transmitted to both the patient and the family. Rehabilitation staff who take a more optimistic approach are in a better position to help the newly injured SCI individual to transcend (Phillips, Ozer, Axelson, & Chizeck, 1987).
   d. A rehabilitation program that focuses on control, challenge, and commitment (Pollack, 1987) fosters "hardiness" and ability to withstand societal prejudices and physical barriers present in the community.
   e. Flexible treatment programs, capable of emphasizing the uniqueness of each individual, are needed.

3. Process for Transcending:
   a. Begin the transcending process for both the patient and the family during the initial rehabilitation program so that preconceived notions about what is proper for someone with a disability does not limit goals and life plans.
   b. Humanize hospital routines and environment.
   c. Socialize staff to reject the negative cultural stereotypes about persons with disabilities.
   d. Make dependency invisible. Dependency is one aspect of SCI that is difficult to accept. Experienced SCI nurses can make dependency invisible through subtle efforts to distract patients while efficiently completing necessary procedures. On the other hand, new or unskilled staff become so task-oriented that they exaggerate dependency. When dependency is magnified, patients respond with embarrassment, hostility, detachment, or apathy.

C. **Toughening** is the process of physically and emotionally preparing the individual for community re-entry.

1. Expected outcomes of toughening:
   a. Physical: Increasing endurance and independence in activities of daily living (ADLs), and learning to manage architectural barriers.
   b. Social: learning to put people at ease, managing unwanted assistance, asserting oneself, venturing out in public, and managing accessibility problems at movies and restaurants.
   c. Psychological: learning to live with the disability and what it means in terms of life dreams and ambitions.
   d. Material: learning to survive the changes in income, and costs of supplies and caregivers. Toughening also includes how to survive with as few adaptive devices as possible and to be creative in inventing ways to make oneself more independent.

2. Conditions for toughening:
   a. Experienced, well-trained staff.
   b. Continuity of staff.
   c. High visibility of patient-staff interactions.
   d. Unit philosophy that pushes self-care.
   e. High level of activity and work on goals.

3. Process for toughening:
   a. Begin when the patient is able to get out of bed and independently move about unit. Start slowly, with subtle teasing and coaxing; strategies may vary based on the extent of disability and how long the patient has been injured.
   b. Strategies for toughening include:

      (1) Critical feedback on behavior
      (2) Use of humor, teasing
      (3) Fostering hard work and competition
      (4) Praise
      (5) Exposure to outside world
      (6) Discharge is the ultimate toughening strategy.

  c. Peer counselors are most skilled at toughening those with a new SCI diagnosis. Critical feedback on behavior is provided to minimize conflict between individuals with SCI and family members or the staff. Criticism can be buffered through appropriate use of humor.

  d. Not all rehabilitation team members toughen patients at the same time. While nursing staff may be toughening by insisting that the person do his/her own bowel and bladder care, the social worker may be buffering the same individual in relation to family stressors brought on by the SCI. Individuals may use this discrepancy to play one staff member against another saying one is supportive and kind, while another is demanding and insistent.

D. **Launching:** Vulnerability is defined as the susceptibility to destruction and defeat (Henry, 1975). Our society fosters vulnerability by playing on fears of economic insecurity, and fears of outsiders. The function of vulnerability is to promote dependency and exaggerate the image of those who could harm us or protect us. One of the goals of launching is for individuals to say, "I may be stronger than I think" as opposed to "I am afraid" (Henry, 1975). Launching is the process of exposing rehabilitation patients to the real world, exploring the range of options for living in the community, promoting patient autonomy and decision making, and facilitating the discharge of the patient from the rehabilitation program.

1. Expected outcomes of launching:
  a. Launching can be described in terms of readiness:
      (1) Appropriate launching occurs when the patient, family, and staff are in agreement about the timing of the discharge.
      (2) Delayed launching is typically the result of one or more individuals who have conflicting goals for discharge.
      (3) The staff may initiate premature launching if the patient refuses to participate in the rehabilitation program.
  b. The individual is socialized to believe that successfully rehabilitated individuals can manage most situations outside the hospital with effective planning, foresight, and a good sense of humor.
  c. Other expected outcomes of the launching process include adapting a realistic appraisal of the injury, maintaining hope while effectively functioning day-to-day, and planning for accessible housing, vocation, social relationships, leisure activities, and family reintegration.

2. Conditions for launching:
  a. A staff who communicate in a timely and effective manner.
  b. A program that fosters patient autonomy, promotes goal-setting behaviors, and provides markers for measuring success.
  c. A unit environment that is linked to the real world.

3. Process for launching:
  a. Exposing persons in rehabilitation to the real world, allowing them to make mistakes, confronting fears, and discharging them even though they have not achieved every goal. Beginning with the first therapeutic pass, patients start getting glimpses of what life will be like after discharge.
  b. Exploring the range of options for living in the community and providing anticipatory guidance.
  c. Promoting individual autonomy and decision making.
  d. Facilitating the discharge of the patient from the rehabilitation program.

IX. Process of Rehabilitation (Nelson, 1990)

A. **Selecting the Appropriate Approach:** The process of rehabilitation encompasses all four nursing approaches. The challenge rehabilitation staff must accept is to learn when to protect and buffer the patient and when to be tough and unwavering. Individuals progress through the buffering, transcending, toughening, and launching phases at different speeds. Davis (1980) explored various organizational, interactional, and care-oriented conditions for patient participation and continuity of care on a rehabilitation unit. These conditions included positive staff-patient interaction, high visibility of staff, explicit unit philosophy, explicit staff expectations for patients, and effective and informal communication among staff.

B. **Socializing New Staff in Rehabilitation:** Much of what experienced staff members do to enhance rehabilitation outcomes is intuitive and difficult to articulate to newer staff members. When new staff are being oriented, they may observe the physical tasks being performed but fail to see, or perhaps misinterpret, the very powerful informal interactions taking place. Timing is the critical determinant as to whether a staff member is buffering or promoting dependency when intervening with a patient. It is difficult, if not impossible, for staff to help individuals transcend negative cultural stereotypes, if they themselves harbor negative attitudes about persons with disabilities. Frequently, newer staff perceive toughening behaviors as mean, hostile, uncaring, and unprofessional.

C. **Dimensions of Rehabilitation:** There are four dimensions of reintegration: physical, social, emotional, and material.
1. The physical dimension includes safety, comfort, and health. For example, wheelchair mobility and strategies to manage physical barriers are taught.
2. The social dimension includes efforts to decrease isolation and enhance the support system.
3. The emotional dimension involves efforts to allay anxiety and fears, demonstrate caring, and assign value to the patient as a unique individual.
4. The material dimension deals with financial issues as well as efforts to provide necessary adaptive equipment and supplies to facilitate independence.

D. **Extent of Rehabilitation Services:**
1. A special report from the World Health Organization (WHO) succinctly states the problem of predicting which individuals will benefit from rehabilitation: Since rehabilitation can be costly, the development of improved criteria for selecting patients for intensive rehabilitation is of the utmost importance (WHO, 1980). Such selection should be based on classification according to the prognosis of recovery of function(s):
   a. Individuals who spontaneously make good recovery without rehabilitation
   b. Individuals who can make satisfactory recovery only through intensive rehabilitation;
   c. Individuals with little likelihood of significant recovery of function, irrespective of type of rehabilitation.
2. Operationally, rehabilitation encompasses a broad array of biomedical, social, educational, and vocational interventions that can be provided in a variety of institutional and community settings. Services are often provided by an interdisciplinary team, in which the specific participation will depend on the patient's physical, cognitive, and emotional disabilities and the availability of rehabilitation resources in the community.

E. **Trajectory of Rehabilitation Services:** Rehabilitation has a definitive beginning and end. However, securing ongoing services may be necessary to sustain the goals of rehabilitation, e.g., prevention of secondary complications; remediation, or treatment to reduce neurological deficits; compensation to offset and adapt to residual disabilities; and maintenance of function and health promotion throughout the life span.

References and Selected Bibliography

Albrecht, G. (Ed). (1976). *The sociology of physical disability and rehabilitation.* Pittsburgh, PA: University of Pittsburgh Press.

Albrecht, G., & Higgins, P. (1978). Rehabilitation success: The interrelationships of multiple criteria. *Journal of Health and Social Behavior, 18*(1), 36-45.

Alderfer, C., & Smith, K. (1982). Studying intergroup relations embedded in organizations. *Administrative Science Quarterly, 27,* 35-65.

Anthony, W. (1977). Societal rehabilitation: Changing society's attitudes toward the physically and mentally disabled. In J. Stubbins (Ed.), *Social and psychological aspects of disability* (pp. 269-278). Baltimore, MD: University Park Press.

Asch, A. (1984). The experience of disability. *American Psychologist, 39*(5), 529-536.

Barker, R. (1948). The social psychology of physical disability. *Journal of Social Issues, 4*(4), 28-39.

Bartol, G. (1978). Psychological needs of a spinal cord injured person. *Journal of Neurosurgical Nursing, 10*(4), 171-175.

Bedbrook, G., & Sedgley, G. (1980). The management of spinal cord injuries - past and present. *International Rehabilitation Medicine, 2*(2), 45-61.

Belgrave, F. (1984). The effectiveness of strategies for increasing social interaction with a physically disabled person. *Journal of Applied Social Psychology, 14*(2), 147-161.

Belgrave, F., & Mills, J. (1981). Effect upon desire for social interaction with a physically disabled person of mentioning the disability in different contexts. *Journal of Applied Social Psychology, 11*(1), 44-57.

Bell, A. (1962). Attitudes of selected rehabilitation workers and other hospital employees toward the physically disabled. *Psychological Reports, 10,* 183-186.

Berkowitz, E. (1984). Professionals as providers: Some thoughts on disability and ideology. *Rehabilitation Psychology, 29*(4), 211-216.

Betz, R., & Mulcahey, M.J. (Eds.). (1994). *The child with a spinal cord injury.* Rosemont, IL: American Academy of Orthopaedic Surgeons.

Bleiberg, J., & Merbitz, C. (1983). Learning goals during initial rehabilitation hospitalization. *Archives of Physical Medicine and Rehabilitation, 64*(10), 448-450.

Bodehnamer, E. (1983). Staff and patient perceptions of the psychosocial concerns of spinal cord injured persons. *American Journal of Physical Medicine, 62*(4), 182-193.

Bracken, M., & Bernstein, M. (1980). Adaptation to and coping with disability one year after spinal cord injury: An epidemiological study. *Social Psychiatry, 15*(1), 33-41.

Bracken, M., & Shepard, M. (1980). Coping and adaptation following acute spinal cord injury: A theoretical analysis. *Paraplegia, 18*(2), 74-85.

Brodsky C., & Platt, R. (1978). *The rehabilitation environment.* Lexington, MA: Lexington Books.

Brown, D., Judd, F., & Ungar, G. (1987). Continuing care of the spinal cord injured. *Paraplegia, 25*(3), 296-300.

Buckholdt, D., & Gubrium, J. (1980). The underlife of behavior modification. *American Journal of Orthopsychiatry, 50*(2), 279-290.

Cirillo, S., & Sorrentino, A. (1986). Handicap and rehabilitation: Two types of information upsetting family organization. *Family Process, 24*(2), 283-292.

Cleveland, M. (1980). Family adaptation to traumatic spinal cord injury: Response to crisis. *Family Relations, 29*(4), 558-565.

Cloerkes, G. (1981). Are prejudices against disabled persons determined by personality characteristics? *International Journal of Rehabilitation Research, 4*(1), 35-46.

Cogswell, B. (1967). Rehabilitation of the paraplegic: Processes of socialization. *Sociological Inquiry, 37*, 11-26.

Cogswell, B. (1968a). Self-socialization: Readjustment of paraplegics in the community. *Journal of Rehabilitation, 34*(3), 11-35.

Cogswell, B. (1968b). Some structural properties influencing socialization. *Administrative Science Quarterly, 13*(3), 417-440.

Cogswell, B. (1977). Self-socialization: Readjustment of paraplegics in the community. In J. Stubbins (Ed.), *Social and psychological aspects of disability* (pp. 123-130). Baltimore: University Park Press.

Cohn, N. (1961). Understanding the process of adjustment to disability. *Journal of Rehabilitation, 27*(6), 16-18.

Comer, R., & Piliavin, J. (1972). The effects of physical deviance upon face-to-face interaction: The other side. *Journal of Personality and Social Psychology, 23*(1), 33-39.

Comer, R., & Piliavin, J. (1975). As others see us: Attitudes of physically handicapped and normals toward own and other groups. *Rehabilitation Literature, 36*(7), 206-225.

Conomy, J. (1973). Disorders of body image after spinal cord injury. *Neurology, 23*(8), 842-850.

Cook, D. (1982). Dimensions and correlates of postservice adjustment to spinal cord injury: A longitudinal inquiry. *International Journal of Rehabilitative Research, 5*(3), 373-375.

Cook, D. (1983). Postservice adjustment of former rehabilitation center clients: A longitudinal analysis. *Rehabilitation Literature, 44*(7-8), 194-200.

Corbin, J., & Strauss, A. (1988). *Unending work and care: Managing chronic illness at home*. San Francisco, CA: Jossey-Bass.

Davis, M. (1980). The organizational, interactional and care-oriented conditions for patient participation in continuity of care: A framework for staff intervention. *Social Science Medicine, 14A*(1), 39-47.

DeJong, G., Branch, L., & Corcoran, P. (1984). Independent living outcomes in spinal cord injury: Multivariate analysis. *Archives of Physical Medicine and Rehabilitation, 65*(2), 66-73.

Diamond, M., Weiss, A., & Grynbaum, B. (1968). The unmotivated patient. *Archives of Physical Medicine and Rehabilitation, 49*(5), 281-284.

Diehl, L. (1989). Client and family learning in the rehabilitation setting. *Nursing Clinics of North America, 24*(1), 257-64.

Dinardo, Q. (1971). *Psychological adjustment to spinal cord injury.* Unpublished doctoral dissertation, University of Houston.

Dunn, M. (1975). Psychological intervention in a spinal cord injury center: An introduction. *Rehabilitation Psychology, 22*(4), 165-178.

Dunn, M. (1977). Social discomfort in the patient with spinal cord injury. *Archives of Physical Medicine and Rehabilitation, 58*(6), 257-260.

Dunn, M. (1982). *Social relationships and interpersonal skills: A guide for people with sensory and physical limitations.* Richmond, VA: Institute for Information Studies.

Dunn, M. (1983). *The rehabilitation situations inventory: An instrument to assess discomfort in rehabilitation staff.* Unpublished manuscript.

Edwards, P. (1992). The evolution of rehabilitation facilities for children. *Rehabilitation Nursing, 17*(4), 191-2

English, R. (1977). Correlates of stigma towards physically disabled persons. In J. Stubbins (Ed.), *Social and psychological aspects of disability.* (pp. 207-224). Baltimore: University Park Press.

Ford, M. (1981). *Nurse professionals and the caring process.* Unpublished doctoral dissertation. University of Northern Colorado.

Fordyce, W. (1978). Behavioral methods for engaging the spinal cord injured patient in the rehabilitation process. In M.G. Eisenberg & J.A. Falconer (Eds.), *Treatment of the spinal cord injured: An interdisciplinary perspective* (pp. 82-100). Springfield, IL: Charles C. Thomas.

Forsyth, G., Delaney, K., & Gresham, M. (1984). Vying for a winning position: Management style of the chronically ill. *Research in Nursing and Health, 7*(3), 181-188.

Frank, R., & Elliott, J. (1987). Life stress and psychological adjustment following spinal cord injury. *Archives of Physical Medicine and Rehabilitation, 68*(6), 344-347.

French, D., McDowell, R., & Keith, R. (1972). Participant observation as a patient in a rehabilitation hospital. *Rehabilitation Psychology, 19*(2), 89-95.

Friedman-Campbell, M., & Hart, C. (1984). Theoretical strategies and nursing interventions to promote psychosocial adaptation to spinal cord injuries and disability. *Neuroscience Nursing, 16*(6), 335-342.

Gellman, W. (1977). Roots of prejudice against the handicapped. In J. Stubbins (Ed.), *Social and psychological aspects of disability* (pp. 173-174). Baltimore: University Park Press.

Glasser, P., & Glasser, L. (1970). Illness and disability. In P. Glasser & L. Glasser (Eds.), *Families in crises* (pp. 216-360). New York: Harper & Row.

Graham, P. (1985). Bridge building: Linking a spinal cord injury unit to a skilled nursing facility. *Rehabilitation Nursing,10*(5), 22-27.

Gray, R., Kesler, J., & Newman, W. (1964). Social factors influencing the decision of severely disabled older persons to participate in a rehabilitation program. *Rehabilitation Literature, 25*(6), 162-167.

Grayson, M. (1951). Concept of "acceptance" in physical rehabilitation. *Journal of the American Medical Association, 145*(12), 893-96.

Gritzer, G., & Arluke, A. (1985). *The making of rehabilitation: A political economy of medical specialization, 1890-1980*. Los Angeles: University of California Press.

Gubrium, J., & Buckholdt, D. (1982). *Describing care: Image and practice in rehabilitation*. Cambridge, MA: Oelgeschlager, Gunn & Hain.

Halstead, L., Rintala, D., Kanellos, M., Griffin, B., Higgins, L., Rheinecker, S., Whiteside, W., & Healy, J. (1986). The innovative rehabilitation team: An experiment in team building. *Archives of Physical Medicine and Rehabilitation, 67*(6), 357-361.

Hamric, A. (1981). A teaching tool for spinal cord injured patients. *Journal of Neurosurgical Nursing, 13*(5), 234-238.

Hastorf, A. (1979). Acknowledgment of handicap as a tactic in social interaction. *Journal of Personality and Social Psychology, 37*(10), 1790-1797.

Henry, D. (1975). *Nurse behaviors perceived by patients as indicators of caring*. Unpublished doctoral dissertation, Washington, DC: Catholic University of America.

Hoeman, S. (Ed.). (1996). *Rehabilitation Nursing: Process and Application*. St. Louis, MO: Mosby.

Kaiser, S., Wingate, S., Freeman C., & Chandler, J. (1987). Acceptance of physical disability and attitudes towards personal appearance. *Rehabilitation Psychology, 32*(1), 51-58.

Kalb, M. (1971). *An examination of the relationship between hospital ward behaviors and post-discharge behaviors in spinal cord injury patients*. Unpublished doctoral dissertation, University of Houston, TX.

Katz, A. (1977). Self-help in rehabilitation: Some theoretical aspects. In J. Stubbins (Ed.), *Social and psychological aspects of disability* (pp. 181-186). Baltimore: University Park Press.

Katz, I., Farber, J., Glass, D., Lucido, D., & Emswiller, T. (1978). When courtesy offends: Effects of positive and negative behavior by the physically disabled on altruism and anger in normals. *Journal of Personality, 46*(3), 506-518.

Katz, S., & Shurka, E. (1977). The influence of contextual variables on evaluation of the physically disabled by the nondisabled. *Rehabilitation Literature, 38*(11-12), 369-373.

Kazak, A. (1986). Families with physically handicapped children: Social ecology and family systems. *Family Process, 25*(2), 265-281.

Keane, S., Chastain, B., & Rudisill, K. (1987). Caring: Nurse-patient perceptions. *Rehabilitation Nursing, 12*(4), 182-184.

Keith, R. (1988). Observations in the rehabilitation hospital: Twenty years of research. *Archives of Physical Medicine and Rehabilitation, 69*(8), 625-631.

Keller, M., Ward, S., & Baumann, L. (1989). Processes of self-care: Monitoring sensations and symptoms. *Advances In Nursing Science, 12*(1), 54-66.

Kelman, H., & Wilner, A. (1962). Problems in measurement and evaluation of rehabilitation. *Archives of Physical Medicine and Rehabilitation, 43*(1), 174-80.

Kennedy, P., Fisher, K., & Pearson, E. (1988). Ecological evaluation of a rehabilitative environment for spinal cord injured people: Behavioral mapping and feedback. *British Journal of Clinical Psychology, 27*(Pt 3), 239-246.

Kerr, J. (1985). Space use, privacy, and territoriality. *Western Journal of Nursing Research, 7*(2), 199-219.

Kerr, K. (1977). Understanding the process of adjustment to disability. In J. Stubbins (Ed.), *Social and psychological aspects of disability* (pp. 317-324). Baltimore: University Park Press.

Kerr, N. (1970). Staff expectations for disabled persons: Helpful or harmful. *Rehabilitation Counseling Bulletin*, 85-94.

Kerr, N. (1977). Staff expectations for disabled persons: Helpful or harmful. In J. Stubbins (Ed.), *Social and psychological aspects of disability* (pp. 47-54). Baltimore: University Park Press.

Kerr, W., & Thompson, M. (1972). Acceptance of disability of sudden onset paraplegia. *Paraplegia, 10*(1), 94-102.

Klas, L. (1970). *A study of the relationship between depression and factors in the rehabilitation process of the hospitalized spinal cord injured patient*. Unpublished doctoral dissertation, University of Utah.

Kowalsky, E. (1985). The nurse's role in health maintenance of the physically disabled client. *Rehabilitation Nursing, 10*(1), 9-14.

Lawson, N. (1976). *Depression after spinal cord injury: A multimeasure longitudinal study*. Unpublished doctoral dissertation, Houston, TX: University of Houston.

Lawson, N. (1978). Significant events in the rehabilitation process: The spinal cord patient's point of view. *Archives of Physical Medicine and Rehabilitation, 59*(12), 573-579.

Leviton, G. (1970). Professional-client relations in a rehabilitation hospital setting. In W.S. Neff (Ed.), *Rehabilitation Psychology* (pp. 215-247). Washington, DC: American Psychological Association.

Ludwig, E., & Adams, S. (1977). Patient cooperation in a rehabilitation center: Assumption of the client role. In J. Stubbins (Ed.), *Social and psychological aspects of disability* (pp. 225-236). Baltimore: University Park Press.

MacDonald, M., Nielson, W., & Cameron, M. (1987). Depression and activity patterns of spinal cord injured persons living in the community. *Archives of Physical Medicine and Rehabilitation, 68*(6), 339-343.

Mailick, M. (1979). The impact of severe illness on the individual and family: An overview. *Social Work in Health Care, 5*(2), 117-128.

Malec, J., & Neimeyer, R. (1983). Psychological prediction of duration of inpatient spinal cord injury rehabilitation and performance of self-care. *Archives of Physical Medicine and Rehabilitation, 64*(8), 359-363.

Matthews, P., & Carlson, C. (Eds.). (1987). *Spinal cord injury: A guide to rehabilitation nursing*. Rockville, MD: Aspen Publications.

Mayers, A., Feltin, M., Master, R., Dicastro, D., Cupples, A., Lederman, R., & Branch, L. (1985). Rehospitalization and spinal cord injury: Cross-sectional survey of adults living independently. *Archives of Physical Medicine and Rehabilitation, 66*,(10), 704-708.

Miller, R., & Keith, R. (1973). Behavioral mapping in a rehabilitation hospital. *Rehabilitation Psychology, 20*(4), 148-155.

Nelson, A. (1987). Normalization: The key to integrating the spinal cord injured patient into the community. *SCI Nursing, 4*(1), 3-6.

Nelson, A. (1990). Patients' perspectives of a spinal cord injury unit. *SCI Nursing, 7*(3), 44-64.

Nelson, A. (1992). A model for nursing practice in SCI rehabilitation. In C. Zejdlik (Ed.), *Management of spinal cord injury*. (2nd Ed., pp. 213-227.) Boston: Jones & Bartlett.

Norris-Baker, C., Stephens, M., Rintala, D., & Willems, E. (1981). Patient behavior as a predictor of outcomes in spinal cord injury. *Archives of Physical Medicine and Rehabilitation, 62*(12), 602-608.

Phillips, L., Ozer, M., Axelson, P., & Chizeck, H. (1987). *Spinal cord injury: A guide for patient and family*. New York: Raven Press.

Pollack, N. (1987). Adaptation to chronic illness: Analysis of nursing research. *Nursing Clinics of North America 22* (3), 631-643.

Ray, C., & West, J. (1984). Coping with spinal cord injury. *Parpalegia, 22*(4), 249-259.

Richards, J. (1986). Psychologic adjustment to spinal cord injury during first postdischarge year. *Archives of Physical Medicine and Rehabilitation, 67*(6), 362-365.

Richardson, C., & Robinson, S. (1989). Neonatal intensive care and pediatric rehabilitation: a joint program for care of chronically ill infants. *Journal of Perinatology, 9*(1), 52-5.

Rintala, D., & Willems, E. (1987). Behavioral and demographic predictors of postdischarge outcomes in spinal cord injury. *Archives of Physical Medicine and Rehabilitation, 68*(6), 357-362.

Rintala, D., Willems, E., & Halstead, L. (1986). Spinal cord injury: The relationship between time out of bed and significant events. *Rehabilitation Nursing, 11*(3), 15-18.

Safilios-Rothschild, C. (1970). *The sociology and psychology of disability and rehabilitation*. New York: Random House.

Safilios-Rothschild, C. (1977). Prejudice against the disabled and some means to combat it. In J. Stubbins (Ed.), *Social and psychological aspects of disability* (pp. 261-268). Baltimore: University Park Press.

Sawyer, H., & Baker, R. (1978). The development of personal, social and community adjustment programs: A legitimate mandate for rehabilitation professionals. *Journal of Rehabilitation, 44*(1), 35-38.

Schlesinger, L. (1977). Staff authority and patient participation in rehabilitation. In J. Stubbins (Ed.), *Social and psychological aspects of disability* (pp. 167-172). Baltimore: University Park Press.

Selekman, J. (1991). Pediatric rehabilitation: from concepts to practice. *Pediatric Nursing, 17*(1), 11-4.

Shapiro, L., & McMahon, A. (1966). Rehabilitation stalemate: problems in patient-staff interaction. *Archives of General Psychiatry, 15*(2), 173-177.

Trieschmann, R. (1980). *Spinal cord injuries: Psychological, social, and vocational adjustment*. New York: Pergamon Press.

Tucker, S. (1980). The psychology of spinal cord injury: Patient-staff interaction. *Rehabilitation Literature, 41*(5-6), 114-160.

Vash, C. (1978). Disability as transcendental experience: A personal perspective on learning to live with a disability. In M. Eisenberg & J. Falconer (Eds.), *Treatment of the spinal cord injured - An interdisciplinary perspective* (pp. 101-111). Springfield, IL: Charles C. Thomas.

Willems, E., & Alexander, J. (1982). Behavioral indicators of client progress after spinal cord injury: In T. Millon, C. Green, & R. Meagher, (Eds.), *Handbook of Clinical Health and Psychology*, (pp. 401 - 416). New York: Plenum Press.

Woodrich, F., & Patterson, J. (1983). Variables related to acceptance of disability in persons with spinal cord injuries. *Journal of Rehabilitation, 49*(3), 26-30.

World Health Organization (WHO). (1980). International classification of impairments, disabilities, and handicaps. Geneva, Switzerland: Author.

Yuker, H. (1988). *Attitudes toward persons with disabilities*. New York: Springer

Zahn, M. (1973). Incapacity, impotence and invisible impairment: Their effects upon interpersonal relations. *Journal of Health and Social Behavior, 14*(2), 115-123.

Zejdlik, C. (Ed) (1992). *Management of spinal cord injury.*(2nd Ed.) Boston: Jones & Bartlett.

Zola, I. (1982a). *Missing pieces: A chronicle of living with a disability*. Philadelphia: Temple University Press.

Zola, I. (1982b). *Ordinary lives: Voices of disability and disease*. Cambridge, MA: Apple-wood Books.

Zola, I. (1982c). Social and cultural incentives to independent living. *Archives of Physical Medicine and Rehabilitation, 63*(8), 394-397.

CHAPTER

Caregivers: Training and Support

Fina Canave-Jimenez, M. Ed, RN

I. Learning Objectives

A. Explain the importance of caregiver training and support in spinal cord impairment (SCI) nursing practice.

B. Describe the major theories and concepts of learning that are most influential in caregiver training.

C. Differentiate the three domains of learning.

D. Identify key characteristics of adult learners.

E. Explain the teaching/learning process and its application to training caregivers.

F. Identify teaching strategies for each type of learning and its characteristics.

G. Describe the different approaches to learning needs assessment.

H. Identify guidelines for planning, implementing, and evaluating caregiver training.

I. Identify nursing interventions for providing caregiver support.

II. Introduction

A. **Scope:** Nurses have long recognized how important teaching is for individuals, families, and caregivers. Successful training of caregivers significantly contributes to the rehabilitation process. Teaching and learning processes require great skills under the best circumstances, but they take on new demands and require expanded competencies in health care. Competent nurses have learned to communicate and teach in varying situations; they are forced to use themselves, their attitudes, tone of voice, humor, skill, and a variety of approaches (Benner, 1984). This chapter describes critical components of caregiver training and support in SCI. The significance of this responsibility requires nurses to understand the nature of learning and its three domains: cognitive, affective, and psychomotor, as well as theories and concepts related to learning. Included are guidelines to assist nurses in the training and support of caregivers.

B. **Background:** The impact of SCI is devastating for the individual and family. Promoting adaptation and adjustment to changes brought about by SCI requires learning new competencies (skills, knowledge, and attitudes). Caregiver training and support are integral to the achievement of successful adaptation and adjustment for many reasons.

1. Medical and technological advances have now made a normal life span possible for persons with disabilities. This will give rise to a greater demand for training and support of caregivers (Gender, 1993).
2. Nursing standards frequently have included teaching as a major function of nursing.
3. The need for training of health care providers has been brought to the forefront by the Joint Commission on Accreditation of Health Care Organizations (JCAHO, 1993). The standards emphasize that caregivers must be competent.
4. In 1995, the Commission on Accreditation of Rehabilitation Facilities (CARF) stressed the need for an education plan, identifying content and method for teaching, and criteria for measuring learning.
5. The University of Iowa Nursing Interventions Classification (NIC) Project has identified teaching as one of 38 core interventions of nurses (Iowa Intervention Project Research Team, 1996; Iowa College of Nursing, 1996).
6. Of all professional disciplines involved in the care of rehabilitation clients, nursing had the highest proportion of chart entries focusing on teaching/learning activities (Mumma, 1987).
7. Most families know little about SCI until the moment they learn their family member's diagnosis. From that point on, education of the family is an integral part of the treatment program and care plan (Anderson, 1994).
8. Caregiver training is a key element of health care reform increasing in significance as the length of hospital stays continues to decrease. The average length of stay for patients in freestanding hospitals and rehabilitation centers in 1978 was 52.2; days in 1990, it was 29.1 days (McCourt, 1993). More efficient and effective ways of teaching patients, families, and other caregivers will become necessary.
9. Average annual costs for attendant care are the highest expense incurred by persons with SCI during the first year post-injury (Stover, Delisa, & Whiteneck, 1995).

III. Definitions

A. **Learning:** acquisition of knowledge and information resulting in change of behavior.

B. **Teaching:** system of activities that includes a plan of action designed to produce learning.

C. **Teaching/learning process:** dynamic interaction between the teacher and the learner.

D. **Training:** instructing in a particular skill.

E. **Competency:** ability to integrate and apply the knowledge, skills, and behaviors required for actual performance in a designated role and setting.

F. **Competency-based training:** educational approach that emphasizes a learner's ability to demonstrate the knowledge, skills, and attitudes that are of central importance to a given task, activity, or job.

G. **Caregiver:** person other than a health care professional who provides care or assistance to an individual with SCI. This may include attendants or family members.

H. **Continuum of care:** health care services in acute, rehabilitation, and community reintegration phases. Training is an integral part of these services.

IV. Domains of Learning

Bloom (1969) has identified three domains of learning: cognitive, affective, and psychomotor. Each domain has specific behavior components arranged in levels of mastery. The teacher provides the means for this process to take place. For example, learning the proper technique for application of an external urinary catheter requires that the learner observes the demonstration (cognitive domain), practice the skill (psychomotor domain), repeat the demonstration (psychomotor domain), and appreciate the impact of urinary incontinence to an individual with SCI (affective domain).

A. **Cognitive Domain:**
   1. The cognitive domain includes intellectual skills such as thinking, knowing, and understanding. It is divided into a hierarchical classification of behaviors known as taxonomy. Learners master each behavior in order of complexity. For example, mastery for a caregiver includes having adequate judgement to notify the nurse of any significant changes or observations based on a client-specific baseline. Table 30-1 describes these levels of mastery and Table 30-2 illustrates the critical role that the domains of learning play in client outcomes.

Table 30-1: Cognitive Domain: Levels of Mastery

Level	Description	Example
Knowledge	Recalling facts, methods, procedures	Caregiver is able to list symptoms of autonomic dysreflexia (AD)
Comprehension	Combining recall and understanding; to grasp the meaning of the information	Caregiver describes relationship of urinary retention to AD
Application	Using information in new, specific, and concrete situation	Caregiver describes client's bladder programand specifies methods for prevention of urinary retention
Analysis	Distinguishing between parts of information and understanding relationship among them	Caregiver is able to determine factors causing AD
Synthesis	Putting the parts of information together in a unified whole	When AD occurs, caregiver can describe precipitating factors and measures to handle such a situation
Evaluation	Judging the value of ideas, procedures, and methods by using appropriate criteria	Caregiver can judge how effectively and quickly removal of cause (e.g. urine blockage) relieves symptoms of AD.

Adapted from *Community Health Nursing Process and Practice for Promoting Health* (p.193), by M. Stanhope and J. Lancaster, 1992, St. Louis: Mosby Year Book. Reprinted with permission.

Table 30-2: Outcome Concept System (OCS) Functional Categories For Client Outcomes Measurement

Health Status	Patient's physiological condition
Skill function	Ability of the patient or caregiver to perform tasks and activities necessary to restore or maintain health
Knowledge function	Evaluates what the patient or caregiver needs to know to safely manage care within the limits of their ability.
Psychosocial function	Ability to cope with the demands imposed by the healthcare problems

Adapted from "Outcome data analysis: Putting results to practice," by J. Herzog and M. Schoen, 1997, p. 24, in C. Adams and A. Anthony (Eds.), *Home Health Outcomes and Resource Utilization: Integrating Today's Critical Priorities,* New York: National League for Nursing: Jones & Bartlett Publishers, Sudbury, MA.

    2. Implications for teaching/learning
       a. Assess the learner's cognitive abilities.
       b. Tailor teaching to learner's level of understanding.
       c. Use teaching strategies including lecture, demonstration, and use of audiovisual resources and printed materials.

B. **Affective Domain**
    1. The affective domain emphasizes feelings, emotions, values, attitudes, and appreciations.
    2. Implications for teaching/learning
       a. Listen carefully to identify cues to feelings of learners that would influence learning.
       b. Recognize that values, attitudes, and beliefs are difficult to change.
       c. Use teaching strategies including participative learning, values clarification, and use of case scenarios.

C. **Psychomotor Domain**
    1. The psychomotor domain includes the performance of skills. This requires manual dexterity, coordination, and opportunities to practice the skill.
    2. Implications for teaching/learning
       a. Facilitate learning by skill demonstration.
       b. Allow the learner to practice skill.
       c. Provide immediate feedback on any errors in performing the skill.
       d. Use teaching strategies including demonstrations, return demonstrations, and simulation exercises.

V. Theories of Learning

Fundamental to every professional discipline is the ability to develop and refine a body of knowledge that can be applied to its practice (Huckabay, 1991; Torres, 1990). This body of knowledge is expressed in terms of concepts and theories. SCI nurses should be skillful in applying learning theories as they teach caregivers. Many principles related to teaching and learning have evolved from these theories. Each theory has a specific focus and applications.

A. **Purpose.** The application of learning theories in SCI nursing practice serves several purposes:
    1. Provide a framework for the teaching/learning process.
    2. Assess and guide the development of teaching plans and strategies.
    3. Explain the dynamics of the teaching and learning transactions.
    4. Establish training objectives based on assessed learning needs.
    5. Predict and evaluate training outcomes.

B. **Conditioning Theories**
1. Behavioral (stimulus-response) theorists focus on behaviors that can be observed and measured.
2. Learning is a series of stimulus-response connections, which may be strengthened or weakened.
3. Conditioning aims to change or reinforce behavior.
4. The environment enhances learning.
5. Approaches for teaching/learning situations include:
   a. Positive reinforcers to promote learning, (e.g. recognition, tangible rewards, additional responsibilities)
   b. Systematic approach with stimulus situations planned to achieve specific responses (outcomes)
   c. Maximal participative learning through active involvement of learners.
   d. Repetition and feedback for skill mastery and retention
   e. Use of teaching strategies such as computer-assisted instruction, games, or problem-based learning

C. **Cognitive View of Learning**
1. Theorists focus on the cognitive processes in learning, which involve not only understanding of facts but also the relationships among them.
2. Cognition or thinking is an active and interactive process with the environment and with readiness to learn.
3. Learning is facilitated when it has meaning.
4. Approaches for teaching/learning situations include:
   a. Systematic (i.e., from simple to complex, and from concrete to abstract.)
   b. Searching for key ideas that can be used to organize bodies of information.
   c. Teaching strategies such as creative thinking, problem-solving techniques, and multi-modal approach. Memorizing lists of information is of little value.

D. **Humanistic View of Learning**
1. Theorists emphasize that learners are basically self-determining and capable of identifying their own needs.
2. Learner's emotions and feelings are acknowledged in the teaching/learning process.
3. Each learner is treated as a unique individual with personality variables (temperament types) that may influence learning.
4. Approaches for teaching/learning situations include:
   a. Emphasis on learner-centered approach to training.
   b. Facilitation of learning through partnership of learner and educator whereby educators provide resources and support, while learners assume responsibility for learning.
   c. Consideration of learning styles and personality variables that may influence learning.
   d. Use of teaching strategies such as learning contracts and self-directed learning.

E. **Other Theories**
1. Knowles (1987) Concepts of Adult Learning: Education can be explained as a set of assumptions that adults:
   a. Have a need to know why they should learn something.
   b. Have a deep need to be self-directed.
   c. Have a greater volume and different quality of experience than youth.
   d. Become ready to learn when they experience in their life situations a need to know.
   e. Enter into a learning experience with a task-centered, problem-centered, or life-centered orientation to learning.
   f. Are motivated to learn by both extrinsic and intrinsic motivators.
2. Benner's (1984) Concepts of Levels of Practice include: novice, advanced beginner, competent, proficient, and expert. These different levels reflect changes in general aspects of skilled performance. A caregiver who is new to the activity is, likely to focus initially, more on tasks, rules, and skills that are components of a process (e.g., physical care) than on the

activity itself (e.g., providing psychosocial care.) However, caregivers need opportunities to learn what is meaningful for care of the individual with SCI and how a task or skill relates to a broader goal. As skills develop, learners change their intellectual orientation, increase their knowledge, and refocus their decision-making processes based on perceptual awareness rather than on process-oriented foundations. Teaching/learning strategies are tailored to each level of competency.

3. Brookfield's Concepts of Critical Thinking: Brookfield (1987, 1993) advocates methods of encouraging learners to identify and challenge assumptions, to explore alternative ways of thinking and acting, and to set priorities. These skills are needed to develop knowledge that is comprehensive, regularly updated, and flexibly applied. For caregivers who choose to work with individuals with SCI, these skills are crucial to facilitate provision of assistance within the process and context of care. Teaching strategies include use of media, case studies, role-playing, discussions, brainstorming, games, and simulations. Interaction with individuals with SCI and their families must be an integral part of training.

4. Competency-Based Training (CBT): CBT is an educational approach popularized by Del Bueno, Weeks, & Brown-Stewart (1987) that emphasizes the learner's ability to demonstrate the proficiencies (knowledge, skills, and attitudes) that are of central importance to a designated role and setting. Fundamental to this approach is the identification of competency standards (Abruzzese, 1992; Bard, Jimenez, & Tomack, 1994; Carnevale, Gainer, & Meltzer, 1990; Del Bueno et al., 1987;). The critical elements of the competency-based approach include:
   a. A clear definition of knowledge and skills
   b. Emphasis on end results (performance of tasks)
   c. A focus on the learner's ability to demonstrate the proficiencies that are of central importance to a given task
   d. Acquisition of knowledge as demonstrated in its application to performance of skill
   e. Integration of prior learning or experience
   f. Standards for successful achievement of skills that are clearly stated and measured
   g. Maintenance and monitoring of competencies

VI. Principles Related to Teaching and Learning Process

Caregivers vary in experiences, learning needs, and competencies. SCI nurses must be knowledgeable about these differences in order to choose appropriate instructional content and teaching methods. In addition, nurses must understand those factors that facilitate or inhibit learning.

A. **Learner's Characteristics**
   There are four major characteristics of the learner that are important for SCI nurses to consider in teaching/learning situations (Duffy, 1997; Knowles 1987; Stanhope & Lancaster, 1992;).
   1. Self-concept
      a. Adult learners are self-directed, doers rather than passive receivers of information, and they make their own decisions.
      b. Effective teaching emphasizes participation in learning and provision of educational resources rather than directing learning activities.
   2. Experience
      a. Adult learners' past experiences, level of education and previous knowledge affect learning.
      b. Teachers must acknowledge and value the learner's past experiences and provide experiential learning activities that capture their competencies.
   3. Motivation and readiness to learn
      a. Readiness to learn and motivation are prerequisites to learning. In Knowles' (1980) view, learners become ready to learn when they experience a "need to know" "need to perform" more effectively.
      b. Teachers can best facilitate learning by involving learners in assessing their own needs and in planning how to meet those needs. Use of learning needs tools, (e.g., competency

rating scale or a pretest) are recommended.

4. Individual differences
   a. Learners vary in learning style, perception, culture, and language—all of which affect learning. Perception is influenced by values, age, past experiences, education, and sociocultural factors. Teachers need to be culturally competent by acknowledging and integrating the beliefs, practices, and values of cultural groups into the training plan. In particular, diets and health attitudes vary considerably. Learners from diverse backgrounds and life experiences provide a rich, and thereby useful, context for learning.
   b. Individual learning style refers to the way the learner receives and processes information in learning situations. There are three types of learners each of whom benefit most from a specific type of learning activity (McCourt, 1993):
      (1) Visual learners learn best by seeing or reading printed and audiovisual materials, including journal writing.
      (2) Auditory learners learn best by listening to mini-lectures, group and panel discussions, brainstorming, case studies, and dialogue.
      (3) Tactile or psychomotor learners learn best by doing skills demonstrations, role-playing, simulation games, and clinical experiences.
   c. Teachers should be aware of individual differences, which can influence teaching/learning situations and outcomes.

B. **Trainer's Competencies:** SCI nurses frequently train families/caregivers who provide direct care in various settings. The ability to provide care does not always translate into the ability to train others to provide care. Therefore, competency guidelines for trainers are critical. The following competencies for trainers are recommended:
   1. Demonstrates commitment to the care of individuals with SCI.
   2. Possesses extensive experience in caring for individuals with SCI.
   3. Communicates effectively.
   4. Demonstrates competence in problem solving concerning care issues for individuals with SCI.
   5. Demonstrates knowledge of the teaching/learning process.
   6. Individualizes methods and style of training to maximize skills and knowledge of the trainee.
   7. Responds appropriately to questions posed during the training sessions.
   8. Creates a supportive and nonthreatening learning environment.
   9. Uses evaluation methods based on defined, measurable, and observable training outcomes.
   10. Documents trainee's performance at defined intervals during training and follow-up period.

VII. Learning Needs Assessment

A. **Purpose:** Assessment of the learner's needs is the first step in the design of educational activities. The emphasis is on the knowledge, skills, and attitudes that learners must have to perform an expected and defined standard. Primarily, needs assessment serves to seek information regarding (Rosetti, 1989):
   1. Optimal performance or knowledge.
   2. Actual or current performance or knowledge.
   3. Perceptions about the task or competence related to a need.

B. **Needs Assessment Strategies:** The process of conducting a learning needs assessment involves the use of various data collection methods, choosing those most reliable and suited to the learner's characteristics. Training activities are targeted toward those identified competencies that are performed often and have the following characteristics: complex, high-risk, problem-prone, and high-cost. Caregivers of individuals with SCI require sufficient knowledge and skills to perform safely in specific situations and to use technical/electronic equipment or devices proficiently. Among the most commonly used learning needs assessment strategies are questionnaires, checklists/inventories, interviews, direct observation, and focus groups.

1. Questionnaire items focus on assessing the difference between actual and optimal performance. Rosetti (1989) suggests it is important to find out:
   a. How well the learner can perform a specific competency.
   b. How important it is that the learner perform that competency.
   c. How often the learner is called on to perform the competency.
2. Checklists /Competency Inventories provide readily available data that indicate learning needs such as:
   a. Identifying skills, knowledge, and attitudes
   b. Identifying topics for learning
   c. Prioritizing aspects of care that are most important
3. Interviews provide an opportunity for learners to share in-depth views of the training content or areas of particular concern.
4. Observation focuses on an individual's needs through direct observation of work performance. Standards are used to determine the adequacy of performance.
5. Focus groups are designed to provide more comprehensive information on a specific topic and can provide an informal but targeted discussion about what experienced caregivers and learners define as needs.

VIII. Planning and Implementation

A. **Expected Outcomes:** The training program for family/caregivers of the individual with SCI includes the following expected outcomes:
1. Demonstration of knowledge and skills that family/caregiver needs in order to assist the individual with SCI to return home and resume life as fully as possible. The family/caregiver is able to:
   a. Describe client's needs, developmental age, level, type and etiology of injury/disorder, associated injuries, potential problems/complications, and SCI related conditions, (e.g., spasticity, autonomic dysreflexia, pain, cardiovascular and thermoregulatory dysfunction, sexuality needs, and life long effects.)
   b. Describe individual's basic health and maintenance requirements related to SCI. The description should include knowledge of structure and function of the health system and requirements for follow up.
   c. Demonstrate 100 percent competency in the performance of health care procedures related to the day-to-day care of the individual with SCI (e.g., personal care, bowel/bladder, respiratory and skin care, mobility/transfers, medications, types of equipment/devices, range of motion, nutrition, and handling spasticity).
   d. Demonstrate knowledge of technology commonly used with individuals with SCI (e.g., wheelchairs, lifts, orthoses, pressure-reducing devices, respiratory treatments/assistive devices, tracheostomy care and management, environmental control units).
   e. Use a guideline to review the individual's baseline health status, including self-care abilities, respiratory status, and degree of independent breathing, as appropriate.
   f. Describe warning signs and symptoms and precautions specific to SCI, such as health care procedures, abnormal physiological responses, and equipment failure.
   g. Demonstrate ability to troubleshoot, recognize problems, and initiate and carry out emergency procedures in cases of equipment malfunction and/or abnormal physiological responses of the individual with SCI.
   h. Demonstrate knowledge of concepts on health promotion, community reintegration, family-centered care, and individual care planning.
   i. Demonstrate competencies related to communication, collaboration, accessing resources, and documentation.
   j. Respond appropriately to "what if" questions posed during training.

B. **Key Concepts**
1. The primary goal of training caregivers is to assess, maintain, and develop the caregiver's competence to meet the expectations and standards of performance in a given role, setting, and level of practice (e.g., novice vs. skilled). Caregivers can function in skilled nursing facilities, residential facilities, care agencies, and private homes.

2. The training program includes components to ensure that caregivers have had the opportunity to gain the knowledge and skill necessary to perform and to practice newly developed skills

3. The range of requisite knowledge and skills of caregivers will determine the content of the training program. It is essential to differentiate the "must know" from the "nice to know." The training content should be broken into in learning modules.

4. Training caregivers should reflect a commitment to provide care within a nursing practice framework.

5. Training is best accomplished when it is interactive and involves active participation of learners. Health care professionals are facilitators and enablers of learning.

6. Training recognizes the value of partnerships with patients/families and caregivers during the teaching/learning process.

7. Training should utilize a variety of methods including appropriate pacing suited to the learners, to the content to be learned, and to the teacher. (Refer to Table 30-3 for a sample of an interactive game-based education tool.)

Table 30-3: Team Jeopardy!®* Sample Questions

Categories	Questions and Responses
Physical Well-Being	A: The process of examining skin twice a day for possible problems.
	Q: What are skin checks?
Self-Care	A: Do not use these substances to clean latex leg bags as they will corrode the bag.
	Q: What is vinegar and bleach?
Community Living	A: Provincial organization that provides services to members with SCI.
	Q: Who is the British Columbia Paraplegia Association?
Social and Emotional Adjustment	A: Feelings such as intense sadness, frustration, and anger.
	Q: What are common feelings after SCI?
Grab Bag	Questions selected here could be from any of the above categories.

Adapted from Team Jeopardy!® Learning about living with spinal cord injury. (June 1999) by C. Heenan, *SCI Nursing, 16* (2), p. 59. Reprinted with permission.

* Jeopardy!® is a registered trademark of Sony Pictures Entertainment, Inc.

8. Training outcomes will be specified as demonstrable, measurable, and observable behavior, (e.g., increase in knowledge, performance of skill, or change in attitudes.) These involve both knowing and doing. A statement such as "understands the caregiver's role in client's bladder program" is neither observable nor measurable. A statement such as "follows protocol for clean intermittent catheterization" meets both of these attributes. These clearly defined competency standards, integrated with each care procedure, provide the criteria by which the learner's performance is evaluated and monitored. For example:

a. Knowledge: Explains importance of adhering to client-specific bladder program.

b. Skill: Demonstrates client-specific catheterization techniques, which help ensure that all urine is drained from bladder.

c. Attitude: Appreciates the significance of maintenance of urinary continence in client's quality of life.

9. The evaluation and documentation of competence are critical to ensure that the caregiver has sufficient knowledge and skill to carry out the assigned responsibilities for safe and effective care.

10. Support for caregivers is based on the belief that the best training tools are good role models and preceptors.

C. **The Teaching Plan:** The basic components of the teaching plan are (Gatens, Herbert, Dischene, Gleason, & Hays, 1993; Hanak, 1991; Zejdlik, 1992):

1. Learning objectives will be specified as measurable behaviors based on the skills, tasks, and competencies that the family/caregiver must perform within a specific time frame.

2. Subject content must be individualized to achieve learning objectives and reflect priorities and long-term learning needs.

3. Teaching methods and tools should be tailored to the learner, the subject content, and the teacher. Organize learning experiences in a systematic way.

4. Evaluation will be a shared process by which the teacher and the family/caregiver can determine whether learning goals have been achieved.

D. **Implementation:** The intent in the implementation of family/caregiver training program is that the defined training outcomes will be achieved. Resources and circumstances unique to each situation or setting will influence how the outcomes are achieved and how teaching/learning processes are selected and applied. The following guidelines for implementation are based on concepts critical to the care of individuals with SCI, assumptions on the nature of SCI care, and where and how it is delivered; and assumptions regarding learning, what it involves, and how it is supported and evaluated.

1. Ensure that theory and practice are inextricably linked through classroom and hands-on practice in client-specific situations. Be aware of how content will be applied in client's home environment, routines, and lifestyle. What the caregiver learns in the hospital setting is invalid if it cannot be adapted to the home environment.

2. Facilitate caregiver's active participation in care activities to foster learning and commitment to the activity. Include out-trips or weekend passes, in which caregivers accompany the client on trips outside the health facility as part of the training program.

3. Provide opportunities for caregivers to work with more experienced caregivers/nurses as preceptors who can help them with competency development and serve as role models. Preceptors should be selected for their commitment to teaching caregivers and expert level of knowledge and skills in caring for individuals with SCI.

4. Provide information in an organized, carefully paced manner to facilitate learning based on learner's abilities.

5. Encourage client and family to participate in the teaching/learning process.

6. Individualize the teaching to the particular social, emotional, cultural, and training needs of each family/caregiver.

7. Provide information in a supportive and sensitive manner, realizing that the stress of SCI may be disruptive to the usual learning process. Be aware of the barriers and factors influencing learning.

8. Inform family/caregivers about available SCI training resources such as, *Yes, You Can! A Guide to Self-Care for Persons with SCI* (Hammond, Umlauf, Matteson, & Perduta-Fulginiti, 1989), and the American Spinal Cord Injury Nurses (AASCIN) or Educational Guide for Spinal Cord Injury Nurses: *A Manual for Teaching Patients, Families and Caregivers* (Hanak, 1991). A free service cataloging all SCI audiovisual materials is available through Texas Institute for Rehabilitation and Research in Houston, TX. Helpful websites include:

   http://www.pva.org
   http://www.aascin.org
   http://www.nmss.org/eduprog.html
   http://www.rehabnurse.org/index.htm
   http://www.nim.nih.gov/pubs/resources.html
   http://www.vard.org
   http://www.paralysis.org

9. Organize the training program based on the principles of continuity, sequence, and integration.
   a. Continuity involves placing repeated emphasis on particular components of the educational experience.
   b. Sequence means that each learning experience builds on the previous one.
   c. Integration of the various components of the teaching plan shows how each aspect fits into the big picture.
10. Consider learner's educational level, literacy, and fluency with English in teaching and in selection of learning materials.

E. **Training During Continuum of Care:** The content of a family/caregiver training program relates to the phases of care from acute care and rehabilitation to community reintegration. Training is central to this continuum of care.
   1. Although education actually begins during the acute phase, most of the hands-on training takes place during rehabilitation. During this phase, education may play a critical role in reducing anxiety, alleviating misconceptions, and fostering a sense of control among family members. They need to be informed observers. The rationale for focusing on education during the acute phase is to:
      a. Increase knowledge and understanding of the effects of SCI on physical, vocational, social, and psychological functioning.
      b. Increase the participation of family members in the individual's rehabilitation program and decrease feelings of isolation, hopelessness, and anxiety.
      c. Maintain or reestablish communication channels among family members and enhance mutual support in emotionally dealing with disability.
      d. Direct the family toward planning for an independent future (Zejdlik, 1992).
   2. During the rehabilitation phase, the teaching is designed so that training and support are provided and expected outcomes are achieved in a timely fashion. In this context, rehabilitation is viewed as a learning process that involves active participation of the individual, family, and caregivers. The content of family/caregiver training programs typically includes topics listed in Tables 30-4, 30-5, and 30-6.
   3. During community reintegration, all efforts of care, training, and support are increasingly important in helping individuals with SCI and their families to maintain health, manage the effects of disability, and reintegrate into community life. Interventions to promote training and support of caregivers in the community include:
      a. Providing in-service education
      b. Consulting one-on-one with care providers regarding ways to manage health care needs, and promoting access to health care services
      c. Encouraging family/caregiver involvement early in the rehabilitation process regarding equipment, care procedures, medications, and emergency management
      d. Coordinating a home visit by the rehabilitation team to evaluate the need for home modifications and equipment, and ways to improve safety
      e. Providing information on community resources and linking families with SCI groups, such as the National SCI Association, for ongoing information and peer support
      f. Providing written materials for future reference
      g. Promoting interagency communication regarding ongoing rehabilitation and learning needs
      h. Providing current information on resources, equipment, and technological advances as they become available (Buchanan, 1993; Zejdlik, 1992)

F. **Teaching Family Members as Caregivers**
   1. Zejdlik (1992) described family health education as any information or knowledge, skills, and attitudes needed to understand and manage the effects of the disability and maintain health.
   2. Gatens, Herbert, Duchene, Gleason, & Hays, (1993) and Anderson (1994) make the following recommendations in teaching family members:
      a. Establish family's readiness to learn.
      b. Select family member who spends the most time with the patient.

Table 30-4: Content of Sample Family/Caregivers Education Program

A. General Overview of SCI and Related Care
1. Anatomy and physiology of the spinal cord
2. Spinal cord injury
3. Skin management
4. Bladder management
5. Bowel management
6. Autonomic dysreflexia
7. Sexuality
8. Nutrition
9. Medications
10. Warning signs of impending problems
11. Resources

B. Treatments and Equipment
1. Types of physical and occupational therapy needed
2. Training
3. Equipment needed and resources

C. School and vocational information
1. Educational laws, rights, advocacy, and resources
2. School reentry information
3. Specific grade-related information
   a. Early intervention
   b. Preschool
   c. Elementary/high school
   d. College
4. Vocational/career services and training

D. Transportation and accessibility
1. Resources
2. Rights
3. Advocacy

E. Social, recreational, and community issues
1. Mainstreamed versus adapted activities
2. Resources

F. Psychosocial issues
1. Adjustment to trauma from a family perspective
   a. Parents/marriage
   b. Siblings
   c. Grandparents, relatives, and friends
2. Parenting a child with a disability
   a Fostering independence
   b. Advocating
   c. Promoting self-esteem and confidence
   d. Sexuality
3. Obtaining support
   a. Individual and family counseling
   b. Community support
   c. Support groups
   d. Respite care

Adapted from Family Education, by C. Anderson, 1994, in R.R. Betz & M.J. Mulcahey (Eds.), *The Child with a Spinal Cord Injury.* (p.584), Rosemont, IL: American Academy of Orthopedic Surgeons. Reprinted with permission.

Table 30-5: Spinal Cord Injury Education Workshop

You will learn...
- General management of a person with spinal cord injury at the SCI center and at home
- Some of the problems associated with spinal cord injury
- About community and home supports available to you
- Ideas for leisure activities
- About considerations for return to work or further education
- About coping with change and stress

The Program...
- What is spinal cord injury?
- Effects and research
- Physical and emotional needs: how do we address them?
- Managing the physical effects of SCI and mobility
- Self-care, home management, and home modifications
- Coping with disability and dealing with behavior changes
- Community reintegration: community resources, home supports, leisure and vocational planning, sexual rehabilitation

The Format...
- Short educational sessions presented by members of the spinal cord program team
- Questions, group discussion, sharing and problem solving with other families
- Family members are encouraged to follow their family member through his or her individual program following the workshop
- Opportunities are provided to discuss and practice specific procedures/methods for assisting/caring for family member during individual therapy sessions.

Adapted from *Spinal Cord Injury Program*, by G.F. Strong Rehabilitation Centre, 1996, Vancouver. Author. Reprinted with permission.

Table 30-6: Caregiver Training Program: Care of Ventilator-Dependent Individuals

Unit 1:
General overview of SCI (high quadriplegia) and care
Related anatomical structures and functions
Client-centered care
Personal care
Transfers/mobility/wheelchair
Nutrition
Bladder and bowel care
Infection control

Unit 2:
Client-specific respiratory care
Tracheostomy care and management
Suctioning (clean technique)
Bronchial hygiene techniques
Portable ventilators/circuitry

Unit 3:
Equipment/devices care and management
Disinfection/sterilization
Maintenance and care
Humidifiers, portable suction machines, resuscitator bag, speaking valves
Power wheelchairs
Environmental control units
Other client-specific technical aids

Unit 4:
Management of emergencies
Airway patency
Respiratory emergencies
Ventilator malfunction/failure
Other clinical problems (e.g., autonomic dysreflexia)
Emergency preparedness

Adapted from Attendant Training Manual: Care of the Ventilator-Dependent Quadriplegic Individual in the Community, by George Pearson Center, 1995, Vancouver: Author. Reprinted with permission.

    c. Teach one, at most two, persons. This reduces misunderstandings of several members about what should be done and makes for a more time-effective teaching schedule.

    d. Choose content and appropriate method of teaching based on needs. Patient and family workshops are recommended, particularly when families must travel long distances (Nelson & Kelley, 1983).

    e. Focus on potential problems and what actions to take, (e.g., when to call the physician, sources of help, telephone numbers).

    f. Consider various social, cultural, and educational backgrounds in planning content and teaching methods.

    g. Document what was taught, by whom, and to whom. Include resources used and response to teaching. Provide feedback mechanism in which family members discuss their understanding of information and/or demonstrate caregiving skills.

    h. Engage the cooperation of parents/family members/peers with the training as soon as possible. Support groups for families with similar diagnoses can be helpful to provide opportunities to learn from and support each other (Nelson, Tilbor, Frieden, & Smith, 1994).

G. **Skills Training for Caregivers**

    1. Steps for skills demonstration: When designing a training program in which performance of psychomotor skills is the expected outcome, focus on the "what", "why", and "how" of the skill. Miller (1992) suggests the following steps:

        a. Focus on the task at hand and why it is to be learned.

        b. Demonstrate the task from start to finish without interruption.

        c. Demonstrate each step in the skill again with an explanation and pause for questions and clarification.

        d. Repeat the demonstration as a "master" or "model".

        e. Immediately assign learners to a practice period with simulation models, if available.

        f. Supervise and assist learners through the practice session.

        g. Allow each learner to perform a return demonstration.

    2. Tools and resources: The keys to well-planned skills training sessions include:

        a. Adequate space

        b. Appropriate facilities

        c. Simulation aids

        d. Equipment and supplies

        e. Tools such as performance checklists

        f. Adequate number of trainers to supervise and check off learners as they acquire the skill

IX. Promoting Training and Support of Caregivers

A. **Caregiver Support.** Caregiver support refers to the provision of the necessary information, advocacy, and support to facilitate patient care (McCloskey & Bulechek, 1992).

B. **Nursing Interventions**

    1. Determine caregiver's level of knowledge.

    2. Determine caregiver's acceptance of role.

    3. Accept expressions of negative emotion.

    4. Explore with the caregiver his/her strengths and weaknesses.

    5. Encourage caregiver to assume responsibility as appropriate.

    6. Provide information about client's condition in accordance with client's preferences.

    7. Teach caregiver the client's therapy in accordance with client's preferences.

    8. Provide for follow-up caregiver assistance through phone calls and/or community nursing care.

    9. Monitor for indicators of stress. Include activities that help family members /caregivers identify potential sources of stress, mobilize strengths, and find resources.

   10. Teach caregiver stress management techniques.

   11. Educate caregiver about the rehabilitation process.

12. Support caregiver through rehabilitation process.
13. Teach caregiver health care maintenance strategies to sustain own physical and mental health.
14. Inform caregiver of health care and community resources.
15. Teach caregiver strategies to access and maximize health care and community resources.
16. Provide respite care as needed.

X. Evaluation of Teaching

A learner's achievement of competencies can be evaluated in a variety of ways during and at the end of the training program. Specific competency measures should be identified and developed. Clark and DiFilippo (1994) recommend the following methods of measuring competence:

A. **Cognitive domain:** a learner's knowledge in this area can be demonstrated through paper-and-pencil testing, pre-and post-tests, and individual dialogue with teacher.

B. **Affective domain:** a learner's acquisition and identification of values can be measured through discussions with teacher. Affective competency also can be evaluated by observational data, (e.g., avoidance behaviors.)

C. **Psychomotor domain:** a learner's abilities to perform certain functions and/or activities can be observed by the teacher in simulated or actual clinical situations. Use of performance checklist will be helpful.

Practical Application

M.J., a 27-year-old single male, was admitted for rehabilitation after acute hospitalization for C5-C6 fracture with a complete spinal cord lesion as a result of a fall from a porch. He uses a power wheelchair with hand controls, and requires assistance with personal care, transfers, and bowel and bladder management. Before this accident, M.J. worked for eight years in construction. He was being prepared for discharge four months after his injury.

The primary nurse at the rehabilitation unit had been working with M.J. in planning for his needs upon discharge. M.J. was looking forward to going home to an apartment that was wheelchair accessible and had an environmental control unit. During M.J.'s care conference it was noted that he planned to hire personal care attendants (PCAs) to provide assistance with many of his daily routines: bowel/bladder care, bathing, dressing, grooming, and transfers. These caregivers needed to learn skills in these areas prior to his discharge.

Planning for the caregivers' training program began during rehabilitation. Assessments of M.J.'s educational needs as well as caregiver's roles and needs, were done. The primary nurse arranged a goal conference with M.J. and the rehabilitation team to determine training goals, plan, teaching content, methods, and appropriate time frames. To monitor the progress of the caregivers' training program, a checklist was developed with the dates of actual teaching and the target dates for specific knowledge or skills to be mastered. Regular feedback mechanisms were included to monitor progress and outcomes. Consultations with the caregivers were held to assess their confidence in managing every aspect of M.J.'s care. A discharge conference with M.J. and the team was arranged to review the training goals and their completion. Prior to discharge, a weekend pass provided a "trial run." In the months and years following discharge from the rehabilitation program, training needs were reassessed and updated.

References and Selected Bibliography

Abruzzese, R.S. (1992) *Nursing staff development strategies for success* (pp.30-43). St. Louis, MO: Mosby Year Book.

Anderson, C. (1994). Family education. In R. R. Betz & M.J. Mulcahey (Eds.), *The child with a spinal cord injury* (p. 584). Rosemont, IL: American Academy of Orthopedic Surgeons.

Bard, J., Jimenez, F.C., & Tornack, R. (1994). *Integration with school setting. Outcome based health support program* (p.56). Vancouver, CAN: British Columbia Rehabilitation Society.

Benner, P. (1984). From novice to expert. Menlo Park, NJ: Addison-Wesley.

Bloom, B. (1969). *Taxonomy of educational objectives*. New York: David McKay.

Brookfield, S. (1987). *Developing critical thinkers*. San Franscisco: Jossey-Bass.

Brookfield, S.D. (1993). On impostorship, cultural suicide, and other dangers: How nurses learn critical thinking. *Journal of Continuing Education in Nursing, 24*(5), 197-205.

Buchanan, L.C. (1993). Life skills and community living. In A. E. McCourt (Ed.), *The specialty practice of rehabilitation nursing: A core curriculum* (3rd. ed.,p. 218). Skokie, IL: Rehabilitation Nursing Foundation of the Association of Rehabilitation Nurses.

Clark B., & DiFilippo, J. (1994). *Basic competencies for rehabilitation nursing practice* Skokie, IL: Rehabilitation Nursing Foundation of the Association of Rehabilitation Nurses.

Commission on Accreditation of Rehabilitation Facilities (CARF). (1995). *Standards manual for organizations serving people with disabilities*. Tucson, AZ: Author.

Del Bueno, D., Weeks, L., & Brown-Stewart, P. (1987). Clinical assessment centers: A cost effective alternative for competency development. *Nursing Economics, 5*(1), 21-26.

Duffy, B. (1997). Using a creative teaching process with adult patients. *Home Health Care Nurse, 15*(2), 102-108.

G.F. Strong Rehabilitation Centre. (1996). *Spinal cord injury program*. Vancouver, CAN: Author.

Gatens, C., Herbert, R., Duchene, P., Gleason, C., & Hays, S. (1993). Cognitive - Perceptual pattern. In A. E. McCourt (Ed.), *The specialty practice of rehabilitation nursing: A core curriculum* (3rd ed.). Skokie, IL: Rehabilitation Nursing Foundation of the Association of Rehabilitation Nurses.

Gender A. (1993). Future challenges for the specialty practice of rehabilitation nursing. In A.E. McCourt (Ed.), *The specialty practice of rehabilitation nursing: A core curriculum* (3rd. ed. p.239). Skokie, IL: Rehabilitation Nursing Foundation of the American Rehabilitation Nurses.

George Pearson Centre. (1995). *Attendant training manual: Care of the ventilator-dependent quadriplegic individual in the community*. Vancouver, CAN: Author.

Hammond, M.C., Umlauf, R.L., Matteson, B., & Perduta-Fulginiti. (Eds.) (1989). *Yes, you can: A guide to self-care for persons with spinal cord injury*. Washington, DC: Paralyzed Veterans of America.

Hanak, M. (Ed.). (1991). *Educational guide for spinal cord injury nurses: A manual for teaching patients, families and caregivers*. Jackson Heights, NY: American Association of Spinal Cord Injury Nurses.

Heenan, C. (1999). Team Jeopardy! Learning about living with spinal cord injury. *SCI Nursing, 16*(2), 59.

Herzog, J., & Schoen, M. (1997). Outcome data analysis: Putting results to practice. In C. Adams & A. Anthony, (Eds.). *Home health outcomes and resource utilization: Integrating today's critical priorities* (p. 24). New York: National League for Nursing.

Huckabay, L. (1991). The role of conceptual frameworks in nursing practice, administration, education & research. *Nursing Administration Quarterly, 15*(3), 17-28.

Iowa Intervention Project Research Team. (1996). Core interventions by specialty nursing intervention classification (NIC). Iowa City, IA: University of Iowa College of Nursing.

Johnson, K. (Ed.). *(1994)Spinal cord injury: Educational content for professional nursing practice* (2nd ed.). Jackson Heights, NY: American Association of Spinal Cord Injury Nurses.

Joint Commission for Accreditation of Healthcare Organizations (p.419) (JCAHO). (1993). *1994 Accreditation standards manual for hospitals* (Vol. I., p. 54). Oakbrook Terrace: Author.

Knowles, M.S. (1980) *The modern practice of adult education: Andragogy versus pedagogy* (2nd ed.). Chicago: Follett.

Knowles, M.S. (1987). Adult learning. In R.L. Craig, (Ed.) *Training and development handbook* (3rd ed.). New York: McGraw Hill.

Kozier, B., & Erb, G. (1987). *Fundamentals of nursing concepts and procedures* (3rd. ed. p. 615). Reading: Addison-Wesley.

McCloskey, J.C., & Bulechk, G. (1992). Iowa intervention project. *Nursing Interventions Classification* (NIC), 161, 492-494.

McCourt, A.E. (Ed.). (1993). *The specialty practice of rehabilitation nursing: A core curriculum* (3rd ed.). Skokie, IL: Rehabilitation Nursing Foundation of the Association of Rehabilitation Nurses.

Miller, P.J. (1992). Planning programs: Strategies for success. In K. J. Kelly (Ed.), *Nursing staff development current competence, future focus* (pp. 122-123). Philadelphia: J.B. Lippincott.

Mumma, C. (1987). Rehabilitation nursing concepts and practice: A Core Curriculum (2nd. ed., p.53). Skokie, IL: Rehabilitation Nursing Foundation of the Association of Rehabilitation Nurses.

Nelson, A. L., & Kelley, B. (1983). Patient and family workshops: A new teaching approach for spinal cord injury. *Rehabilitation Nursing, 8*(6), 13-16.

Nelson, M.R., Tilbor, A., Frieden, L., & Smith, W.(1994). Introduction to pediatric rehabilitation. In R. R. Betz & M.J. Mulcahey (Eds.), *The child with a spinal cord injury* (p. 465). Rosemont, IL: American Academy of Orthopedic Surgeons.

Rosetti A. (1989). Assess for success. *Training, 26*(4), 55-59.

Stanhope, M., & Lancaster, J. (1992). *Community health nursing process and practice for promoting health* (p. 193). St. Louis, MO: Mosby Year Book.

Stover, S., DeLisa J., & Whiteneck, G. (1995). *Spinal cord injury clinical outcomes from the model systems* (pp. 246-247). Rockville, MD: Aspen.

University of Iowa College of Nursing, Iowa Intervention Project Research Team. (1996). *Core interventions by specialty.* (p. 47). Iowa City, IA. Author.

Zejdlik, C. (1992). *Management of spinal cord injury* (2nd ed., pp. 203-210, 661-679). Boston: Jones & Bartlett.

CHAPTER

Community Re-entry and Independent Living
Donna L. Stultz, MS, RN

I. Learning Objectives

A. Define community reintegration and independent living.

B. Describe examples of community reintegration programs and resources.

II. Introduction

A. **Scope:** One of the principal rehabilitation goals of the rehabilitation team is to help the individual with spinal cord impairment (SCI) look ahead to life after discharge from a rehabilitation program. The aim is to help the patient become as independent as possible and reenter the community. Nurses are involved in coordinating follow-up health care and support through rehabilitation programs in the community. These actions are critical and affect the success of community re-entry. This chapter provides nurses with an understanding of the role of community reintegration and independent living programs. It also provides information about how to find and develop resources to facilitate community re-entry and independent living.

B. **Overview**

1. Independent living is defined as the process of making decisions that affect one's own life, always within the context of the individual's circumstances. For people with severe limitations in mobility, for example, independent living may depend upon the availability of accessible public transportation. For an individual with functional deficits secondary to SCI, independent living may depend upon sufficient social supports in living arrangements, and occupational and social environments. Independent living may mean independence in the sense that a person lives alone with very few ancillary support services, or it may mean that one simply has control of his or her environment through assistance provided by support services and caregivers.

2. Community reintegration is defined as the process of adaptation into the community and achievement of the greatest possible degree of independence. It includes social integration, community participation, and utilization of community resources. Community reintegration programs are designed to assist individuals with disabilities in this process. For example, independent living programs are geared toward providing essential community support services, including peer counseling, information and referral, personal assistance services, housing, transportation, and other services as necessary.

3. Theoretically, every person with a disability is a candidate for community reintegration and independent living. People who have experienced traumatic disabilities are most likely to require structured community programs, since they have had few, if any, opportunities to acquire knowledge about living with a disability during the natural developmental process.

4. Within the rehabilitation process, it is important to educate the individual about several areas related to independent living. One of the major areas is community support services. Persons with SCI need to know what vocational rehabilitation services, public and private support services, and medical services are available. It is also important to identify advocacy organizations and social and recreational groups in their geographical area. Having individuals with disabilities who lead active, full lives visit with a person with a newly diagnosed SCI can also be a way to promote independent living. Finally, sharing consumer magazines (e.g., *Sports and Spokes*, *Paraplegia News*) and other literature that promotes a full, active life can be beneficial.

III. Assessment

Assessment of the needs of an individual with a disability may be appropriate at several stages during rehabilitation.

A. **Initial Rehabilitation:** Early in the inpatient comprehensive rehabilitation phase, the rehabilitation team may use diagnostic information to predict the individual's future as it relates to community reintegration and independent living. At this point, the assessment may lead to developing realistic options for the person following his or her discharge from the inpatient facility. This early assessment may be useful to assisting the individual and/or caregivers in making transition back into the community shortly prior to the discharge from the inpatient rehabilitation program.

B. **Community Rehabilitation:** Most organized community reintegration and independent living programs will provide an additional assessment prior to initiating services to the individual with a disability. These assessments are used to fashion an appropriate array of services to educate the individual in choosing among the available options. Thorough assessments must look at functional, as well as psychosocial, issues. Failure to do so could result in the inability to provide the individual with comprehensive feedback regarding abilities and resources for reintegrating into the community. Important information includes, but is not limited to: expenses, bills or insurance, community resources, housing, ability to provide for daily needs, and/or the availability of a caregiver, equipment, supplies, transportation, driving, recreation, employment, follow-up appointment(s), and plans for emergencies. The goal of the assessment is to provide needed information about options to the individual. This information can then be used by the individual to make decisions about the available resources in the home and community.

IV. Goals

A. **Similar to rehabilitation:** The goals of community reintegration and independent living mirror the goals of rehabilitation. Rehabilitation aims to facilitate optimal functional status and a quality of life consistent with unique functional abilities and desires.

B. **Formal and informal approaches:** These goals can be reached through either informal methods or organized, structured programs that facilitate community reintegration and independent living. For some individuals, the formal programs are necessary to ensure that the person has access to the kind of structured support necessary to reach the goals of independent living.

C. **Lack of Progress:** Finally, some individuals may either be unwilling to embrace the concept of independent living or, in some cases, are frustrated by a dearth of caregivers or other vital services, which may prevent them from achieving independent living.

V. Community Reintegration Programs and Resources

A. **Organized Programs:** Currently, the most common route to independent living and community reintegration for people with disabilities appears to be through organized programs. Such programs are widely available in larger communities throughout the nation, and to a lesser extent in some smaller communities or rural areas. Programs are typically sponsored and operated by agencies that recognize their responsibility to ensure that persons with disabilities have opportunities to live as independently as possible in the community, and have the opportunity to reintegrate into the community following the onset of SCI.

1. Government agencies: Some programs are sponsored and operated by federal agencies. The Department of Veterans Affairs is one such agency, and some of its resources are available to non-veterans as well. Another large federally funded program that provides support for independent living is the state/federal vocational rehabilitation program. State vocational agencies focus on developing employment opportunities for people with disabilities. However, they also sponsor independent living programs and may pay for some medical treatment, education, training, and a variety of other services for eligible persons.

2. Service organizations: Some programs are operated by chapters of national not-for-profit service agencies such as the National Easter Seal Society, Inc., and the United Cerebral Palsy Association. Other programs are operated by local organizations that provide inpatient rehabilitation services and seek to ensure an appropriate transition for individuals following discharge from inpatient hospitalization. Programs of this nature may offer counseling, training, or assistance in negotiating legal and administrative issues. They may also provide information about rehabilitation services and rights of the person with a SCI, referrals to programs and services, and independent living skills training.

3. Peer support groups: Local chapters of the Paralyzed Veterans of America (PVA) and National Spinal Cord Injury Association (NSCIA) may run support groups for people with spinal cord injuries. Peer support is one of the most important aspects of independent living. Other programs are sponsored by freestanding, community-based, not-for-profit human service organizations. Such programs manifest themselves frequently as centers for independent living. These centers are typically run by consumers with disabilities and provide services organized around a core service mix, which includes information and referral, independent living skills training, peer counseling, and advocacy.

B. **Other Resources**

1. Written materials: For communities with no independent living programs, there are written materials that can be obtained that address community living during the rehabilitation process. Both published and unpublished educational resources on SCI are available for use.

2. Nurses: Nurses knowledgeable about the local, state, and national programs and resources can provide an invaluable service to the patient undergoing rehabilitation. The nurse can often help the individual identify the appropriate agency or program, and provide the necessary information to contact the organization. Nurses might also work together with independent living specialists to make the patient's transition from the hospital to the community more satisfactory.

3. Community support services: Independent living, from a practical standpoint, is generally facilitated by an array of community support services. In most communities, public transportation will provide some mobility assistance to people with disabilities. Vocational rehabilitation agencies are widely available and capable of providing support necessary for people who choose to seek vocational goals. Some local agencies, such as home health agencies, provide personal assistance services. Housing assistance may be available to

individuals through local housing bureaus, congregate housing, or community home loan funds. Meals on Wheels may be an essential part of the independent living network for some individuals. Communities may have agencies that provide assistive animals or technology. Assistance such as reader services or sign language interpreter services may be available in the community for persons who have visual or hearing impairments.

C. **Self-Direction:**

The objective of a program should be to empower the individual with a sense of autonomy, personal self-confidence, and independence. Nurses should not underestimate their influence in helping individuals reintegrate into the community and live independently. However, everyone involved in the process of rehabilitation must realize that ultimately, the responsibility for independence and self-direction must rest with the person with a disability, and all efforts should be directed towards empowering the individual. In order to facilitate independence, caregivers, family members, support network participants, nurses, and other health care workers should make appropriate recommendations toward maximizing utilization of resources, both local and national.

Practical Application

S.T. is a 30-year-old male with a T1-T2 spinal cord injury, which occurred when a tree fell on him while he was jogging. He was admitted to a comprehensive rehabilitation hospital 10 days post-injury. He is the divorced father of two children, ages six and four. He shares custody of the children with his ex-wife. S.T. was extremely depressed upon admission to the rehabilitation hospital. He was accustomed to a physically active lifestyle. He did not believe he would be able to live a "useful, fun" life, since he would have to depend on others to meet his needs. He was also very worried about being able to take care of his children.

At admission, his nurse began looking ahead to discharge and preparing S.T. for a life of independence and full community integration by assessing important areas. S.T. owned his own home, was financially stable, had health insurance through a health maintenance organization, and had worked at the same company for six years. S.T. doubted whether he could return to the same job, since it entailed climbing to do electrical work. He had begun training for a triathlon when his injury occurred. He had never attended college and had no other skills. He had no major debts at the time of his injury. S.T. lived in the suburbs of a large metropolitan area, just outside the area covered by public transportation. His car was appropriate for adaptation.

The nurse shared this information with the treatment team, and the proper referrals were initiated. The social worker referred the patient to the state's rehabilitation commission, based on the nurse's report that S.T. had expressed an interest in getting more job retraining and possibly returning to school. The therapists ordered adaptive equipment needed for S.T.'s home. The nurse began discussing with S.T. the supplies he would need upon discharge. She kept a list, deleting things no longer needed as he made progress.

The nurse also contacted a representative from a local wheelchair sports organization. This person visited S.T. in the hospital and took him to see a wheelchair track and field event during an evening pass. S.T. signed up to train for long distance races before he left the hospital.

The day of discharge, the nurse and S.T. reviewed all the supplies ordered for him. She helped him make the follow-up appointment, and gave him written instructions for emergencies.

After discharge, S.T. wrote a thank-you note to the treatment team. He thanked everyone, but singled out his nurse. He said that without her attention to detail and her communication with the rest of the team about the things that he would need "to get on with his life," he wouldn't be where he was at that time. He said the biggest thing she did for him was give him hope; she made that first contact to an outside sports group that gave him reason to think his life was not over.

A year later, S.T. was attending the university on a scholarship sponsored by the state's rehabilitation commission. He had also created a part-time job for himself as trainer for wheelchair athletes.

References and Selected Bibliography

Baker, D. (1994). Independent living in communities: The role of the independence fund in Vermont. *American Rehabilitation, 20*(1), 39-41.

Chappell, J. A., Jr. (1994). The whole is greater than the sum of its parts. *American Rehabilitation, 20*(1), 23-29.

Clay, J.A. (1992). Native American independent living. *Rural Special Education Quarterly, 11*(1), 41-50.

Curl, R.M., Hall, S.M., Chisholm, L.A., & Rule, S. (1992). Co-workers as trainers for entry-level workers: A competitive employment model for individuals with disabilities. *Rural Special Education Quarterly, 11*(1), 31-35.

Daugherty, T., Daugherty, D., & Daugherty, J. (1994). The effects of insurance benefits coverage: Does it affect persons with spinal cord injury? *OSERS 6*(2), 19-22.

DeJong, G. (1981). *Environmental accessibility and independent living outcomes: Directions for disability policy and research.* East Lansing; MI: University Center for International Rehabilitation.

DeJong, G. (1983). Physical disability and public policy. *Scientific American, 248*(6), 40-49.

DeJong, G., & Hughes, J. (1981). Report of the Sturbridge Conference on independent living services. Boston: Tufts Medical Rehabilitation Research and Training Center.

The Disability Rag. A bi-monthly publication reflecting ideas and discussions in the disability rights movement. Available at $12 for a one-year subscription. Write to: Subscriptions, The Disability Rag, 1962 Roanoke Ave, Louisville, KY 40205 (502) 459-5343 (V/TTY/fax).

French, D. (1994). Independent living: Driven by principles of democracy. *OSERS, 6*(2), 37-38.

Giordiano, G., & D'Alonzo, B.J. (1994). The link between transition and independent living. *American Rehabilitation, 20*(1), 2-7.

Veterans Benefits Administration, *Handbook for design: Specially adapted housing*, 1978 VA Pamphlet 26-13, Washington DC: Author.

Kafka, B. (1994). Perspectives on personal assistance services. *OSERS, 6*(2), 11-13.

Kailes, J.I. (1993). *Disability pride: The interrelationship of self-worth, self-empowerment, & disability culture.* Houston, TX: ILRU Program.

Kailes, J.I., & Jones, D. (1993). *A guide to planning accessible meetings.* Houston, TX: ILRU Program.

Kennedy, J., Zukas, H., & Litvak, S. (1994). Independent living and personal assistance services: The research, training, and technical assistance programs at the world institute on disability. *OSERS, 6*(2), 43-45.

Lachat, M. A.. (1988a). *An evaluation and management information system for independent living.* Staying on track: ILRU Management Support Series. Houston, TX: ILRU Program.

Lachat, M. A.. (1988b). *The independent living service model: Historical roots, core elements, and current practice.* Hampton: Center for Resource Management.

Lachat, M.A. (1994). Using the power of management information system technology to support the goals of centers for independent living. *American Rehabilitation, 20*(1), 42-48.

Lougheed, V., Hunter, B., & Wilson, S. (1994). Partners for independence: A team approach to community-based rehabilitation. *American Rehabilitation, 20*(1), 37-38.

Maddox, S. (1994). *Spinal network* (2nd ed.). Malibu: Spinal Network and Miramar Communications.

Mathews, M. R. (1994). Learning from the experts: Best practices in rural independent living. *OSERS, 6*(2), 23-29.

McCourt, A.E. (Ed.). (1993). *The specialty practice of rehabilitation nursing - A core curriculum* (3rd ed.). Skokie, IL: Rehabilitation Nursing Foundation of the Association of Rehabilitation Nurses.

Michaels, R.E. (1994). Title VII: A major step forward. *OSERS, 6*(2), 8-10.

Montagano, T. (1994). Bringing the rehabilitation family together: An IL-VR partnership. *American Rehabilitation, 20*(1), 35-36.

Moore, J. E., & Stephens, B.C. (1994). Independent living services for older individuals who are blind: Issues and practices. *American Rehabilitation, 20*(1), 30-34.

National Council on the Handicapped (NCD). (February 1986). *Toward independence: An assessment of federal laws and programs affecting persons with disabilities - With legislative recommendations.* Washington, DC: Author.

National Council on the Handicapped (NCD). January 1988. *On the threshold of independence: A report to the president and the congress of the United States.* Washington, DC: Author.

Nelson, J. (1994). Changes in the Rehabilitation Act of 1973 and Federal Regulations. *OSERS, 6*(2), 4-8.

Nosek, M. (1992). The personal assistance dilemma for people with disabilities living in rural areas. *Rural Special Education Quarterly, 11*(1), 36-40.

Nosek, P., Narita, Y., Dart, Y., & Dart, J. (1982). *A philosophical foundation for the independent living and disability rights movement.* Occasional Paper No. 1. Houston, TX: ILRU Program.

Potter, C.G., Smith, Q.W., Quan, H., & Nosek, M.A. (1992). Delivering independent living services in rural communities: Options and alternatives. *Rural Special Education Quarterly 11*(1), 16-23.

Richards, L., & Smith, Q. (1992). Independent living centers in rural communities. *Rural Special Education Quarterly, 11*(1), 5-10.

Seekins, T., Revesloot, C., & Maffit, B. (1992). Extending the independent living center model to rural areas: Expanding services through state and local efforts. *Rural Special Education Quarterly, 11*(1), 11-15.

Shapiro, J.P. (1992). *No pity.* New York: Random House.

Smith, L.W., Smith, Q.W., Richards, L., Frieden, L., & King, K. (1994). Independent living centers: Moving into the 21st century. *American Rehabilitation, 20*(1), 14-22.

Smith, Q., Frieden, L., Richards, L., & Redd, L.G. (1994). Improving management effectiveness in independent living centers through research and training. *OSERS, 6*(2), 30-36.

Smith, Q., Smith, L.W., King, K., Frieden, L., & Richards, L. (1993). *Health care reform, independent living, and people with disabilities*. Houston, TX: ILRU Program.

Smith, Q. W., Fasser, C.E., Wallace, S., Richards, L.K., & Potter, C.G. (1992). Children with disabilities in rural areas: The critical role of the special education teacher in promoting independence. *Rural Special Education Quarterly, 11*(1), 24-30.

Smith, R., Smith, L., & Smith, Q. (1987). *An orientation to independent living centers*. Houston, TX: ILRU Program.

United States Department of Education. (1986). *Comprehensive evaluation of the Title VII, Part B of the Rehabilitation Act of 1973, as amended*. Centers for Independent Living Program. University of Kansas.

We Won't Go Away, videocassette. Sells for $20 each, including postage, from the World Institute on Disability, 510 16th Street, Suite 100, Oakland, CA 94612 (510) 763-4100 (V), 208-9493 (TTY).

Westbrook, J.D. (1994). Consumer-driven supported employment: Consolidating services for people with significant disabilities. *OSERS, 6*(2), 14-18.

Willig, C.L. (1988). *A people's history of independent living*. Research and Training Center on Independent Living: University of Kansas.

Zejdlik, C. (1992). *Management of spinal cord injury* (2nd ed.). Boston: Jones and Bartlett.

Ziegler, M. (1994). How parent networks are working with independent living centers. *OSERS, 6*(2), 39-42.

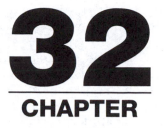

CHAPTER

Prevention and Management of Secondary Disability in Persons With Spinal Cord Injury

Sheila M. Sparks, DNSc, RN, CS

I. Learning Objectives

A. Describe measures to prevent secondary disabilities in individuals with spinal cord injury (SCI).

B. Discuss management of secondary disabilities.

II. Introduction

A. **Scope**

Secondary disabilities are "health complications that result in additional functional difficulties superimposed on the original functional losses that resulted from the spinal cord injury (SCI) itself" (Lanig, Chase, Butt, Hulse, & Johnson, 1996, p.8). These complications may affect persons with SCI vascular, inflammatory, or congenital and developmental disorders of the spinal cord; and diseases of the spine. "Spinal cord disease, especially injury to the cervical portion of the cord, can affect virtually every body system by impairing voluntary motor and autonomic nervous system functions" (Schmitt, Midha, & McKenzie, 1995, p.297). A framework of secondary disabilities (Fuhrer, 1991), organized in five areas: cardiovascular/cardiopulmonary, genitourinary and bowel, psychosocial, skin, and neuromusculoskeletal, is used to cover the essential elements for the prevention and management of secondary disability in the SCI population (Refer to Table 32-1). Each area addresses commonly occurring secondary disabilities, and their assessment, diagnostic studies, and treatment. This is followed by selected nursing diagnoses, desired outcomes, and interventions used in managing secondary disabilities. Immobility is associated with many of the secondary disabilities experienced by individuals with SCI; Risk for Disuse Syndrome, is a nursing diagnosis that provides a framework for the assessment, establishment of outcomes, and selection of interventions to deal with several of these problems (Sparks & Taylor, 1995; Sparks, Taylor, & Dyer, 1996) (Refer to Table 32-2). Finally, a summary of health education tips to prevent and minimize secondary disabilities is presented.

B. Demographics

1. Acute and long-term survival rates for persons with SCI have improved in the last 50 years (DeVivo & Stover, 1995). The occurrence of secondary disabilities reduces survival; "the most significant prognostic factors related to survival are age and measures of injury severity such as neurologic level, degree of injury completeness, and ventilator dependency" (DeVivo & Stover, 1995, p.289).

2. Pulmonary complications are the most common cause of death in the acute and chronic phases after SCI; pneumonia was the primary cause of death in every age group and in both incomplete and complete lesions for a group of clients followed for 12 years after injury (Ragnarsson, Hall, Wilmot, & Carter, 1995).

3. Cardiovascular conditions such as deep vein thrombosis, pulmonary embolus, and autonomic dysreflexia are also major causes of morbidity and mortality (Ragnarsson et al., 1995).

4. Metabolic dysfunctions in SCI are associated with altered endocrine function, sedentary lifestyle, and impaired neurogenic influence; these include heterotopic ossification, osteoporosis, pathologic bone fractures, and immobilization hypercalcemia (Ragnarsson et al., 1995).

5. Pressure ulcers are a frequent complication of SCI.

6. Urinary tract infections are the most common secondary complication of SCI (Cardenas, Farrell-Roberts, Sipski, & Rubner, 1995). Upper tract urologic complications are more of a risk to long-term health and survival.

7. Secondary neuromusculoskeletal disabilities include spasticity, contractures, pain, post-traumatic syringomyelia, osteoporosis with limb fracture, and heterotopic ossification (Maynard, Karunas, Adkins, Richards, & Waring, 1995).

8. Psychosocial secondary disabilities were not described adequately in literature reviewed for this chapter, although a reference is made to "a decrease in depression and an increase in reported adjustment in personal, familial, social, and vocational areas" (Dijkers, Abela, Gans, & Gordon, 1995, p.206). Suicide rates were higher than expected in several studies; it is most common in the first few years after injury.

Table 32-1: Summary of Secondary Disabilities, Prevention/Health Promotion Strategies, Medical Management, and Nursing Management

Secondary Disability	Prevention/Health Promotion Strategies	Medical Management	Nursing Management
Pulmonary embolism (PE)	Avoid immobility, trauma, obesity, cardiovascular disease; cautious use of oral contraceptives	Anticoagulant therapy Monitoring for side effects Thrombolytic therapy Oxygen therapy	Early mobility Compression stockings Leg exercises Education: avoid constriction of venous return, hazards of immobility, treatment regimen, smoking cessation
Deep vein thrombosis (DVT)	Same as PE	Anticoagulant therapy Thrombolytic agents Venous thrombectomy	Same as PE Warm, moist compresses Bedrest as ordered No exercises to affected limb.
Reflex sympathetic dystrophy (RSD)	Avoid musculoskeletal trauma	Sympathetic nervous system blocking agent	Pain management Mobility therapy

continued on page 451

Table 32-1: Continued

Secondary Disability	Prevention/Health Promotion Strategies	Medical Management	Nursing Management
Pneumonia medication	Recognition of early signs and symptoms; identification of organism; pneumococcal and influenza vaccine for at risk populations; smoking cessation	Antibiotics Bronchodilators Liquefying agents Oxygen therapy Increased fluid intake Chest physiotherapy Suctioning Pneumococcal vaccine Influenza vaccine	Pulmonary toilet Monitor medications Ensure fluid intake Suction Education: benefits of immunization; regimen; signs and symptoms to report; energy conservation; smoking cessation
Aspiration	Upright position for eating and drinking; avoid ingesting large boluses of food; chew food well; avoid heavy alcohol use; emergency intervention for respiratory distress; knowledge of CPR in caretakers	Management of respiratory complications Referral to dysphagia team Enteral feedings if appropriate	Monitor for signs and symptoms of aspiration Check swallow and gag reflexes Position at 90° for eating and drinking Suction equipment available Educate: CPR, suctioning, monitoring
Atelectasis clearance	Avoid immobility and infections; smoking cessation; monitoring of mechanical ventilation	Chest physiotherapy Bronchoscopy Antibiotic therapy	Positioning Maintain airway Encourage fluids Educate: fluids, cough and deep breathing, pulmonary care, avoiding infections

Ventilatory failure
 	
clearance
	Avoid physical fatigue; increase strength and excursion of diaphragm; monitor vital capacity; adopt
	
	a healthy lifestyle; smoking cessation; immunizations
		Ventilator support:
		  Static ventilator
		  Portable ventilator
		  Pneumobelt
		
		Phrenic nerve stimulator
		Treat respiratory infections and other conditions
			Pulmonary toilet
			Immunizations
			Ventilator care
			Effective airway
			
			Assist with cough, turn, deep breathing, and suctioning

Urinary tract infection	Complete bladder emptying; maintain acid urine; minimize urethral trauma; avoid urinary stasis; monitor prostate, diabetes, and other chronic conditions	Antimicrobial therapy Urinary anti-infectives Urinary analgesics Surgery (removal of calculi, ureteral stent, cystoscopy) Pain management	Monitor intake and output Pain management Urinary care program Bladder management regimen
Upper urinary tract complications	Baseline urologic studies and routine follow-up	Management of urinary tract infections Urinary management Surgery (external sphincterotomy or bladder neck resection, ileal conduit)	Bladder management regimen Monitor intake and output Urinary care program

continued on page 452

Table 32-1: Continued

Secondary Disability	Prevention/Health Promotion Strategies	Medical Management	Nursing Management
Gallstone disease	Avoid high-fat foods; avoid obesity	Pharmacologic: oral bile acids, bile acid agents Surgery (cholecystectomy, conventional or laproscopic) Extracorporeal shock wave lithotripsy (ESWL) Diet therapy	Monitor medications Diet management Symptom management Pain management
Esophageal dysfunction	Avoid foods that cause heartburn; sitting position for eating and drinking; avoid obesity, smoking, use of alcohol or caffeine	Pharmacologic: antacids, histamine2-receptor antagonist Diet modification	Diet management Lifestyle modification Weight reduction Smoking cessation
Altered bowel elimination	High fiber content diet; adequate fluid intake; avoid overuse of laxatives, cathartics, or enemas; maintain regular bowel pattern; maintain activity level	Bowel regimen Diet modifications	Perform and educate about bowel regimen Diet modifications Monitor laxative, enema, cathartic usage Encourage activity to level of tolerance
Suicide \n\n making	Avoid alcohol and drug use; seek counseling for depression and/or suicidal ideation; \n\n participate in peer support groups	Suicide risk analysis Referral for counseling Alcohol and drug use \n\n screening Monitor accidental injuries	Suicide risk analysis Coping techniques Facilitate decision \n\n Encourage participation in peer support groups Refer for counseling
Spasticity	Avoidance of bowel, bladder, and skin complications	Pharmacologic: antispasticity drugs Local nerve block Ablative surgical procedures (rhizotomy or myelotomy) Dorsal column stimulator Intrathecal infusion pump	Range-of-motion exercises Positioning Bowel, bladder, and skin regimens Monitor medications Discuss impact of spasticity on functional outcomes
Syringomyelia	Regular monitoring for cystic changes in the spinal cord	Surgery: drainage of spinal cord cyst Regular neurologic imaging of spinal cord	Monitor for decreasing levels of functioning, spasticity, motor and sensory loss
Pain exercises	Neurogenic: lowers \n\n quality of life Musculoskeletal: more common in shoulder and hand, then wrist: avoid chronic overuse of muscles and joints, use assistive and/or adaptive equipment; maintain range of motion; avoid contractures	Pharmacologic: \n\n Nonsteroid anti-inflammatory drugs, anticonvulsants, tricyclic antidepressants. TENS unit Pain management surgery (myelotomy, cordotomy, rhizotomy) Carpal tunnel treatment Median neuropathy treatment Elbow pain treatment	Range-of-motion \n\n Prevent contractures Move and position gently and in correct alignment Pain management: nonpharmacologic measures such as imagery, diversional activities, and relaxation techniques Referrals to behavioral management resources

continued on page 453

452

Table 32-1: Continued

Secondary Disability	Prevention/Health Promotion Strategies	Medical Management	Nursing Management
Contractures exercises	Maintain joint range of motion.	Pain management Surgical correction Cold or heat therapy Splinting	Therapeutic positioning Positioning aids Range-of-motion Therapeutic exercises Activity to tolerance level Consultation with PT and OT
Heterotopic ossification	Joint range of motion; avoid flexion positions	Pharmacologic: anti-inflammatory agents, disodium etidronate Regular monitoring of joint and mobility status	Range of motion exercises Management of spasticity and avoidance of contractures
Immobilization hypercalcemia	Early mobilization; low calcium diet	Pharmacologic: calcitonin Diet: low calcium	Monitor diet Avoid immobilization
Acquired scoliosis	Avoid obesity; maintain activity level	Stretching exercises to improve posture and maintain flexibility Wheelchair, cushions, accessories (seatbelts, chest straps, thoracic supports, posture panels)	Monitor neuromusculoskeletal status Maintain exercise program Evaluate weight
Fractures from osteoporosis cessation,	No smoking; maintain activity levels; adequate calcium intake; estrogen replacement therapy; avoid alcohol and caffeine	Pharmacologic: calcium supplements, Vitamin D, calcitonin, sodium fluoride estrogen replacement therapy Fracture therapy Pain management	Educate about calcium intake, smoking estrogen replacement therapy, benefits of regular exercise, limiting caffeine and alcohol intake, safety and fall precautions Maintain activity level to tolerance, use of assistive devices Pain management, including nonpharmacologic treatments

C. **Etiology/Precipitating Factors**

The etiology of secondary disabilities is related to the effects of aging with a SCI; physiologic changes that accompany paralysis include losses in the areas of sensation, movement, bone density, and bowel and bladder function (Menter & Hudson, 1995). Some secondary disabilities increase with age: pneumonia, contractures, pressure ulcers, acquired scoliosis, pain, and dependence in self-care activities. Others decrease with time since onset of SCI: spasticity, fevers, and urinary tract infections; this decrease may be due to the greater incidence of incomplete injuries in the older age population (Menter & Hudson).

III. Cardiovascular and Cardiopulmonary Secondary Disabilities

A. **Cardiovascular secondary disabilities include pulmonary embolus (PE) and deep vein thrombosis (DVT) and autonomic dysreflexia (AD)** (See Chapter 13).

1. PE, the sudden occlusion of a pulmonary artery, causes decreased blood supply to the lung. A frequent cause is thromboemboli from the right side of heart associated with DVT. Risk factors include stasis of blood, immobility, trauma, heart disease, obesity, age, and use of oral contraceptives (LeMone & Burke, 1996). Treatment includes respiratory management and anticoagulant therapy (Schmitt et al., 1995). Recurrent PE may require placement of a Greenfield filter in the vena cava; an increased risk of complications from the filters has been reported in this population.
   a. Assessment: includes history of risk factors: respiratory status: abrupt onset of dyspnea, tachycardia, tachypnea, crackles, hemoptysis, cough, shortness of breath, chest pain, anxiety, apprehension, and low-grade fever.
   b. Diagnostic studies: Chest x-ray, electrocardiogram, lung scan, and pulmonary angiography.
   c. Laboratory tests: arterial blood gases and coagulation studies.
2. DVT is a clot in the deep veins with complete or partial occlusion of blood flow; primary cause is venous stasis, also associated with trauma and increased blood coagulation. Preventive strategies include prophylactic anticoagulation, external pneumatic calf compression, and electrical stimulation of the calf (Schmitt et al., 1995). Anticoagulant therapy is more aggressive when DVT occurs.
   a. Assessment: history of risk factors (see PE above), pain, fever, chills, edema, and cyanosis along the affected vein (Monahan & Neighbors, 1994).
   b. Diagnostic studies: venography, impedance plethysmography, and duplex ultrasonography;
   c. Laboratory tests: arterial blood gases and coagulation studies.
3. Nursing diagnoses/outcomes/interventions:
   a. Ineffective breathing pattern
      (1) Outcomes: Respiratory rate ±5 breaths/minute of baseline, arterial blood gases normal, no crackles, fever, or cyanosis
      (2) Interventions: The key to success is bronchial hygiene - Monitoring respiratory status every 4 hours, maximizing chest expansion by positioning, assisting with use of incentive spirometer, performing chest physiotherapy, monitoring anticoagulant therapy, and use of relaxation techniques to reduce anxiety.
   b. Tissue perfusion alteration (cardiovascular)
      (1) Outcomes: Pulse and blood pressure within parameters; no arrhythmias; skin warm and dry; verbalization measures to modify lifestyle to minimize decreased perfusion.
      (2) Interventions: Monitoring vital signs every 2 hours; EKG, oxygen therapy as ordered; repositioning and bronchial hygiene; monitoring laboratory values and pulse oximetry; instructing client and family about risk factors, use of medications, and lifestyle changes.
   c. Tissue perfusion alteration (peripheral)
      (1) Outcomes: No further emboli, improved venous blood flow, clotting studies within therapeutic range, demonstration measures to prevent pooling of blood in lower extremities, verbalization risk factors that impede venous flow.
      (2) Interventions: Monitoring vital signs and breath sounds every 4 hours, reporting deviations; administering and monitoring anticoagulant therapy as ordered; applying antiembolic stockings (remove once every 8 hours and observe skin condition); instructing client in proper positioning to avoid constriction of peripheral blood flow, use of anticoagulant therapy, and antiembolic stockings.

B. **Cardiopulmonary secondary disabilities include atelectasis, pneumonia, aspiration, and respiratory failure.**
   1. Atelectasis is incomplete expansion or collapse of lung tissue; there is an increased incidence with higher level of injury. With complete tetraplegia, the incidence averaged 2.6 percent. There is no apparent correlation associated with years post-injury (Ragnarsson et al., 1995). Preventive strategies focus on pulmonary hygiene, breathing humidified air, taking deep breaths to expand lungs, and use of an incentive spirometer.
      a. Assessment: Evaluation of respiratory status (dyspnea), breath sounds (diminished), skin

color (cyanosis).

   b. Diagnostic studies: Chest x-ray, pulse oximetry, pulmonary function tests.

2. Pneumonia is an infection of the lung parenchyma by bacteria, viruses, fungi, protozoa (infectious), or aspiration or inhalation of toxic gases (noninfectious) (LeMone & Burke, 2000). It is correlated with level of injury; incomplete paraplegia has the lowest incidence (<1 percent) and complete tetraplegia has the highest (4.7 percent) (Ragnarsson et al., 1995). Prevention includes pneumoccal vaccine and annual influenza vaccinations, performing the "quad" cough, and vigorous pulmonary toilet. Treatment of pneumonia includes use of appropriate antibiotics, humidified oxygen therapy, hydration, and if necessary, bronchoscopy to remove mucous plugs.

   a. Assessment: History of respiratory symptoms, fever, chills, chest pain, cough, sputum, and auscultation of breath sounds.

   b. Diagnostic studies: Chest x-ray; arterial blood gases; sputum gram stain, culture and sensitivity; complete blood count; pulse oximetry; blood cultures; pulmonary function studies; fiberoptic bronchoscopy; and vital capacity.

3. Aspiration is drainage of fluid, mucus, saliva, or blood into the airway. The incidence is relatively low, but of some concern in tetraplegia. A side-lying, prone, or semi-sitting position may help in preventing aspiration. If aspiration occurs, treatment centers on relieving respiratory distress and instituting measures to prevent recurrence.

   a. Assessment: Evaluation of swallowing and gag reflex, breath sounds, dyspnea, shortness of breath, vital signs, and skin color.

   b. Diagnostic studies: Arterial blood gases, pulse oximetry, swallowing video fluoroscopy, barium swallow.

4. Respiratory Failure is the need for partial or total ventilator support for more than seven days. It is correlated with level of injury; paraplegia has the lowest incidence, followed by incomplete tetraplegia (<1 percent), and complete tetraplegia (0.5-2.3 percent) (Ragnarsson et al., 1995). Persons with high cervical cord lesions (>C3-C5) require mechanical ventilation or phrenic nerve pacing.

   a. Assessment: Evaluation of respiratory status, chest expansion, and neurologic status.

   b. Diagnostic studies: Arterial blood gases, pulse oximetry, and pulmonary function tests.

5. Nursing diagnoses/outcomes/interventions:

   a. Ineffective airway clearance

      (1) Outcomes: Effective and expectoration of sputum; clear breath sounds; arterial blood gases within parameters; demonstration and verbalization of understanding of hydration, sputum monitoring, controlled cough techniques, and chest physiotherapy.

      (2) Interventions: Monitoring respiratory status; assisting with positioning, turning, coughing, and deep breathing; suctioning, providing adequate humidification and fluid intake; performing chest physiotherapy; encouraging mobility; instructing about hydration, monitoring sputum, staying active, and controlled coughing techniques.

   b. Ineffective breathing pattern

      (1) Outcomes: Respiratory rate within ± 5 breaths/minute of baseline, arterial blood gases within normal limits, no adventitious breath sounds, and demonstration of correct breathing techniques.

      (2) Interventions: Monitoring respiratory status, oxygen therapy, need for ventilator support, and pain status every 4 hours; administering and assessing the effectiveness of pain medications; instructing in the use of incentive spirometer, performing chest physiotherapy, use of relaxation techniques, need for periods to avoid fatigue, and deep breathing exercises.

   c. Gas exchange impairment

      (1) Outcomes: Ability to perform activities of daily living to level of tolerance without fatigue, respiratory rate within ± 5 breaths/minute of baseline, no adventitious breath sounds, arterial blood gases within parameters, effective cough and expectoration of sputum.

      (2) Interventions: Monitoring pulmonary status, respiratory therapy every 4 hours,

positioning to facilitate chest expansion and breathing every 2 hours, assisting with activities of daily living as necessary, reducing oxygen demand by coordinating rest and activity, instructing to cough and breathe deeply every 2-4 hours.

d. Inability to sustain spontaneous ventilation
   (1) Outcomes: Respiratory rate within ± 5 breaths/minute of baseline; arterial blood gases within normal limits; ability to perform to limits of activity tolerance; no use of accessory muscles for breathing; no evidence of respiratory muscle fatigue; pulmonary function tests within parameters for patient; smooth transition on and off ventilator if needed.
   (2) Interventions: Monitoring vital signs, signs of respiratory distress, arterial blood gases, pulse oximetry, performance of activities of daily living; reducing patient's anxiety; instructing patient to monitor respiratory distress and to recognize symptoms that require treatment; and being prepared for use of mechanical ventilation.

IV. Genitourinary and Bowel Secondary Disabilities

A. **Urinary tract infections and upper tract urologic complications**
   1. Urinary tract infections are characterized by bacteriuria (colony count of 1 to 100,000 colonies or >100,000 colonies) (Cardenas et al., 1995). It is the most common secondary complication after initial hospital discharge. Bacteriuria may be symptomatic or asymptomatic. Antibiotic treatment is usually given for "the first episode of bacteriuria, with or without pyuria, or in the situation of actually symptomatic infections" (Stover, Lloyd, Waites & Jackson, 1995, p. 206). Antibiotic treatment of asymptomatic bacteriuria is not recommended in long-term management. Reinfections are evaluated; treatment is dependent upon causative factors. Use of intermittent catheterization, reflex voiding or external condom catheters has reduced colonization of the urinary tract and subsequent infections.
      a. Assessment: Urologic history, voiding patterns, change in continence or retention of urine, characteristics of urine, fever, inspection of genitalia, bladder management practices, and use of urinary equipment. Other signs in the person with SCI include "increased sweating, abdominal discomfort, costovertebral angle pain or tenderness, and foul-smelling urine" (Stover et al., 1995, p. 201).
      b. Diagnostic studies: Urinalysis, urine culture and sensitivity, and urodynamic studies.
   2. Upper tract urinary complications: Vesicoureteral reflex, hydronephrosis, pyelocaliectasis, renal calculi (increased incidence in individuals with indwelling catheters; incidence increases with years post-injury), renal and perirenal infection, and renal insufficiency and failure (Cardenas et al., 1995).
      a. Assessment: Urologic history; bladder management practices; history of previous calculi, infections, or renal failure.
      b. Diagnostic studies: Glomerular filtration rate, excretory urogram/intravenous pyelogram, cystoscopy, renal scan, renal ultrasound, urinalysis, blood cultures, characteristics of calculi, BUN, creatinine, urinalysis, urine culture and sensitivity, and urodynamic studies.
   3. Nursing diagnoses/outcomes/interventions:
      a. Urinary elimination pattern alteration
         (1) Outcomes: Maintenance of fluid balance, clear urine, no fever, demonstration of bladder management techniques, verbalization of understanding of food/fluids that impact on urinary status, urodynamic studies within normal parameters for patient.
         (2) Interventions: Monitoring characteristics of urine and effectiveness of pain medications and antibiotics; recording intake and output; adjusting fluid intake to output, carrying out the usual bladder management regimen; straining urine-reporting and obtaining analysis of any particles passed; instructing patient in dietary management of urinary tract infections and/or calculi; referring for nutrition consultation; and administering medications or antibiotics as ordered.
      b. Urinary retention
         (1) Outcomes: Maintenance of fluid balance; demonstration of bladder management

regimen (intermittent catheterization, voiding techniques such as Credé, suprapubic tapping, Valsalva maneuver, indwelling catheter); urinalysis within normal parameters; no bladder distention; verbalization understanding of symptoms and management of urinary retention, signs and symptoms of autonomic dysreflexia, and drug regimen.

    (2) Interventions: Recording intake and output; instructing patient in, and having return demonstration of, bladder management regimen; encouraging appropriate fluid intake; instructing the patient in signs, symptoms, and management of urinary retention; monitoring characteristics of urine; treatment and management of autonomic dysreflexia; and making referrals to appropriate agencies for continuity of care.

  c. Urinary Incontinence

    (1) Outcomes: Maintenance of fluid balance and continence; demonstration of bladder management regimen (external catheter, indwelling catheter, suprapubic catheter, transurethral sphincterotomy, augmentation enterocystoplasty, continent diversion); verbalization of understanding of drug regimen (anticholinergics/spasmodics, alpha-adrenergic agonists, conjugated estrogens, or cholinergic agonists); return to usual lifestyle; no skin breakdown; and decreased incidence of infections.

    (2) Interventions: Monitoring voiding pattern, recording intake and output; instructing to follow usual bladder management regimen; administering and monitoring the effectiveness of and instructing in the use of drugs used for urinary incontinence (see outcomes above); restricting intake of caffeine, alcohol, and carbonated beverages; encouraging discussion about the impact of incontinence on the patient and family.

B. Gallstone disease, esophageal dysfunction, and altered bowel elimination

1. Gallstone disease is the development of cholelithiasis (formation of stones), that leads to obstruction of bile in the hepatic, cystic, or common bile duct and inflammation of the gallbladder (cholecystitis). Clinical manifestations include abdominal pain or cramping (may be referred to subscapular area), nausea, vomiting, bile reflux, jaundice, pancreatitis, intolerance to fatty foods, fever, and changes in laboratory values (high white blood count, elevated serum bilirubin, alkaline phosphatase, and serum amylase). Persons with SCI may be asymptomatic or have no reports of pain. Treatment includes diet therapy, use of pharmacologic agents, and removal of the gallbladder and gallstones.

  a. Assessment: Tolerance to fatty foods, nausea, vomiting, pain, vital signs, skin characteristics.

  b. Diagnostic studies: Laboratory studies (complete blood count, serum bilirubin, serum amylase, alkaline phosphatase), oral cholecystogram, ultrasonography of gallbladder, cholescintigraphy).

2. Esophageal dysfunction includes esophagitis, heartburn, and dysphagia.

  a. Assessment: Nutritional status, swallowing and gag reflex, throat examination, complaints related to heartburn or chest pain.

  b. Diagnostic studies: Esophageal videofluoroscopy, barium swallow, endoscopy, esophagogastroduodenoscopy (EGD).

3. Altered bowel elimination may be related to poor dietary management, chronic constipation, bowel incontinence, or impaired transit time (Cardenas et al., 1995).

  a. Assessment: Bowel patterns, nutritional status, characteristics of stool, bloating, abdominal distension, gas, and presence of hemorrhoids.

  b. Diagnostic studies: Stool for gross and microscopic examination, stool culture, sigmoidoscopy, rectal biopsy, barium enema, serum electrolytes, and gastrointestinal transit time studies.

4. Nursing diagnoses/outcomes/interventions:

  a. Bowel incontinence

    (1) Outcomes: Maintenance a regular bowel regimen, no episodes of incontinence, demonstration bowel care, regulation food and fluids to tolerance.

    (2) Interventions: Establishing of a bowel care program (suppository, digital removal of

stool, stool softeners, bulking agents), documenting of results, maintaining of bowel record, encouraging adequate fluid intake, instructing client in bowel care program with return demonstration, timing bowel care program to accommodate patient's schedule and usual bowel habits, using protective padding as necessary, providing nutritionally balanced diet, and avoiding foods that aggravate incontinence.

 b. Chronic constipation
  (1) Outcomes: Maintenance elimination pattern, complete evacuation of stool, demonstration of bowel care program, verbalization of understanding of measures to manage constipation, maintenance activity level.
  (2) Interventions: (see above) Encouraging intake of high fiber foods and adequate fluids, encouraging regular participation in exercise/ activity programs. If impaction occurs, a mineral oil retention enema may be needed to soften the stool; watch persons with high paraplegia or quadriplegia closely for autonomic dysreflexia.
 c. Swallowing impairment
  (1) Outcomes: No aspiration pneumonia, clear breath sounds, maintenance of weight within parameters, demonstration of correct eating or feeding techniques to maximize swallowing.
  (2) Interventions: Elevating the head of the bed 90 degrees (or having the patient sit upright) during meals and for 30 minutes afterwards; monitoring intake, output, and weight; providing oral hygiene; instructing individual in feeding techniques to stimulate swallowing.

V. Psychosocial Secondary Disabilities

Psychosocial secondary disabilities relate to adaptation, adjustment, and quality of life issues following SCI. The psychosocial rehabilitation model addresses behavioral and psychological adaptation to disability (Lanig et al, 1996). Although employment, marital status, living arrangements, and educational level are part of psychosocial adjustment, this section is limited to a discussion of suicide and coping following SCI.

A. **Suicide:** Suicide is the taking of one's own life. For some individuals with SCI the suicide attempt may be obvious, as in self-inflicted gunshot wounds, overdoses or putting oneself in danger. Less obvious attempts may involve substance abuse, self-neglect (lack of skin maintenance or nutritional balance), or refusal of care (operations or rehabilitation). Suicide rates are higher than average during first few years after injury. After 5-10 years they approach those of the general population. (Dijkers et al., 1995).
 1. Assessment: History of previous suicide attempts; psychiatric disorders; criminal activities; substance abuse; family dysfunction; physical examination (neurologic status); psychosocial status, self-care status, skin status, nutritional status, suicidal ideation, plan, and access.
 2. Diagnostic studies: Alcohol and drug levels, suicide risk analysis.

B. **Coping:** Coping is the process of learning to adapt and adjust to changes. Generally, quality of life and life satisfaction are high in persons with SCI. Pre-injury personality, social support systems, and the quality of rehabilitation are related to the coping abilities and satisfaction level with life after SCI. Long-term management and follow-up are needed to enhance coping, socialization, and adjustment.
 1. Assessment: Cultural status, neurologic status, psychosocial status, self-care status, social status, and family status.
 2. Diagnostic studies: Locus of control, coping styles, self-care scales, role and social scales.

C. **Nursing diagnoses/outcomes/interventions:**
 1. Adjustment impairment
  a. Outcomes: Individual identifies inability to cope and adjust, participates in health care regimen, demonstrates management of health, verbalizes the ability to accept and adapt to new health status.
  b. Interventions: Encouraging the individual to express feelings in a safe environment,

supporting normal grieving process, providing reassurance, instructing individual in health regimen activities, incorporating the individual in decision making and maintenance of control, facilitating meeting with individuals with similar disabilities, referring to support groups or psychological follow-up.

2. Ineffective individual coping
   a. Outcomes: Individual verbalizes feelings, develops therapeutic relationship with health care team, participates in self-care activities, identifies and uses usual coping techniques, implements new coping techniques, practices assertive behaviors.
   b. Interventions: Active listening, providing gradual incorporation of self-care activities, instructing in cognitive and behavioral coping techniques, assisting individual to use coping techniques, encouraging evaluation of effectiveness, referring for psychological counseling if necessary.

3. Social isolation
   a. Outcomes: Individual interacts with health team members and family, identifies barriers to social interaction and ways to minimize their effect, participates in social activities, verbalizes increased social interaction.
   b. Interventions: Providing assistive devices and equipment to maximize mobility and communication (wheelchair, computer, phone, transportation), encouraging participation in social activities (outings, movie, club or organization, parties), welcoming visitors and family (providing visiting area), incorporating social events in daily schedule.

4. Social interaction impairment
   a. Outcomes: Individual identifies needs and communicates if needs are met, participates in planning care, uses culturally and socially appropriate social skills, verbalizes satisfaction with social interactions, uses social networks.
   b. Interventions: Understanding the sociocultural background of the individual, using interpreter if needed to enhance interactions, instructing patient in effective social-interaction behaviors, demonstrating respect for privacy and cultural practices, referring to social worker for additional suggestions.

5. Self-directed violence
   a. Outcomes: Individual does not injure self, discusses feelings, contracts not to harm self, verbalizes need for support, and plans to use support systems.
   b. Interventions: Initiating of appropriate safety protocols (one-to-one, seclusion, restraints) as necessary to control behavior; removing of self-injury items (razors, belts, glass, pills, gun, knife, etc.); monitoring feelings (ask "Have you thought of killing yourself?" If so, "What do you plan to do?"), developing a short-term written contract not to harm self; supervising administration of prescribed medications, instructing individual to contact staff if feelings intensify or become overwhelming; assisting to identify source of discomfort, but placing limits on excessive talk about suicide; assisting patient to identify positive qualities in self; referring to mental health professional for long-term help; providing numbers and information about crisis centers, hot lines, counselors, and other emergency services.

6. Risk for self-mutilation
   a. Outcomes: Individual does not injure self; verbalizes self-destructive or suicidal thoughts; explores adaptive methods of coping with anger and frustration; demonstrates ability to cope with impulses, anxiety, or self-destructive ideas; verbalizes understanding of community support and emergency systems.
   b. Interventions: Removing hazardous items from environment; limiting the number of staff interacting with the individual and making the interactions frequent and short; developing short-term verbal contracts not to harm self; decreasing stimulation if mutilation thoughts increase; developing a behavior-modification program to reward self-control; instructing patient in cognitive techniques to manage fear, anxiety, stress, and depression; referring individual to appropriate agencies.

7. Ineffective management of therapeutic regimen
   a. Outcomes: Individual verbalizes personal thoughts about management of regimen; develops plans for integrating therapeutic regimen into daily routine; selects activities to support goals of regimen, achieves therapeutic goals, reduces risk factors, and uses

appropriate support services.

    b. Interventions: Discussing the individual's personal beliefs and values; instructing regarding the pathophysiology of the injury and its relationship to the therapeutic regimen; assisting to clarify values associated with lifestyle; establishing and carrying out a daily routine to achieve therapeutic goals while being congruent with patient's values and beliefs; assisting to identify and modify risk factors that interfere with therapeutic management; encouraging health promotion activities; referring to support services; consulting with primary health care practitioner to monitor the patient and prevent complications.

8. Body image disturbance

    a. Outcomes: Individual verbalizes change in body image; participates in decisions and aspects of care; communicates feelings about change; participates in rehabilitation program; expresses positive feelings about self; engages in social interaction; discusses disability or limitations.

    b. Interventions: Providing an environment conducive to expressing feelings; assisting person to identify positive aspects about appearance; providing positive feedback; encouraging the keeping of a journal or tape for recording feelings, goals, concerns, and progress; facilitating participation in support group or individual interactions; instructing and assisting to practice healthful coping strategies; referring to support services; encouraging participation in activities and hobbies that the individual enjoys.

Table 32-2: Risk for Disuse Syndrome

Assessment	Outcomes	Interventions
Age Sex History of disability, immobility	Maintains reality orientation	Provide orienting materials (clock, radio, and calendar); encourage contact with staff, family, and friends.
Neurologic status Cardiovascular status Respiratory status Gastrointestinal status Nutritional status	No evidence of thrombus formation, venous stasis, or altered cardiovascular function.	Change position at least every 2 hours; inspect for signs of thrombus or stasis; use antiembolic stockings; monitor clotting profile.
Fluid status Genitourinary status Musculoskeletal status Integumentary status Psychosocial status	No evidence of decreased chest movement, cough stimulus, or depth of ventilation; and shows no pooling of secretions or signs and symptoms of infection. Effective ventilation restored and maintained.	Monitor breath sounds and respiratory status; instruct about pulmonary toilet, use of incentive spirometer, relaxation techniques, respiratory muscle training, mechanical ventilation, ventilator support devices, or electrical phrenic pacing.
Risk Factors Altered level of consciousness Mechanical immobilization Paralysis Prescribed immobilization Severe Pain	Maintains adequate dietary intake, hydration, and weight.	Weigh routinely, compare with baseline data, refer for dietary counseling if weight loss or gain occurs; encourage fluid intake to 3 quarts/day unless contraindicated; monitor hydration status, gag and swallowing reflexes; use dysphagia feeding techniques if necessary; provide adaptive equipment to facilitate independence.
	No signs of urinary retention, infections, or renal calculi.	Maintain a voiding record, perform bladder management program - have patient assume responsibility

continued on page 461

Table 32-2: Continued

Assessment	Outcomes	Interventions
		when appropriate; monitor characteristics of urine; provide high fluid intake if appropriate; monitor for signs of urinary infection, retention, or calculi.
	Maintains muscle strength and tone; joint range of motion, no evidence of contractures.	Perform active or passive range-of-motion exercises at least once/8 hours. Instruct in isometric and isotonic exercises as appropriate; refer to PT and OT for exercise program and adaptive equipment; encourage activity to tolerance level, use of adaptive equipment and supplies.
	No signs of skin breakdown.	Inspect skin each shift, protect areas subject to irritation; use pressure-reducing, pressure-relieving, or support services as indicated (bed, wheelchair); provide or assist with daily hygiene, keep skin clean and dry (mild soap, warm water, no harsh cleansers), use moisturizers (no irritants), humidity >40%, follow pressure ulcer prevention and treatment guidelines presented in Chapter 17.
	Maintains bowel pattern, no constipation or incontinence.	Keep a bowel record, follow bowel management program (stool softeners, laxative, suppository, enema, digital or manual removal of stool); consult with dietician to plan and provide a high fiber, high protein and high Vitamin C diet, and adequate intake of calcium.
	Carries out self-care activities to highest level (specify).	Record self-care status on a regular basis, use to set goals for highest level of independent functioning; consult with OT regarding adaptive equipment and assistive devices to maximize function; encourage participation in self-care activities, provide assistance when necessary.
	Verbalizes relationship between inactivity and secondary disabilities.	Discuss impact of inactivity and immobility on the body and measures to reduce the impact. Establish regular follow-up to monitor for occurrence of secondary disabilities and make early interventions, refer for regular health visits with primary health care provider, dentist, and other health professionals.

From Validation of Risk Factors for Disuse Syndrome, by K. V. Hayes, 1995, in M. J. Rantz & P. LeMone (Eds.), *Classification of Nursing Diagnoses: Proceedings of the Eleventh Conference* (pp. 244-245), Glendale, IL: CINAHL Information Systems; *Nursing Diagnosis Reference Manual* (3rd ed.), by S. M. Sparks & C. M. Taylor, 1998, Springhouse: Springhouse Corporation; *Nursing Diagnosis Pocket Manual*, by S. M. Sparks, C. M. Taylor, & J. G. Dyer, 1998, Springhouse : Springhouse Corporation.

VI. Skin Secondary Disabilities (Refer to Chapter 17)

A. **Outcomes:** No signs of skin breakdown.

B. **Interventions:** Inspecting skin each shift, and protecting areas subject to irritation; using pressure-reducing, pressure-relieving, or support services as indicated (bed, wheelchair); providing or assisting with daily hygiene; keeping skin clean and dry (mild soap, warm water, no harsh cleansers); using moisturizers (no irritants); humidity >40 percent, following pressure ulcer prevention and treatment guidelines presented in Chapter 17.

VII. Neuromusculoskeletal Secondary Disabilities

A. **Spasticity, syringomyelia, reflex sympathetic dystrophy, and pain**
1. Spasticity is characterized by hyperactive deep tendon reflexes and increased muscle tone. It is expected to occur as a result of the pathophysiology of injury to the spinal cord above the conus medullaris (Maynard et al., Richards, & Waring, 1995). Spasticity has some benefit for health and functioning, but becomes problematic when it is severe enough to interfere with daily functioning, and requiring medication or surgical treatment. Spasticity occurs in 32.2 percent of persons in the National SCI database before discharge from initial hospitalization, increases to 42.7 percent by end of first year after injury, decreases to 35 percent by 10 years post-injury (Maynard et al., 1995). Treatment includes antispasticity medications, passive stretching of spastic muscles, local nerve block, ablative surgical procedures such as rhizotomy or myelotomy (very low in SCI database), dorsal column stimulators, intrathecal drug infusion pumps.
   a. Assessment: Neuromusculoskeletal status, pain, self-care abilities, and functional status.
   b. Diagnostic studies: Multichannel electromyographic (EMG) analysis; ruling out problems that increase spasticity, (e.g., urinary tract infection, pressure ulcer, or use of non-tricyclic antidepressant.)
2. Syringomyelia is characterized by a fluid-filled cystic cavity in the central intramedullary gray matter; it causes pain, motor weakness, loss of sensation, and spasticity. Treatment may be with surgical drainage and/or placement of permanent shunts. Incidence varies from 1 percent to 3 percent in those with symptoms, may be 67 percent in those with cysts but no symptoms (Maynard et al., 1995). More research is needed to determine the natural course of these cysts and their development into symptomatic cysts.
   a. Assessment: Neuromusculoskeletal status, self-care and functional abilities, and pain.
   b. Diagnostic studies: Magnetic resonance imaging (MRI), and contrast CT scan with delayed imaging.
3. Reflex sympathetic dystrophy is pain and autonomic dysfunction in the shoulder, hand, and arm of the affected side; clinical manifestations include edema; pain; altered sweating, temperature, and skin color. Later on, there is atrophy of the skin, and bone contractures form. This is also called shoulder-hand syndrome.
   a. Assessment: Pain status, mobility status, skin condition, neurovascular status, and range of motion.
   b. Diagnostic studies: X-ray of affected extremity, thermography, bone scan, and evaluation of sympathetic block
4. Pain (neurogenic and musculoskeletal) is neurogenic in nature (central pain, phantom pain, deafferentation pain, dysesthetic pain, central dysesthetic syndrome, spinal cord pain). Symptoms include "burning, tingling, or aching diffuse pain below the level of injury" (Maynard et al., 1995, p. 154). Pain impulses ascend within the lateral spinothalamic tract to the thalamus and cerebral cortex where the perception of pain is moderated.

B. **Contractures, heterotopic ossification, osteoporosis, immobilization hypercalcemia, acquired scoliosis, and fractures.**
1. Contractures are characterized by permanent shortening of connective tissue; after contracture develops, inelasticity limits body movement. Considered a preventable complication, prevention includes positioning and repositioning, splinting, and regular range-of-motion and stretching exercises. Rates are lower in those treated in Model SCI

Systems. Incidence increases following injury with higher rates in tetraplegia, and in those with spasticity and heterotopic ossification (Maynard et al., 1995). Increase range-of-motion exercises to counteract contractures; use padding to prevent skin breakdown; surgery may be needed later.

   a. Assessment: Neuromusculoskeletal status, range of motion, self-care status, and pain.

   b. Diagnostic studies: Goniometer (assesses angle of flexion in a joint).

2. Heterotopic Ossification is a collection of calcium, especially in joints distal to the level of injury. It occurs most frequently in the hips (60-70 percent) and knees (20-30 percent) (Ashford, 1995). It restricts joint range of motion, limits functional abilities, and may lead to pressure ulcers. Treatment includes etidronate disodium and indomethacin; early initiation of stretching and joint range-of-motion exercises, and avoidance of flexion positions. If incomplete range of motion or joint ankylosis is present, surgery may be performed to prevent potential pathologic fractures. Incidence is about 3 percent of persons with SCI (Maynard et al., 1995).

   a. Assessment: Level of injury, neuromusculoskeletal status, pain, spasticity, skin status, joint range of motion, functional status.

   b. Diagnostic studies: X-ray or bone scan, elevation of serum alkaline phosphatase.

3. Osteoporosis is a metabolic bone disorder characterized by bone reabsorption greater than bone formation, reduction in bone mass, risk for bone fractures, and other degenerative changes. Osteoporosis resulting in fractures is coded in the National SCI Database. The estimated incidence is around 1 percent (probably low). Rapid bone loss occurs early after injury; and further bone loss continues over time, possibly related to aging. Treatment consists of Vitamin D, calcium supplement, and activity. In SCI, "standard treatments such as sitting exercises or standing frames, [may be] ineffective for bone gain" (Ashford, 1995, p. 350).

   a. Assessment: Musculoskeletal status, mobility status, range of motion, risk factors (age, female, postmenopausal, Caucasian, calcium or estrogen deficiency, smoking, high caffeine or alcohol intake, sedentary).

   b. Diagnostic studies: X-rays (osteoporotic changes not seen until >30 percent bone mass is lost), computed tomography, dual photon absorptiometry, urinary hydroxyproline level, serum bone GLA-protein, bone biopsy, bone density studies.

4. Immobilization Hypercalcemia is increased reabsorption of calcium from bones leading to muscle weakness, fatigue, altered mental status, ataxia, personality changes, decrease in level of consciousness, abdominal pain, nausea and vomiting, constipation, weight loss, and dysrhythmias. Treated with a low calcium diet, calcitonin, and acutely with intravenous sodium phosphate or potassium phosphate.

   a. Assessment: Symptoms listed immediately above, evidence of immobility, musculoskeletal status.

   b. Diagnostic studies: Serum electrolytes-(serum calcium above 10.0 mg/dl.), parathyroid hormone (PTH), electrocardiogram.

5. Acquired scoliosis is lateral curvature of the spine occurring after an injury. May lead to pain, shortness of breath, gastrointestinal disturbances, and pressure ulcers. In children treated with braces, electrical stimulation, surgery, and traction; in adults, weight reduction, active and passive exercises, use of braces. Surgical insertion of metal straightening rods may be used to reduce the curvature and provide rotational stability. In children, the incidence of scoliosis occurring after SCI may be 98 percent; treatment is with a thoracolumbar sacral orthosis (Zejdlik, 1992).

   a. Assessment: Neuromusculoskeletal status, self-care status, functional status, respiratory status, inspection of the spine, and skin status.

   b. Diagnostic studies: Upright posteroanterior and lateral x-rays.

6. Fractures are characterized by a break in the continuity of a bone. They may result from trauma, or disease (cancer or osteoporosis). They are classified as open or closed, complete or incomplete, stable or unstable. They are treated with traction, surgery to perform internal or external fixation or to visualize and correct problems.

   a. Assessment: Neurovascular status, musculoskeletal status, pain, and range of motion.

   b. Diagnostic studies: X-rays, bone scan, complete blood count, coagulation studies, urine myoglobin.

C. Nursing Diagnoses/Outcomes/Interventions

1. Mobility impairment
   a. Outcomes: Verbalization of pain relief, maintenance of muscle strength and joint range of motion, no evidence of complications (contractures, venous stasis, thrombus, or skin breakdown), return to pre-fracture level of mobility, implementation of mobility regimen, verbalization of plans to reduce risk factors and incorporate safety practices.
   b. Interventions: Immobilizing fracture site; providing of traction, splint, or brace care; conducting neurovascular exam every 4 hours until stable; monitoring skin and muscle status daily; providing progressive mobilization in consultation with physical therapy; encouraging attendance at physical therapy sessions; discussing fracture risk and measures to reduce injury; obtaining adaptive equipment or assistive devices to maximize independence; assisting with performance of activities of daily living.

2. Risk for injury
   a. Outcomes: Maintenance of safety measures, no occurrence of injury, verbalization of relationship between level of disability and necessary safety measures.
   b. Interventions: Assisting the individual to identify risk factors for injury and measures to improve safety; using safety devices (seat belts, side rails, transfer belts); instructing in use of safety devices, test of bath water before bathing, avoidance of open heaters, skin inspection, and removal of safety hazards from environment.

3. Tactile sensory/perceptual alteration
   a. Outcomes: No falls or injury, no skin breakdown, use of safety precautions, safely maneuvering in environment, receipt of appropriate tactile stimulation.
   b. Interventions: Instructing in safety measures, and regular skin inspection; using safety precautions; providing tactile stimulation to areas of preserved sensation (arms, top of shoulder, face) as appropriate.

4. Risk for neurovascular dysfunction
   a. Outcomes: Maintenance of circulation in extremities, no evidence of neurovascular dysfunction, demonstration of correct body positioning techniques, verbalization of relationship between neurovascular status and damage, attendance at a smoking cessation program or verbalization of risk of smoking, recognition of symptoms of neurovascular dysfunction.
   b. Interventions: Immobilizing of joints above and below site of fracture; monitoring neurovascular status in any area with a brace, cast, or splint; positioning the extremity to maximize blood flow and reduce edema; avoiding flexion of the affected extremity; monitoring effectiveness of vasodilators; encouraging attendance at smoking cessation program; instructing in recognition of symptoms of neurovascular dysfunction and measures to relieve it.

5. Risk for activity intolerance
   a. Outcomes: Heart rate, rhythm, and blood within normal parameters for the patient; implementation of self-care activities without fatigue; maintenance muscle mass, strength, and joint range of motion.
   b. Interventions: Using range of motion exercises, turning and repositioning, maintaining proper body alignment, monitoring physiologic responses to increased activity (increase or decrease as appropriate), providing assistive devices and adaptive equipment to maximize independence and promote activity, encouraging performance of self-care activities to tolerance, establishing a realistic exercise program, instructing about how to take pulse and blood pressure.

6. Chronic pain
   a. Outcomes: Management pain program, adjustment of behavior and participation in activities, use of pain-relieving techniques (diversion, relaxation, imagery, biofeedback, self-hypnosis), desire for ongoing counseling.
   b. Interventions: Monitoring pain symptoms and effectiveness of relief measures; instructing individual in pain-relieving techniques; developing a pain management plan; consulting with chronic pain experts; instructing in body mechanics, posture, and positioning to minimize effects of pain; monitoring effectiveness of pain medications; protecting patient from injury due to sensory/perceptual deficits; referring for counseling and long-term follow-up.

Table 32-3: Health Education Tips To Prevent/Minimize Secondary Disabilities

Body System	Prevention Strategies	Minimize Effect Of Disability
Cardiovascular	Maintain weight at norm Avoid alcohol, drug abuse, caffeine, high fat and high cholesterol diet, immobility Maintain activity level to tolerance Avoid venous stasis Use antiembolic stockings	Follow cardiovascular treatment regimen Initiate further lifestyle changes Position to avoid vascular compromise
Cardiopulmonary	Coordinate activity and rest periods to maximize oxygenation Avoid persons with respiratory infections Seek health care intervention for signs and symptoms of respiratory problems Maintain adequate hydration and humidification Perform pulmonary toilet Monitor respiratory status Get pneumococcal and influenza immunizations	Use incentive spirometer Relaxation techniques Use controlled cough techniques Perform chest physiotherapy Follow cardiopulmonary treatment regimen Reduce oxygen demand
Genitourinary	Empty bladder completely every 2-4 hours Maintain adequate fluid intake and monitor intake/output Use clean intermittent catheter technique Maintain acid urine Avoid urinary stasis Minimize urethral trauma Get baseline and follow-up urologic studies Monitor prostate, diabetes, and other chronic conditions	Follow urinary treatment regimen Incorporate new urinary care programs into regular care regimen
Gastrointestinal	Avoid high fat, high cholesterol foods Maintain weight at norm Sit upright when eating or drinking Avoid smoking, alcohol, or caffeine Eat a high fiber diet Avoid overuse of laxatives, enemas, or cathartics Maintain regular bowel program Maintain activity level	Make additional diet modifications as recommended Follow bowel program Follow gastrointestinal treatment program
Psychosocial	Avoid alcohol and drug use Seek counseling for psychological or social problems Participate in support groups Use coping techniques Seek individual, group, or family therapy to improve relationships Participate in spiritual activities according to your beliefs	Learn new coping techniques Attend group or individual therapy sessions Enroll in alcohol or drug cessation programs Explore other therapists, spiritual support personnel, or support groups until one meets your needs Seek additional help if initial efforts do not work
Skin	Perform regular skin inspection Change position frequently enough	Incorporate skin care regimen into daily routine

continued on page 466

Table 32-3: Continued

Body System	Prevention Strategies	Minimize Effect Of Disability
Skin	to avoid pressure areas Maintain adequate nutrition Maintain activity level to tolerance Seek health care assistance at the first sign of skin breakdown or other problem Use assistive devices and aids to minimize pressure	Change skin care products Evaluate wheelchair, bed, wheelchair cushion, etc. on a regular basis Increase frequency of position changes Avoid pressure on fragile skin
Musculoskeletal	Avoid bowel, bladder, and skin complications Maintain joint range of motion Avoid contractures Avoid flexion positions Activity level to tolerance Early mobilization Low calcium diet (if recommended) Adequate calcium intake Estrogen replacement therapy (for postmenopausal females) Maintain weight at norm Avoid smoking, alcohol, and caffeine Follow a safety program	Incorporate new exercise regimen into daily routine Follow musculoskeletal treatment regimen Use pain management techniques including imagery, relaxation therapy, and diversional activities Therapeutic positioning Positioning aids

References and Selected Bibliography

Cardenas, D.D., Farrell-Roberts, L., Sipski, M.L., & Rubner, D. (1995). Management of gastrointestinal, genitourinary, and sexual function. In I.S. Lanig, T.M. Chase, L.M. Butt, K.L. Hulse, & K.M.M. Johnson (Eds.), *A practical guide to health promotion after spinal cord injury* (pp. 120-144). Gaithersburg, MD: Aspen.

DeVivo, M.J., & Stover, S.L. (1995). Long-term survival and causes of death. In S.L. Stover, J.A. DeLisa, & G.G. Whiteneck (Eds.), *Spinal cord injury: Clinical outcomes from the model systems* (pp. 289-316). Gaithersburg, MD: Aspen.

Dijkers, M.P., Abela, M.B., Gans, B.M., & Gordon, W.A. (1995). The aftermath of spinal cord injury. In S.L. Stover, J.A. DeLisa, & G.G. Whiteneck (Eds.) *Spinal cord injury: Clinical outcomes from the model systems* (pp. 185-212). Gaithersburg, MD: Aspen.

Fuhrer, M.F. (1991). Setting the conceptual landscape. In P.L. Graitcer & F.M. Maynard (Eds.), *Proceedings from the first colloquium on preventing secondary disabilities among people with spinal cord injuries, February 27-28, 1990,* (pp. 37-46). Atlanta, GA: U.S. Department of Health and Human Services, Centers for Disease Control and Prevention.

Hayes, K. V. (1995). Validation of risk factors for disuse syndrome. In M.J. Rantz & P. LeMone (Eds.), *Classification of nursing diagnoses: Proceedings of the eleventh conference* (pp. 244-245). Glendale: CINAHL Information Systems.

Hoeman, S.P. (Ed.). (1996). *Rehabilitation nursing: Process and application.* St. Louis, MO: Mosby.

Lanig, I.S., Chase, Butt, Hulse & Johnson, (1996). Historical perspectives. In I.S. Lanig, T.M. Chase, L.M. Butt, K.L. Hulse, & K.M.M. Johnson (Eds.), *A practical guide to health promotion after spinal cord injury* (pp. 5-11). Gaithersburg, MD: Aspen.

LeMone, P., & Burke, K.M. (Eds.). (2000). *Medical-surgical nursing: Critical thinking in client care.* (2nd ed) Menlo Park: Addison-Wesley.

Maynard, F.M., Karunas, R.S., Adkins, R.H., Richards, J.S., & Waring III, W.P. (1995). Management of the neuromusculoskeletal systems. In S.L. Stover, J.A. DeLisa, & G.G. Whiteneck (Eds.), *Spinal cord injury: Clinical outcomes from the model systems* (pp. 145-169). Gaithersburg, MD: Aspen.

Menter, R.M., & Hudson, L.M. (1995). Effects of age at injury and the aging process. In S.L. Stover, J.A. DeLisa, & G.G. Whiteneck (Eds.), *Spinal cord injury: Clinical outcomes from the model systems* (pp. 272-288). Gaithersburg, MD: Aspen.).

Monahan, F.D., & Neighbors, M. (1994). *Pocket companion for nursing care of adults.* Philadelphia: W.B. Saunders.

Ragnarsson, K.T., Hall, K.M., Wilmot, C.B., & Carter, R.E. (1995). Management of pulmonary, cardiovascular, and metabolic conditions after spinal cord injury. In I.S. Lanig, T.M. Chase, L.M. Butt, K.L. Hulse, & K.M.M. Johnson (Eds.), *A practical guide to health promotion after spinal cord injury* (pp. 79-99). Gaithersburg, MD: Aspen.

Schmitt, J., Midha, M;, & McKenizie, N. (1995). Medical complications of spinal cord disease. In R. R. Young & R. M. Woolsey (Eds.), *Diagnosis and management of disorders of the spinal cord* (pp. 297-315). Philadelphia: W.B. Saunders.

Sparks, S.M., & Taylor, C.M. (1998). *Nursing diagnosis reference manual* (4th ed.). Springhouse IL: Springhouse Corporation.

Sparks, S.M., Taylor, C.M., & Dyer, J.G. (*1996*). *Nursing diagnosis pocket manual*. Springhouse IL: Springhouse Corporation.

Stover, S. L., Lloyd, L.K., Waites, K. B., & Jackson, A. B. (1995). In R. R. Young & R. M. Woolsey (Eds.), *Diagnosis and management of spinal cord disease* (pp. 198-210). Philadelphia: W. B. Saunders Co.

Trieschmann, R. (1987). *Aging with a disability*. New York: Demos Publications.

Yarkony, G.M., & Heinemann, A.W. (1995). Pressure ulcers. In S.L. Stover, J.A. DeLisa, & G.G. Whiteneck (Eds.), *Spinal cord injury: Clinical outcomes from the model systems* (pp. 100-119). Gaithersburg: Aspen.

Zejdlik, C. P. (1992). *Management of spinal cord injury* (2nd ed.). Boston: Jones and Bartlett.

CHAPTER

Aging with a Disability

Grace Nolde-Lopez, MS, RN, CRRN

I.   Learning Objectives

A. Discuss normal changes that occur with aging.

B. Identify changes that occur when aging with spinal cord impairment (SCI), including physical and emotional changes.

C. Discuss nursing diagnoses common for aging individuals with SCI, and identify appropriate interventions.

D. Apply knowledge regarding the aging process of individuals with SCI.

II.   Introduction

Aging is a natural process and frequently involves many losses that may by physical, sociocultural, and psychological. Aging with SCI may create new problems, and during times of loss, people can either stagnate or grow (Ebersole & Hess, 1985). Nurses are frequently in contact with persons during vulnerable and changing times and can use their knowledge and caring interventions to influence individuals to develop and grow.

A. **Scope**

This chapter describes the losses and changes that occur in the aging of persons with SCI and delineate interventions to prepare and cope with them.

B. **Demographics**
1. Survival of persons with spinal cord injury (SCI)
   a. Prior to World War II, survival following SCI was rare.
   b. During 1940's, some individuals with paraplegia survived with the goal of a sedentary life. Survival increased due to development of sulfa drugs.
   c. During 1950's and 1960's, survival improved with development of antibiotics.

    d. In the late 1960's and 1970's, there was an increase in the number of survivors with higher level injuries primarily due to emergency medical system (EMS).

    e. During the 1970's and 1980's, ventilator support resulted in survival of individuals with high level tetraplegia.

    f. The early 1990's saw the first group of long-term SCI survivors, and the effects of aging with a disability were noted.

  2. Aging with SCI

    a. Twenty years post-injury is the point when aging problems begin to increase (Menter, 1993).

    b. In 1988, 25 percent of all SCI survivors were over 20 years post-injury, and 40 percent of SCI survivors were over 45 years old (Paralyzed Veterans of America, 1991).

    c. In 1990 the Centers for Disease Control made recommendations for studying aging in SCI to:

      (1) Develop wellness programs for persons with SCI to promote health and prevent related disease and rehospitalizations.

      (2) Train health care professionals to educate patients about ways to prevent complications from becoming major medical problems.

    d. In 1993, the first National Institute on Disability and Rehabilitation Research and Training Center on Aging with Spinal Cord Injury was established as a joint project between Craig Hospital and the Department of Rehabilitation Medicine at the University of Colorado Health Science Center (Hulse, 1996). Its goals include:

      (1) Identify risk factors for secondary impairments, disabilities, and handicaps.

      (2) Establish health-promoting strategies and health-protecting interventions.

      (3) Study the relationship of actual health and health-related quality-of-life issues for those with SCI.

  3. Age at time of injury: Older individuals have a greater physiological risk following SCI and develop problems sooner (Devivo, M., Kartus, P., Rutt, R., Stover, S., & Fine, P., 1990).

C. Etiology

Individuals have unique predispositions that determine their response to the aging process. Factors that influence the aging process include:

1. Genetics
2. Lifestyle
3. Adaptation to stress
4. Sociological role
5. Trauma
6. Gender
7. Living and working environment

D. Physical and Psychosocial Changes of Normal Aging

Some physical changes of aging are obvious, such as the telltale gray hair or crow's feet around the eyes. However, it is important for the nurse to be aware of less overt physical and psychosocial changes.

1. Physical changes

    a. Skin

      (1) Precipitating factors

        (a) Diet

        (b) Sun exposure

        (c) Intrinsic factors

        (d) Biological aging (Yarkony, 1993)

      (2) Skin becomes thinner and pigment changes

      (3) Decreased rate of cell replacement

      (4) Loss of subcutaneous fat (decreased padding)

      (5) Decreased moisture content

      (6) Frank degradation of collagen in the dermis

      (7)   Increased susceptibility to shearing forces for older skin, this can be more disastrous than vertical pressure (Yarkony, 1993).

      (8)   Decreased sweat gland activity

  b. Strength, endurance, and flexibility

      (1)   Decreased stamina

      (2)   Decreased strength and flexibility

      (3)   Decreased muscle mass and range of motion

  c. Bone Density/Osteoporosis

      (1)   A normal phenomenon of aging, but accelerated by inactivity and lack of weight bearing.

      (2)   Causes loss of bone mass with increased risk for fractures and collapsed vertebrae

      (3)   Four times more prevalent in women, especially with declining estrogen levels (Ebersole & Hess, 1985)

      (4)   Causes kyphosis and posture changes

  d. Joints and connective tissue

      (1)   Vertebral disks become thin, causing a shortening of the trunk.

      (2)   Average loss of 1.2 cm of height every 20 years as aging occurs (Jacobs, 1981).

      (3)   Decreased tissue elasticity more prevalent due to damage and overuse syndrome

  e. Gastrointestinal (GI)

      (1)   Decreased peristaltic action affects absorption and blood flow to the GI tract.

      (2)   Vitamin and mineral deficiencies due to faulty absorption and inadequate diet

      (3)   Slower transmission of neural impulses and a decreased awareness of bowel evacuation (Ebersole & Hess, 1985)

      (4)   Increased problems with constipation and increased concern about bowel function

  f. Cardiovascular changes

      (1)   Reduced efficiency and contractile strength

      (2)   Decreased physical conditioning can lead to stiffening of heart muscle fibers and prolonged contraction duration.

      (3)   Elasticity and integrity of blood vessels decrease.

      (4)   Increased risk of orthostatic hypotension

  g. Respiratory changes

      (1)   Decreased ability to expand lungs due to thoracic changes

      (2)   Lungs become more rigid.

      (3)   Due to structural changes, a cough may be less effective (Ebersole & Hess, 1985).

  h. Genitourinary/Reproductive

      (1)   Renal function declines with age, and kidneys lose nephrons over time, causing fluid regulatory function impairment.

      (2)   Prostatic enlargement can cause vesicoureteral reflux. Seminal pathway infections can evolve into epididymitis or prostatitis.

  i. Other

      (1)   Body fat content increases by 16 percent, from age 25 to 75, while water weight decreases by 8 percent (Jacobs, 1981).

      (2)   Sweat glands decrease in size and also, inactivity causes a decrease in the body's cooling mechanism (Ebersole and Hess, 1985).

      (3)   Increased risk for diabetes due to decreased ability to metabolize glucose

      (4)   Thyroid activity decreases and pituitary gland shrinks.

2. Psychosocial changes

  a. Diminished financial resources

  b. Aging family and caregivers

  c. Death of a spouse

  d. "Empty" nest syndrome

  e. Changes in coping behavior

      (1)   Increased abuse of alcohol and/or drugs

      (2)   Suicide rates increase concomitantly with age until about 80 years old (Ebersole & Hess, 1985).

E. **Effects of SCI on the Aging Process**

Just as all individuals have their own unique responses to aging, persons with a disability find they age sooner and with greater intensity. Nurses should be aware of these changes, so they can educate and troubleshoot problems for individuals with SCI.

1. Factors that influence aging of individuals with SCI.
   a. Type and severity of injury
   b. Age at injury and duration of injury
   c. Pre-existing injuries and concomitant injuries
   d. Social and environmental support
2. Aspects of SCI that promote aging
   a. Decreased ability to regulate body temperature
   b. Decreased lung capacity and decreased cough effort, depending on level of spinal cord lesion
   c. Decreased gastrointestinal motility
   d. Rapid decrease in total bone mineral content in first four months following injury.
3. Physical changes
   a. Skin
      (1) Decreased sitting tolerance
      (2) Increased need for pressure relief
      (3) Greater prevalence of skin sores, which may respond to supplemental vitamin A, vitamin C, and zinc.
   b. Musculoskeletal
      (1) Persons with SCI have 63 percent of normal bone density (Walters, Sie, and Adkins, 1993).
      (2) Pathological fractures are 10 times more common in persons with complete SCI than in those with incomplete SCI (Walters et al., 1993).
      (3) Heterotropic Ossification (HO): "Late" onset can occur at any time in response to trauma; peaks at two months following trauma. HO in hip joints may cause increased compensation and stress in lumbar spine.
      (4) Upper Extremities: Most vulnerable areas: shoulder, elbow, and wrist. Shoulder pain is a problem in 51 percent of persons with long-term SCI. Over-use syndrome is one of the common problems that cause upper extremity degeneration. Inactivity can also cause degenerative changes. It is important to find a balance between enough activity to protect the joint and too much activity.
   c. Strength, endurance, and fatigue
      (1) Decreases with the increasing years of SCI.
      (2) Aging individuals with SCI may have only enough endurance to do personal care activities.
      (3) Decline of energy with aging reduces the ability to handle the daily stress of life with a disability (Trieschmann, 1987).
   d. Cardiovascular
      (1) Sedentary lifestyle, obesity, and decreased lean body mass all increase the risk of cardiovascular problems; individuals with SCI are at high risk (Ragnarsson, 1993).
      (2) Arteriosclerotic degeneration of the spinal cord's small arteries may cause further neurological damage.
      (3) Emotional stress and depression can cause increased risk for heart attack and stroke. SCI survivors can have excessive emotional stress accumulate over time, as a result of various life changes. Depression may also be affected by an endocrine dysfunction, such as increased secretion of cortisol and decreased secretion of endorphins (Ragnarsson, 1993).
      (4) Cardiovascular disease has been the number one cause of death in some studies of SCI, but difficult this varies depending on how broad a definition of cardiovascular disease was used (Trieschmann, 1987).
      (5) Risk of hypertension for injuries below level of T7.

e. Respiratory
   (1) Most common cause of death one year after injury are respiratory problems (Wilmot & Hall, 1993).
   (2) Progressive scoliosis and kyphosis can be deleterious to the respiratory system. Individuals with high quadriplegia are especially at risk.
   (3) Spasticity can impair the expansion of the diaphragm, due to markedly increased intra-abdominal pressure.
   (4) Abdominal distention or bloating from gas can impair respiratory function significantly (to the point of death) (Cosman, Stone, & Perkash, 1993).
   (5) Acute gastric dilation (air swallowed into the stomach during rapid respiration and becoming trapped.) can act as a splint against the diaphragm.
   (6) Other infections can present as respiratory difficulty, due to bronchiolar asthmatic reaction to an infection.

f. Neurologic
   (1) Post Traumatic Syringomyelia
       (a) Occurs in 6 percent of cases (Wilmot & Hall, 1993).
       (b) Initially presents as increased spasticity, sweating, and progressive loss of sensation.
       (c) If original lesion is cervical and syrinx is progressive and left untreated, vital capacity may decrease.
   (2) Autonomic nervous system becomes less efficient with aging.
       (a) Increased difficulties with bowel program
       (b) Increased problems with orthostatic hypotension and thermoregulation.
   (3) Nerve entrapment neuropathies due to over-use syndrome (Lammertse, 1993).
   (4) Post-Traumatic cystic myelopathy

g. Genitourinary
   (1) Renal function declines with age and kidneys lose nephrons over time, causing fluid regulatory function impairment.
   (2) Pyelonephritis, the most common renal disease in the elderly, also occurs frequently among persons aging with SCI (Lanig, 1993).
   (3) Increased risk of urinary tract infection
   (4) Prostatic enlargement can cause:
       (a) Vesicoureteral reflux
       (b) Seminal pathway infections that can evolve into epididymitis or prostatitis
       (c) Increased risk for of autonomic dysreflexia
   (5) Estrogen deficiencies and physical changes can cause:
       (a) Conversion the vaginal environment to alkaline environment, predisposing to infection
       (b) Urethral prolapse
       (c) Urethritis and urethrocili irritated by indwelling catheter
   (6) Bladder cancer
       (a) Increased incidence of bladder cancer in the SCI population (Lanig, 1993).
       (b) Possible connection between chronic cystitis and bladder cancer (Lanig, 1993).
       (c) Possible increased risk of squamous cell carcinoma with long term use of indwelling catheters and irritation from catheter tip (Lanig, 1993).

h. Immune system
   (1) Immune system becomes less efficient with aging, causing increased susceptibility to infections and neoplastic disease.
   (2) Persons aging with SCI are at a greater risk for developing immune dysfunction due to:
       (a) Sleep deprivation/interruption
       (b) Drug use/abuse
       (c) Constant pain
       (d) Consequences of loss of central nervous system control over lymphoid organs
       (e) Depression (Nash & Fletcher, 1993).

       (3)   Repeated infections of urinary tract, respiratory system, and skin can diminish the defense system of individuals with SCI.

   i. Metabolic
      (1)   Glucose intolerance associated with aging may occur sooner in SCI (Bauman, 1993).
      (2)   Prolonged inactivity can impair glucose tolerance associated with hyperinsulinemia.
      (3)   Basal energy expenditure (BEE) is depressed.
      (4)   Depressed BEE can lead to weight gain even with minimal overeating on a daily basis.
      (5)   Individuals with SCI have lipid levels similar to those of persons with obesity and diabetes (Bauman, 1993).

   j. Gastrointestinal
      (1)   High rate of gallstone disease in persons with SCI above T10 level (Cosman et al., 1993).
      (2)   Chronic gastric dilation may occur in quadriplegics with chronic abdominal distention/mega-colon.
      (3)   Gastric motility is decreased.
      (4)   Increased problems with bowel evacuation and constipation
      (5)   High risk for symptomatic hemorrhoids due to sedentary lifestyle, constipation, and trauma during bowel program (Cosman et al., 1993).

   k. Chronic pain
      (1)   Pain is typically described as burning, tingling, electric shock, vise-like, or pins and needles.
      (2)   90 percent of the SCI population experiences chronic pain (Lammertse, 1993).
      (3)   SCI pain is believed to be of neurologic origin (Lammertse, 1993).
      (4)   Categories of chronic SCI pain:
         (a) Central spinal cord pain
         (b) Functional pain
         (c) Spinal cord dysethetic pain syndrome
         (d) Phantom pain
         (e) Deafferentation pain

4. Functional Changes: The aging process profoundly affects functional levels. Functional changes affect vocation, living arrangements, and relationships.
   a. Personal assistance needs increase with aging due to problems of over-use and increased fatigue. Problems of costs and availability may limit access to such assistance.
   b. Environmental and equipment needs
      (1)   Accessibility needs will increase, perhaps requiring a wheelchair or van with a lift; cost may be prohibitive.
      (2)   Psychosocial support systems frequently decrease with aging
   c. Mobility changes.

5. Psychosocial Changes: Psychosocial changes may not be obvious, but they can have a profound impact on a person's response to aging. When discussing the aging process in SCI, it is important to involve family, especially if they provide care.
   a. Psychological
      (1)   Quality of life and will to live are strongly correlated with the need to be free to make one's own decisions. Living in an institution is a great fear of many persons with SCI (Trieschmann, 1987).
      (2)   Depression does not seem to be as high as in the non-disabled aging population. Many individuals living with a disability for 20 years or more had a very positive outlook (Trieschmann, 1987).
      (3)   Stress management skills may need to be used, due to changes of aging.
   b. Social
      (1)   Spouses may develop their own medical problems related to aging and be unable to provide care, as they have done in the past.
      (2)   Number of friends may decrease, along with their social support.
      (3)   Involvement in activities or social groups may decrease due to fatigue, and may lead to social isolation.

III. Nursing Assessment

A. **Initial and Ongoing Assessment**

The initial nursing assessment is helpful in identifying current or past problems related to aging.

1. Skin
   a. History of previous or current skin problems; scars have only 80 percent of the strength of the original skin.
   b. Nutritional deficiencies, especially of Vitamin C, may predispose the individual to pressure ulcers (Yarkony, 1993).
   c. Nicotine use is a risk factor for skin breakdown.
   d. Adequate hydration is essential to skin health.
   e. Examine for any areas of skin breakdown and determine the cause. Identify ways to modify activity and eliminate causes of skin breakdown.
   f. Albumin, hematocrit and hemoglobin levels may be evaluated.
2. Osteoporosis
   a. History of previous fractures
   b. Nutritional assessment of calcium intake. Adequate calcium intake should be maintained throughout life to preserve bone mineral content (Bauman, 1993).
3. Heterotropic ossification: History of decreased joint range of motion (ROM), localized swelling, joint erythema, warmth, pain, and history of recent trauma
4. Upper extremities (UE)
   a. Assess for any significant pain in UE.
   b. Check patient's current ROM in UE.
   c. Try to identify specific structures causing the pain.
5. Strength and endurance
   a. Assess level of fatigue at end of the day.
   b. Assess individual's resources to assist with activities of daily living to allow preservation of strength for social or work interactions.
   c. Assess cause of fatigue:
      (1) Lack of sleep
      (2) Poor nutrition
      (3) Loss of attendant help
      (4) Inadequate stress management
      (5) Infections
      (6) Current medication regime
6. Cardiovascular
   a. Basic assessment of adequacy of cardiovascular function
   b. Assessment of risk factors for cardiovascular disease
   c. History of autonomic dysreflexia
   d. Assess for excess emotion, stress, or personality characteristics that may predispose to cardiac problems.
   e. Cardiac work-up according to patient's symptoms and risk for cardiac disease
7. Respiratory
   a. History of shortness of breath and upper respiratory infection
   b. Smoking history (past and present)
   c. Assess use of chest and accessory muscles of thorax and neck to see if they are being used to compensate.
   d. Assess for history/problems with sleep apnea.
   e. Assess vital capacity
8. Neurological
   a. Assess cognition and orientation.
   b. Assess for neurological deficits, including decreased sensation and strength.
   c. Assess spasticity.
9. Genitourinary
   a. Regular follow-up of neurogenic bladder over the life span

b. BUN and creatinine level may not show moderate renal dysfunction; determine glomeruli filtration rate and renal plasma flow.

c. Assess frequency of infection and effectiveness of treatment.

10. Metabolic
   a. Body weight
   b. Serum glucose level or tolerance

11. Gastrointestinal
   a. Assess for problems with bowel evacuation or management
   b. Assess elements of bowel program: diet, medications, timing, and frequency.
   c. Cancer screening
      (1) Fecal occult blood has high number of false positive results in the SCI population.
      (2) Sigmoidoscopic exam yields more accurate results.
   d. If problems with incontinence are due to anal sphincter changes, may need to change bowel program.

12. Chronic pain
   a. Dorsal Root Entry Zone (DREZ) procedure may be done to eliminate and treat deafferent pain.
   b. Treatment of chronic SCI pain requires an interdisciplinary team approach.

IV. Expected Outcomes/Interventions

A. **Nursing Diagnoses**
   1. Fatigue related to aging with a disability, as manifested by inability to participate in usual activities or exhaustion at the end of the day.
      a. Expected outcomes:
         (1) Individual will be able to discuss causes of fatigue and share feelings regarding impact of fatigue.
         (2) Individual will prioritize activities.
         (3) Individual will investigate resources for personal assistance care.
         (4) Individual will participate in activities that stimulate and balance physical, cognitive, affective, and social domains.
      b. Interventions:
         (1) Discuss causes of fatigue.
         (2) Allow individual to express feelings of frustration concerning fatigue.
         (3) Assist individuals to identify the time of day they have the most energy and evaluate ways to rearrange their schedules, identify tasks that can be delegated, or explore options related to personal care attendants.
         (4) Teach/discuss energy conservation techniques.
         (5) Assist with stress management techniques.

   2. Over-use Syndrome, as manifested by pain and decreased strength in joints and extremities frequently used in daily activities.
      a. Expected outcomes:
         (1) Individuals will demonstrate exercise program and use of adaptive devices to increase mobility or avoid over-use.
         (2) Individuals will have decreased symptoms of over-use syndrome after interventions applied.
         (3) Individuals will be able to verbalize what activities aggravate their over-use syndrome.
      b. Interventions:
         (1) Institute UE exercise programs to prevent degenerative problems and pain.
         (2) Identify causative and contributing factors that may be aggravating condition.
         (3) Investigate if surgical procedure is an option.
         (4) Use pain and anti inflammatory medications as indicated.
         (5) Identify alternative treatment to alleviate discomfort, (e.g., heat, cold, massage.) Involve the patient in identifying these methods.
         (6) Avoid activities or prolonged positioning that aggravate the condition, (e.g., proving

the prone position can increase stress on upper extremity).

    (7)   Recommend adaptive devices and equipment, (e.g., sliding board, electric wheelchair).

    (8)   Allow individual to verbalize feelings of loss in having to utilize increased amount of adaptive equipment.

V. Health Education Tips

Education about general health and type of lifestyle is important for persons with SCI. These individuals have rates of death from cardiovascular disease equal to or greater than those of the general population (Trieschmann, 1987). Health education should include:

A. Good nutrition

B. Routine exercise program

C. Promotion of self-actualization during the aging process

D. Assessment of adequate coping skills and positive self-talk (Hulse, 1996).

E. Importance of following through with routine health maintenance and screening.

Practical Application

J.M. is a 55-year-old retired professor of biology who sustained a C6 spinal injury in a diving accident in 1961. He is now 39 years post injury and has retired because his physical problems are increasing with age and he has chronic fatigue.

Urologic: Bladder management was with an indwelling catheter. In 1966, J.M. had an ileo-conduit procedure performed because of recurrent urinary tract infections and stone encrustation of a thick-walled contracted bladder. In 1990, on ultrasound examination, he was found to have a 1.2 centimeter stone in the left kidney and a smaller stone in the right kidney. In 1991, he developed increasing spasticity in his legs and abdomen, which improved with antibiotic management. The left kidney stone was then removed.

Bowel: For years, J.M. managed his bowels with a warm soap suds enema once every four days. In recent years, he has had increasing frequency of bowel incontinence, ranging from mucus discharge, to hard solid stool, to diarrhea. In addition, he has had excessive flatulence and an increase in waist size from 36 to 48 inches. He has attempted to take more fiber but this does not seem to resolve the problem. A recent x-ray of the abdomen showed diffused impaction of the large bowel. Magnesium citrate was taken, followed by massive stool results. He now continues to have bowel irregularity and spontaneous stools.

Skin: In 1961, J.M. developed a sacral pressure ulcer, which was treated with flap closure that never completely healed. For 32 years, he had a chronic fistula track draining serous fluid, which required dressings. In 1993, an infection occurred underneath the flap and surgical revision was necessary. An extensive myocutaneous flap was successful with no subsequent problems.

Extremity Edema: For many years, J.M. has had very severe edema in the feet and ankles. Elastic stockings were not successful in controlling the problem. Recently, he has been using compression inflation boots, which squeeze the legs in a peristaltic fashion every ten to twenty seconds. J.M. uses the boots for 30 minutes before arising and again for 30 minutes after getting into bed at night.

Respiratory: J.M.'s last reported respiratory infection was in 1985. He receives a yearly influenza vaccine and has had the pneumococcal vaccination.

Nursing Assessment and Interventions: J.M. has had numerous medical problems since his spinal cord injury. To further investigate whether appropriate interventions are needed, the nurse should ask the following questions: Age 55 is earlier than most people are able to retire. Will this affect his current standard of living? What about his insurance benefits? Is he having any additional problems with urinary infections or kidney stones, and how regularly will he need urological evaluations in the future? Increasing his bowel program from every four days to every other day may decrease the frequency of bowel incontinence. He should also use a combination of fiber, stool softener, and stimulant to maintain bowel regularity. Is his increase in waist measurement related to megacolon or obesity? What is his weight and is it controlled? Since J.M. has had flap surgery, his skin is at risk at the scar area. What steps is he taking to prevent breakdown in the future? How long is he sitting each day? How are his weight shifts done? Does he use a power recline wheelchair? Is he maintaining good nutrition? An evaluation of his usual diet may be helpful. For his respiratory status, J.M. has been proactive by receiving his yearly flu shots. Further investigation should be done to see if he is having any problems with his respiratory status related to increasing abdominal girth. J.M. should also be counseled on the importance of receiving his routine health screening as appropriate for his age.

References and Selected Bibliography

Bauman, W. (1993). The endocrine system. In G. Whiteneck, S. Charlifue, K. Gerhardt, D. Lammertse, S. Manley, R. Menter, K. Seedroff, (Eds.), *Aging with spinal cord injury* (pp. 139-157). New York: Demos.

Bortz, W. (1982). Disuse and aging. *Journal of the American Medical Association*, 248(10), 1203-1207.

Brenes, G., Dearwater, S., Shapera, R., LaPorta, R., & Collins, E. (1986). High density lipoprotein cholesterol concentrations in physically active and sedentary spinal cord injured patients. *Archives of Physical Medicine and Rehabilitation*, 67(7), 445-450.

Breslow, L., & Somers, A. (1977). A lifetime health-monitoring program. *The New England Journal of Medicine, 296*(11), 601-608.

Butt, L., & Fitting, M. (1993). Psychological adaptation. In G. Whiteneck, S. Charlifue, K. Gerhardt, D. Lammertse, S. Manley, R. Menter, K. Seedroff, (Eds.), *Aging with spinal cord injury* (pp. 199-210). New York: Demos.

Carpentino, L. (1989). *Nursing diagnosis application to clinical practice* (3rd ed.). Philadelphia: J.B. Lippincott.

Cosman, B., Stone, J., & Perkash, I. (1993). The gastrointestinal system. In G. Whiteneck, S. Charlifue, K. Gerhardt, D. Lammertse, S. Manley, R. Menter, K. Seedroff, (Eds.), *Aging with spinal cord injury* (pp. 117-127). New York: Demos.

Crewe, N., Athelstan, G., & Krumberger, J. (1979). Spinal cord injury: A comparison of preinjury and postinjury marriages. *Archives of Physical Medicine and Rehabilitation*, 60(6), 252-256.

DeVivo, M., Kartus, P., Rutt, R., Stover, S., & Fine, P. (1990). The influence of age at time of spinal cord injury on rehabilitation outcome. *Archives of Neurology, 47*(6), 687-693.

Donovan, W., Dimitrijevic, M., Dahm, L., & Dimitrijevic, M. (1982). Neurophysiological approaches to chronic pain following spinal cord injury. *Paraplegia, 20*, 135-146.

Ebersole, P. & Hess, P. (1985). *Toward healthy aging human needs and nursing response*. St. Louis, MO: C.V. Mosby.

Hackler, R. (1977). A 25-year prospective mortality study in the spinal cord injured patient: Comparison with the long-term living paraplegic. *The Journal of Urology, 117*(4), 486-488.

Hall, D., Blackett, A., Zajac, A., Switala, S., & Airey, C. (1981). Changes in skinfold thickness with increasing age. *Age and Aging, 10*, 19-23.

Hulse, K. (1996). Promoting emotional, social, intellectual, and spiritual health. In I. Lanig, T. Chase, L. Butt, K. Hulse, & K. Johnson, *A practical guide to health promotion* (pp. 81-133). Gaithersburg, MD: Aspen.

Jacobs, R. (1981). Physical changes in aged. In M.O. Devereaux, L.H. Andrus, C.D. Scott, M.I. Gary. (Eds.), Eldercare: *A guide to clinical geriatrics* (pp. 31-47). New York: Grune and Stratton.

Krause, J., & Crewe, N. (1991). Chronological age, time since injury and time of measurement: Effect on adjustment after spinal cord injury. *Archives of Physical Medicine and Rehabilitation, 72*(2), 91-100.

Lammertse, D. (1993). The nervous system. In G. Whiteneck, S. Charlifue, K. Gerhardt, D. Lammertse, S. Manley, R. Menter, K. Seedroff, (Eds.), *Aging with spinal cord injury* (pp. 129-137). New York: Demos.

Lanig, I. (1993). The genitourinary system. In G. Whiteneck , S. Charlifue, K. Gerhardt, D. Lammertse, S. Manley, R. Menter, K. Seedroff, (Eds.), *Aging with spinal cord injury* (pp. 105-115). New York: Demos.

Lanig, I., Chase, T., Butt, L., Hulse, K., & Johnson, K., (1996). *A practical guide to health promotion after spinal cord injury.* Gathersburg, MD: Aspen.

Madersbacher, G., & Oberwalder, M. (1987). The elderly para- and tetraplegic: Special aspects of the urological care. *Paraplegia, 25,* 318-323.

Menter, R. (1993). Issues of aging with a spinal cord injury. In G. Whiteneck , S. Charlifue, K. Gerhardt, D. Lammertse, S. Manley, R. Menter, K. Seedroff, (Eds.), *Aging with spinal cord injury* (pp. 1-8). New York: Demos.

Nash, M., & Fletcher, M. (1993). The immune system. In G. Whiteneck, S. Charlifue, K. Gerhardt, D. Lammertse, S. Manley, R. Menter, K. Seedroff. (Eds.), *Aging with spinal cord injury* (pp. 159-181). New York: Demos.

Nepomuceno, C., Richards, J., Gowens, H., Stover, S., Rantanuabol, U., & Houston, R. (1979). Pain in patients with spinal cord injury. *Archives of Physical Medicine and Rehabilitation, 60*(12), 605-609.

Paralyzed Veterans of America. (1991). *Study on the economic consequences of traumatic spinal cord injury.* (From Aging with SCI. Whiteneck et.al. 1993, p. 1).

Pender, N. (1987). *Health promotion in nursing practice* (2nd ed.). Norwalk: Appleton and Lange.

Ragnarsson, K. (1993). The cardiovascular system. In G. Whiteneck , S. Charlifue, K. Gerhardt, D. Lammertse, S. Manley, R. Menter, K. Seedroff, (Eds.), *Aging with spinal cord injury* (pp. 79-92). New York: Demos.

Silfverskiold, J., & Waters, R. (1991). Shoulder pain and functional disability in spinal cord injury patients. *Clinical Orthopaedics and Related Research, 272*(11), 141-145.

Trieschmann, R. (1987). *Aging with a disability.* New York: Demos.

Walters, R., Sie, I., & Adkins, R. (1993). The musculoskeletal system. In G. Whiteneck, S. Charlifue, K. Gerhardt, D. Lammertse, S. Manley, R. Menter, K. Seedroff, (Eds.), *Aging with spinal cord injury* (pp. 53-71). New York: Demos.

Whiteneck, G. (1993). Learning from recent empirical investigations. In G. Whiteneck, S. Charlifue, K. Gerhardt, D. Lammertse, S. Manley, R. Menter, K. Seedroff, (Eds.), *Aging with spinal cord injury* (pp. 23-37). New York: Demos.

Whiteneck, G., Charlifue, S., Frankel, M., Fraser, M., Gardner, B., Gerhart, K., Kirshman, K., Menter, R., Nuseibeh, I., Short, D., & Silver, J. (1992). Mortality, morbidity, and psychosocial outcomes of persons spinal cord injured more than 20 years ago. *Paraplegia, 30,* 617-630.

Whiteneck, G., Charlifue, S., Gerhart, K., Lammertse, D., Manely, S., Menter, R., & Seedroff, K. (Eds.). *Aging with spinal cord injury.* New York: Demos.

Wilmot, C., & Hall, K. (1993). The respiratory system. In G. Whiteneck , S. Charlifue, K. Gerhardt, D. Lammertse, S. Manley, R. Menter, K. Seedroff, (Eds.), *Aging with spinal cord injury* (pp. 93-104). New York: Demos.

Wylie, E. & Chakera, T. (1988). Degenerative joint abnormalities in patients with paraplegia of duration greater than 20 years. *Paraplegia, 26,* 101-106.

Yarkony, G. (1993). Aging skin, pressure ulcerations, and spinal cord injury. In G. Whiteneck, S. Charlifue, K. Gerhardt, D. Lammertse, S. Manley, R. Menter, K. Seedroff, (Eds.), *Aging with spinal cord injury* (pp. 39-52). New York: Demos.

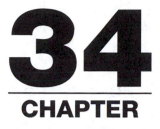

CHAPTER

Quality Improvement and Outcome Evaluation

Andrea Kaye Hixon, MS, RN, C, CNAA

I. Learning Objectives

A. Compare and contrast the traditional Quality Assurance (QA) approach to approaches utilizing the principles of Continuous Quality Improvement (CQI).

B. List three domains of quality.

C. Differentiate the purpose and methods for developing standards and practice guidelines.

D. Identify three advantages of clinical pathways.

II. Introduction

Professional nursing has a rich history related to improving the quality of health care. Florence Nightingale gathered data and utilized mortality and morbidity measures to evaluate and publicize outcomes of care provided to soldiers during the Crimean War. She also developed standards to improve clinical care and environmental conditions during that time (Lang & Marek, 1991).

Nightingale's approach remains the foundation for improving quality in healthcare. The American Nurses' Association (ANA) advocated development and implementation of quality assurance programs more than 15 years before such activities were mandated by external accreditation agencies such as the Joint Commission for Accreditation of Healthcare Organizations (JCAHO) or the Commission on Accreditation of Rehabilitation Facilities (CARF).

In 1966, the ANA advocated development of standards for nursing practice. ANA's leadership to ensure safety and quality practice resulted in national professional standards of care and practice (Smeltzer, 1988). The adoption of these standards foundation led to practice, education, and research guidelines for nurses, health care teams, and specialty nursing organizations such as the American Association of Spinal Cord Injury Nurses (AASCIN), to link quality practice to health outcomes.

This chapter provides information on strengthening the role of the professional nurse to measure, assess, and improve care. These concepts and principles are applicable to any phase of spinal cord impairment (SCI) practice, useful in a variety of practice settings, and dependent upon strong health care team collaboration.

III. Background/Evolution of Quality Programs

A. **Quality Assurance** (QA) refers to programs with a primary goal of improving care, which are often driven by external accreditation agencies (CARF, 1993; JCAHO, 1995).
   1. Focus: Typical QA programs included concurrent or retrospective audits, medical record reviews, and observations of the care delivered. Measures are often limited to the nursing unit and cannot be compared or benchmarked externally.
   2. Limitations: Typical QA approaches are limited to a single nursing unit or department and are not multidisciplinary in scope. Data gathering is time-consuming and results shared infrequently with other care providers. Activities are problem-focused, rather than focused on the needs and expectations of customers. Frequently, departments cast blame on one another rather than working collaboratively. QA efforts and activities are often not supported nor viewed favorably by employees (Masters & Schmele, 1991).
   3. Scope: Traditional nursing QA approaches have been criticized as limited in scope and lacking an organizational perspective (Patton & Stanley, 1993).

B. **Domains of Quality**
   1. During the past three decades, the focus of health care policy and accreditation efforts has shifted among three domains of quality -- process, structure, and outcomes (Lang & Marek, 1991).
   2. Norma Lang, RN, and Avedis Donabedian, MD are prominent healthcare quality theorists. Their work describes and categorizes evaluation measures (Hegyvary, 1991; Holden, 1989).
   3. "Using Donabedian's conceptual framework, indicators are developed to measure the structure, processes, and outcomes of care" (Patton & Stanley, 1993; p. 19).
      a. Process Indicators: Measures with a focus on the manner (sequence of steps) in which care or services are delivered. SCI examples include: functional assessment, provision of health education, discharge planning, performance of diagnostic tests, consultations, and referrals.
      b. Structure Indicators: Measures reflecting the SCI environment of care settings such as staffing, staff qualifications, preparation of equipment, and availability of supplies.
      c. Outcomes Indicators: Measures used to evaluate the end results of care. In SCI settings, functional assessment is a key clinical outcome.
         (1) "Outcome is defined as a measurable change in a client's health status related to the receipt of nursing care" (Marek, 1989; p. 3). Marek's framework identifies eight categories for consideration in measuring patient outcomes.). Table 34-1 describes the framework for outcome indicators.
         (2) The ANA is currently conducting research to demonstrate causal relationships between nursing care and health outcomes. "Outcome Indicators focus on how patients, and their conditions, are affected by their interactions with nursing staff" (ANA, 1995a).
   4. Lang and Donabedian stress the need for measurements in each of the domains. Outcomes are dependent upon structures and processes to deliver care. Therefore, outcomes must be measured in relation to the process and structure domains (Patton & Stanley, 1993

C. **Spinal Cord Injury Program Evaluation**
   1. Functional status measures are the primary focus for efforts to evaluate outcomes of rehabilitation, home health care, and long-term care.

Table 34-1: Framework for Outcome Indicators

Outcome	Description	Examples
Physiological Status	Processes that maintain life	Blood pressure, pulse, temperature, lung sounds, skin integrity, weight
Psychosocial	Examines a client's patterns of behavior	Mentation, emotion, attitude, mood, affect, social functioning
Functional Measures	Examines a client's level of self-care	Activities of daily living, mobility, communication, external support for care
Behavior Domain	Concerns activities, skills, and actions of a client	Application of knowledge and skills, level of compliance, motivation, and competence
Knowledge	Cognitive level of understanding	Knowledge of diagnosis, diet, medications, and treatments
Symptom Control	(closely related to physiological)	Pain, level of comfort, fatigue, nausea, constipation, and diarrhea
Home Maintenance	Refers to functioning of family in the home environment	Family living patterns, environment support, safety issues, family roles
Patient Satisfaction	Useful but difficult outcome to measure	Art of care, technical aspects of care

From "Outline Measurement in Nursing," by K. Marek, 1989, *Journal of Nursing Quality Assurance*, 4 (1), pp. 1-9.

2. CARF requires rehabilitation facilities to conduct formal program evaluation and report performance (outcome measurements) to consumers.
3. The Uniform Data System for Medical Rehabilitation (1990) is one of several systems of measures of functional status used in SCI programs. The system defines six categories and outlines 18 areas for evaluating function. The Functional Independence Measure (FIM) is included. Each functional area is evaluated using a seven-level scale, with a rating of "1" indicating need for total assistance and a rating of "7" denoting total independence. As the FIM is more widely utilized and results are reported, outcomes may be used to compare program effectiveness and to identify program excellence ("benchmarking"). The FIM includes:
   a. Self-care: eating, grooming, bathing, upper body dressing, lower body dressing, toileting
   b. Sphincter control: bladder management, bowel management
   c. Mobility: transfers to/from bed/wheelchair/chair; transfers to tub/shower; transfer to toilet
   d. Locomotion: walking/wheelchair; stair climbing
   e. Communication: comprehension and expression
   f. Social cognition: social interaction, problem-solving, memory

D. **Promoting Quality Nursing Care**
   1. Since Nightingale, there has been concern for defining, standardizing, and evaluating nursing care. Current efforts reflect an interdisciplinary approach to standardizing care. Highlights of efforts to promote quality are depicted in Table 34-2.
   2. Standardization efforts continue as interdisciplinary groups of SCI professionals collaborate in the development of practice guidelines to improve the processes, structure, and outcomes of care.

E. **Quality Assurance versus Research**

Table 34-2: Quality Improvement Timeline

Year	Event
1856	Nightingale's "Notes on Nursing"
1946	Minimum standards for nurses in hospitals (American College of Surgeons)
1953	Joint Commission on Accreditation of Hospitals (JCAH) published first *Standards for Hospital Accreditation*
1967	Evaluation was defined as one element of the nursing process (Yura & Walsh, 1967)
1973	American Nurses Association (ANA) published general *Standards of Nursing Practice*
1977	ANA published specialty standards: Standards of Rehabilitation Nursing Practice
1986	ANA & Association of Rehabilitation Nurses (ARN) published joint standards: *Standards of Rehabilitation Nursing Practice*
1990	Agency for Health Care Policy & Research (AHCPR) established
1994	American Association of Spinal Cord Injury Nurses (AASCIN) published *Standards of Spinal Cord Injury Nursing Practice*
1994	JCAHO published criteria supporting concepts of continuous quality improvement, standards for *Improving Organizational Performance* (IOP)
1996	AASCIN published *Clinical Practice Guidelines: Autonomic Dysreflexia*

1. Quality improvement and research both use systematic methods to collect and measure data.
   a. Similarities:
      (1) Systematic data collection processes.
      (2) Analysis of data to draw conclusions.
      (3) Recommendations to improve care.
      (4) Wide dissemination of results and feedback.
   b. Differences:
      (1) QA usually limited to clinical practice. Research has a broader scope to include nursing education and administration.
      (2) QA traditionally focuses on problems.
      (3) Research focus is on the testing of hypotheses or generating of new knowledge that can be generalized beyond the current focus of study.
2. Both quality assurance and research are utilized by professionals to improve the quality and effectiveness of nursing care.

IV. Concepts of Continuous Quality Improvement (CQI)/ Total Quality Management (TQM)

During the 1990s, quality assurance methods have undergone a transition to embrace the principles of continuous quality improvement (CQI). The JCAHO's *Agenda for Change* also influenced this evolution (Nadzam, 1991; Patterson, 1993). JCAHO's accreditation standards promote the use of health outcome measurements and advocate that CQI concepts be systematically introduced throughout the organization.

A. **Definitions of CQI** (also known as "TQM -- total quality management")
   1. "A top-down management philosophy that implies an organizationwide, continuous commitment to the improvement of quality" (Masters & Schmele, 1991, p. 8).
   2. "The proactive approach that minimizes the potential for future errors rather than focusing on the resolution of problems after they have occurred --- quality is designed into services" (Dressman, 1993, p. 73).

3. "A long-term customer oriented cultural change ... may require several years to achieve quality and productivity gains" (Masters & Schmele, 1991, p. 15).

B. **Goal**: To change the processes and systems of health care organizations toward improved health care delivery and health outcomes. "QA provided a solid base upon which quality improvement can be built. Continuous quality improvement incorporates the strengths of QA, while broadening its scope, refining its approach, and utilizing tools used by industries to improve quality of products and services" (JCAHO, 1993).

C. **Paradigm Shift** (Refer Table 34-3)
   1. CQI/TQM requires new assumptions. Hospital leaders must establish a vision and identify priorities for quality improvement. Their mission and goals must be communicated throughout the organization.
   2. Most problems in the organization are due to systems and processes of care, not individual incompetence. Deming, a pioneer in the field of CQI, hypothesized that 85-95 percent of all errors in an organization are due to the system, and not the employees (Deming, 1982; Lopresti & Whetstone, 1993).
   3. Healthcare organizations can improve care regardless of their present performance.
   4. Healthcare organizations must embrace CQI in order to survive the current, competitive environment. Estimates are that 30 - 40 percent of all healthcare expenditures are the result of poor quality (Ernst, 1994; Lopresti & Whetstone, 1993; Masters & Schmele, 1991).
   5. CQI principles and methods can work in health care organizations. Berwick, et al, (1991) demonstrated the success of CQI methods at Yale-New Haven Hospital with strong physician and employee commitment.

D. **Guiding Principles of Organizational Quality Improvement**
   1. Organization defines the needs and expectations of internal and external customers. The basis for defining quality and establishing goals is the needs and expectations of external customers.
   2. Leaders of the organization define and communicate the mission, vision, and strategic goals of the organization after a consideration of customer needs.

Table 34-3: Comparison of Quality Assurance (QA) to Continuous Quality Improvement (CQI)/Total Quality Management (TQM)

QA	CQI/TQM
Planning for quality at the unit or department level	Organization's leaders responsible for planning throughout the organization
Problem-focused	System/process-focused
Individuals, managers, or small groups within the service or unit work on problem	Cross-functional teams established with broad organizational representation; widespread employee involvement
Monitors practitioners	Measures organizational processes that cross department lines
Practitioners determine priorities	Priorities identified based upon assessment of customer needs and expectations
Medical record reviews; observation of care/patient outcomes	Expanded tools and methods to include flowcharting, Pareto diagrams, histograms, cause-and-effect charts
Individuals/departments are responsible for competency	Organization assumes responsibility for competency of all employees and professional staff

3. Analysis and improvement efforts are focused on processes and systems. Employee teams use CQI philosophy and tools such as flowcharting, Pareto diagrams, fishbone charts, and graphic data presentations to analyze and improve processes.
4. Data provide the basis for decision-making.
5. Empowered employee teams survey customer needs, study and improve processes, and pilot new services.
6. Systems of performance evaluation and rewards are linked to success in meeting the strategic goals of organization.
7. Employee teams are recognized and rewarded.

V. Nursing Leadership for Accreditation

Healthcare providers and organizations are increasingly involved in assuring that programs are in compliance with established standards and regulatory mandates. The accreditation process is closely linked to an organization's quality improvement program. Accreditation now extends to virtually all practice settings and disciplines. Accreditation is linked to a high level of excellence and may be required for reimbursement or academic affiliations

A. **Joint Commission for Accreditation of Healthcare Organizations (JCAHO)**
1. Mission: "To improve quality of care provided to the public" (JCAHO, 1995, p. ii)
2. History: At the turn of the century, there was great variability in clinical practice and hospital conditions.
   a. 1917: the American Medical Association (AMA) and the American College of Surgeons agreed to work together to improve quality of care
   b. 1951: Joint Commission formed
   c. 1953: Joint Commission first published standards for accreditation
   d. 1980s: JCAHO broadened its accreditation focus to include long-term care, ambulatory care, home care, hospice, mental health, and managed care.
   e. 1996: specific standards for rehabilitation are included in JCAHO's chapters on Patient Assessment, Patient Education, and Care of Patients.
3. JCAHO is the nation's largest healthcare accrediting body, with nearly 8,300 healthcare organizations accredited.
4. Accredited organizations undergo formal review every three years.
5. Organizations voluntarily seek JCAHO accreditation to:
   a. Enhance medical staff recruitment
   b. Enhance community confidence
   c. Fulfill partial requirements for state and/or federal licensure
   d. Facilitate third-party payment for services provided
6. *Agenda for Change* promotes dual role: accreditation as well as education and consultation for promoting quality.
7. JCAHO's Standards for Improving Organizational Performance (IOP)
   a. Requirements for quality improvement focus on the organization rather than individual departments. "There must be a planned, systematic organization-wide approach to design, measure, assess, and improve performance... which shifts the primary focus from performance of individuals to the performance of the organization's systems and processes..." (JCAHO, 1994)
   b. The standards for IOP promote integration of the concepts of continuous quality improvement without mandating use of any particular management style or tools, or approaches. (Refer to Table 34-4).
      IOP requirements:
      (1) Measurement of organization's systems and processes to assess present level of performance
      (2) Establishment of organizational priorities for improvement
      (3) Comparison of level of performance with that of other organizations (benchmarking)
      (4) Design of new processes or systems
      (5) Measurement of outcomes

Table 34-4: Framework for Improving Organization Performance (IOP)

Required Element	IOP Activity
Measurement	Organization collects baseline data concerning performance: Process and outcome indicators Customer needs and expectations Customer satisfaction with current services Infection control Safety/Risk management Utilization information
Assessment	Organization compares data internally over time, compares data to accreditation standards and practice guidelines, compares data/benchmarks performance to other facilities
Planning	Leaders guide performance improvement efforts Leaders ensure that processes are implemented and structures created Written organizational plan guides efforts All departments and disciplines collaborate in carrying out IOP
Design and Improvement	Leaders assure that process, function, and service of the organization are consistent with mission Design/redesign incorporates consideration of customer needs Information about the performance of similar processes, functions, or service in other facilities is considered in design

  c. IOP must measure performance of processes in all patient care functions, such as Assessment, Patient/Family Education, and Care of Patients. Improvements are evaluated over time, rather than according to arbitrarily assigned thresholds. Example: The admission process to a SCI facility takes four days. A team works to simplify paperwork and improve communication. The plan of care is now finalized in less than 3 days.

B. **Commission on Accreditation of Rehabilitation Facilities (CARF)**
 1. Mission: "To serve as the preeminent standards-setting and accrediting body promoting quality services to people with disabilities" (CARF, 1993, p. vii).
  a. Formed in 1966 as a not-for-profit organization for promoting outcomes of rehabilitation
   (1) Involves consumers, providers, and purchasers of all types of rehabilitative services
   (2) Has adapted specialized standards for programs addressing needs of individuals with SCI
  b. Types of Standards
   (1) Organizational standards: Leadership, information management, consumer-based planning, human resources, staff competency, safety, staffing methodologies
   (2) Program standards: General standards for inpatient comprehensive rehabilitation; address admission and orientation, assessment of client's needs, individualized program planning and referrals, discharge planning, and follow-up measurement of patient outcomes
   (3) Specific program standards: Specialized standards applicable to special populations (such as SCI), chronic pain management, brain injury, and vocational training
 2. Accreditation Process
  a. Organization completes a self-study
  b. After completion of self-study, organization applies to CARF
  c. CARF sends site survey team consisting of an administrator, a nurse, and physiatrist
  d. Full CARF accreditation is granted for three-year period
  e. Team conducts survey activities: opening orientation with administrators, tour of facility, interview with staff members and clients, review of required documents, and exit conference

    f. The decision for accreditation is made based upon the organization's compliance with CARF standards

3. Unlike JCAHO, CARF includes nursing on its Advisory Board.

4. There are many similarities in the standards, composition of site team, and survey activities for both accrediting organizations. The current philosophy and frameworks for both organizations are closely linked to the Malcolm Baldrige National Quality Criteria.

VI. Professional Standards and Guidelines

Healthcare professionals embrace a variety of activities to improve healthcare delivery. Professional organizations such as the American Nurses' Association (ANA) and the Association of Rehabilitation Nurses (ARN) have been in the forefront of standards development. AASCIN established a systematic process to support development of practice guidelines.

A. **Quality**
1. Quality: a subjective perception of the structure, process, or outcome components of health care (Duchane, 1996).
2. Clinical Indicator is "A quantitative measure that can be used as a guide to monitor and evaluate the quality of important patient care and support service activities" (Williams, 1991, 1). Interdisciplinary indicators are effective and powerful collaborative tools.

B. **Standards**
1. Standards: "Authoritative statements promulgated by the profession by which the quality of practice, service, or education can be judged" (ANA, 1991, p. 7).
2. Standards of Nursing Practice: "Authoritative statements that describe a level of care or performance common to the profession of nursing by which the quality of nursing practice can be judged" (McDonald, 1993, p. 130). The ANA's model for standards development includes both standards of care and stet of professional performance. Standards apply to all registered nurses engaged in clinical practice regardless of practice setting or level of preparation.

C. **Guidelines**
1. Practice Guidelines are "Systematically developed statements based on available scientific evidence and expert opinion, ...assist practitioner and patient decisions about appropriate health care for specific clinical conditions" (McDonald, 1993, p. 130).
2. Guidelines are being developed and promoted by the Agency for Health Care Policy and Research (AHCPR) and by specialty practice organizations such as AASCIN. Guidelines focus on a clinical condition or diagnosis.
    a. AHCPR's methodology for guideline development:
        (1) Conduct extensive literature review of the topic, diagnosis or clinical condition selected.
        (2) Analyze information for empirical evidence.
        (3) Identify health outcomes.
        (4) Utilize peer and field reviews to test the validity, reliability, and usefulness of the draft guideline.
    b. Guidelines should reflect the professional judgment and consensus of experts in that particular practice areas if the literature is incomplete or not research based.
    c. Guidelines should be disseminated for field use.
    d. Guidelines should be updated periodically with new information or practice changes.

D. **Development**
AASCIN promotes development of standards and guidelines to improve the quality of care of individuals with spinal cord injury.
1. "The function of established standards in an evaluation process is to organize professionally desirable criterion against which performance and outcomes can be measured" (AASCIN, 1994: p. 2).
2. AASCIN's standards of Spinal Cord Injury Nursing Practice (AASCIN, 1994) includes:

Purpose, Philosophy, Mission Statement, Scope of Practice, Code for Nurses, Standards of Care, and Standards of Professional Performance. The document is supported by a glossary and definition of terms.

3. AASCIN membership was queried in 1993 to elicit its ranking of diagnoses or clinical conditions for practice guideline development. Twelve topics were identified.
   a. Autonomic Dysreflexia (AD) was chosen as the top priority for guideline development. The guideline has been developed, field-tested, and refined by two consensus forums. The AD guideline was disseminated to all AASCIN members and the collaborating professional organizations in 1996.
   b. Clinical practice guidelines have been developed for Bladder Management.

4. AASCIN supports the Consortium for Spinal Cord Medicine Clinical Practice Guidelines. AASCIN is represented on the steering committee and provides clinical experts to serve as Panel Members for guideline development and review.

E. **Evaluation of Nurse Competency**
   1. JCAHO and CARF standards address the organization's responsibility for assuring competence of all staff who provide care. Determination of competence for nurses may be categorized in several stages (Patterson, 1993);
      a. Pre-Employment: Nurses are evaluated based upon educational preparation, licensure, and previous clinical experience. Organizational standards vary, but there is a growing trend to verify all information provided by nurse applicants.
      b. Orientation: Specialized training is provided at the time of employment and entry to duty. Orientation must be individualized to the needs of the nurse, the expectations of the position, and current skills. In the SCI practice setting, nurses may be expected to demonstrate the wide range of skills appropriate to rehabilitation of SCI individuals and families. Evaluation of competence is ongoing throughout this phase.
      c. Staff development: The provision of ongoing education in the workplace is driven by external standards, nursing licensure requirements, new technology, and organizational policy. There should be a dynamic, continuous process for assuring ongoing nurse competence. In the SCI setting, inservice education may be related to clinical care, equipment or products, newly introduced medications, research-based changes in practice, and team skills.
   2. Advanced education, experience, or responsibility for providing care may be addressed by certification. In 1973, the ANA developed a comprehensive program for identifying and formally recognizing nurses with specialized knowledge and application of nursing theory. The certification process includes formal testing and evaluation. Nurses who attain certification have demonstrated a high level of professional achievement.
   3. AASCIN has funded model projects related to SCI nurse competencies (Thomason, Binard, Gregg, Padios, & Trotman, 1996).

VII. Clinical Pathways

In many organizations, health care providers are developing their own protocols to guide treatment of specific clinical conditions. Development of clinical pathways, also known as "critical paths," "CareMap"™, or "managed care plans" is being driven by the managed care environment. Managed care is "An organized system of care that seeks to influence the selection and utilization of health services of an enrolled population and ensures that care is provided in a high-quality, cost effective manner" (Phoon, Corder, & Barter, 1996). In the past, clinical algorithms and plans of care were discipline-specific and may have led to divergent approaches or fragmenting of patient care.

A. **Development**
Clinical pathways were first developed at the New England Medical Center Hospital in the 1980's.
   1. Definition: "Clinical pathways reflect the accumulated knowledge from many disciplines and in effect map out the progression of suggested interventions expected to promote optimal outcomes for patients with similar problems" (Ebener, Baugh, & Formella, 1996)

2. Clinical pathways reflect the essential activities / interventions that must be done and time frames for their measurement.

B. **Advantages of Clinical Pathways**
   1. Clinical pathways are closely linked to CQI. The goal is focus on improving processes and reducing variation in care (Spath, 1993).
   2. Pathways delineate roles of each member of the healthcare team.
   3. The needs of internal and external customers are assessed.
   4. Ongoing measures of performance are incorporated.
   5. Progress is systematically assessed, and patient outcomes are utilized as evaluation measures, at predetermined intervals.
   6. Health education is enhanced.
   7. Most organizations report improved medical record documentation.
   8. Clinical pathways drive team collaboration for providing and evaluating care.

C. **Limitations:**
   1. Some professionals disdain additional limitation or restriction of their professional autonomy.
   2. Implementation fails when key health care team members are not involved.
   3. May be criticized as being concerned only with financial performance.
   4. There is anecdotal reporting, but little empirical evidence, of effectiveness in improving quality or producing cost savings (Ebener et al., 1996).

VIII. Opportunities for the Professional Nurse

There are multiple quality improvement roles and responsibilities for the nurse in the SCI setting. Nurses should incorporate standards of their professional and specialty practice organizations in their education and daily practice. There are many opportunities for professional nurses to participate locally and nationally in the development of clinical practice guidelines.

Within their practice settings, nurses can contribute to all aspects of the organization's plan for improving performance by gathering data, comparing data, and supporting process improvements. Nurses have long been advocates for assessing client needs and expectations as well as measuring consumer and family satisfaction with service provided. Nurses have been in the forefront of the transition to managed care and development of clinical pathways.

Practical Application

The Northside Rehabilitation Center is a 115-bed facility providing comprehensive rehabilitation. The program is accredited by JCAHO and is seeking CARF accreditation. The quality program has been centralized to an eight-person quality assurance committee representing nursing and medicine. The activities of the committee have been limited to medical record reviews and some observations of care. The other disciplines periodically gather data as related to the care they provide. The center recently developed a patient satisfaction survey which will be given to all clients and their families.

Increasingly, staff have been concerned about the frequent problem of skin breakdown in both children and adults, particularly those with spinal cord injury. The center's leadership and staff have recently committed themselves to a program of continuous quality improvement in this area. Table 34-5 outlines the quality improvement process for this practical application.

Table 34-5: Summary of Case Study

CQI Principles	How utilized by Northside staff to improve skin care:
Employee TQM involvement	The Quality Improvement (QI) committee was restructured to include representatives of all disciplines; all committee members received comprehensive training in CQI/TQM methods and quality tools.
	The staff contributed to a review of the literature for existing standards and practice guidelines. There was a commitment to involve all staff by using clinical rounds, case presentations, and widespread sharing of data.
Definition of Quality	The QI committee proposed a definition of quality skin care and established performance goals. Staff supported the idea of preventing any nosocomial skin breakdown and committed themselves to state-of-the-art wound healing. Leadership supported the goals and pledged to assure adequate resources.
Analysis of Process	Committee studied the processes affecting skin care. Assessment of skin integrity was flowcharted. A cause and effect (fishbone) diagram was developed by staff to identify possible causes of skin breakdown. A Pareto chart was developed to demonstrate the most commonly occurring sites of anatomic skin breakdown.
Assessment of customer needs	The QI committee identified the internal customers (employees) who were involved in this process and held focus groups to identify their needs and concerns. Each discipline was asked for strengths and barriers to providing high-quality skin care.
	External customers (clients, families, caregivers) were also involved in focus groups discussing skin care. Questions regarding their perception of the quality of skin care and additional concerns in the definition of quality were addressed.
Accumulation and measurement particularly of data	Staff had varied assumptions about the quality of skin care; several complicated wound cases had recently been observed and several nosocomial breakdowns had occurred in the SCI population. The committee established guidelines for measuring all skin breakdown and adopted a staging system - all staff were trained.
	There is a program for continuous monitoring of all skin care.
Assessment of data	Initial data revealed an incidence rate of nosocomial breakdown lower than that reported for similar facilities. Although no causal relationships could be established, there were several breakdowns attributed to the use of braces and other prosthetic devices. The largest number of pressure areas were on the heels. This fact was consistent with information from the literature review.
Design	The process for initial skin integrity assessment was revised and added to the admission clinical pathway. Skin care is now included in the treatment plan.
	Clients with braces or special prosthetic equipment are to be assessed more frequently. Clinical staff consulted with different product vendors and manufacturers to explore alternative devices; extra padding was added to the devices causing skin breakdown. Staff education was provided concerning use of prosthetic devices.
	Interdisciplinary staff developed treatment approaches for each stage of skin breakdown. Client and family/caregiver education was broadened to include shared responsibilities for skin integrity.
Teamwork	All disciplines were involved in each phase of the improvement process-- review of the literature, assessment of customer needs, measurement, and design of treatment approaches. The shared responsibility was recognized by center leaders at the annual awards banquet. There is increased pride in the high quality of skin care being provided by the center.

References and Selected Bibliography

American Association of Spinal Cord Injury Nurses (AASCIN). (1994). *Standards of spinal cord injury nursing practice*. Jackson Heights, NY: Author.

American Nurses' Association (ANA). (1973). *Standards of nursing practice*. Kansas City, KS: Author.

American Nurses' Association (ANA) and Association of Rehabilitation Nurses (ARN). (1986). *Standards of rehabilitation nursing practice*. Kansas City, KS: Author.

American Nurses' Association (ANA). (1977). *Standards of rehabilitation nursing practice*. Kansas City, KS: Author.

American Nurses' Association. (ANA) (1991a). *Standards of clinical nursing practice*. Kansas City, KS: Author.

American Nurses' Association. (ANA) (1991b). Task force on nursing practice standards and guidelines: Working paper. *Journal of Nursing Quality Assurance*, 5(3), 1-17.

American Nurses' Association (ANA). (1994). *Standards for nursing professional development: Continuing education and staff development*. Washington, DC: Author.

American Nurses' Association (ANA). (1995a). *Nursing care report card for acute care*. Washington, DC: Author.

American Nurses' Association (ANA). (1995b). *Nursing data systems: The emerging framework*. Washington, DC: Author.

Berwick, D., Godfrey, A., Roessner, J. (1991). *Curing health care: New strategies on quality improvement*. San Francisco: Jossey-Bass.

Brown, M. G. (1994). *Baldrige award winning quality: How to interpret the Malcolm Baldrige award criteria* (4th ed.). White Plains, NY: Quality Resources.

Commission on Accreditation of Rehabilitation Facilities (CARF). (1993). *Standards manual for organizations serving people with disabilities*. Tucson, AZ: Author.

Crosby, P. (1979). *Quality is free*. New York: New American Library.

Deming, W. (1982). *Out of the crisis*. New York: New American Library.

Donabedian, A. (1980). *The definition of quality and approaches to its assessment*. Ann Arbor, MI: Health Administration Press.

Dressman, K. (1993). Lessons learned from an early TQM effort: Surgical prophylaxis. *Journal of Nursing Care Quality*, 7(4), 73-81.

Duchane, P. (1996). Total quality management and outcome evaluation. In S. Hoeman, (Ed)., *Rehabilitation nursing: Process and application* (pp. 2, 87-98). St. Louis, MI: Mosby

Ebener, M., Baugh, K., & Formella, N. (1996). Proving that less is more: Linking resources to outcomes. *Journal of Nursing Care Quality*, 10(2), 1-9.

Ernst, D. (1994). Total quality management in the hospital setting. *Journal of Nursing Care Quality*, 8(2), 1-8.

Fields, W., & Siroky, K. (1994). Converting data into information. *Journal of Nursing Care Quality*, 8(3), 1-11.

Gillem, T. (1988). Deming's 14 points and hospital quality: Responding to the consumer's demand for the best value health care. *Journal of Nursing Care Quality*, 2(3), 70-78.

Heacock, D., & Brobst, R. (1994). A multidisciplinary approach to critical path development: A valuable CQI tool. *Journal of Nursing Care Quality*, 8(4), 38-41.

Hegyvary, S. (1991). Issues in outcomes research. *Journal of Nursing Quality Assurance*, 5(2), 1-6.

Holden, L. (1989). Quality, standards, and criteria: A physician and nurse perspective. *Journal of Nursing Quality Assurance*, 3(2), 27-33.

Hoyman, K., & Gruber, N. (1992). A case study of interdepartmental cooperation: Operating room acquired pressure ulcers. *Journal of Nursing Care Quality, Special Report*, Supp l: 12-17.

Joint Commission on Accreditation of Healthcare Organizations (JCAHO). (1993). *1994 Comprehensive accreditation manual for hospitals*. Oakbrook Terrace, IL: Author.

Joint Commission on Accreditation of Healthcare Organizations (JCAHO). (1994). *1995 Comprehensive accreditation manual for hospitals*. Oakbrook Terrace, IL: Author.

Joint Commission on Accreditation of Healthcare Organizations (JCAHO). (1995). *1996 Comprehensive accreditation manual for hospitals*. Oakbrook Terrace, IL: Author.

Katz, J., & Green, E. (1992). *Managing quality: A guide to monitoring and evaluating nursing services*. St. Louis, MO: Mosby.

Lang, N. & Marek, K. (1991). The policy and politics of patient outcomes. *Journal of Nursing Quality Assurance*, 5(2), 7-12.

Lopresti, J., & Whetstone, W. (1993). Total quality management: Doing things right. *Nursing Management*, 24(1), 34-36.

Marek, K. (1989). Outcome measurement in nursing. *Journal of Nursing Quality Assurance*, 4(1), 1-9.

Masters, F., & Schmele, J. (1991). Total quality management: An idea whose time has come. *Journal of Nursing Quality Assurance*, 5(4), 7-16.

McDonald, S. (1993). Standards and guidelines. *SCI Nursing*, 10(4), 130-131.

Nadzam, D. (1991). The agenda for change: Update on indicator development and possible implications for the nursing profession. *Journal of Nursing Quality Assurance*, 5(2), 18-22.

Patterson, C. (1993). Joint commission nursing care standards: The framework for a comprehensive program to assess and improve quality. *Journal of Nursing Care Quality*, 7(2), 1-14.

Patton, S., & Stanley, J. (1993). Bridging quality assurance and continuous quality improvement. *Journal of Nursing Care Quality*, 7(2), 15-23.

Peters, D., & Pearlson, J. (1989). Clinical evaluation: Research or quality assurance. *Journal of Nursing Quality Assurance*, 3(3), 1-6.

Phoon, J., Corder, K., & Barter, M. (1996). Managed care and total quality management: A necessary integration. *Journal of Nursing Care Quality*, 10(2), 25-32.

Rehabilitation Nursing Foundation. (1987). *Concepts and practice: A core curriculum* (2nd ed.). Evanston, IL: Author.

Ribnick, P., & Carrano, V. (1995). Understanding the new era in health care accountability: Report cards. *Journal of Nursing Care Quality, 10*(1), 1-8.

Scholte, P. (1991). *The team handbook*. Madison, WI: Joiner Associates.

Smeltzer, C. (1988). Evaluating a successful quality assurance program: The process. *Journal of Nursing Quality Assurance, 2*(4), 1-10.

Spath, P. (1993). *Critical path management: New approaches for you to manage cost and quality*. San Diego, CA: Medical Management Development Associates

Thomason, S., Binard, J., Gregg, B., Padios, E., Trotman, J. (1996). Paradigm for SCI nurse competency on Adult-Geriatric SCI Rehabilitation Unit. *SCI Nursing, 13*(4), 101-104.

Uniform Data System for Medical Rehabilitation. (1990). *Guide for the use of the uniform data set for medical rehabilitation in the functional independence measure*. Buffalo, NY: State University of New York.

Williams, A. (1991). Development and application of clinical indicators for nursing. *Journal of Nursing Care Quality, 6*(1), 1-5.

Woodyard, L., & Sheetz, J. (1993). Critical pathway patient outcomes: The missing standard. *Journal of Nursing Care Quality, 8*(1), 51-57.

Yura, H., & Walsh, M. (1967). *The nursing process: Assessing, planning, implementing, and evaluating*. New York: Appleton-Century Crofts.

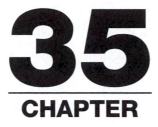

CHAPTER

Priorities for Research Related to SCI Nursing

Audrey Nelson, Ph.D., RN, FAAN

I. Introduction

The conduct of research and application of research findings to practice will: (1) Create an intellectually stimulating professional environment that ultimately facilitates professional growth and enhances clinical skills, (2) Enhance the professionalism and foster collegial relationships with other disciplines, (3) Improve the quality of life and health care delivery for patients, and (4) Promote a practice environment that fosters innovation.

II. Goals of Nursing Research in Spinal Cord Impairment (SCI)

A. Examine the effect of the organization, financing, and management of health care on delivery, quality, cost, access, and health outcomes.

B. Develop or design devices or equipment to improve nursing practice and the quality of life for persons with disabilities.

C. Advance knowledge leading to improvements in prevention, assessment, and interventions of nursing diagnoses or patient care problems.

D. Identify and develop ways to improve quality of care.

III. Nurses' Roles Related to Research

A. **Conduct of Research**: Not all nurses have the skills, knowledge, or interest necessary for developing and implementing research studies. However, all nurses are responsible for developing the skills and knowledge needed to become "consumers" of research.

B. **Research Dissemination**: Research as an isolated activity has little value in practice unless the findings are shared with others. Findings from research can be disseminated through:

1. Presentations, both within and outside the nursing profession.
2. Publications, including professional journals and books and lay publications targeted to the consumer.
3. Development of products, such as teaching guides, models of care delivery, staffing guidelines, and clinical practice guidelines.

C. **Research Utilization**: In this ever-changing, technology-driven society, the quick and effective application of research findings is critical to the establishment of the nursing profession as a research-based practice. Research utilization has implications for improved patient outcomes, nursing standards, policies and procedures, quality improvement, and care delivery systems.
1. Research utilization is defined as the process of analyzing and synthesizing research findings with the goal of implementing and refining a change in practice.
2. Research utilization process:
   a. Identify problem.
   b. Conduct literature search.
   c. Read and critique studies.
   d. Analyze and synthesize findings.
   e. Select change to be instituted.
   f. Obtain support for innovation.
   g. Institute pilot program.
   h. Refine innovation based on evaluation data.

IV. Historical Overview of the Contributions of Research in SCI

A. **Emergency/Trauma.** Goal: improving chances for survival of trauma.
1. Prior to the 1940's, surviving trauma was a major focus of research (DeJong & Batavia, 1991)
2. Sulfa drugs and penicillin dramatically improved survival from secondary complications such as urinary and respiratory tract infections (DeJong & Batavia, 1991)
3. Trauma researchers have developed tools to measure severity of injury, such as Injury Severity Scale (Baker, O'Neill, Haddon, & Long, 1974)) and Revised Trauma Score (Champion, Sacco, Carnazzo, Copes, & Fouty, 1981).
4. Use of high dose methylprednisolone (Bracken, Shepard, Collins, Holford, Young, Baskin, Eisenberg, Flamm, Leo-Summers, Maroon, et al. 1990) and GM-I ganglioside (Geisler, Dorsey, & Coleman, 1991; Paice & Magolan, 1991) to reduce effects of trauma.

B. **Acute Rehabilitation 1950's-1980's.** Goals: enhance recovery, reduce secondary complications, and maximize function and independence (DeLisa, 1992).
1. Specialized treatment of persons with SCI developed after WWII; focusing on reducing the functional limitations of disabilities and increasing ability to live independently and productively. The independent living movement (1970's) promoted research related to rehabilitation (DeJong & Batavia, 1991).
2. Renal disease was no longer a leading cause of death in persons with SCI due to careful monitoring using renal scans, ultrasound, urodynamic tests, and lithotripsy (DeLisa, 1992).
3. Intrathecal catheters and pumps allow for administration of neuroactive and possibly neurotropic agents directly onto the spinal cord for treatment of spasticity and pain (DeLisa, 1992; Paice & Magolan, 1991).
4. Decreased incidence of deep vein thrombosis, pulmonary embolism, and death in SCI due to use of low dosage heparin, external pneumatic compression, and electrical stimulation (DeLisa, 1992; Merli, et al., 1988; Merli et al., 1990).
5. Sexuality was male focused: improved technology for sperm collection, processing, and artificial insemination (DeLisa, 1992).

C. **Physical Restoration**
1. Functional electrical stimulation
   a. Neuromuscular electrical stimulation, also known as functional electrical stimulation (FES), has been used since the 1970's to restore purposeful movement to muscles

paralyzed by upper motor neuron lesions. FES is a means of eliciting activation of the nervous system in order to achieve a therapeutic functional effect.

    b. Documented functional use of FES for persons with SCI include ambulation (Mauritz &Peckham, 1987; Marsolais & Kobetic, 1983; Cybulski, Penn, & Jaeger, 1984), grasp/release of hand (Peckham, Marsolais, Mortimer, 1980), sensation, activation of diaphragm for respiratory pacing, control of urinary bladder, and fitness through an FES exercise cycle (Ragnarsson, Pollack, O'Daniel, Edgar, Petrofsky, & Nash, 1988).

    c. Documented therapeutic use of FES for persons with SCI include muscle strengthening, relief of spasticity, reversal of joint contractures, reversal of muscle adhesions, and correction of spinal curvature (Peckham, 1987).

    d. Although still in the experimental stage, this technology offers possible solutions to functional deficits.

  2. Regeneration:

    a. Progress is being made in neural regeneration on animal models (Harris, 1991). Scientists believe that SCI could be cured by first identifying genes that control growth and differentiation and then reconstructing the complex connections necessary for the central nervous system to function.

    b. Over 40 basic research studies were funded by the Department of Veteran Affairs (DVA) related to regeneration; 16 of them were in SCI (Seil, 1988)

D. Psychosocial Rehabilitation

  1. Violence: Using data from the Model Spinal Cord Injury Care System of the National Institute of Disability and Rehabilitation Research (NIDRR), it was determined that 1,732 cases were attributed to violent acts; African American individuals and persons of Hispanic origin represent an increasing percentage of new cases of injury due to violence (Seelman, 1995).

  2. Psychological consequences of SCI: There is considerable debate concerning the extent of psychological reaction to SCI (Craig, Hancock, Dickson, Martin, Chang, 1990).

E. Development /Technology

  1. Equipment design for mobility and independence

    a. Wheelchair sports led to aesthetically-pleasing designs of lighter and stronger wheelchairs.

    b. One-handed joy stick control drive cams

    c. Voice controlled wheelchairs and beds

    d. Environmental control systems

    e. Articulated prone carts, bowel care chairs

    f. Standing and walking aids: therapeutic and functional standing could be achieved in a greater number of individuals using existing technology; however, barriers still exist, which prevent the equipment from being more widely used (Jaeger, Yarkony, & Roth, 1989).

  2. Fitness equipment

    a. Voluntary arm-crank and wheelchair ergometry (Figoni, 1990)

    b. Electrical stimulation leg-cycle ergometry, including models such as the ES-LCE, ERGYS 1 and REGYS 1 (Figoni, 1990) which provide the SCI population with an aerobic exercise mode comparable to able-bodied bicycling or jogging (Glaser, 1990).

    c. Combined voluntary arm-crank and wheelchair ergometry and electrical stimulation leg-cycle ergometry (hybrid) (Figoni, 1990).

F. Health Services

  1. Changes in payment of health care services have resulted in new types of health care delivery systems (DeJong & Batavia, 1991).

  2. Goals have changed to increasing chances for long term survival and prospects for living an independent and productive life (DeJong & Batavia, 1991).

  3. National Spinal Cord Injury Database facilitates empirical research-- particularly in evaluation of outcomes. The National SCI Database originally was located in Phoenix, but

was moved to Birmingham (DeJong & Batavia, 1991). The Uniform Data System (UDS) for Medical Rehabilitation located in Buffalo, serves as a repository for outcome data, including data related to SCI (DeJong & Batavia, 1991).

4. Future health services research needs include (DeJong & Batavia, 1991, pp. 379, 387):

   a. How advances in emergency medical management and trauma care are changing the chances of survival for persons with SCI for given level of injury severity.

   b. How trauma care is affecting the degree of residual disability among survivors, especially among new survivors with high-level injuries.

   c. How trauma care is altering the mix of patients with SCI in medical rehabilitation, such as the proportion of patients who require permanent use of a ventilator.

   d. How trauma care may be reshaping the post-rehabilitation health care needs of selected survivors.

   e. Ways to improve access to rehabilitative care.

   f. Effects of payment mechanisms on rehabilitation utilization and outcome.

   g. Relative effectiveness of various outpatient modalities.

   h. Impact of health maintenance education on subsequent care utilization.

   i. Effective strategies to decrease high rate of unscheduled rehospitalizations; identification of causes and predictors of rehospitalizations.

   j. Lack of access to primary care for persons with SCI.

   k. Effects of aging with a disability.

   l. How many and what types of persons need and want user-directed attendant services.

   m. Whether a user-directed model of attendant services can foster a more independent and productive lifestyle.

   n. Whether user-directed attendant services foster health maintenance behaviors that help avert complications leading to rehospitalizations.

   o. Whether user-defined criteria can be developed whereby the quality of attendant service programs can be evaluated and alternative models can be critiqued.

   p. How eligibility and income requirements for attendant services affect incentives for work, and how disincentives can be averted.

   q. How attendant services should be financed.

   r. How much a national attendant care program would cost.

V. Research-Based Practice Guidelines

Research-based practice is facilitated through the implementation of Clinical Practice Guidelines. Several guidelines applicable to SCI have been published over the past seven years. The Agency for Health Care Policy and Research has published guidelines on urinary incontinence and pressure ulcers. The Consortium for Spinal Cord Medicine has developed a series of clinical practice guidelines for spinal cord injury and multiple sclerosis. Topics include autonomic dysreflexia, neurogenic bowel, depression, deep vein thrombosis, and pressure ulcers. Each guideline has a companion consumer guide. Copies of the guidelines are available through the Internet. Clinicians can benefit from these concise presentations of research findings and tools for applying research to practice.

VI. National Research Priorities

A. **AASCIN**: Research priorities were identified through a Delphi Study (Nelson, Goltry, Loewenhardt, & Moody, 1993).

   1. Effectiveness of home care, outpatient, or other community-based programs.

   2. Effective teaching programs for SCI patients/significant others.

   3. Aging in SCI and quality-of-life issues.

   4. Effective discharge planning.

   5. Define and promote community re-entry.

   6. Effectiveness of rehabilitation post-discharge.

   7. Define and promote quality of life post-discharge.

   8. Effective teaching programs for SCI nurses.

   9. Attributes of SCI centers with quality patient outcomes.

   10. Nursing's contribution to SCI patients' success at home.

11. Attendant care or caregiver strain/problems.
12. Rehabilitation outcome studies.
13. Defining and fostering community independence.
14. Home management of pressure sores.
15. Nursing interventions to decrease depression and self-neglect.
16. Prevention/treatment of pressure sores.
17. Wellness/fitness programs for SCI patients.
18. Nursing interventions to humanize hospital routines on SCI units.
19. Effective interdisciplinary team collaboration and role of nurse.
20. Prediction of outcomes in SCI nursing interventions.
21. Impact of health care policy reform on SCI nursing practice and patient care.

B. **Association of Rehabilitation Nurses** (ARN) established its first research agenda in 1996 through the use of an interactive computer technology . The following five research priorities were identified:
   1. Health promotion, and primary and secondary prevention, to facilitate management of self-care and independence for persons with or at risk for chronic illness and/or disability.
   2. Interventions and symptom management for persons with disabilities to maximize function.
   3. Community context of care for persons at risk or with a chronic illness and/or disability and their quality of life.
   4. Rehabilitation-nurse-sensitive outcomes and costs in the continuum of care and interdisciplinary setting(s).
   5. Rehabilitation practice and roles in the changing health care system.

C. **NIDRR.**
   Consensus Validation Conference on Prevention and Management of Urinary Tract Infections Among People with Spinal Cord Injuries (January, 1992) (NIDRR, 1991, pp. 203-204). Research priorities identified include:
   1. Identify the best methods for teaching people with SCI; to observe, monitor, and respond quickly to their bodies' prodromal warning signs that urinary tract infections may be developing.
   2. Determine strategies to integrate the expertise of the professional and the experienced person with SCI to improve bladder management techniques and reduce medical complications of the neurogenic bladder.
   3. Assess the impact of peer counseling on management of the neurogenic bladder and on reducing the incidence of UTIs.
   4. Determine effective strategies to provide holistic information to interdisciplinary health professionals, with an emphasis on enhancing consumer choices and responsibilities to promote desired outcomes.
   5. Identify critical factors and establish practice parameters for physicians treating UTIs among people with SCI. These parameters must include patient-physician relationship factors, as well as medical knowledge and skill factors.
   6. Changes in bladder system function over time after onset of SCI (including both the effects of age at onset and the time since onset).
   7. The extent to which esthetic issues influence adherence to bladder management techniques that minimize UTIs.
   8. The advantages and disadvantages of various bladder management methods as they affect fertility and sexual pleasure.
   9. Determine which strategies that facilitate accommodation to people with SCI and their independent functions reduce the burden to caregivers, and are more emotionally acceptable to those in the older generation.
   10. The relationship between health status and degree of involvement in normal life activities. Support needs to be obtained for the hypothesis that well-being and attitude toward life have an important impact on the frequency and severity of UTIs in people with SCI.
   11. Whether activity levels of people with spinal cord injuries change the frequency of infection;

12. Differences in how people with SCI in rural areas manage urinary tract infections versus those in metropolitan areas.

13. Determine if treatment of symptomatic bacteria or prophylaxis reduces morbidity (including fever, bladder function abnormalities, calculi, epididymitis, renal changes), improves patient well-being, or leads to fewer visits to clinics and hospitals.

14. Develop tests to determine tissue invasion (e.g., antibodies, C-reactive protein, or interleukin-6).

15. Determine whether any bacterial species or strains are more or less virulent.

16. Determine the results of treatment of symptomatic and asymptomatic infection more than six months after injury.

17. Determine if acidification or other methods, such as irrigation, prevent calculi or other complications of indwelling catheters.

18. Determine whether immunization against various established microorganisms has potential.

19. Determine whether increase in the length of antibiotic use would reduce the risk of reoccurrence.

20. Identify predictors of bacterial invasion in people with SCI.

21. Compare the suitability of bladder management strategies for people with SCI, including psychosocial consequences of the various strategies to manage the neurogenic bladder. For example, which strategies permit children with SCI to develop social skills without the hindrance of unpredictability in daily life activities? Which strategies permit children to have maximum flexibility and freedom to live a normal life, develop the skills needed for successful adult social and vocational endeavors, and reduce the burden on caregivers ?

22. Determine the psychosocial impact of a neurogenic bladder in childhood and the impact of incontinence on social skills development, emotional response of the child to the disability, and on family stress.

23. Determine methods to prevent leakage of urine in women.

24. Identify ways in which optimal bladder management may differ for women and men.

25. Study the use of intermittent catheterization in women to determine its medical and social advantages/disadvantages as well as its cost/benefit ratio.

26. Promote the development of new products (such as catheter coatings) that may minimize UTIs.

27. Evaluate treatment with antibiotics, surgical procedures, and various methods of bladder drainage through long-term follow-up studies.

28. Determine the frequency of incontinence across various types of bladder management.

29. Determine whether sphincterotomy increases longevity and reduces morbidity.

30. Evaluate effectiveness of new alternative methods (stents, balloon dilatation, etc.) to surgical sphincterotomy.

31. Study the effects of using the bowel to augment bladder function and the long-term implications on carcinoma of the bladder; determine whether these operations preserve upper urinary tract function.

32. Further investigate the relationships between bladder pressure and risk of UTI.

33. Compare UTI methods across the lifetime of SCI people with SCI, with regard to the prevention of future problems and increasing longevity.

34. Study the impact of bladder management procedures on the quality of life of people with SCI.

35. Compare the effectiveness of functional electrical stimulation with traditional methods for bladder emptying and continence.

D. **National Institute of Neurological Disorders and Stroke (NINDS)**

NINDS has developed an implementation plan for the Decade of the Brain (1990's). Within this plan, several research priorities are related to SCI (NINDS Report, 1993, p. 321)

1. Continue multicenter clinical trials to evaluate the next generation of drugs and optimal timing of administration to treat SCI.

2. Use animal models to test agents that block specific mechanisms of immediate and secondary nerve tissue damage in the traumatized spinal cord.

3. Support innovative research on transplantation, including transplantation immunology, which offers hope of restoring movement and sensation to disabled patients.
4. Investigate the molecular biology of the natural chemicals that promote regeneration within the nervous system following trauma.
5. Study animal and human models to find the most effective ways to maximize function of surviving spinal cord nerves following injury.
6. Initiate new efforts to define the long-term impact of SCI and foster the new field of restorative neurology, so that new therapies will be devised to alleviate long-term consequences and improve quality of life.
7. Work with citizen organizations to educate health professionals and the general public about injury prevention and treatment.

E. **Miscellaneous Research Priorities:**
1. Determine which exercises will enable high-level, yet safe, cardiac volume-loading in SCI individuals (Figoni, 1990, p. 68).
2. Determine whether the sympathetic nervous system can be stimulated to provide appropriate support of high level aerobic metabolism (Figoni, 1990, p. 68).
3. Examine central versus peripheral trainability in quadriplegics and paraplegics for various modes of voluntary and/or electrically induced exercise training (Figoni, 1990, p. 69).
4. Explore the clinical benefits of increased cardiovascular fitness in SCI (Figoni, 1990, p. 69).

VII. Future Directions for Research in SCI Nursing.

There is little doubt that research has played a significant role in advancing knowledge in the field of spinal cord impairment. Nursing has participated as part of interdisciplinary teams responsible for a small part of this research. The future holds many opportunities for nurses to conduct studies and apply research to practice. Research provides the key for providing cost-effective nursing care delivery, and improving the quality of services provided, access to services and care, technology, and health outcomes for the patients.

References and Selected Bibliography

Baker, S., O'Neill, B., Haddon, W. Jr., & Lang, W. (1974). The injury severity score: a method for describing patients with multiple injuries and evaluating emergency care. *Journal of Trama*, 14(3), 187-196

Berninger, V., Gans, B., St. James, P., & Connors, T. (1988). Modified WAIS-R for patients with speech and/or hand dysfunction. *Archives of Physical Medicine and Rehabilitation, 69*(4), 250-255.

Bracken, M., Shepard, M., Collins, W., Holford, T., Young, W., Baskin, D., Eisenberg, H., Flamm, E., Leo-Summers, L., Maroon, J., Baskin, D., Eisenberg, H., Flamm, E., Leo-Summers, L., Maroon, J. (1990). A randomized, controlled trial of methylprednisolone or naloxone in the treatment of acute spinal cord injury; results of the second national acute spinal cord injury study. *New England Journal of Medicine, 322*(20), 1405-1411.

Brenes, G., Dearwater, S., Shapera, R., LaPorte, R., & Collins, E. (1986). High density lipoprotein cholesterol concentrations in physically active and sedentary spinal cord injured patients. *Archives of Physical Medicine and Rehabilitation, 67*(7), 445-450.

Champion, H., Sacco, W., Carnazo, A., Copes, W. & Fouty, W. (1981). Trauma Score. *Critical Care Medicine,* 9(9): 672-676.

Charlifue, S., Gerhart, K., Menter, R., Whiteneck, G., & Manley, M. (1992). Sexual issues of women with spinal cord injuries. *Paraplegia, 30*(3), 192-199.

Chiu, W., Dearwater, S., McCarty, D., Songer, T., & LaPorte, R. (1993). Establishment of accurate incidence rates for head and spinal cord injuries in developing and developed countries: A capture-recapture approach. *Journal of Trauma, 35*(2), 206-211.

Craig, A., Hancock, K., Dickson, H., Martin, J., Chang, E. (1990). Psychological Consequences of Spinal Injury: A review of the literature. *Australia/New Zealand Journal of Psychiatry,* 24(3), 418-425.

Cumming, W., Tompkins, W., Jones, R., & Marglis, S. (1986). Microprocessor-based weight shift monitors for paraplegic patients. *Archives of Physical Medicine and Rehabilitation, 67*(3), 172-174.

Cybulski, G., Penn, R., & Jaeger, R. (1984). Lower extremity functional neuromuscular stimulation in cases of spinal cord injury. *Neurosurgery, 15*(1), 132-146.

DeJong, G., & Batavia, A. (1991). Toward a health services research capacity in spinal cord injury. [Review] *Paraplegia, 29*(6), 373-389.

DeLisa, J. (1992). Clinical rehabilitation research advances in spinal cord injury. *Paraplegia, 30*(1), 73-74.

Ernst, F. (1987). Contrasting perceptions of distress by research personnel and their spinal cord injured subjects. *American Journal of Physical Medicine, 66*(1), 12-15.

Figoni, S. (1990). Perspectives on cardiovascular fitness and SCI. [Review] [Published erratum appears in Journal of American Paraplegia Society, 1991; 14 (1), 21.] *Journal of the American Paraplegia Society, 13*(4) 63-71.

Geisler, F., Dorsey, F., & Coleman, W. (1991). Recovery of motor function after spinal cord injury: A randomized, placebo-controlled trial with GM-I ganglioside. *New England Journal of Medicine, 324*, 1829-1838.

Glaser, R. (1990). Functional neuromuscular stimulation for physical fitness training for the disabled. In Kaneko M., (Ed.), *Fitness for the aged, disabled and industrial worker: International series on sport sciences.* (pp. 127-134.). Champaign, IL: Human Kinetics Books.

Hambrecht, F., & Reswick, J. (1977). *Functional electrical stimulation: Applications in neural prostheses.* New York: Marcel Dekker.

Handa, Y., Ichie, M., Handa, T., et al. (1985). Control of the paralyzed hand by a computer-controlled FES system. *Proceedings of the seventh IEEE-EMBS conference.* 322-326.

Harris, P. (1991). Spinal cord injuries in the 21st century. *Journal of the American Paraplegia Society, 14*(2), 55-57.

Hinderer, S. (1990). The supraspinal anxiolytic effect of baclofen for spasticity reduction. *Archives of Physical Medicine and Rehabilitation, 69*(5), 254-258.

Holle, J., Frey, M., & Gruber, H., et al. (1984). Functional electrostimulation of paraplegics: Experimental investigations and first clinical experience with an implantable stimulation device. *Orthopaedics, 7*(7), 1145-1160.

Jaeger, R., Yarkony, G., & Roth, E. (1989). Rehabilitation technology for standing and walking after spinal cord injury [Review] *Archives of Physical Medicine and Rehabilitation, 68*(3), 128-133.

Kakulas, B. (1987). The clinical neuropathology of spinal cord injury. A guide to the future. *Paraplegia, 25* (3), 212-216.

Keith, R. (1988). Observations in the rehabilitation hospital: twenty years of research. *Archives of Physical Medicine and Rehabilitation, 69*(8), 625-631.

Krause, J., & Crewe, N. (1991). Chronologic age, time since injury, and time of measurement: Effect on adjustment after spinal cord injury. *Archives of Physical Medicine and Rehabilitation, 72*(2), 91-100.

Langbein, W., & Fehr, L. (1993). Research device to preproduction prototype: A chronology. *Journal of Rehabilitation Research and Development, 30*(4), 436-442.

Lavallee, D., Lapierre, N., Henwood, P., Pivik, J., Best, M., Springthorpe, V., & Sattar, S. (1995). Catheter cleaning for re-use in intermittent catheterization: new light on an old problem. *SCI Nursing, 12*(1), 10-12.

Levi, R., Hultling, C., & Westgren, N. (1994). A computer assisted follow up system for spinal cord injury patients. *Paraplegia, 32*(11), 736-742.

Little, J. (1990). The decade of the spinal cord [Editorial]. *Journal of the American Paraplegia Society, 13*(3), 32.

Malassigne, P., Nelson, A., Amerson, T., Salzstein, R., & Binard, J. (1993). Toward the design of a new bowel care chair for the spinal cord injured: A pilot study. *SCI Nursing, 10*(3), 84-90.

Marsolais, E., & Kobetic, R. (1983). Functional walking in paralyzed patients by means of electrical stimulation. *Clinical Orthopaedics, 175*, 30-36.

Marsolais, E., & Kobetic, R. (1986) Implantation techniques and experience with percutaneous intramuscular electrodes in the lower extremeties. *Journal of Rehabilitation Research and Development, 23*(6), 1-8.

Marsolais, E., & Kobetic, R. (1987). Functional Electrical Stimulation for Walking in Paraplegia. *Journal of Bone and Joint Surgery, 69*(5), 728-733.

Mauritz, K. & Peckham, P. (1987). Restoration of grasping functions in quadriplegic patients by functional electrical stimulation (FES). *International Journal of Rehabilitation Research,* 10(4 Suppl.5), 57-61

Merli, G., Herbison, G., Ditunno, J., Weitz, H., Henzes, J., Park, C., Jaweed, M. (1988). Deep-vein thrombosis: Prophylaxis in acute spinal cord injured patients. *Archives of Physical Medicine and Rehabilitation, 69,*661-664.

Merli, G., Rensman, B., Doyle, L., et al (1990). Prophylaxis for deep-vein thrombosis in acute spinal cord injury comparing two doses of low molecular weight heparinoid (ORG 10172) in combination with either external pneumatic compression or electrical stimulation. *American Spinal Injury Association Abstracts Digest 16th Annual Scientific Meeting, 8.*

Mulcahey, M. (1992). Returning to school after a spinal cord injury: Perspectives from four adolescents. *American Journal of Occupational Therapy, 46*(4), 305-312.

National Institute on Disability and Rehabilitation Research (NIDRR) (1991). The prevention and management of urinary tract infections among people with spinal cord injuries: NIDRR consensus statement. *Journal of the American Paraplegia Society, 15*(3), 194-204.

National Institute on Disability and Rehabilitation Research (NIDRR) (1991). The prevention and management of urinary tract infections among people with spinal cord injuries consensus statement. *SCI Nursing, 10*(2), 49-61.

National Institute of Neurological Disease and Stroke (NINDS) Report (1991). Progress and promise 1992: A status report on the NINDS. Implementation plan for the decade of the brain. *Annals of Neurology, 33*(3), 320-324.

Paice, J., & Magolan, J. (1991). Intraspinal drug therapy [Review]. *Nursing Clinics of North America, 26*(2), 477-498.

Peckham, P., Marsolais, E., & Mortimer, J. (1980). Restoration of key grip and release in the C6 tetraplegic patient through functional electrical stimulation. *Journal of Hand Surgery, 5*(5), 462-469.

Peckham, P. (1988). Functional electrical stimulation: Current status and future prospects of applications to the neuromuscular system in spinal cord injury. *Paraplegia, 25*(3), 279-288.

Ragnarsson, K., Pollack, S., O'Daniel, W., Jr., Edgar, R., Petrofsky, J., & Nash, M. (1988). Clinical evaluation of computerized functional electrical stimulation after spinal cord injury: A multicenter pilot study. *Archives of Physical Medicine and Rehabilitation, 69*(9), 672-677.

Richards, J., Osuna, F., Jaworski, T., Novack, T., Leli, D., & Boll, T. (1991). The effectiveness of different methods of defining traumatic brain injury in predicting postdischarge adjustment in a spinal cord injury population. *Archives of Physical Medicine and Rehabilitation, 72*(5), 275-279.

Richards, J., Seitz, M., & Eisele, W. (1986). Auditory processing in spinal cord injury: A preliminary investigation from a sensory deprivation perspective. *Archives of Physical Medicine and Rehabilitation, 67*(2), 115-117.

Rodriquez, G., Claus-Walker, J., Kent, M., & Stal, S. (1986). Adrenergic receptors in insensitive skin of spinal cord injured patients. *Archives of Physical Medicine and Rehabilitation, 67*(3), 177-180.

Salzberg, C., Harmatz, A., & Byrne, D. (1990). Development of a computerized data base to evaluate pressure ulcers. *Decubitus, 3*(3), 29-36.

Seelman, K. (1995). Physical rehabilitation and violence: Initiatives. *Journal of Health Care for the Poor and Underserved, 6*(2), 217-233.

Seil, F. (1988). Spinal cord injury research in the Veterans Administration. *Journal of the American Paraplegia Society, 11*(1), 16-17.

Sipski, M. (1991). The impact of spinal cord injury on female sexuality, menstruation and pregnancy: A review of the literature. *Journal of American Paraplegia Society, 14*(3), 122-126.

Treischmann, R. (1978). The psychological, social, and vocational adjustment to spinal cord injury. *U.S. Department of Commerce Final Report.* RSA 13-P-59011/9-01.

Triolo, R., Betz, R., Mulcahey, M., & Gardner, E. (1994). Application of functional neuromuscular stimulation to children with spinal cord injuries: Candidate selection for upper and lower extremity research. *Paraplegia, 32* (12), 824-843.

Urey, J., & Henggeler, S. (1987). Marital adjustment following spinal cord injury. *Archives of Physical Medicine and Rehabilitation, 68*(2), 69-74.

Yerxa, E., & Locker, S. (1990). Quality of time use by adults with spinal cord injuries. *American Journal of Occupational Therapy, 44*(4), 318-326.

Glossary

Abdominal binder: An elasticized wrap that is applied around the lower part of the torso to support the abdomen.

Abscess: A cavity containing pus and surrounded by inflamed tissue, formed as a result of suppuration in a localized infection.

Accessory nerve: Either of a pair of cranial nerves; essential for speech, swallowing, and certain movements of the head and shoulders.

Accreditation: A process whereby a professional association or nongovernmental agency grants recognition to a school or institution for demonstrated ability in a special area of practice or training.

Acculturation: The modification of the culture of a group or an individual as a result of contact with a different culture; the process by which the culture of a particular society is instilled in a human being from infancy onward.

Acute care: A pattern of health care in which a patient is treated for an abrupt episode of illness, for the sequelae of an accident or other trauma, or during recovery form surgery.

Acute respiratory distress syndrome (ARDS): A respiratory emergency characterized by respiratory insufficiency and failure; usually after aspiration of a foreign body, cardiopulmonary bypass surgery, gram-negative sepsis, multiple blood transfusions, oxygen toxicity, trauma, pneumonia, or other respiratory infection. It may also occur in such diseases as Guillain-Barré syndrome, muscular dystrophy, myasthenia gravis, emphysema, asthma, or poliomyelitis.

Adaptation: A change or response to stress of any kind; the dynamic process wherein the thoughts, feelings, behavior, and biophysiologic mechanisms of change to adjust to a constantly changing environment.

Affective learning: The acquisition of behaviors involved in expressing feelings in attitudes, appreciations, and values.

Altered thermoregulation: A state in which an individual is unable to maintain a steady internal body temperature and may assume the temperature of the environment.

Ambulatory health care: Health services provided on an outpatient basis to those who visit a hospital or other health care facility and depart after treatment on the same day.

Amyotrophic lateral sclerosis (ALS): A degenerative disease of the motor neurons; characterized by atrophy of the muscles of the hands, forearms, and legs, and spreading to involve most of the body.

Anal tone reflex: Contraction of the internal anal muscle over the examiner's finger upon digital stimulation.

Anal wink reflex: Contraction of the external anal sphincter in response to stroking or pricking the skin or nervous membrane in the perianal regions.

Anesthesia: Loss of sensation resulting from pharmacologic depression of nerve function or from neurological dysfunction.

Angiography: The x-ray visualization of the internal anatomy of the heart and blood vessels after the intravascular introduction of radiopaque contrast medium.

Ankylosing spondylitis: A chronic inflammatory disease of unknown origin; first affecting the spine and adjacent structures, and commonly progressing to eventual fusion (ankylosis) of the involved joints.

Ankylosis: Stiffening or fixation of a joint as the result of a disease process, with fibrous or bony union across the joint, as occurs in rheumatoid arthritis.

Anterior cord injury: A lesion that produces variable loss of motor function and of sensitivity to pain and temperature while preserving posterior column functions (proprioception, pressure, and vibration).

Anterior spinothalamic tract: The more anterior or ventral part of the spinothalamic tract, involved in tactile sensation.

Antiembolism hose: Elasticized stockings worn to prevent the formation of emboli and thrombi, especially in patients after surgery or in those with restricted mobility.

Apnea: An absence of spontaneous respiration. Types of apnea include cardiac apnea, deglutition apnea, periodic apnea of the newborn, primary apnea, reflex apnea, secondary apnea, and sleep apnea.

Architectural barriers: Architectural features of homes, buildings, and structures that limit access and mobility of persons with disabilities.

Arterial blood gas: The oxygen and carbon dioxide in arterial blood; measured by various methods to assess the adequacy of ventilation and oxygenation and the acid base status.

Arterial pressure: The stress exerted by the circulating blood on the walls of the arteries. The amount of arterial pressure in an individual is the product of the cardiac output and the systemic vascular resistance.

Artificial airway: A plastic or rubber device that can be inserted into the upper or lower respiratory tract to facilitate ventilation or the removal of secretions.

Aspiration pneumonia: An inflammatory condition of the lungs and bronchi caused by the inhalation of foreign material or vomitus containing acid gastric contents.

Atelectasis: An abnormal condition characterized by the collapse of lung tissue, preventing the respiratory exchange of carbon dioxide and oxygen.

Atlantoaxial subluxation: An incomplete dislocation of the joint between the first two cervical vertebrae, pertaining to the atlas and the axis.

Autonomic dysreflexia: A life-threatening condition that can occur in persons with a spinal cord injury at T7 or above, resulting from an uninhibited sympathetic response of the nervous system to a noxious stimulus. Specifically, a discharge of uninhibited sympathetic nervous system impulses as a result of noxious stimulation of sensory receptors below the level of spinal cord injury, resulting in a hypertensive episode. See also autonomic hyperreflexia or dysreflexia.

Autonomic hyperreflexia: See autonomic dysreflexia.

Autonomy: The quality or state of being self-governing; of having the ability or tendency to function independently.

Bacteriuria: Presence of any of the small unicellular microorganisms in the urine.

Barium swallow: The ingestion of barium sulfate, a radiopaque contrast medium, for the radiographic examination of the esophagus, stomach, and intestinal tract used in the diagnosis of such conditions as dysphagia, peptic ulcer, and fistulas.

Basal energy expenditure: The minimal energy expended for the maintenance of respiration, circulation, peristalsis, muscle tone, body temperature, glandular activity, and the other vegetative functions of the body.

Biofeedback: A training technique that enables an individual to gain some element of voluntary control over autonomic body functions such as blood pressure, muscle tension, and brain wave activity, usually through use of instrumentation.

Biomechanics: The study of mechanical laws and their application to living organisms, especially the human body and its locomotor system.

Bladder distention: The state of the bladder being stretched or distended when unable to pass urine.

Bladder reconditioning program: See bladder training program. Bladder training program: Method by which the bladder is trained to empty without an indwelling catheter. See also bladder reconditioning program.

Body image: A person's subjective concept of his or her physical appearance.

Bone density: The mass per unit volume of the largely calcareous connective tissue of the skeleton of a vertebrate.

Bowel training: A method of establishing regular bowel evacuation by reflex conditioning used in the treatment of altered bowel elimination. Also called timed toileting.

Brown-Séquard syndrome: A traumatic neurologic disorder resulting from damage to of one side of the spinal cord, above the tenth thoracic vertebrae, characterized by spastic paralysis on the injured side of the body and loss of postural sense, pain, and temperature on the opposite side of the body.

Buffering: The nurturing and protective process of helping patients to gather the physical and emotional strength necessary for a strenuous rehabilitation program.

Bulbocavernosus reflex: A sharp contraction of the bulbocavernosus and ischiocavernosus muscles when the glans penis or clitoris is suddenly compressed or tapped.

Caliectasis: Dilation of a flower-shaped or funnel-shaped structure; specifically, one of the branches or recesses of the pelvis of the kidney, usually due to obstruction or infection. Also called pyelocaliectasis.

Case management: The assignment of a health care provider to assist a patient in assessing health and social service systems and to assure that all required services are coordinated and obtained.

Case manager: Person who functions as an integrator of health services with a focus on high quality, cost-efficient care.

Cauda equina syndrome: A condition characterized by dull pain in upper sacral region with anesthesia or analgesia in buttocks, genitalia, or thigh, accompanied by disturbed bowel and bladder function; due to a cauda equina injury.

Centers for Disease Control (CDC): A federal agency that provides facilities and services for the investigation, identification, prevention, and control of disease. It is concerned with all aspects of the epidemiology and laboratory diagnosis of disease.

Central cord syndrome: Quadriparesis most severely involving the distal upper extremities, with or without sensory loss and bladder dysfunction; usually due to ischemia from osteophytic or traumatic compression of the central part of the cervical spinal cord and/or artery.

Cerebrovascular accident (CVA): An abnormal condition of the blood vessels of the brain; characterized by occlusion by an embolus or cerebrovascular hemorrhage, and resulting in ischemia of the brain tissues normally perfused by the damaged vessels.

Cervical disk syndrome: Pain, paresthesia, and sometimes weakness in the area of distribution of one or more cervical roots, due to pressure of a protruded cervical intervertebral disc.

Chest physiotherapy: The procedures to help remove mucus and fluid from the lungs by the use of the clinical nursing techniques of manual percussion and vibration or to dislodge and mobilize the secretions. Also called cupping and vibrating.

Chiari malformation: Malformed posterior fossa structures, resulting from caudal traction and displacement of the rhombencephalon caused by tethering of the spinal cord.

Cholecystectomy: Surgical removal of the gallbladder.

Cholescintigraphy: Examination of the gallbladder and bile ducts by nuclear medicine scanning.

Chronic illness: An abnormal process lasting more than six months in which aspects of the social, physical, emotional, or intellectual condition and function of a person are diminished or impaired, compared with that person's previous condition.

Chronic pain: A condition in which the individual experiences pain that continues for more than 6 months in duration.

Clinical pathway: A systematically organized program that highlights those tasks that must be accomplished within a given timeframe in order for the overall outcome to be achieved. Also called critical pathway.

Cognitive learning: Learning that is concerned with acquisition of problem-solving abilities and with intelligence and conscious thought; a theory that defines learning as behavioral change based on the acquisition of information about the environment.

Cold-blooded: See Poikilothermic.

Colonoscopy: The examination of the mucosal lining of the colon using a colonoscope, an elongated endoscope.

Commission on Accreditation of Rehabilitation Facilities (CARF): The standard accrediting authority for organizations providing services to people with disabilities.

Community reintegration: The return and acceptance of an individual with a disability as a participating member of the community.

Complete spinal cord injury: Total disruption of the cord, with complete loss of motor and sensory function below level of injury.

Conscious sedation: An anesthetic procedure in which analgesia and anesthesia are accomplished without loss of consciousness and the concomitant need for life-support equipment, personnel, and expertise.

Constipation: Difficulty in passing stools or an incomplete or infrequent passage of hard stools.

Consumer based planning: The establishment of goals, policies, and procedures to satisfy human wants.

Continent urinary reservoir: Construction of internal pouch using segments of detubularized ileum or colon.

Contractures: Shortening muscle or scar tissue, producing distortions, deformity, or abnormal limitations of movement of a joint.

Conus medullaris syndrome: A group of signs and symptoms that occur together and characterize a particular abnormality in the cone-shaped lower end of the spinal cord, at the level of the upper lumbar vertebrae.

Coping ability: The degree to which an individual is able to adapt to any stress encountered in the activities of daily life, whether of a physical or psychological nature, through the use of both conscious and unconscious mechanisms.

Coping: A process by which a person deals with stress, solves problems, and makes decisions.

Coronary artery disease: Any one of the abnormal conditions that may affect the arteries of the heart and produce various pathologic effects, especially the reduced flow of oxygen and nutrients to the myocardium.

Credé method: A manual method of emptying the bladder by exerting firm pressure on the abdomen in the area of the bladder with the hands to push urine out of the bladder.

Cricothyrotomy: An emergency incision into the larynx, performed to open the airway in a person who is choking.

Critical pathway: See clinical pathway.

Crutchfield tongs: An instrument inserted into the skull to hyperextend the head and neck of patients with fractured cervical vertebrae.

Cultural assimilation: A process by which members of an ethnic minority group lose cultural characteristics that distinguish them from the dominant cultural group.

Cultural diversity: The variations among cultural groups due to differences in ways of life, language, values, norms, and other cultural aspects.

Cultural relativism: The uniqueness of a culture and the need for that culture to be evaluated by its own values and standards.

Cultural values: Refers to the powerful internal and external directive forces that give meaning and order to individual's or group's thinking, decisions, and actions.

Culture: A set of learned values, beliefs, customs, and behavior that is shared by a group of interacting individuals.

Cyanosis: Bluish discoloration of the skin and mucous membranes; caused by an excess of deoxygenated hemoglobin in the blood or a structural defect in the hemoglobin molecule, such as in methemoglobin.

Cystometrogram (CMG): A graphic recording of urinary bladder pressure at various volumes.

Cystoplasty: Any reconstructive operation on the urinary bladder.

Cystoscopy: The direct visualization of the urinary tract by means of a cystoscope inserted in the urethra.

Deafferentation: A loss of the sensory input from a portion of the body, usually caused by interruption of the peripheral sensory fibers.

Debridement: Removal of dirt, foreign objects, damaged tissue, and cellular debris from a wound or a burn to prevent infection and to promote healing.

Decubitus ulcer: See Pressure ulcer.

Deep abdominal reflex: Contraction of abdominal muscles elicited by stimulation, such as tapping a deep structure.

Deep tendon reflex (DTR): A brisk contraction of a muscle in response to a sudden stretch induced by a sharp tap by a finger or rubber hammer on the tendon of insertion of the muscle. Absence of the reflex may have been caused by damage to the muscle, the peripheral nerve roots, or the spinal cord at that level.

Deep vein thrombosis (DVT): Formation or presence of a clot (thrombus) within a blood vessel, which may cause infarction of tissues supplied by the vessel.

Demyelination: The process of destruction or loss of the myelin sheath from a nerve or nerve fiber.

Dermatome: An area on the surface of a body innervated by afferent fibers from one spinal root.

Detrusor pressure: The component of intravesical pressure created by the tension (active and passive) exerted by the bladder wall; the transmural pressure across the bladder wall, estimated by subtracting abdominal pressure from intravesical pressure.

Detrusor sphincter dyssynergia (DSD): A disturbance of the normal relationship between bladder (detrusor) contraction and sphincter relaxation during voluntary or involuntary voiding efforts.

Diaphoresis: The secretion of sweat, especially the profuse secretion associated with an elevated body temperature, physical exertion, exposure to heat, and mental or emotional stress.

Diaphragm: A dome-shaped musculofibrous partition that separates the thoracic and the abdominal cavities. The diaphragm aids respiration by moving up and down. During inspiration it moves down and increases the volume of the thoracic cavity; during expiration it moves up, decreasing the volume.

Diaphragmatic pacemaker: A device that paces the diaphragm, used in patients with chronic ventilatory insufficiency resulting from malfunction of the respiratory control center, for certain types of phrenic nerve malfunction. Also called Phrenic nerve pacemaker.

Diarrhea: The frequent passage of loose watery stools, generally the result of increased motility in the colon.

Diastematomyelia: Complete or incomplete sagittal division of the spinal cord by an osseous or fibrocartilaginous septum, usually in spina bifida.

Digital stimulation: A maneuver used to stimulate the bowel, by rotating one finger in a circular movement inside the rectum.

Dignity: The quality or state of being worthy, honored, or esteemed.

Disk disease: A constellation of symptoms and signs; including pain, paresthesias, sensory loss, weakness, and impaired reflexes, due to a compressive radiculopathy caused by intervertebral disk pressure.

Disuse phenomena: The physical and psychological changes, usually degenerative, that result from the lack of use of a part of the body or a body system. The defining characteristics are the presence of risk factors such as paralysis, mechanical immobilization, severe pain, and altered level of consciousness.

Dysesthesia: A common effect of spinal cord injury, characterized by sensations of numbness, tingling, burning, or pain felt below the level of the lesion; abnormal sensations experienced in the absence of stimulation; impairment of sensation short of anesthesia.

Dysreflexia: See autonomic dysreflexia.

Dysuria: Painful urination, usually the result of a bacterial infection or obstructive condition in the urinary tract.

Ejaculation: The sudden emission of semen from the male urethra, usually occurring during copulation, masturbation, and nocturnal emission.

Ejaculatory dysfunction: Impairment, disturbance, or abnormality in expulsion of the semen from the male urethra.

Electromyogram (EMG): A record of the intrinsic electric activity in a skeletal muscle. Such data helps diagnose neuromuscular problems and pinpoints lesions of motor nerves.Electromyograms also measure electric potentials induced by voluntary muscular contraction.

Emotional dimension of rehabilitation: Involves efforts to allay anxiety and fears, demonstrate caring, and assign value to the patient as a unique individual.

Endourethral prosthesis: See Urethral stent.

Endurance: The ability to continue an activity despite increasing physical or psychological stress; as in the effort to perform additional numbers of muscle contractions before the onset of fatigue.

Enteral administration: Within or by way of the intestine or gastrointestinal tract, especially as distinguished from parenteral.

Erectile dysfunction: Impairment, disturbance, or abnormality inability to become rigid and elevated, as erectile tissue.

Ergometry: The study of physical work activity, including work performed by specific muscles or muscle groups.

Erogenous zones: Any part of the body which causes sexual feelings when touched.

Esophageal dysfunction: Any disturbance, impairment, or abnormality that interferes with the normal functioning of the esophagus, such as dysphagia, esophagitis, or sphincter incompetence. The condition is one of the primary symptoms of scleroderma.

Esophagogastroduodenoscopy (EGD): Endoscopic examination of the esophagus, stomach, and duodenum usually performed using a fiberoptic instrument.

Ethnicity: The state of belonging or relating to a religious, racial, national, or cultural group; ethnic pride.

Ethnocentrism: A belief in the inherent superiority of the "race" or group to which one belongs; a proclivity to consider other ethnic groups in terms of one's own racial origins.

Expiratory reserve volume (ERV): The maximal volume of air (about 1000 ml) that can be expelled from the lungs after a normal expiration.

Extended care facility: An institution devoted to providing medical, nursing, or custodial care for an individual over a prolonged period of time, such as during the course of a chronic disease or during the rehabilitation phase after an acute illness.

External anal sphincter: A fusiform ring of striated muscular fibers surrounding the anus, attached posteriorly to the coccyx and anteriorly to the central tendon of the perineum.

External sphincter: Striated skeletal muscle surrounding the urethra, which can be voluntarily relaxed and contracted.

Failure to empty: See Urinary retention.

Failure to store: See Urinary incontinence.

Family-centered care: Primary health care that includes an assessment of the health of an entire family, identification of actual or potential factors that might influence the health of its members, and implementation of actions needed to maintain or improve the health of the unit and its members.

Fasciculation: A localized, uncoordinated, uncontrollable twitching of a single muscle group innervated by a single motor nerve fiber or filament that may be palpated and seen under the skin.

Fatigue: A state, following a period of mental or bodily activity, characterized by a lessened capacity for work and reduced efficiency of accomplishment; usually accompanied by a feeling of weariness, sleepiness, or irritability.

Fecal Impaction: An immovable collection of compressed or hardened feces in the colon or rectum.

Fertility: The capacity to conceive or to induce conception.

Fiberoptic bronchoscopy: The visual examination of the tracheobronchial tree through a fiberoptic bronchoscope.

Fiberoptics: The technical process by which an internal organ or cavity can be viewed, using glass or plastic fibers to transmit light through a specially designed tube and reflect a magnified image.

Flaccid paralysis: An abnormal condition characterized by the weakening or loss of muscle tone.

Flaccid rectum: Relaxed, flabby, or without tone, terminal portion of the digestive tube, extending from the rectosigmoid junction to the anal canal.

Flexibility: The capability of being turned, bowed, or twisted without breaking; not invincibly rigid.

Fluoroscopy: A technique in radiology for visually examining a part of the body or the function of an organ using a fluoroscope.

Functional electrical stimulation (FES): The production of functional movement or activity by the electrical stimulation of muscles and nerves.

Gallstone: A stone formed in the biliary tract, consisting of bile pigments and calcium salts. Biliary calculi may cause jaundice, right upper quadrant pain, obstruction, and inflammation of the gallbladder.

Gastric ulcer: A circumscribed erosion of the mucosal layer of the stomach that may penetrate the muscle layer and perforate the stomach wall.

Gastrocolic reflex: A mass movement of the contents of the colon, frequently preceded by a similar movement in the small intestine, which sometimes occurs immediately following the entrance of food into the stomach.

Gastroesophageal reflux: Regurgitation of the contents of the stomach into the esophagus, and possibly into the pharynx, where they can be aspirated between the vocal cords and down into the trachea.

Glasgow Coma Scale: A quick, practical, and standardized system for assessing the degree of conscious impairment in the critically ill and for predicting the duration and ultimate outcome of coma, primarily in patients with head injuries.

Glossopharyngeal breathing (GPB): Respiration unaided by the usual primary muscles of respiration; the air is forced into the lungs by use of the tongue and muscles of the pharynx.

Glossopharyngeal nerve: Either of a pair of cranial nerves essential for the sense of taste, sensation in some viscera, and for secretion from certain glands.

Goniometer: An instrument for measuring angles.

Goose flesh: Goose bumps and a roughness of the skin produced by erection of its papillae especially from cold, fear, or a sudden feeling of excitement. Also called pilomotor reflex.

Greenfield filter: A multistrutted, spring-styled filter, usually placed in the inferior vena cava to prevent venous emboli from reaching the pulmonary circulation from the lower extremity.

Guillain-Barré syndrome: An idiopathic, peripheral polyneuritis, occurring between one and three weeks after a mild episode of fever, and associated with a viral infection or with immunization. Results in demyelination of the peripheral nerves.

Habilitation: The process of supplying a person with the means to develop maximum independence in activities of daily living through training or treatment.

Habit training: The process of acquiring, developing, educating, establishing, learning, or training new responses in an individual. Used to describe both respondent and operant behavior; in both usages, refers to a change in the frequency or form of behavior as a result of the influence of the environment.

Halo brace: An orthopedic device used to help immobilize the neck and head. It incorporates the trunk, usually with shoulder straps and an apparatus by means of an outrigger within the cast to secure pins to a band around the skull.

Hand splint: Material or device used to protect and immobilize the hand.

Handedness: Voluntary or involuntary preference for use of either the left or right hand. The preference is related to cerebral dominance, with left-handedness corresponding to dominance of the right side of the brain and vice versa.

Hangman's fracture: An extension fracture through the pedicles of C2, causing the separation of the neural arch from the body of the axis. Also called traumatic spondylolisthesis of the axis.

Head injury: Any traumatic damage to the head resulting from penetration of the skull or from too-rapid inertial acceleration or deceleration of the brain within the skull.

Health belief model: A conceptual framework that describes a person's health behavior as an expression of health beliefs. The model was designed to predict a person's health behavior, including the use of health services, and to justify intervention to alter maladaptive health behavior.

Health maintenance organization (HMO): A type of group health care practice that provides basic and supplemental health maintenance and treatment services to voluntary enrollees who prepay a fixed periodic fee that is set without regard to the amount or kind of services received.

Health promotion: The process of enabling people to increase control over and improve their health; it involves the population as a whole in the context of their everyday lives, rather than focusing on people at risk for specific diseases, and is directed toward action on the determinants of health.

Health resources: All materials, personnel, facilities, funds, and anything else that can be used for providing health care and services.

Health: A state of physical, mental, and social well-being.

Heat cramps: A condition marked by sudden development of cramps in skeletal muscles, accompanied by profuse perspiration with loss of serum sodium, results from prolonged activity in high environment temperatures.

Heat exhaustion: A condition marked by weakness, nausea, dizziness, and profuse sweating that results from physical exertion in a hot environment.

Heat stroke: A condition marked especially by cessation of sweating, extremely high body temperature, and collapse that results from prolonged exposure to high temperature.

Hemoptysis: Coughing up blood from the respiratory tract. Blood-streaked sputum often occurs in minor upper respiratory infections or in bronchitis. More profuse bleeding may indicate infection, lung abscess, tuberculosis, or bronchogenic carcinoma.

Hemothorax: An accumulation of blood and fluid in the pleural cavity, between the parietal and visceral pleura, usually the result of trauma.

Herniated disk: A rupture of the fibrocartilage surrounding an intervertebral disk, releasing the nucleus pulposus that cushions the vertebrae above and below. The resultant pressure on spinal nerve roots may cause considerable pain and damage the nerves. The condition most frequently occurs in the lumbar region. Also called a herniated nucleus pulposus.

Herniated nucleus pulposus (HNP): See Herniated disk.

Heterotopic ossification (HO): A nonmalignant overgrowth of bone, frequently occurring after a fracture or around joints of paralyzed limbs.

Home care: Health service provided in the individual's place of residence for the purpose of promoting, maintaining, or restoring health or minimizing the effects of illness and disability.

Homeostasis: A relative constancy in the internal environment of the body, naturally maintained by adaptive responses that promote healthy survival.

Hospice: An institution that provides a centralized program of palliative and supportive services to dying persons and their families in the form of physical, psychological, social, and spiritual care.

Hydromyelia: An increase of fluid in the dilated central canal of the spinal cord, or in congenital cavities elsewhere in the cord substance.

Hydronephrosis: Distention of the pelvis and calyces of the kidney secondary to urinary tract obstruction.

Hypercapnia: Greater than normal amounts of carbon dioxide in the blood.

Hyperesthesia: Abnormal acuteness or sensitivity to touch, pain, or other sensory stimuli.

Hyperextension hyperflexion injury: Violence to the body causing the unsupported head to hyperextend and hyperflex the neck rapidly.

Hypertension: A common, often asymptomatic disorder characterized by elevated blood pressure.

Hyperthermia: An extreme elevation of body temperature.

Hypoglossal nerve: Either of a pair of cranial nerves essential for swallowing and for moving the tongue. Each nerve has four major branches, communicates with the vagus nerve, and connects to nucleus XII in the brain. Also called twelfth cranial nerve.

Hypothermia: A subnormal temperature of the body usually caused by prolonged exposure to cold.

Ileal conduit: An isolated segment of the ileum serving as a replacement for another tubular organ; specifically, the use of this segment as a urinary conduit into which ureters can be implanted following total cystectomy or other loss of normal bladder function requiring supravesical diversion.

Immune dysfunction: Condition in which a body organ or system is unable to resist the possibility of acquiring a given infectious disease.

Impairment: Any disorder in structure or function resulting from anatomic, physiologic, or psychological abnormalities that interfere with normal activities.

Impedance plethysmography: A technique for detecting blood vessel occlusion that determines volumetric changes in the limb by measuring changes in its girth as indicated by changes in the electric impedance of mercury- containing silastic tubes in a pressure cuff.

Incomplete spinal cord injury: Partial preservation of the motor and sensory functions which are intact below the level of injury.

Incontinence: The inability to control urination or defecation.

Independent living centers: Rehabilitation facilities in which persons with disabilities can receive special education and training in the performance of activities of daily living.

Infarct: A localized area of necrosis in a tissue, vessel, organ, or par; resulting from tissue anoxia caused by an interruption in the blood supply to the area, or less frequently, by circulatory stasis produced by the occlusion of a vein that ordinarily carries blood away from the area.

Inspiratory reserve volume (IRV): The maximal volume of air that can be inspired after a normal inspiration.

Interdisciplinary team: A mix of health and human service professionals who collaborate to identify client goals and strive to avoid duplication or conflict in goals.

Intermittent assisted ventilation (IAV): In respiratory therapy, a system in which an assisted rate is combined with spontaneous breathing. Also called intermittent demand ventilation (IDV).

Intermittent catheterization program (ICP): A routine program by which the bladder is emptied of urine at regular intervals by straight urethral catheter.

Intermittent positive pressure breathing (IPPB): A form of assisted or controlled respiration produced, by a ventilatory apparatus in which compressed gas is delivered under positive pressure into the person's airways until a preset pressure is reached.

Intermittent positive pressure ventilation (IPPV): Artificial ventilation in which all inspirations are provided by positive pressure applied to the airway.

Internal anal sphincter: A smooth muscle ring, formed by an increase of the circular fibers of the rectum, situated at the upper end of the anal canal, internal to the outer voluntary external anal sphincter.

Internal sphincter: located at the bladder neck, functions include closing off the bladder neck in the resting state and maintaining continence.

Intradisciplinary team: Members from different levels of expertise or different specializations within the same discipline, working together to deliver quality care.

Intravenous urogram (IVU): Radiography of kidneys, ureters, and bladder following injection of contrast medium into a peripheral vein.

Jaw thrust: The lifting of the lower jaw by placing the fingers behind the angles of the jaw in front of the earlobes and displacing it upward.

Joint Commission on Accreditation of Health Care Organizations (JCAHO): A private, nongovernmental agency that establishes guidelines for the operation of hospitals and other health care facilities, conducts accreditation programs and surveys, and encourages the attainment of high standards of institutional medical care.

Kidney stones: See Renal calculi.

Kinesitherapy: Physical therapy involving movement and range-of- motion exercises.

KUB: Radiographic examination of the kidneys, ureter, and bladder.

Kugelberg-Welander disease: Slowly progressive proximal muscular weakness and wasting, beginning in childhood, caused by degeneration of motor neurons in the anterior horns of the spinal cord; juvenile spinal muscular atrophy.

Kyphosis: A deformity of the spine characterized by extensive flexion.

Lamina of vertebral arch: The flattened posterior portion or the vertebral arch extending between the pedicles and midline, forming the dorsal wall of the vertebral foramen, and from the midline junction of which the spinous process extends.

Laminectomy: Surgical chipping away of the bony arches of one or more vertebrae; performed to relieve compression of the spinal cord, (caused by a bone displaced in an injury or as the result of degeneration of a disk), or to reach and remove a displaced intervertebral disk.

Laparoscopy: Examination of the contents of the peritoneum with a laparoscope (type of endoscope) passed through the abdominal wall.

Latex sensitivity: Condition in which the skin is easily irritated or affected by an emulsion of rubber or plastic globules in water, which is used in paints, adhesives, and various synthetic rubber products (gloves).

Launching: Process of exposing rehabilitation patients to the real world, exploring the range of options for living in the community, promoting patient autonomy and decision making, and facilitating the discharge of the patient from the rehabilitation program.

Life care planning: A continuous plan or process to ensure that care is consistent with the individual's needs and progress toward self-care.

Lithotripsy: The crushing of a stone in the renal pelvis, ureter, or bladder by mechanical force or sound waves.

Long term care: The provision of medical, social, and personal care services on a recurring or continuing basis to persons with chronic physical or mental disorders.

Lordosis: An abnormal extension deformity; antero-posterior curvature of the spine, generally lumbar with the convexity looking anteriorly. Also called hollow back, saddle back, bending backward.

Lower motor neuron (LMN) lesion: Injury to lower motor neurons, generally involving the sacral segments of the spinal cord, characterized by a flaccid paralysis.

Magnetic resonance imaging (MRI): Medical imaging that uses nuclear magnetic resonance as its source of energy.

Managed care: An arrangement whereby a third party payer (e.g., insurance company, federal government, or corporation) mediates between physicians and patients, negotiating fees for service and overseeing the types of treatment given.

Manual assisted coughing: Application of pressure under the patient's sternum/rib cage during expiration to expel secretions from the deep air sacs of the lungs.

Material dimension of rehabilitation: Focus on financial issues and efforts to provide necessary adaptive equipment and supplies to facilitate independence.

Mechanical ventilation: Use of automatic cycling devices to generate airway pressures; employed in assisted or controlled ventilation.

Meningocele: Protrusion of the membranes of the brain or spinal cord through a defect in the skull or spinal column. It forms a hernial cyst that is filled with cerebrospinal fluid but does not contain neural tissue.

Meningomyelocele: A developmental defect of the central nervous system in which a hernial sac containing a portion of the spinal cord, its meninges and cerebrospinal fluid protrude through a congenital cleft in the vertebral column. Also called Myelomeningocele.

Meningomyelohydrocele: The accumulation of fluid in any sac-like cavity or duct in the brain or spinal cord.

Minerva brace: An orthopedic cast applied to the trunk and head with spaces cut out for the face area and the ears. The cast is used for immobilizing the head and trunk in the treatment of torticollis, cervical and thoracic injuries, and cervical spinal infections.

Motor domain: Client's ability to perform physical skills within the parameters set by the state of their neuromuscular systems. In addition, learning to perform a skill depends upon the ability to envision mentally how the skill is performed.

Multidisciplinary team: A team that is characterized by discipline-specific goals, clear boundaries between disciplines, and outcomes that are the sum of each discipline's efforts.

Multiple sclerosis: A progressive disease characterized by demyelination of nerve fibers of the brain and spinal cord.

Myelocele: Protrusion of the spinal cord in spina bifida; a sac-like protrusion of the spinal cord through a congenital defect in the vertebral column.

Myelomeningocele: See Meningomyelocele.

Nerve entrapment: An abnormal condition and type of mononeuropathy, characterized by nerve damage and muscle weakness or atrophy.

Nervous system: The extensive, intricate network of structures that activates, coordinates, and controls all the functions of the body.

Neural arch: The posterior projection from the body of a vertebra that encloses the vertebral foramen; it consists of paired pedicles and laminae; the spinous, transverse, and articular processes arise from the arch.

Neural tube defect (NDT): Any of a group of congenital malformations involving defects in the skull and spinal column that are caused primarily by the failure of the neural tube to close during embryonic development.

Neurofibromatosis: A congenital condition transmitted as an autosomal dominant trait, characterized by numerous neurofibromas of the nerves and skin, café-au-lait spots on the skin and, in some cases, developmental anomalies of the muscles, bones, and viscera. Also called NF-1 NF-2 Von Recklinghausen disease.

Neurogenic bladder: Dysfunctional urinary bladder caused by lesions of the central or peripheral nervous system.

Neurogenic bowel: Bowel dysfunction caused by lesions of the central or peripheral nervous system.

Neurogenic shock: A form of shock that results from peripheral vascular dilatation as a result of neurologic injury.

Neuropathic ulcers: A lesion of the skin or mucous membrane resulting from an abnormal condition characterized by inflammation and degeneration of the peripheral nerves.

NF-1 NF-2 Von Recklinghausen disease: See Neurofibromatosis.

Numbness: A partial or total lack of sensation in a part of the body, resulting from any factor that interrupts the transmission of impulses from the sensory nerve fibers.

Nursing process: The process that serves as an organizational framework for the practice of nursing.

Nursing theory: An organized framework of concepts and purposes designed to guide the practice of nursing.

Orthosis: A force system designed to control, correct, or compensate for a bone deformity, deforming forces, or forces absent from the body.

Osteomyelitis: Local or generalized infection of bone and bone marrow, usually caused by bacteria introduced by trauma or surgery, by direct extension from a nearby infection, or via the bloodstream.

Osteoporosis: Deossification with absolute decrease in bone tissue resulting in bone trabeculae that are scanty, thin, weak, and without osteoclastic resorption.

Outcome: The condition of a client at the end of therapy or a disease process, including the degree of wellness and the need for continuing care, medication, support, counseling, or education.

Oximeter: Any of several devices used to measure oxyhemoglobin in blood.

Pain: An unpleasant sensation caused by noxious stimulation of the sensory nerve endings.

Pallor: An unnatural paleness or absence of color in the skin.

Paradoxical breathing: A condition in which a part of the lung deflates during inspiration and inflates during expiration.

Paralysis: An abnormal condition characterized by the loss of muscle function or the loss of sensation, or both.

Paralytic ileus: A decrease in or absence of intestinal peristalsis in the small bowel, which allows fluid and gas to accumulate.

Paraparesis: A partial paralysis of the lower extremities.

Paraplegia: A condition characterized by motor or sensory loss in the lower limbs; paralysis of both lower extremities and generally, the lower trunk.

Parenteral administration: By some means other than through the gastrointestinal tract; referring particularly to the introduction of substances into an organism by intravenous, subcutaneous, intramuscular, or intramedullary injection.

Paresthesia: Any subjective sensation experienced as numbness, tingling, or a "pins and needles" feeling.

Parkinson's Disease: A neurological syndrome, usually resulting from deficiency of the neurotransmitter dopamine, as the consequence of degenerative, vascular, or inflammatory changes in the basal ganglia; characterized by rhythmical muscular tremors, rigidity of movement, festination, drooping posture, and mask-like facies.

Pathologic fracture: The breaking of a bone that has occurred at a site weakened by preexisting disease, especially neoplasm or necrosis of the bone.

Pedicle of arch of vertebra: The constricted portion of the arch on either side extending from the body to the lamina; bound to the intervertebral foramina superiorly and inferiorly.

Percussion: A technique in physical examination used to evaluate the size, borders, and consistency of some of the internal organs and to discover the presence and evaluate the amount of fluid in a cavity of the body.

Peristalsis: The coordinated, rhythmic, serial contraction of smooth muscle that forces food through the digestive tract, bile through the bile duct, and urine through the ureters.

Phantom limb pain: The sensation that an amputated limb is still present; often associated with painful paresthesia.

Phrenic nerve pacemaker: See Diaphragmatic pacemaker

Physical dimension of rehabilitation: Includes safety, comfort, and health (e.g., wheelchair mobility and strategies to manage physical barriers).

Physical fitness: The ability to carry out daily tasks with alertness and vigor, without undue fatigue, and with enough energy reserve to meet emergencies or to enjoy leisure time pursuits.

Physical therapy: The treatment of disorders with physical agents and methods such as massage, manipulation, therapeutic exercises, cold, heat, hydrotherapy, electric stimulation, and light, to assist in rehabilitating individuals and restoring function after an illness or injury. Also called physiotherapy.

Pilomotor reflex: See Goose flesh.

Plethysmograph: An instrument for measuring and recording changes in the sizes and volumes of extremities and organs by measuring changes in their blood volumes.

Pleural effusion: An abnormal accumulation of fluid in the interstitial and air spaces of the lungs, characterized by fever, chest pain, dyspnea, and non-productive cough.

Pneumatic antishock garment: An inflatable suit used to apply pressure to the peripheral circulation, thus reducing blood flow and fluid exudation into tissues, to maintain central blood flow in the presence of shock.

Pneumobelt: A corset with an inflatable bladder that fits over the abdominal area. The bladder is connected by a hose to a ventilator that delivers positive pressure at an adjustable rate and pressure. It is used to assist in the respiratory rehabilitation of individuals with high cervical injuries so that the neck muscle effort can be spared for other activities.

Pneumonia: Inflammation of the lung parenchyma characterized by consolidation of the affected part; the alveolar air spaces become filled with exudate, inflammatory cells, and fibrin.

Pneumothorax: A collection of air or gas in the pleural space causing the lung to collapse.

Poikilothermic: Having a variable body temperature; as fish, reptiles, and amphibians that have internal temperatures, close to the temperatures of the environments in which they live. Also called cold-blooded.

Post-traumatic malnutrition: Any disorder concerning nutrition that may result from an unbalanced, insufficient, or excessive diet, or to the impaired absorption, assimilation, or use of foods.

Post-traumatic syringomyelia: Cystic degeneration of the spinal cord resulting in a fluid-filled cavity, causing an enlarging cavitation up and down the spinal cord.

Postural hypotension: A form of low blood pressure that occurs in an upright posture.

Pressure ulcer: Skin and underlying tissue damage due to prolonged pressure that disrupts the flow of blood to susceptible areas.

Priapism: An abnormal condition of prolonged or constant penile erection, often painful, and seldom associated with sexual arousal.

Primary health care: A basic level of health care that includes programs directed at the promotion of health, early diagnosis of disease or disability, and prevention of disease.

Primary prevention: A program of activities directed toward improvement of the general well-being, while also involving specific protection for selected diseases, such as immunization against measles.

Problem-solving approach to patient-centered care: A conceptual framework in nursing that incorporates the overt physical needs of a patient with covert psychological, emotional, and social needs.

Process standards: Defined actions and behaviors in providing care; may have a variety of formats, including job descriptions, procedures, protocols, guidelines for using nursing tools, standards of performance, and statements of standardized care plans.

Process: A series of related events that follow in sequence from a particular state or condition to a conclusion or resolution.

Proctitis: Inflammation of the rectum and anus caused by infection, trauma, drugs, allergy, or radiation injury.

Prophylaxis: Prevention of or protection against disease; often involving the use of biological, chemical, or mechanical agents to destroy or prevent the entry of infectious organisms.

Proprioception: A sense or perception, usually at a subconscious level, independent of vision of the movements and position of the body and especially its limbs.

Prostatectomy: Surgical removal of a portion of the prostate gland that surrounds the neck of the bladder and urethra and elaborates a secretion that liquefies coagulated semen.

Psychogenic erection: The condition of hardness, swelling and elevation observed in the penis, resulting from the interaction of the mind or psyche and the body

Psychogenic pain disorders: Disorders characterized by persistent and severe pain for which there is no apparent organic cause.

Psychomotor domain: The area of observable performance of skills that require some degree of neuromuscular coordination.

Ptosis: An abnormal condition of one or both upper eyelids, in which the eyelid droops because of a congenital or acquired weakness of the levator muscle or paralysis of the third cranial nerve.

Pulmonary embolism (PE): The blockage of a pulmonary artery by foreign matter such as fat, air, tumor tissue, or a thrombus that usually arises from a peripheral vein.

Pyelocaliectasis: See caliectasis.

Pyelogram: A radiograph or series of radiographs of the renal pelvis and ureter, following injection of contrast medium.

Quadriplegia: See tetraplegia.

Quality assurance: Providing the best possible care within available resources; a program designed to objectively and systematically monitor and evaluate the quality and appropriateness of patient care, and resolve identified problems.

Reflex bladder: See Spastic bladder.

Reflexogenic erection: The condition of hardness, swelling, and elevation observed in the penis, resulting from an involuntary reaction in response to a stimulus applied to the periphery and transmitted to the nervous centers in the brain or spinal cord.

Regeneration: Renewal or restoration of a body or bodily part after injury or as a normal process.

Rehabilitation: Restoration to the fullest physical, mental, social, vocational, and economic capacity of which the individual is capable.

Renal calculi: Concretions occurring in the kidney. Also called kidney stones.

Renal scan: A scan of the kidneys to determine their size, shape, position, and function; performed after the intravenous injection of a radioactive substance.

Residual volume (RV): The volume of air remaining in the lungs after a maximal expiratory effort.

Respiratory failure: The inability of the cardiac and pulmonary systems to maintain an adequate exchange of oxygen and carbon dioxide in the lungs.

Respiratory tract infection: Any infectious disease of the upper or lower respiratory tract. Upper respiratory tract infections include the common cold, laryngitis, pharyngitis, rhinitus, sinusitis, and tonsillitis. Lower respiratory tract infections include bronchitis, bronchiolitis, pneumonia, and tracheitis.

Retrograde ejaculation: Ejaculation with discharge of the semen into the bladder rather than through the uretha to the outside.

Rheumatoid arthritis: A chronic, destructive, sometimes deforming, collagen disease that has an autoimmune component. Rheumatoid arthritis is characterized by symmetric inflammation of the synovium and increased synovial exudate, leading to thickening of the synovium and swelling of the joint.

Rigidity: A condition of hardness, stiffness, or inflexibility.

Romberg's test: An indication of loss of the sense of position, in which the individual loses balance when standing erect, feet together, and eyes closed.

Scoliosis: Abnormal lateral curvature of the vertebral column.

Secondary prevention: A level of preventive medicine that focuses on early diagnosis, use of referral services, and rapid initiation of treatment to stop the progress of disease processes or handicapping disabilities.

Sedentary lifestyle: A style of living characterized by little or no exercise.

Self-care: The personal and health care performed by the patient, usually in collaboration with and after instruction by, a health professional.

Self-esteem: The degree of worth and competency one attributes to oneself.

Self-image: The total concept, idea, or mental image one has of oneself and of one's role in society; the person one believes oneself to be.

Self-neglect: Failure to care for or give proper attention to one's own well-being.

Shear: An applied force or pressure exerted against the surface and layers of the skin as tissues slide in opposite but parallel planes.

Shunt: To redirect the flow of a body fluid from one cavity or vessel to another; a tube or device implanted in the body to redirect a body fluid from one cavity or vessel to another.

Sigmoidoscopy: The inspection of the rectum and sigmoid colon by the aid of sigmoidoscope.

Skin tear: A torn or jagged wound, or an accidental cut wound.

Sleep deprivation: A loss of or lack of the needed hours for sleep; a state marked by reduced consciousness, diminished activity of the skeletal muscles, and depressed metabolism.

Social dimension of rehabilitation: Includes efforts to decrease isolation and enhance the individual's support system.

Social isolation: A condition in which a feeling of aloneness is experienced; and seen by the client as a negative or threatening state imposed by self or others.

Somatosensory evoked potential (SEP): Evoked potential elicited by repeated stimulation of the pain and touch systems.

Spastic bladder: A form of neurogenic bladder caused by a lesion of the spinal cord above the voiding reflex center. It is marked by loss of bladder control and bladder sensation, incontinence, and automatic, interrupted, incomplete voiding. Also called reflex bladder.

Spastic sphincter: A muscle that encircles a duct, tube or orifice in such a way that its contraction constricts the lumen or orifice, causing a greater degree of tension.

Spasticity: A form of muscular hypertonicity with increased resistance to stretch.

Sphincter control: Conscious limitation or suppression of impulses that cause muscle fibers to constrict a passage or close a natural opening in the body.

Sphincterotomy: Incision or division of a circular band of muscle fibers that constrict a passage or close a natural opening in the body.

Spina bifida: Congenital neural tube defect characterized by a developmental anomaly in the posterior vertebral arch; a congenital neural tube defect with defective closure of the vertebral column.

Spinal cord injury: Occurs when the delicate spinal cord is compressed, contused, severed, distracted, transected, or dissected, or suffers an interruption of the blood supply; any traumatic disruption of the spinal cord, often associated with extensive musculoskeletal involvement.

Spinal cord tumor: A neoplasm of the spinal cord; over 50 percent are extramedullary, about 25 percent are intramedullary, and the rest are extradural.

Spinal fusion: The fixation of an unstable segment of the spine, can be accomplished by skeletal traction or immobilization of the patient in a body cast, but is most frequently accomplished by a surgical procedure.

Spinal manipulation: The forced passive flexion, extension, and rotation of vertebral segments carrying the elements of articulation beyond the usual range of movement to the limit of anatomic range.

Spinal shock: Transient depression or abolition of reflex activity below the level of an acute spinal cord injury or transection.

Spinal tract: Any one of the ascending and descending pathways for motor or sensory nerve impulses that is found in the white matter of the spinal cord.

Spondylolisthesis: The partial forward dislocation of one vertebra over the one below it; most commonly the fifth lumbar vertebra over the first sacral vertebra.

Spondylolysis: Degeneration or deficient development of the articulating part of a vertebra.

Spondylosis: A condition of the spine characterized by fixation or stiffness of a vertebral joint.

Stagnate: To fail to progress or develop; to remain motionless.

Stasis ulcer: A necrotic crater-like lesion of the skin of the lower leg, caused by chronic venous congestion.

Stimulation: The application of a stimulus to a responsive structure, such as a nerve or muscle, regardless of whether the strength of the stimulus is sufficient to produce excitation.

Stress management: Methods of controlling factors that require a response or change within a person by identifying the stressors, eliminating negative stressors, and developing effective coping mechanisms to counteract the response constructively.

Stress ulcer: A gastric or duodenal ulcer that develops in previously unaffected individuals subjected to severe stress, such as when burned, or other severe bodily injuries.

Stress: Any emotional, physical, social, economical, or other factor that requires a response or change.

Stretching: Useful in maintaining or improving flexibility; can be incorporated into warm-up and cool-down activities or done as part of a daily workout; an exercise of extending beyond ordinary or normal limits.

Structural standards: Defined set of conditions and mechanisms basic to the provision of care under the identified criteria; defined conditions and mechanisms that facilitate desired staff functioning systems operation, and patient care delivery.

Substance abuse: The overindulgence in and dependence on a stimulant, depressant, or other chemical substance, leading to effects that are detrimental to the individual's physical or mental health, or the welfare of others.

Suprapubic catheter: A hollow flexible tube that is inserted above the symphysis pubis to withdraw or to instill fluids.

Suprapubic tapping: Rapid, short taps over the abdomen, done over the bladder area to assist with voiding.

Swan-Ganz catheter: A long, thin cardiac catheter with a tiny balloon at the tip, used during anesthesia for open heart surgery to determine left ventricular function by measuring left atrial wedge pressure.

Syncope: A brief lapse in consciousness caused by transient cerebral hypoxia.

Syringomyelia: The presence in the spinal cord of longitudinal cavities, which are not caused by vascular insufficiency, lined by dense, gliogenous tissue.i

Syrinx: A pathologic tube-shaped cavity in the brain or spinal cord. Plural is syringes.

Taxonomy: A system for classifying organisms on the basis of natural relationships and assigning them appropriate names.

Teamwork: Cooperative effort by the members of a group or team to achieve a common goal.

Tethered Cord syndrome: Abnormal low positioning (below L2) of the distal spinal cord (conus medullaris) by the filum terminal. May be associated with incontinence, progressive motor and sensory impairment in the legs, pain, and scoliosis.

Tetraplegia: A condition characterized by paralysis of the arms, the legs, and the trunk of the body below the level of an associated injury to the spinal cord. Also called quadriplegia.

Thermoregulation: The control of heat production and heat loss; specifically, the maintenance of body temperature through physiologic mechanisms activated by the hypothalamus.

Thrombophlebitis: Inflammation of a vein often accompanied by formation of a clot.

Tidal volume: The volume of air that is inspired or expired in a single breath during regular breathing. Also called VT.

Tilt table: A tool for diagnosing neurocardiogenic syncope in adults; also aids in progression to an upright position for individuals with orthostatic hypotension.

Timed toileting: See bowel training.

Tissue perfusion alteration: Nursing diagnosis for the interruption of the venous or arterial circulation to the affected part of the body (hypovolemia or hypervolemia), or a condition that causes abnormal exchange of fluids and nutrients to or from the cells to the circulation.

Tissue tolerance: Ability of the skin and tissue to redistribute applied pressure.

Total quality management (TQM): A concept that defines quality in the context of a customer's experience. It is a hospital-wide concept embedded in every aspect of patient care.

Toughening: Process of physically and emotionally preparing the individual for community re-entry.

Tracheostomy: An opening through the neck into the trachea through which an indwelling tube may be inserted.

Tracheotomy: An incision made into the trachea through the neck below the larynx, performed to gain access to the airway below a blockage due to a foreign body, tumor, or edema of the glottis.

Traction: The process of putting a limb, bone, or group of muscles under tension by means of weights and pulleys to align or immobilize the part, or to relieve pressure on it.

Transcending: The process of rising above the negative, stereotypical beliefs about people with disabilities.

Transcultural nursing: A field of nursing in which the nurse transcends ethnocentricity and practices nursing in other cultural environments. Because current nursing process and theory are not culturally bound, and the needs of each person are considered individually, transcultural nursing is a part of all nursing practice.

Transdisciplinary team: Characterized by blurring of boundaries between disciplines; cross training and flexibility minimize duplication toward client goal attainment.

Transurethral sphincterotomy: Incision or division of external urethral sphincter.

Transverse myelitis: Acute inflammation and softening of the spinal cord; involves the entire thickness of the spinal cord but is of limited longitudinal extent.

Trauma: Physical injury caused by violent or disruptive action, or by the introduction into the body of a toxic substance.

Traumatic spondylolisthesis: An extension fracture through the pedicles of C2, causing the separation of the nueral arch from the body of the axis.

Triplegic: Paralysis of three extremities (e.g., both legs and one arm).

Ultrasound: The use of high frequency sound to image internal structures by the differing reflection signals produced when a beam of sound waves is projected into the body and bounces back at interfaces between those structures. Also called Ultrasound imaging.

Unidisciplinary team: Group of providers from one disciplinary background.

Upper motor neuron disease (UMND): A general term including progressive spinal muscular atrophy (infantile, juvenile, and adult), amyotrophic lateral sclerosis, progressive bulbar paralysis, and primary lateral sclerosis; frequently a familial disease.

Upper motor neuron lesion (UMNL): A lesion injury above the sacral spinal cord segments, resulting in hypertonic (spastic) paralysis.

Ureterocele: A prolapse of the terminal portion of the ureter into the bladder; may lead to obstruction of the flow of urine, hydronephrosis, and loss of renal function.

Urethal pressure profile: An index of urethral resistance to bladder output; assists in the assessment of urinary incontinence, provides a distinction between a distensible and fibrotic urethral segment, and contributes information regarding coordination of the detrusor muscle and the external urinary sphincter.

Urethral prolapse: The falling, sinking, or sliding of the urethra from its normal position or location in the body.

Urethral stent: Placement of a mesh stent over the external urinary sphincter to facilitate bladder emptying. Also called Endourethral prosthesis.

Urethrocele: A herniation of the urethra.

Urinary diversion: Ureters are implanted in a section of dissected ileum that is then sewed to an ostomy in the abdominal wall, where a collecting device is attached.

Urinary incontinence: Involuntary passage of urine, with the failure of voluntary control over bladder and urethral sphincters. Also called failure to store.

Urinary retention: Incomplete emptying of the bladder. Also called failure to empty.

Urinary sphincters: There are two urinary sphincters, internal and external. The external sphincter is a striated skeletal muscle surrounding the urethra, which can be voluntarily relaxed and contracted. The internal sphincter is located at the bladder neck and has the function of closing off the bladder neck in the resting state, maintaining continence.

Urinary tract infection (UTI): Bacteriuria with tissue invasion and resultant tissue response, signs, and/or symptoms.

Urodynamics studies: The study of the storage of urine within, and the flow of urine through and from, the urinary tract.

Vagus nerve: Either of the longest pair of cranial nerves essential for speech, swallowing and the sensibilities and functions of many parts of the body. The vagus nerves communicate through 13 main branches, connecting to four areas in the brain. Also called tenth cranial nerve.

Valsalva leak point pressure: Storage pressure in bladder at which urine leakage occurs passively, usually in individuals with neurogenic bladder.

Valsalva maneuver: Any forced expiratory effort ("strain") against a closed airway, whether at the nose and mouth or at the glottis.

Venography: The technique of preparing an x-ray image of veins injected with a radiopaque contrast medium.

Venous pressure: The stress exerted by circulating blood on the walls of veins, normally 60 to 120 mm of water in peripheral veins, but elevated in congestive heart failure, acute or chronic constrictive pericarditis, and in venous obstruction caused by a clot or external pressure against a vein.

Ventilatory failure: The inability of the cardiac and pulmonary systems to maintain an adequate exchange of oxygen and carbon dioxide in the lung.

Vesicoureteral reflux: An abnormal backflow of urine from the bladder to the ureter, resulting from a congenital defect, obstruction of the outlet of the bladder, or infection of the lower urinary tract.

Vital capacity (VC): A measurement of the amount of air that can be expelled slowly after a maximum inspiration, representing the greatest possible breathing capacity; the vital capacity equals the inspiratory reserve volume plus the tidal volume plus the expiratory reserve volume.

Voiding cystourethrogram: Cystourethrograms combine simple cystography with urethrography to visualize abnormalities of the bladder and urethra. Radiopaque dye is instilled in the bladder through a catheter. With the catheter clamped off, an x-ray film is taken to determine presence of ureteral reflux. The catheter is then removed and the client is asked to void. When voiding occurs, an x-ray film is taken to visualize the urethra.

Werdnig-Hoffman disease: A genetic disorder beginning in infancy or young childhood, characterized by progressive atrophy of the skeletal muscle resulting from degeneration of the cells in the anterior horn of the spinal cord and the motor nuclei in the brainstem.

World Health Organization (WHO): An agency of the United Nations that is primarily concerned with worldwide or regional health problems; in emergencies, it is authorized to render local assistance on request.

Wrist conservation: Hand function activities or techniques to prevent nerve entrapment syndromes.

SUNY BROCKPORT

3 2815 00896 6155

RD 594 .3 .N864 2001

Nursing practice related to
spinal cord injury and